THE PILL BOOK, 9th REVISED EDITION:
THE ILLUSTRATED GUIDE TO THE MOST PRESCRIBED DRUGS IN THE UNITED STATES
Illustrated with 32 pages of actual-size color photographs

With more than 11 million copies in print, THE PILL BOOK is the best-selling consumer drug reference ever, offering the most up-to-date, comprehensive information, in a format designed for ease of use.

This new 9th edition of *The Pill Book* contains more profiles of commonly prescribed drugs than any other consumer reference. Compiled by a team of eminent pharmacologists, it is based on official, FDA-approved information usually available only to doctors and pharmacists, plus the latest information gathered from computer databases and on-line resources. It synthesizes the most important facts about each drug in a concise, readable, easy-to-understand entry.

Here are complete profiles of more than 1,500 of the most commonly prescribed drugs, including:

- Generic and brand names
- What the drug is for and how it works
- Usual dosages, and what to do if a dose is skipped
- Side effects and possible adverse reactions, highlighted for quick reference
- Interactions with other drugs and foods
- Overdose and addiction potential
- Alcohol-free and sugar-free medications
- Information for seniors, pregnant and breast-feeding women, and others with special needs
- Cautions and warnings, and when to call your doctor

This completely revised and updated 9th edition contains dozens of new brand names and more than 35 important new drugs approved by the FDA in late 1999 that will go on sale for the first time in 2000. A 32-page insert provides actual-size full color photographs of the most-prescribed pills.

THE PILL BOOK

9th EDITION

Editor-in-Chief
HAROLD M. SILVERMAN, Pharm. D.

Production
**CMD PUBLISHING
A DIVISION OF
CURRENT MEDICAL DIRECTIONS/
THREE V HEALTH**

Consultants
**DRUG INFORMATION SERVICE
ROBERT WOOD JOHNSON UNIVERSITY HOSPITAL
AND RUTGERS COLLEGE OF PHARMACY
JUDITH I. BROWN**

Digital Photography and Color Separations
**SEVEN WORLDWIDE
SIGLER AND FLANDERS**

Original Creators of THE PILL BOOK
**LAWRENCE D. CHILNICK
BERT STERN
HAROLD M. SILVERMAN, Pharm. D.
GILBERT I. SIMON, Sc.D.**

BANTAM BOOKS
NEW YORK · TORONTO · LONDON · SYDNEY · AUCKLAND

THE PILL BOOK

A Bantam Book

PUBLISHING HISTORY

Bantam edition published June 1979
Bantam revised edition / October 1982
Bantam 3rd revised edition / March 1986
Bantam 4th revised edition / February 1990
Bantam 5th revised edition / May 1992
Bantam 6th revised edition / June 1994
Bantam 7th revised edition / June 1996
Bantam 8th revised edition / May 1998
Bantam 9th revised edition / May 2000
*This revised edition was published simultaneously in
trade paperback and mass market paperback.*

ISBN: 0-553-57974-6

*Published simultaneously in the United States
and Canada*

*Bantam Books are published by Bantam Books, a division of Random House, Inc.
Its trademark, consisting of the words "Bantam Books" and the portrayal of a
rooster, is Registered in U.S. Patent and Trademark Office and in other countries.
Marca Registrada. Bantam Books, 1540 Broadway, New York, New York 10036.*

PRINTED IN THE UNITED STATES OF AMERICA

OPM   0 9 8 7 6 5 4 3 2

Contents

The purpose of this book is to provide educational information to the public concerning the majority of various types of prescription drugs that are presently utilized by physicians. It is not intended to be complete or exhaustive or in any respect a substitute for personal medical care. *Only a physician may prescribe these drugs and their exact dosages.*

While every effort has been made to reproduce products on the cover and insert of this book in an exact fashion, certain variations of size or color may be expected as a result of the printing process. Furthermore, pictures identified as brand-name drugs should not be confused with their generic counterparts. In any event, the reader should not rely solely upon the photographic image to identify any pills depicted herein, but should rely upon the physician's prescription as dispensed by the pharmacist.

How to Use This Book

How to Find Your Medication in *The Pill Book*

- *The Pill Book* lists most medications in alphabetic order by generic name because a medication may have many brand names but has only 1 generic name. Most generic medications produce the same therapeutic effects as their brand-name equivalents but are much less expensive. Drugs that are available generically are indicated by the Ⓖ symbol.

- When a medication has 2 or more active ingredients, it is listed by the most widely known brand name. In a few cases, pill profiles are listed by drug type (e.g., sulfonylurea antidiabetes drugs).

- *The Pill Book* includes the names of the top 100 brand-name drugs (cross-referenced to their generic name) in alphabetic order with the pill profiles.

- Most over-the-counter (OTC) medications are not included in *The Pill Book*. For complete information on OTC medications, refer to *The Pill Book Guide to Over-the-Counter Medications*.

- All brand and generic names are listed in the Index. Brand names are indicated by boldface.

- Sugar-free and alcohol-free brand-name drugs are indicated by the Ⓢ and Ⓐ symbols in the beginning of each pill profile.

The Pill Book, like pills themselves, should be taken with caution. Used properly, this book may save you money and, perhaps, your life. It contains life-size pictures of the most prescribed brand-name drugs in the U.S. *The Pill Book*'s product identification system is designed to help you check that the medication you are about to take is the one your doctor prescribed. Although many dosage forms are included, not all available forms and strengths of every medication have been shown. While every effort has been made to create accurate photographic reproductions of the products, some variations in size or color may be expected as a result of the printing process. Do not rely solely on the photographic images to identify your pills; check with your pharmacist if you have any product identification questions.

Each pill profile in *The Pill Book* contains the following information:

Generic and Brand Name: The generic name is the common name of the drug approved by the Food and Drug Administration (FDA). It is listed along with the current brand names available for each generic drug. Medications that are available in a generic form are indicated by the G symbol.

Most prescription drugs are sold in more than one strength. Some drugs, such as oral contraceptives, come in packages containing different numbers of pills. A few manufacturers reflect this fact by adding letters or numbers to the basic drug name; others do not. An example: Loestrin 21 1.5/30 and Loestrin 21 1/20. (The numbers here refer to the number of tablets in each monthly packet, 21, and the amount of medication found in the tablets.) Other drugs come in different strengths: This is often indicated by a notation such as "DS" (double strength) or "Forte" (stronger).

The Pill Book lists generic and brand names together only where there are no differences in basic ingredients (e.g., Loestrin). However, the amount of the ingredient (strength) may vary from product to product. In most cases, the brand names and generic versions listed for each medication are interchangeable; you can use any version of the drug and expect that it will work for you. *The Pill Book* identifies those medications for which generic versions are not considered equivalent and which should not be interchanged with a brand-name product or another generic version of the same drug.

Type of Drug: Describes the general pharmacologic class of each drug: "antidepressant," "tranquilizer," "decongestant," "expectorant," and so on.

Prescribed for: All drugs are approved for some symptoms or conditions by federal authorities, but doctors also commonly prescribe drugs for other, as yet unapproved, reasons; these are also listed in *The Pill Book*. Check with your doctor if you are not sure why you have been given a certain pill.

General Information: Information on how the drug works, how long it takes for you to feel its effects, or a description of how this drug is similar to or different from other drugs.

Cautions and Warnings: This information alerts you to important and more dangerous reactions and to physical conditions, such as heart disease, that can have serious consequences if the medication is prescribed for you.

Possible Side Effects: Side effects are generally divided into 4 categories—those that are most common, common, less common, and rare—to help you better understand what to expect from your pills. If you are not sure whether you are experiencing a drug side effect, ask your doctor.

Drug Interactions: Describes what happens when you combine your medication with other drugs and lists what should not be taken at the same time as your medication. Some interactions may be deadly. At every visit, be sure to inform your doctor of any medication you are already taking. Your pharmacist should also keep a record of all your prescription and OTC medications. This listing, called a *Patient Drug Profile,* is used to check for potential problems. You may want to keep your own drug profile and take it to your pharmacist for review whenever a new medication is added.

Food Interactions: Provides information on foods to avoid while taking your medication, whether to take your medication with meals, and other important facts.

Usual Dose: Tells you the largest and smallest doses usually prescribed. You may be given different dosage instructions by your doctor. Do not change the dosage of ANY medication you take without first calling your doctor.

Overdosage: Describes overdose symptoms and what to do.

Special Information: Includes symptoms to watch for, when to call your doctor, what to do if you forget a dose of your medication, and any special instructions.

Special Populations: *Pregnancy/Breast-feeding:* For women who are or might be pregnant, and what to do if you must take a medication during the time you are nursing your baby. *Seniors:* This section presents the special facts an older adult needs to know about every drug and explains how reactions may differ from those of a younger person.

In an Emergency!

Each year over 1 million people experience drug-related poisoning in the U.S., and about 10% of those cases result in death. In fact, drug overdose is a leading cause of fatal poisoning in the U.S.

Although each of the pill profiles in *The Pill Book* has specific information on drug overdose, there are a few general rules to remember if you are faced with an accidental poisoning.

1. Make sure the victim is breathing, and call for medical help immediately.
2. Learn the phone number for your local poison control center and post it near the phone. Call the center in an emergency. When you call, be prepared to explain

   - What drug was taken and how much
   - Status of the victim (e.g., conscious, sleeping, vomiting, or having convulsions)
   - The approximate age and weight of the victim
   - Any chronic medical problems of the victim (e.g., diabetes, epilepsy, or high blood pressure), if you know them
   - What medications, if any, the victim takes regularly

3. Remove anything that might interfere with breathing. A person who is not getting enough oxygen will turn blue (the tongue or the skin under the fingernails changes color first). If this happens, lay the victim on his or her

back, open the collar, place one hand under the neck, and lift, pull, or push the victim's jaw so that it juts outward. This will open the airway between the mouth and lungs as wide as possible. Begin mouth-to-mouth resuscitation ONLY if the victim is not breathing.

4. If the victim is unconscious or having convulsions, call for medical help immediately. While waiting for the ambulance, lay the victim on his or her stomach and turn the head to one side. Should the victim throw up, this will prevent inhalation of vomit. DO NOT give an unconscious victim anything by mouth. Keep the victim warm.

5. If the victim is conscious, call for medical help and give the victim an 8-oz. glass of water to drink. This will dilute the poison.

Only a small number of poisoning victims require hospitalization. Most may be treated with simple actions or need no treatment at all.

The poison control center may tell you to make the person vomit. The best way to do this is to use ipecac syrup, which is available over-the-counter at any pharmacy. Specific instructions on how much to give infants, children, or adults are printed on the label and will also be given by your poison control center. Remember, DO NOT make the victim vomit unless you have been instructed to do so. Never make the victim vomit if the victim is unconscious, is having a convulsion, or is experiencing a painful, burning feeling in the mouth or throat.

Be Prepared

The best way to deal with a poisoning is to be prepared for it. Do the following now:

1. Write the telephone number of your local poison control center next to your other emergency phone numbers.
2. Decide which hospital you will go to, if necessary, and how you will get there.
3. Buy 1 oz. of ipecac syrup from your pharmacy. The pharmacist will tell you how to use it. Remember, this is a potent drug to be used only if directed.
4. Learn to give mouth-to-mouth resuscitation.

Reduce the Risk of Drug-Related Poisoning

1. Keep all medications in a locked place out of the reach of young children.
2. Do not store medications in containers that previously held food.
3. Do not remove the labels from bottles so that the contents are unknown.
4. Discard all medications when you no longer need them.

The Most Commonly Prescribed Drugs in the United States, Generic and Brand Names, with Complete Descriptions of Drugs and Their Effects

Generic Name

Abacavir (uh-BAK-uh-veer)

Brand Name

Ziagen

Type of Drug

Antiviral.

Prescribed for

Human immunodeficiency virus (HIV) infection.

General Information

Abacavir is a man-made nucleoside drug that inhibits the reproduction of the HIV virus. Once inside the HIV-infected cell, abacavir is transformed by enzymes into carbovir triphosphate. Carbovir triphosphate interferes with the activity of HIV reverse transcriptase, an enzyme essential to the virus' ability to reproduce. Abacavir is always given with another anti-HIV antiviral—such as didanosine, lamivudine, stavudine or zalcitabine—to achieve optimum effectiveness. Some of the drug is broken down in the liver, some passes out of the body unchanged in the urine, and some passes out of the body in the stool.

Cautions and Warnings

Stop taking this drug at the first sign of **drug allergy** or **sensitivity** (see "Special Information"). People have died from abacavir sensitivity.

People with **liver disease** should be cautious about using this drug because of the possibility that it can aggravate the condition. Some people have died from liver damage associated with abacavir.

Resistance to abacavir has developed in laboratory versions of HIV also resistant to lamivudine, didanosine, and zalcitabine. HIV that is resistant to protease inhibitors is not likely to be resistant to abacavir.

Abacavir cannot be used in infants under age 3 months.

Possible Side Effects

Because abacavir is always taken with other drugs, the side effects listed here are those of the drugs in combination.

Adults
▼ Most common: nausea, vomiting, diarrhea, and appetite loss.
▼ Common: sleep disturbances.

Children
▼ Most common: nausea, vomiting, fever, headache, diarrhea, and rash.
▼ Common: appetite loss.

Drug Interactions

• Alcohol interferes with the elimination of abacavir through the liver and can lead to a 40% increase in the amount of drug in the blood.

• Abacavir can increase blood levels of acetaminophen, amitriptyline, bumetanide, chloral hydrate, chlorpheniramine, chlorpromazine, chlorzoxazone, dapsone, doxepin, fluconazole, imipramine, ketoconazole, labetalol, lamotrigine, miconazole, morphine, naloxone, non-steroidal anti-inflammatory drugs (NSAIDs), oxazepam, promethazine, propofol, propranolol, and valproic acid.

• Cigarette smoking and clofibrate may reduce the amount of abacavir in the blood.

• Combining abacavir with isoniazid may decrease abacavir levels and increase isoniazid levels in the blood.

• Abacavir levels in the blood may be decreased if you are also taking phenobarbital, phenytoin, or T3 thyroid hormone replacement.

Food Interactions

None known.

Usual Dose

Adult (age 17 and over): 300 mg 2 times a day.
Child (age 3 months–16 years): 3.6 mg per lb. of body weight twice a day, up to a maximum of 300 mg in each dose.

Overdosage

Little is known about the effects of abacavir overdose. Overdose victims should be taken to a hospital emergency room for treatment. ALWAYS bring the prescription bottle or container.

Special Information

Stop taking this drug and call your doctor at the first sign of allergy or drug sensitivity (symptoms include fever, rash, fatigue, nausea, vomiting, diarrhea, and abdominal pain). If you continue to take this drug and are allergic to it, more severe reactions including a life-threatening drop in blood pressure could develop within hours.

Abacavir is not a cure for HIV. People taking the drug may still develop opportunistic infections and other conditions associated with HIV infection.

People taking abacavir can still be infectious and transmit HIV to others.

The long-term effects of abacavir are not known. Report anything unusual to your doctor.

It is very important for you to take abacavir exactly as prescribed. If you forget to take a dose and remember within 2 to 3 hours, take the medication. If you forget until it is almost time for your next dose, skip the forgotten dose and continue with your regular schedule. Remember, every dose of any HIV medication you forget or skip can make it more difficult for the drugs to do their job and can also lead to the development of HIV resistant to abacavir.

Special Populations

Pregnancy/Breast-feeding

Abacavir passes into the fetal circulation. In animal studies, the drug caused low birth weight and increased the risk of stillbirth. The effect of abacavir in pregnant women is not known. When this drug is considered crucial by your doctor, its potential benefits must be carefully weighed against its risks.

It is not known if abacavir passes into breast milk. Women with HIV are advised to bottle-feed their babies to avoid transmitting the drug.

Seniors

Studies of abacavir did not include many seniors. Seniors should use this drug with caution because of the risk that normal reductions in organ function or drug interactions may affect how abacavir works in the body or increase the likelihood of side effects.

Generic Name

Acarbose (uh-CAR-bose)

Brand Name

Precose

Type of Drug

Antidiabetic.

Prescribed for

Type II (non-insulin-dependent) diabetes mellitus.

General Information

Acarbose works in a different way than other antidiabetes drugs. Acarbose interferes with enzymes in the intestine responsible for breaking down the complex carbohydrates found in starchy foods into simple sugars, including glucose. Acarbose lowers blood sugar by delaying the absorption of glucose into the blood after eating. Because it works against diabetes in this way, the blood-sugar-lowering effect of acarbose adds to that of other antidiabetes drugs. Acarbose may also be used by people who are unable to control their blood sugar by diet alone. Most of acarbose's side effects are related directly to the fact that it leaves undigested carbohydrates in the lower intestines.

Cautions and Warnings

Acarbose should not be used if you are **allergic** or **sensitive** to it. People should not use acarbose if they have **diabetic ketoacidosis, cirrhosis, severe kidney disease, inflammatory bowel disease, ulcers of the colon, intestinal obstruction, severe digestive disease,** or **absorption diseases,** or if **intestinal gas** will be a severe problem. Acarbose may lead to liver inflammation.

Possible Side Effects

▼ Most common: stomach gas (in 75% of people who take it), abdominal pain, and diarrhea. These side effects tend to improve or go away after a few weeks.

▼ Rare: liver irritation and minor abnormalities in blood tests.

Drug Interactions

• Acarbose adds to the blood-sugar-lowering effect of sulfonylureas and other antidiabetes drugs.

• Activated charcoal and antacids—and other drugs intended to absorb stomach contents—and digestive enzyme preparations may reduce the effectiveness of acarbose. Separate these drugs from acarbose by at least 2 hours.

Food Interactions

Acarbose must be taken with the first bite of each meal.

Usual Dose

Adult: 25–50 mg (up to 100 mg) 3 times a day.
Child: not recommended.

Overdosage

Acarbose overdose does not cause low blood sugar, but diarrhea, abdominal pain, and intestinal gas can be expected. Call your local poison control center for more information.

Special Information

It is essential to take each dose of acarbose at the beginning of each meal. Since the drug works in the intestines, it has to be there at the same time as the food you are digesting.

As with all antidiabetes drugs, people taking acarbose must follow their doctors' instructions for diet, exercise, and blood sugar testing.

Read product labels carefully or check with your pharmacist before buying any nonprescription drug to be sure it is safe for diabetics to take with acarbose.

If you forget a dose of acarbose, skip it and continue with your regular schedule. Taking a missed dose between meals will not provide any benefit.

Special Populations

Pregnancy/Breast-feeding

Animal studies of acarbose showed no effects on the fetus, but there is no information available on its effect in humans. Blood sugar control is considered essential during pregnancy and insulin is usually prescribed for that purpose. When acarbose is considered crucial by your doctor, its potential benefits must be weighed against its risks.

It is not known if acarbose passes into human breast milk. Nursing mothers who must take this drug should consider bottle-feeding.

Seniors

Blood levels of acarbose are higher in older adults, but this is not considered important. Seniors with severe kidney disease should avoid this medication.

Accupril   see Quinapril, page 864

Generic Name

Acebutolol   (ah-seh-BUTE-uh-lol) Ⓖ

Brand Name

Sectral

Type of Drug

Beta-adrenergic blocking agent.

Prescribed for

High blood pressure and abnormal heart rhythms.

General Information

Acebutolol hydrochloride is one of many beta-adrenergic blocking drugs, or beta blockers, that interfere with the action of a specific part of the nervous system. Beta receptors are found all over the body and affect many body functions. Beta blockers have different characteristics that can make them more suitable for certain conditions or people.

Cautions and Warnings

You should be cautious about taking acebutolol if you have **asthma, severe heart failure,** a **very slow heart rate,** or **heart block** (disruption of the electrical impulses that control heart rate) because the drug may worsen these conditions.

People with **angina** taking acebutolol for high blood pressure risk aggravating their angina if they suddenly stop taking the drug. These patients should have their acebutolol dosage reduced gradually over 1 to 2 weeks.

Acebutolol should be used with caution if you have **liver or kidney disease** because your ability to eliminate this drug from your body may be impaired.

Acebutolol reduces the amount of blood pumped by the heart with each beat. This reduction in blood flow may aggravate the condition of people with **poor circulation** or **circulatory disease.**

If you are undergoing **major surgery,** your doctor may want you to stop taking acebutolol at least 2 days before surgery.

Possible Side Effects

Side effects are relatively uncommon and usually mild; normally they develop early in the course of treatment and are rarely a reason to stop taking acebutolol.

▼ Most common: impotence.

▼ Less common: unusual tiredness or weakness, slow heartbeat, heart failure (symptoms include swelling of the legs, ankles, or feet), dizziness, breathing difficulties, bronchospasm, depression, confusion, anxiety, nervousness, sleeplessness, disorientation, short-term memory loss, emotional instability, cold hands and feet, constipation, diarrhea, nausea, vomiting, upset stomach, increased sweating, urinary difficulties, cramps, blurred vision, rash, hair loss, stuffy nose, facial swelling, aggravation of lupus erythematosus (chronic condition affecting the body's connective tissue), itching, chest pain, back or joint pain, colitis, drug allergy (symptoms include fever and sore throat), and liver toxicity.

Drug Interactions

• Acebutolol may interact with surgical anesthetics to increase the risk of heart problems during surgery. Some anesthesiologists recommend gradually stopping the drug by 2 days before surgery.

• Acebutolol may interfere with the normal signs of low blood sugar and with the action of oral antidiabetes drugs.

• Acebutolol increases the blood-pressure-lowering effects of other blood-pressure-reducing agents, including clonidine, guanabenz, and reserpine; and calcium channel blockers, such as nifedipine.

• Aspirin-containing drugs, indomethacin, sulfinpyrazone, and estrogen drugs may interfere with the blood-pressure-lowering effect of acebutolol.

• Cocaine may reduce the effectiveness of all beta-blockers.

• Acebutolol may worsen the problem of cold hands and feet associated with ergot alkaloids, used to treat migraine. Gangrene is a possibility in people taking both an ergot and acebutolol.

• Acebutolol will counteract thyroid hormone replacements.

• Calcium channel blockers, flecainide, hydralazine, oral contraceptives, propafenone, haloperidol, phenothiazine tranquilizers (molindone and others), quinolone antibacterials, and quinidine may increase the amount of acebutolol in the bloodstream and lead to increased acebutolol effects.

• Acebutolol should not be taken within 2 weeks of taking a monoamine oxidase inhibitor (MAOI) antidepressant.

• Cimetidine increases the amount of acebutolol absorbed into the bloodstream from oral tablets.

• Acebutolol may interfere with the effects of some anti-asthma drugs, including theophylline and aminophylline, and especially ephedrine and isoproterenol.

• Combining acebutolol with phenytoin or digitalis drugs may result in excessive slowing of the heart, possibly causing heart block.

• If you stop smoking while taking acebutolol, your dose may have to be reduced because your liver will break down the drug more slowly afterward.

Food Interactions

None known.

Usual Dose

Adult: starting dose—400 mg a day, taken all at once or in 2 divided doses. The daily dose may be gradually increased. Maintenance dose—400–1200 mg a day.

Senior: Older adults may respond to lower doses and should be treated more cautiously, beginning with 200 mg a day, increasing gradually to a maximum of 800 mg a day.

Overdosage

Symptoms of overdose include changes in heartbeat— unusually slow, unusually fast, or irregular—severe dizziness or fainting, breathing difficulties, bluish-colored fingernails or palms, and seizures. The victim should be taken to a hospital emergency room. ALWAYS bring the prescription bottle or container.

Special Information

Acebutolol is meant to be taken continuously. When ending acebutolol treatment, dosage should be reduced gradually over a period of about 2 weeks. Do not stop taking this drug unless directed to do so by your doctor: Abrupt withdrawal may cause chest pain, breathing difficulties, increased sweating, and unusually fast or irregular heartbeat.

Call your doctor at once if you develop back or joint pain, breathing difficulties, cold hands or feet, depression, rash, or changes in heartbeat. Acebutolol may produce an undesirable lowering of blood pressure, leading to dizziness or fainting; call your doctor if this happens to you. Call your doctor if you experience persistent or bothersome anxiety, diarrhea, constipation, impotence, headache, itching, nausea or vomiting, nightmares or vivid dreams, upset stomach, trouble sleeping, stuffy nose, frequent urination, unusual tiredness, or weakness.

Acebutolol may cause drowsiness, dizziness, light-headedness, or blurred vision. Be careful when driving or performing complex tasks.

It is best to take acebutolol at the same time each day. If you forget a dose, take it as soon as you remember. If you take acebutolol once a day and it is within 8 hours of your next dose, skip the dose you forgot and continue with your regular schedule. If you take acebutolol twice a day and it is within 4 hours of your next dose, skip the missed dose and continue with your regular schedule. Never take a double dose.

Special Populations

Pregnancy/Breast-feeding

Infants born to women who took a beta blocker while pregnant had lower birth weights, low blood pressure, and slow heart rates. Acebutolol should be avoided by pregnant women and women who might become pregnant while taking it.

Large amounts of acebutolol pass into breast milk. Nursing mothers taking acebutolol should bottle-feed.

Seniors

Seniors taking acebutolol may be more likely to suffer from cold hands and feet, reduced body temperature, chest pain, general feelings of ill health, sudden breathing difficulties, increased sweating, or changes in heartbeat.

Generic Name

Acetaminophen (uh-SEE-tuh-MIN-uh-fen) Ⓖ

Brand Names

Acephen	Liquiprin
Aceta	Mapap*
Acetaminophen Uniserts	Maranox
Apacet	Meda Cap/Tab
Aspirin Free Anacin	Neopap
Maximum Strength	Oraphen-PD
Aspirin Free Pain Relief	Panadol*
Childrens' Pain Reliever Ⓐ	Redutemp
Dapacin	Ridenol
Dynafed	Silapap Ⓐ
Feverall	Tapanol
Genapap*	Tempra*
Genebs	Tylenol*
Halenol	Uni-Ace Ⓐ
Infants' Pain Reliever Ⓐ	

Some products in this brand-name group are alcohol- or sugar-free. Consult your pharmacist.

Type of Drug

Antipyretic and analgesic.

Prescribed for

Relief of pain and fever for people who cannot or do not want to take aspirin or a nonsteroidal anti-inflammatory drug

(NSAID). Acetaminophen may be given to children about to receive a DTP vaccination to reduce the fever and pain that commonly follow the vaccination.

General Information

Acetaminophen is generally used to relieve pain and fever associated with the common cold, flu, viral infections, or other disorders where pain or fever may occur. It is also used to relieve pain in people who are allergic to aspirin, or those who cannot take aspirin because of potential interactions with other drugs such as oral anticoagulants. It can be used to relieve pain from a variety of sources, including arthritis, headache, and tooth and periodontic pain, although it does not reduce inflammation.

Cautions and Warnings

Do not take acetaminophen if you are **allergic** or **sensitive** to it. Do not take acetaminophen for **more than 10 days in a row** unless directed by your doctor. Do not take more than is prescribed or recommended on the package.

Use this drug with extreme caution if you have **kidney or liver disease** or **viral infections of the liver**. Large amounts of alcohol increase the liver toxicity of large doses or overdoses of acetaminophen. **Avoid alcohol** if you regularly take acetaminophen. Some people are more sensitive to this effect than others.

Possible Side Effects

This drug is relatively free from side effects when taken in recommended doses. For this reason it has become extremely popular, especially among those who cannot take aspirin.

▼ Rare: large doses or long-term use may cause liver damage, rash, itching, fever, lowered blood sugar, stimulation, yellowing of the skin or whites of the eyes, and/or a change in the composition of your blood.

Drug Interactions

• Acetaminophen's effects may be reduced by long-term use or large doses of barbiturate drugs, carbamazepine, phenytoin and similar drugs, rifampin, and sulfinpyrazone.

These drugs may also increase the chances of liver toxicity if taken with acetaminophen.

• Alcoholic beverages increase the chances for liver toxicity and possible liver failure associated with acetaminophen.

Food Interactions

None known.

Usual Dose

Adult and Child (age 12 and over): 300–600 mg 4 to 6 times a day, or 1000 mg 3 to 4 times a day. Avoid taking more than 2.6 g (eight 325-mg tablets) a day for long periods of time.
Child (age 11): 480 mg 4–5 times a day.
Child (age 9–10): 400 mg 4–5 times a day.
Child (age 6–8): 320 mg 4–5 times a day.
Child (age 4–5): 240 mg 4–5 times a day.
Child (age 3): 160 mg 4–5 times a day.
Child (age 1–2): 120 mg 4–5 times a day.
Child (age 4–11 months): 80 mg 4–5 times a day.
Child (under age 4 months): 40 mg 4–5 times a day.

Overdosage

Acute acetaminophen overdose may cause nausea, vomiting, sweating, appetite loss, drowsiness, confusion, abdominal tenderness, low blood pressure, abnormal heart rhythms, yellowing of the skin and whites of the eyes, and liver and kidney failure. Liver damage has occurred with 12 extra-strength tablets or 18 regular-strength tablets, but most people need larger doses—20 extra-strength or 30 regular-strength tablets—to damage their livers. Regular use of large doses for long periods—3000 to 4000 mg a day for a year—can also cause liver damage, especially if alcohol is involved. In case of overdose, induce vomiting as soon as possible with syrup of ipecac—available at any pharmacy—and take the victim to a hospital emergency room. ALWAYS bring the acetaminophen bottle or container.

Special Information

Unless abused, acetaminophen is a beneficial, effective, and relatively nontoxic drug. Follow package directions and call your doctor if acetaminophen does not work in 10 days for adults or 5 days for children.

Alcoholic beverages will worsen the liver damage that acetaminophen can cause. People who take this drug on a regular basis should limit their alcohol intake.

If you forget to take a dose, take it as soon as you remember. If it is within an hour of your next dose, skip the dose you forgot and continue with your regular schedule. Do not take a double dose.

Special Populations

Pregnancy/Breast-feeding

Acetaminophen is considered safe during pregnancy when taken in usual doses. Taking continuous high doses of the drug may cause birth defects or interfere with fetal development. Three cases of congenital hip dislocation appear to have been associated with acetaminophen. Check with your doctor before taking this drug if you are or might be pregnant.

Small amounts of acetaminophen may pass into breast milk, but the drug is considered harmless to nursing infants.

Seniors

Seniors may take acetaminophen as directed by a doctor.

Generic Name

Acetazolamide (uh-sete-uh-ZOLE-uh-mide) Ⓖ

Brand Names

Dazamide   Diamox Sequels
Diamox

Type of Drug

Carbonic-anhydrase inhibitor.

Prescribed for

Glaucoma and prevention or treatment of mountain sickness; also prescribed for epilepsy, including absence seizures, petit mal and grand mal epilepsy, and tonic-clonic, mixed, or partial seizures.

General Information

By blocking an enzyme in the body called carbonic anhydrase, acetazolamide produces a weak diuretic effect that helps to treat glaucoma by reducing pressure inside the eye. Acetazolamide's antiseizure properties are also produced by its effect on carbonic anhydrase, though exactly how acetazolamide prevents seizure is not well understood.

Cautions and Warnings

Do not take acetazolamide if you have **low blood sodium or potassium** or serious **kidney, liver, or Addison's disease.**

Possible Side Effects

Side effects of short-term therapy are usually minimal.

▼ Most common: nausea or vomiting; tingling feeling in the arms, legs, lips, mouth, or anus; appetite and weight loss; a metallic taste; increased frequency in urination; diarrhea; not feeling well; occasional drowsiness; and weakness. You may also experience rash, drug crystals in the urine, painful urination, low back pain, urinary difficulty, and low urine volume.

▼ Rare: Rare side effects can affect the liver, mental state, blood sugar, muscles, and senses. Contact your doctor if you experience any side effect not listed above.

Drug Interactions

• Avoid over-the-counter drug products that contain stimulants or anticholinergics, which tend to aggravate glaucoma and cardiac disease.

• Acetazolamide may increase blood concentrations of cyclosporine (used to prevent the rejection of transplanted organs).

• Acetazolamide may block or delay the absorption of primidone (prescribed for seizure).

• Avoid aspirin because it may enhance acetazolamide side effects.

• Combining diflunisal and acetazolamide can result in an excessive lowering of eye pressure.

Food Interactions

Acetazolamide may be taken with food if it upsets your stomach. Because acetazolamide can increase potassium loss, take this drug with potassium-rich foods such as bananas, citrus fruits, melons, and tomatoes.

Usual Dose

250–1000 mg a day.

Overdosage

Symptoms of overdose include drowsiness, loss of appetite, nausea, vomiting, dizziness, tingling in the hands or feet, weakness, tremors, or ringing or buzzing in the ears. In case of overdose, induce vomiting as soon as possible with ipecac syrup—available at any pharmacy—and take the victim to a hospital emergency room. ALWAYS bring the prescription bottle or container.

Special Information

Acetazolamide may cause minor drowsiness and confusion, particularly during the first 2 weeks of therapy. Be careful when driving or doing any task that requires concentration.

Call your doctor if you develop sore throat, fever, unusual bleeding or bruises, tingling in the hands or feet, rash, or unusual pains.

Acetazolamide can increase sensitivity to the sun. Avoid prolonged sun exposure and protect your eyes while taking this drug.

If you forget a dose, take it as soon as you remember. If it is almost time for your next dose, skip the dose you forgot and continue with your regular schedule. Do not take a double dose.

Special Populations

Pregnancy/Breast-feeding

High doses of this drug may cause birth defects or interfere with fetal development. When this drug is considered crucial by your doctor, its potential benefits must be carefully weighed against its risks.

Small amounts of acetazolamide may pass into breast milk. Nursing mothers who must take this drug should consider bottle-feeding.

Seniors

Seniors are more sensitive to this drug's side effects.

Generic Name

Acitretin (ah-sih-TREH-tin)

Brand Name

Soriatane

Type of Drug

Antipsoriatic.

Prescribed for

Severe psoriasis; also prescribed for a variety of other skin conditions.

General Information

Acitretin is related to vitamin A and prescription drugs such as etretinate and isotretinoin. Acitretin is produced when etretinate is broken down in the body and its effects are very similar to etretinate. The way that acitretin works is not known. Its effects are not likely to be seen until you have taken it for 2 or 3 months. Your doctor is urged to use this medication only in cases of severe psoriasis that have not responded to other treatments because of the risks associated with acitretin.

Cautions and Warnings

Women who take acitretin must not be pregnant during treatment or for 3 years after the completion of treatment. It is not known if acitretin taken by men before conception is also a risk to the fetus.

A small number of people taking this drug have developed **liver damage** including jaundice (symptoms include yellowing of the skin and whites of the eyes). People with **kidney failure** have much less acitretin in their blood than people with normal kidneys. Caution is advised for people with liver or kidney damage.

Blood fat levels rise in 25% to 50% of people taking acitretin. Very large increases in triglycerides are uncommon but a few cases of **pancreatitis** (pancreas inflammation) have occurred. Your doctor should measure your blood fat levels before you start taking acitretin and monitor them weekly or biweekly until your response to the medication has been determined.

People with **diabetes,** who are **obese,** or who have a **history of these conditions** are at increased risk for high blood fat levels as are people who **drink alcohol excessively**.

Drugs similar to acitretin have been associated with **pseudotumor cerebri** (increased pressure in the brain). Symptoms of pseudotumor cerebri include **visual disturbances, headache, nausea,** and **vomiting**. Report these or any unusual symptoms to your doctor at once.

People taking acitretin who had **spine or bone—including knee or ankle—problems** before starting the drug may find that their problems worsen while on the drug.

People with **diabetes** may find it more difficult to control their blood sugar while on acitretin.

Possible Side Effects

▼ Most common: hair loss, peeling skin, and inflammation of the lips.

▼ Common: dry eyes, chills or stiffness, dry skin, fingernail problems, itching, rash, tingling in the hands or feet, increased sensory awareness, loss of some sections of skin, sticky skin, and runny nose.

▼ Less common: drying and thickening of eye tissue, eye irritation, eyebrow or eye lash loss, changes in appetite, swelling, fatigue, hot flashes, flushing, sinus irritation, headache, pain, Bell's palsy, crusting of the eyelids, blurred vision, conjunctivitis (pinkeye), double vision, itchy eyes or eyelids, cataracts, swelling inside the eye, unusual sensitivity to bright light, dry mouth, nosebleeds, joint pain, and worsening of existing spinal problems.

▼ Rare: Rare side effects can occur in almost any part of the body. Contact your doctor if you experience any side effect not listed above.

Drug Interactions

• People combining acitretin and glyburide (an antidiabetic) may have unusually low blood-sugar levels. Your doctor may have to adjust your diabetic treatment program while you are taking acitretin.

• Combining acitretin with methotrexate increases the risk of liver damage.

• Acitretin reduces the effectiveness of low-progestin oral contraceptives (the "mini-pill"). If you are taking one of these contraceptives, switch to another type of birth control and use at least one other contraceptive method for at least 3 years after treatment is completed.

• Combining alcohol with acitretin produces acitretin's parent compound, etretinate. Etretinate stays in the body much longer than acitretin and may therefore affect the fetus for an even longer period of time than might acitretin. Avoid alcoholic beverages.

• Do not take a vitamin A supplement that has more than the standard minimum daily requirement (1000 mcg). Excess vitamin A plus acitretin exposes you to possible vitamin A toxicity.

Food Interactions

Acitretin is best absorbed when taken with food or meals.

Usual Dose

Adult: 25–50 mg a day with your main meal. Dosage must be individualized to your specific needs.

Child: not recommended.

Overdosage

Little is known about the effects of acitretin overdose, though one person vomited for several hours after taking too much of the drug. Call your local hospital emergency room or local poison control center for more information.

Special Information

Contact your doctor at once if you become pregnant while taking acitretin or in the 3 years following treatment. The risk of birth defects persists as long as the drug is in your body. In one case, small amounts of etretinate were found in blood plasma and fatty tissue more than 5 years after treatment.

Report visual disturbances, headache, nausea, vomiting, or anything unusual to your doctor at once.

Do not drink any alcoholic beverages during acitretin treatment and for at least 2 months after treatment has been completed.

Avoid excess vitamin A (see Drug Interactions).

Some birth control methods, including low-dose progestin contraceptives and tubal ligation may fail while taking this drug. Use at least one additional form of contraception while taking acitretin to avoid pregnancy.

You may have problems tolerating contact lenses while you are taking acitretin.

Do not donate blood while taking acitretin or for 3 years afterwards because your blood might be given to a pregnant woman.

Avoid exposure to excessive sunlight or to sunlamps because of unusual sensitivity caused by acitretin.

If you forget to take a dose of acitretin, take it with food as soon as you remember. If it is almost time for your next dose, skip the one you forgot and continue with your regular schedule. Do not take a double dose.

Special Populations

Pregnancy/Breast-feeding

Acitretin causes birth defects and may damage the fetus. Women who take acitretin must be sure they are not pregnant before starting therapy by using reliable contraception for at least 1 month before starting the drug and taking a pregnancy test within 1 week of starting treatment. Women must use 2 reliable contraceptive methods during treatment and for 3 years following the completion of treatment.

Acitretin may pass into breast milk. Nursing mothers who must take this drug should bottle-feed.

Seniors

Seniors have twice as much acitretin in their blood as do younger adults but may take acitretin without special precaution.

Generic Name

Acyclovir (ae-SYE-kloe-vir) Ⓖ

Brand Name

Zovirax

Type of Drug

Antiviral.

Prescribed for

Serious, frequently recurring herpes simplex infections of the genitals, mucous membrane tissue, and central nervous system; herpes zoster (shingles); varicella (chickenpox); and viral infections including nongenital herpes simplex, herpes simplex, and cytomegalovirus (CMV) in immunocompromised patients, and varicella pneumonia.

General Information

Acyclovir is the only oral drug that reduces growth rates of the herpes virus and the related viruses, Epstein-Barr, varicella, and CMV; both oral acyclovir and oral ganciclovir work against CMV. Intravenous drugs, including acyclovir injection, may also be used for these viral infections; however, intravenous antiviral drugs are usually reserved for patients with AIDS, cancer, or otherwise compromised immune systems.

Acyclovir is selectively absorbed into cells that are infected with the herpes simplex virus, where it is converted into its active form. Acyclovir works by interfering with the reproduction of viral DNA, slowing the growth of existing viruses. It has little effect on recurrent infections. To treat both local and systemic (whole-body) symptoms acyclovir must be given by intravenous injection or taken by mouth. Local symptoms may be treated with the ointment alone. Oral acyclovir may be taken every day to reduce the number and severity of herpes attacks in people who suffer 10 or more attacks a year; it may also be used to treat intermittent attacks as they occur, but treatment must be started as soon as possible to have the greatest effect.

Cautions and Warnings

Do not use acyclovir ointment if you have had an **allergic** reaction to it or to the major component of the ointment base, polyethylene glycol. Do not apply acyclovir ointment inside the vagina because the polyethylene glycol base may cause irritation and swelling of sensitive vaginal tissue. Acyclovir ointment is not intended for use in the eye and should not be used to treat a herpes infection of the eye.

Some people develop **tenderness, swelling, or bleeding of the gums** while taking acyclovir. Regular brushing, flossing, and gum massage may help prevent these conditions.

Possible Side Effects

Ointment

▼ Most common: mild burning, irritation, rash, and itching. These effects are more likely to occur when treating an initial herpes attack than a recurrent attack. Women are 4 times more likely to experience burning than men.

Capsules, Suspension, and Tablets

▼ Most common: dizziness, headache, diarrhea, nausea, and vomiting.

▼ Less common: appetite loss, stomach gas, constipation, fatigue, rash, not feeling well, leg pains, sore throat, a bad taste in the mouth, sleeplessness, and fever.

▼ Rare: aching joints, weakness, and tingling in the hands or feet.

Drug Interactions

• Do not apply acyclovir together with any other ointment or topical medication.

• Oral probenecid may decrease elimination of acyclovir from the body, which increases blood levels of oral or injected acyclovir, increasing the risk of side effects.

• Combining acyclovir and zidovudine (an AIDS drug—also known as AZT) may lead to severe drowsiness and lethargy.

Food Interactions

Acyclovir may be taken with food if it upsets your stomach.

Usual Dose

Capsules, Suspension, and Tablets

Adult: genital herpes attack—200 mg every 4 hours, 5 times a day for 10 days. Recurrent infections—400 mg twice a day or 200 mg 2–5 times a day. Suppressive therapy for chronic herpes—400–800 mg a day, every day. Herpes zoster—800 mg 5 times a day for 7–10 days.

Child (age 2 and over): Acyclovir has been given to children in daily doses as high as 36 mg per lb. of body weight without any unusual side effects.

Child (under age 2): not recommended.

If you have kidney disease, your doctor should adjust your dose according to the degree of functional loss.

Ointment
Apply every 3 hours, 6 times a day for 7 days. Apply enough
medication to cover all visible skin lesions. About ½ in. of ointment should cover about 4 sq. in. of lesions. Your doctor may
prescribe a longer course of treatment to prevent the delayed
formation of new lesions over the duration of an attack.

Overdosage

Overdose of oral acyclovir may lead to kidney damage due to
deposits of acyclovir crystals in the kidneys. The risk of experiencing toxic side effects from swallowing acyclovir ointment is quite small. In the case of overdose or accidental
ingestion, call your poison control center.

Special Information

Use a finger cot or rubber glove when applying acyclovir ointment to protect against inadvertently spreading the virus. Be
sure to apply the medication exactly as directed and to completely cover all lesions. Keep affected areas clean and dry.
Loose-fitting clothing will reduce possible irritation of a healing lesion. If you skip several doses, or a day or more of treatment, the drug will not exert its maximum effect.

Herpes may be transmitted even if you do not have symptoms of active disease. To avoid giving the condition to a sexual partner, do not have intercourse while visible herpes
lesions are present. A condom offers some protection against
transmission of the herpes virus, but spermicidal products
and diaphragms do not. Acyclovir alone will not prevent herpes transmission.

Women with genital herpes have an increased risk of cervical cancer. Speak with your doctor about the need for an
annual Pap smear.

Call your doctor if acyclovir does not relieve your symptoms, if side effects become severe or intolerable, or if you
become pregnant or want to begin breast-feeding. Check with
your dentist if you notice swelling or tenderness of the gums.

Special Populations

Pregnancy/Breast-feeding

Acyclovir crosses into the circulation of the fetus. Animal
studies have shown that large doses—up to 125 times the
human dose—cause damage to both mother and fetus. While
there is no information to indicate that acyclovir affects a
human fetus, do not use it during pregnancy unless it is

specifically prescribed by your doctor and the possible benefit outweighs the risk.

Acyclovir passes into breast milk in concentrations up to 4 times the concentration in blood, and it has been found in the urine of a nursing infant. Although no side effects have been found in nursing babies, mothers who must take acyclovir should consider bottle-feeding.

Seniors
Shingles attacks in people over age 50 tend to be more severe and respond best to acyclovir treatment if the drug is started within 48 to 72 hours of the appearance of the first rash. Seniors with reduced kidney function should be given a lower dose of oral acyclovir than younger adults.

Adalat CC *see Nifedipine, page 728*

Generic Name
Adapalene (uh-DAP-uh-lene)

Brand Name
Differin

Type of Drug
Anti-acne.

Prescribed for
Acne.

General Information
Adapalene is similar to a retinoid. Retinoids are compounds related to vitamin A and are used in acne treatment. When adapalene is applied to an acne lesion, it modifies several of the processes involved in skin cell function. It reduces inflammation in the acne lesion and slows the formation of the material that fills the lesion. Very little adapalene is absorbed through the skin.

Cautions and Warnings
Do not use adapalene if you are **sensitive** or **allergic** to it. If

you are **sunburned,** wait until your sunburn clears before applying adapalene to your skin. **Avoid sun or sunlamp exposure** while using adapalene. If you must be in the sun, be sure to apply sunscreen or wear protective clothing over areas where you have applied adapalene. Extreme wind or cold can also be irritating to skin where adapalene has been applied.

Adapalene can be **highly irritating** if it gets into your eyes or if it is applied to your lips, the angles of your nose, mucous membranes, cuts, abrasions, or sunburned or damaged skin.

Possible Side Effects

▼ Most common: redness, irritation, dryness, scaling, itching, and burning are common after applying adapalene to your skin. These effects usually occur during the first 2 to 4 weeks of adapalene use and may be severe enough to cause you to stop using adapalene; call your doctor if this happens to you.

▼ Rare: skin irritation, stinging sunburn, and worsening acne.

Drug Interactions

None known.

Usual Dose

Adult and Child (age 12 and over): Wash affected areas and apply a thin layer of adapalene at bedtime.

Child (under age 12): not recommended.

Overdosage

Accidental ingestion of adapalene can cause liver toxicity and other side effects associated with swallowing large amounts of vitamin A. Swallowing adapalene gel is extremely dangerous for pregnant women, who should not take more vitamin A than is contained in their prenatal vitamins. Infants who swallow adapalene should be taken to a hospital emergency room for treatment. Ingestion of adapalene may cause symptoms such as headache, facial flushing, abdominal pain, dizziness, and weakness.

Special Information

Stop using adapalene and call your doctor if you develop a

severe skin reaction or any sign of drug allergy or reaction (symptoms include rash, hives, itching, changes in complexion, and breathing difficulties or irregularities).

If you must be in the sun, be sure to apply sunscreen or wear protective clothing over areas to which you have applied adapalene.

Using more than a thin film of adapalene does not produce better results and may be more irritating to the skin.

If you forget to apply a dose of adapalene, apply it as soon as you remember. If it is almost time for your next application of adapalene, skip the dose you forgot and continue with your regular schedule.

Special Populations

Pregnancy/Breast-feeding

Animal studies of adapalene have shown no effects on the fetus. Since the effect of adapalene on pregnant women is not known, the drug should be used only when the possible benefits outweigh the risks.

It is not known if adapalene passes into breast milk. Nursing mothers should consider bottle-feeding.

Seniors

Seniors may use this drug without special precautions.

Brand Name

Adderall

Generic Ingredients

Dextroamphetamine Sulfate + Dextroamphetamine Saccharate + Amphetamine Aspartate + Amphetamine Sulfate

The information in this profile also applies to the following drug:

Generic Ingredient: Dextroamphetamine G
Dexedrine   Dextrostat

Type of Drug

Central-nervous-system stimulant.

Prescribed for

Weight control, attention-deficit hyperactivity disorder (ADHD), and narcolepsy (uncontrollable desire to sleep).

General Information

Amphetamines are stimulants that work on the brain's feeding center. Adderall, which is a mixture of two forms of amphetamine, may be used as a short-term aid in weight reduction. It should not be taken for longer than a few months for this purpose.

Amphetamines may also be prescribed for childhood ADHD. They should be used only after a complete evaluation of the child has been done. Frequency and severity of symptoms and their appropriateness for the age of the child—not solely the presence of certain behavioral characteristics—determine whether drug therapy is required. Many experts believe that amphetamines offer only a temporary solution because they do not permanently change behavioral patterns. Psychological measures must also be taken to ensure successful treatment in the long term.

Cautions and Warnings

Amphetamines should be used with extreme caution because they are highly **addictive** and easily abused.

Do not take this drug if you are **sensitive** or **allergic** to any amphetamine or have **heart disease, high blood pressure, thyroid disease,** or **glaucoma.**

Stimulants like amphetamines are not effective for children whose symptoms are related to environmental factors or primary psychiatric conditions, including psychosis.

Possible Side Effects

▼ Common: heart palpitations, restlessness, overstimulation, dizziness, sleeplessness, increased blood pressure, and rapid heartbeat.

▼ Less common: euphoria (feeling "high"), hallucinations, muscle spasms and tremors, headache, dry mouth, unpleasant taste in the mouth, diarrhea, constipation, upset stomach, itching, and loss of sex drive.

▼ Rare: psychotic drug reactions.

Drug Interactions

• Combining an amphetamine and a monoamine oxidase inhibitor (MAOI) drug may cause a severe increase in blood pressure as well as bleeding inside the skull. Wait at least 2 weeks after stopping an MAOI before taking an amphetamine.

• Amphetamines may reduce guanethidine's effectiveness for high blood pressure.

• Your insulin dosage may need an adjustment if you start taking an amphetamine.

• Tricyclic antidepressants may reduce an amphetamine's effects.

Food Interactions

Take this drug with food if it upsets your stomach.

Usual Dose

Weight Control: 5–30 mg a day in divided doses 30–60 minutes before meals; alternately, a single, long-acting dose may be taken in the morning.

ADHD: 2.5–40 mg a day.

Narcolepsy: 5–60 mg a day.

Overdosage

Symptoms include tremors, muscle spasms, restlessness, exaggerated reflexes, rapid breathing, hallucinations, confusion, panic, and overaggressive behavior. These may be followed by depression, exhaustion, abnormal heart rhythms, blood pressure changes, nausea, vomiting, diarrhea, convulsions, and coma. Take the victim to a hospital emergency room immediately. ALWAYS bring the prescription bottle or container.

Special Information

When taken for weight control, this drug may gradually lose its effectiveness as the body starts breaking it down faster. Do NOT increase your dosage when this occurs. The drug must be discontinued.

To prevent this drug from interfering with sleep, take it at least 6 to 8 hours before bedtime.

Do not crush or chew the sustained-release form.

If you forget your once-daily dose, skip it and go back to your regular schedule the next day. If you take the drug 2 to 3 times a day and miss a dose, take it as soon as you remember. If it is within 3 hours of your next dose, skip the one you forgot and continue with your regular schedule. Never take a double dose.

Special Populations

Pregnancy/Breast-feeding
Use of amphetamines during the early stages of pregnancy may cause birth defects. Amphetamines also increase the risk of premature delivery and low-birth-weight infants and may cause drug withdrawal symptoms in newborns. When this drug is considered crucial by your doctor, its potential benefits must be carefully weighed against its risks.

It is not known if amphetamines pass into breast milk. Nursing mothers who must take them should consider bottle-feeding.

Seniors
Seniors are more sensitive to this drug's effects.

Brand Name

Aggrenox

Generic Ingredients
Dipyridamole + Aspirin

Type of Drug
Antiplatelet.

Prescribed for
Prevention of recurrent stroke or transient ischemic attack (TIA)—"mini-stroke."

General Information
Stroke is often the result of a clot blocking flow in a blood vessel supplying the brain. Aggrenox helps prevent blood clot formation by reducing the "stickiness" of platelets, blood cells that stick together to form the beginnings of all clots.

The combination of ingredients in Aggrenox, which achieve their antiplatelet effects in different ways, prevented 30% more strokes than aspirin in one study.

Cautions and Warnings

Do not use this drug if you are **sensitive** or **allergic** to any of its ingredients or any nonsteroidal anti-inflammatory drug (NSAID). People who have **asthma,** or **nasal polyps and a runny nose,** are likely to be sensitive to aspirin.

The aspirin in Aggrenox can cause Reye's syndrome, a severe reaction (vomiting, lethargy, and belligerence, and possibly worsening to coma) in **children under age 16**.

People with a history of **stomach ulcers or problems** should avoid Aggrenox.

People who have **angina** or have had a recent **heart attack** should be very cautious about taking this drug. It may worsen chest pain.

People with **low blood pressure, liver disease, or kidney failure** should be cautious about taking this drug.

People taking Aggrenox have a higher risk of **bleeding**.

Women being treated for myasthenia gravis should avoid aspirin, because it can interfere with anticholinesterase drugs used to treat that condition.

Possible Side Effects

▼ Most common: headache, upset stomach, abdominal pain, nausea, and diarrhea.

▼ Common: pain, tiredness, and vomiting.

▼ Less common: convulsions, rectal bleeding, blood in the stool, hemorrhoids, back pain, accidental injuries, stomach bleeding, feeling unwell, weakness, fainting, memory loss, arthritis, joint or muscle pain, coughing, and respiratory infection.

▼ Rare: Rare side effects can occur in almost any part of the body. Contact your doctor if you experience any side effect not listed above.

Drug Interactions

• Avoid alcohol. People who take 3 or more drinks a day while using any aspirin-containing product are more likely to develop stomach ulcers or bleeding.

• Aspirin may reduce the blood-pressure-lowering effects of angiotensin-converting enzyme (ACE) inhibitor drugs, beta blockers, and diuretics.

• Aspirin blocks the effects of sulfinpyrazone and probenecid.

• Combining aspirin and acetazolamide or an NSAID can cause kidney problems.

• Aspirin can increase the blood-thinning effects of warfarin. Avoid aspirin- containing products if you are taking warfarin.

• Aspirin can increase blood levels of oral antidiabetes drugs, methotrexate, phenytoin, or valproic acid, possibly leading to drug side effects.

Food Interactions

Aggrenox is best taken on an empty stomach but may be taken with food if it upsets your stomach.

Usual Dose

Adult: 1 capsule morning and evening.

Overdosage

Symptoms include a sensation of warmth, flushing, sweating, restlessness, weakness, dizziness, low blood pressure, and rapid heartbeat. Take the victim to a hospital emergency room. ALWAYS bring the prescription bottle or container.

Special Information

Avoid alcohol while taking this drug.

In people taking Aggrenox, minor cuts may take longer than normal to stop bleeding.

If you forget a dose, take it as soon as you remember. If it is almost time for your next dose, skip the one you forgot and continue with your regular schedule.

Special Populations

Pregnancy/Breast-feeding

Pregnant women should avoid Aggrenox because of its aspirin content. Aspirin can cause bleeding problems in mother and fetus and result in a low-birth-weight infant.

Both ingredients in Aggrenox pass into breast milk. Nursing mothers who must take this drug should bottle-feed.

Seniors

Seniors may take this drug without special precaution.

Generic Name

Albendazole (al-BEN-duh-zole)

Brand Name

Albenza

Type of Drug

Anthelmintic.

Prescribed for

Nervous system infections caused by the pork tapeworm and cysts caused by the dog tapeworm.

General Information

Albendazole fights certain worm infections by interfering with routine functions of the infecting organisms. It is rapidly broken down in the liver and passes out of the body through the intestines. Your doctor will monitor your liver function and blood count while you are taking albendazole.

Cautions and Warnings

Albendazole can cause **liver inflammation,** but liver function usually returns to normal once the drug is stopped. People with **liver obstruction** may have much more albendazole in their blood than those with normal liver function.

Women should have a **pregnancy test** to be sure they are not pregnant before they start taking albendazole.

The drug is **poorly absorbed** unless taken with a high-fat meal.

Few children younger than age 6 have taken albendazole, but those who have taken it have not had special problems.

Possible Side Effects

▼ Most common: liver inflammation and headache.

▼ Common: abdominal pain, nausea, and vomiting.

▼ Less common: dizziness, fainting, increased pressure in the head, and hair loss—which reverses when the medicine is stopped.

▼ Rare: fever, decreases in blood-cell counts, itching, rash, drug allergy, and kidney failure.

Drug Interactions

• Mixing albendazole with dexamethasone, praziquantal—another anthelmintic—or cimetidine increases the amount of albendazole in the blood.

Food Interactions

Eating a high-fat meal—about 40 g of fat—with your dose of albendazole improves the absorption of the drug into the blood.

Usual Dose

Adult and Child (130 lbs. and over): 400 mg twice a day with meals.

Adult and Child (under 130 lbs.): about 7 mg per lb. of body weight a day, divided into 2 doses, up to 800 mg total dose.

For dog tapeworm disease, take the prescribed dose for 28 days and stop for 2 weeks. Repeat this cycle 3 times in a row. For pork tapeworm disease, take the prescribed dose for 8–30 days.

Overdosage

Little is known about the effects of albendazole overdose. Overdose victims should be taken to a hospital emergency room for treatment. ALWAYS bring the prescription bottle or container.

Special Information

Women must have a pregnancy test with a negative result before starting albendazole treatment. Women who are not pregnant must take special care to avoid becoming pregnant while taking albendazole and for 1 month after finishing the drug. Women who become pregnant while taking albendazole must stop taking it at once to avoid possible birth defects.

Take this drug exactly as prescribed. If you forget a dose, take it as soon as you remember. If it is almost time for your next dose, skip the dose you forgot and continue with your regular schedule. Do not take a double dose.

Special Populations

Pregnancy/Breast-feeding

Albendazole causes birth defects in animals. Pregnant women should not take albendazole unless no other treatments are available.

It is not known if albendazole passes into breast milk.

Seniors
Seniors may take this drug without special precaution.

Generic Name

Albuterol (al-BUE-tuh-rawl) Ⓖ

Brand Names

Proventil*   Ventolin*   Volmax

The information in this profile also applies to the following drugs:

Generic Ingredient: Levalbuterol
Xopenex

Generic Ingredient: Pirbuterol
Maxair

Some products in this brand-name group are alcohol- or sugar-free. Consult your pharmacist.

Type of Drug

Bronchodilator.

Prescribed for

Asthma and bronchospasm.

General Information

Albuterol is similar to other bronchodilator drugs, such as metaproterenol and isoetharine, but it has a weaker effect on nerve receptors in the heart and blood vessels; therefore, it is somewhat safer for people with heart conditions. Levalbuterol is a special form of albuterol that carries a lower risk of side effects.

Cautions and Warnings

Albuterol should be used with caution by people with a history of **angina pectoris** (a condition characterized by brief attacks of chest pain), **heart disease, high blood pressure, stroke** or **seizure, diabetes, thyroid disease, prostate disease,** or **glaucoma**. Excessive use of albuterol inhalants may worsen **asthma** or other respiratory conditions, and may increase breathing difficulties rather than relieve them. In the most extreme cases, people have had heart attacks after using excessive amounts of inhalant.

Possible Side Effects

▼ Most common: restlessness, weakness, anxiety, fear, tension, sleeplessness, tremors, convulsions, dizziness, headache, flushing, appetite changes, pallor, sweating, nausea, vomiting, and muscle cramps.

▼ Less common: angina, abnormal heart rhythms, rapid heartbeat and heart palpitations, high blood pressure, not feeling well, irritability and emotional instability, nightmares, aggressive behavior, bronchitis, stuffy nose, nosebleeds, increased sputum, conjunctivitis (pinkeye), tooth discoloration, voice changes, hoarseness, and urinary difficulty.

Drug Interactions

• Albuterol's effects may be increased by monoamine oxidase inhibitors (MAOIs), tricyclic antidepressants, thyroid drugs, other bronchodilator drugs, and some antihistamines.

• The chance of cardiotoxicity may be increased in people taking both albuterol and theophylline.

• Albuterol is antagonized by beta-blocking drugs such as propranolol.

• Albuterol may antagonize the effects of blood-pressure-lowering drugs, especially reserpine, methyldopa, and guanethidine.

• Albuterol may reduce the amount of digoxin in the blood of people taking both drugs. Digoxin dose adjustment may be required.

Food Interactions

Albuterol tablets are more effective when taken on an empty stomach—1 hour before or 2 hours after meals—but can be taken with food if they upset your stomach.

Usual Dose

Albuterol and Pirbuterol Inhalation
   Adult and Child (age 12 and over): 1–2 puffs every 4–6

hours. Asthma triggered by exercise may be prevented by taking 2 puffs 15 minutes before exercising.

Albuterol Inhalation Solution
   Adult and Child (age 12 and over): 2.5 mg 3 or 4 times a day. Dilute 0.5 ml of the 0.5% solution with 2.5 ml of sterile saline. Deliver over 5–15 minutes by nebulizer.

Levalbuterol Inhalation Solution
   Adult and Child (age 12 and over): 0.63 mg 3 times a day every 6 to 8 hours. Some people may benefit from 1.25 mg at each dose. Deliver over 5–15 minutes by nebulizer.

Albuterol Inhalation Capsules
   Adult and Child (age 4 and over): 200–400 mcg inhaled every 4–6 hours using a special Rotahaler device. Adults and adolescents (age 12 and over) may prevent asthma brought on by exercise by inhaling a single 200-mcg dose 15 minutes before exercising.

Albuterol Tablets
   Adult and Child (age 12 and over): starting dose—6–16 mg a day in divided doses. The dosage may slowly be increased to a maximum of 32 mg a day until the asthma is controlled.
   Senior: starting dose—6–8 mg a day in divided doses. Increase to the maximum daily adult dosage, if tolerated.
   Child (age 6–11): starting dose—6–8 mg a day in divided doses. Increase to a maximum daily dose of 24 mg.
   Child (age 2–5): up to 4 mg, 3 times a day.

Albuterol Sustained-Release Tablets
   Adult and Child (age 12 and over): 4–8 mg every 12 hours. Dosage may be cautiously increased to a maximum of 32 mg a day. People being switched from regular to sustained-release tablets generally take the same dosage per day, in fewer tablets—for example, a 4-mg tablet every 12 hours (1 dose) instead of a 2-mg tablet every 6 hours (2 doses).

Overdosage

Overdose of albuterol inhalation usually results in exaggerated side effects, including chest pain and high blood pressure. People who inhale too much albuterol should see a doctor. Overdose of albuterol tablets may lead to changes in heart rate, palpitations, unusual heart rhythm, chest pain, high blood pressure, fever, chills, cold sweats, nausea, vomiting, and dilation of the pupils. Convulsions, sleeplessness, anxiety, and tremors may also develop, and the victim may collapse. If the albuterol overdose was taken within the past half-hour, give the victim syrup of ipecac to induce vomiting. DO NOT GIVE IPECAC IF THE VICTIM IS UNCONSCIOUS OR CONVULSING. If symptoms have already begun to develop, the victim may need to be taken to a hospital emergency room. Call for instructions, and ALWAYS bring the prescription bottle or container.

Special Information

If you are inhaling albuterol, be sure to follow the inhalation instructions that come with the product. The drug should be inhaled during the second half of your inward breath, since this will allow it to reach deeper into your lungs. If you use more than 1 puff per dose, wait about 5 minutes between puffs. Do not inhale albuterol if you have food or anything else in your mouth.

Do not take more albuterol than your doctor prescribes. Taking more than you need can worsen your symptoms. If your condition worsens after taking your medicine, call your doctor at once and stop taking it.

Call your doctor immediately if you develop chest pain, palpitations, rapid heartbeat, muscle tremors, dizziness, headache, facial flushing, or urinary difficulty, or if you continue having breathing difficulties after taking the medicine.

If you forget a dose of albuterol, take it as soon as you remember. If it is almost time for your next dose, skip the one you forgot. Do not take a double dose.

Special Populations

Pregnancy/Breast-feeding

When used during childbirth, albuterol can slow or delay natural labor. It can cause rapid heartbeat and high blood sugar in the mother and rapid heartbeat and low blood sugar in the baby. Albuterol also causes birth defects in animal studies. When your doctor considers this drug crucial, its benefits must be cautiously weighed against its risks.

It is not known if albuterol passes into breast milk. Nursing mothers who must take it should consider bottle-feeding.

Seniors

Seniors are more sensitive to the effects of albuterol.

Generic Name

Alitretinoin (al-ih-TRET-in-oin)

Brand Name

Panretin

Type of Drug

Retinoid.

Prescribed for

Skin lesions of Kaposi's sarcoma (KS).

General Information

Alitretinoin binds to and activates retinoid receptors in human cells. Once activated, these receptors help stimulate the body's natural mechanisms for limiting tissue growth—in this case, the growth of KS cells. KS lesions, which are primarily associated with human immunodeficiency virus (HIV), can respond to alitretinoin in as little as two weeks, but most people do not start to see results for 4 to 8 weeks or, in some cases, 14 weeks or more.

Cautions and Warnings

Do not use alitretinoin if you are **sensitive** or **allergic** to it or any ingredient in this product.

Alitretinoin is applied to individual KS lesions. It does not treat **systemic KS** or prevent **new KS lesions** from forming.

People taking **systemic KS treatment** because they have developed more than 10 new KS lesions in the past year should not use alitretinoin.

People with **swollen lymph glands, KS that affects the lungs,** or **other KS involvement** should not use alitretinoin.

Possible Side Effects

▼ Most common: rash and burning pain.

▼ Common: itchy, flaking, or peeling skin; cracking, oozing, or other skin problems; swelling; and inflammation.

▼ Less common: tingling in the area to which alitretinoin is applied.

Drug Interactions

• Do not use insect repellant products that contain DEET, a widely used chemical repellant. Alitretinoin increases DEET toxicity.

Usual Dose

Adult: Apply 2–4 times a day to KS skin lesions. Seniors should use this drug with caution.

Child: not recommended.

Overdosage

Little is known about the effects of accidental ingestion. Call your local poison control center or a hospital emergency room for information.

Special Information

Apply enough alitretinoin gel to cover the entire skin lesion. Allow the gel to dry for 3 to 5 minutes before covering the area with clothing.

If you use a bandage or dressing, be sure it is not tight and that air can circulate freely over the area.

Avoid applying alitretinoin to unaffected skin because it may be irritated by the drug. Avoid applying near the nose, eyes, or mouth.

Retinoids can cause unusual sensitivity to the sun. While this has not been seen with alitretinoin, you should avoid prolonged exposure to the sun or use sunscreen while taking this drug.

If you forget a dose, apply it as soon as you remember. If it is almost time for your next dose, apply the forgotten dose and then space the rest of your doses throughout the day. Continue with your regular schedule the next day.

Special Populations

Pregnancy/Breast-feeding

Alitretinoin can harm the fetus when sufficient levels of the drug are present in the mother's bloodstream, but it is not known if these levels are achieved during routine use of alitretinoin. Women who are or might be pregnant should only use this drug after discussing its potential benefits and risks with their doctors.

It is not known if alitretinoin passes into breast milk. Nursing mothers who must use alitretinoin should bottle-feed.

Seniors
There is no information on use of alitretinoin by seniors. Seniors should use it with caution.

Allegra   see **Cetirizine**, page 183

Allegra-D   see **Antihistamine-Decongestant Combination Products**, page 81

Allesse   see **Contraceptives**, page 254

Generic Name

Allopurinol   (al-oe-PURE-in-nol) Ⓖ

Brand Name

Zyloprim

Type of Drug

Antigout medication.

Prescribed for

Gout or gouty arthritis; also prescribed for cancer, ulcers, abnormal heart rhythms in heart bypass patients, seizures, and other conditions that may be associated with too much uric acid in the body.

General Information

Unlike other antigout drugs, which affect the elimination of uric acid from the body, allopurinol acts on the system that manufactures uric acid in your body. A high level of uric acid can indicate that you have gout, psoriasis, cancer, or any of a number of other diseases. High levels of uric acid can also be caused by taking certain drugs.

In mouthwash form, allopurinol helps to prevent mouth, stomach, and intestinal ulcers caused by fluorouracil, an antineoplastic drug. Allopurinol may be given before heart bypass surgery to reduce abnormal rhythms and other surgical complications. It can be used to reduce the relapse rates of duodenal ulcers associated with *Helicobacter pylori* infection and to reduce the vomiting of blood from stomach irritation caused by nonsteroidal anti-inflammatory drugs (NSAIDs). Allopurinol has also been used to control seizures in people for whom standard treatments are not effective.

Cautions and Warnings

Do not take this medication if you have ever developed a **severe reaction** to it. Stop taking the medication immediately and contact your doctor if you develop a **rash** or any other adverse effects while taking allopurinol. Do not start taking allopurinol again if you stopped it because of a severe reaction.

Allopurinol should be used by children only if they have high uric acid levels due to neoplastic disease or to rare metabolic conditions.

A few cases of **liver toxicity** have been associated with allopurinol; they improved when the drug was stopped. People taking allopurinol should periodically be tested for liver and kidney function. People with severely **compromised kidney function** should take a reduced dose of allopurinol.

Possible Side Effects

▼ Most common: rash associated with severe, allergic, or sensitivity reaction to allopurinol. If you develop an unusual rash or other sign of drug toxicity, stop taking this medication and contact your doctor.

▼ Less common: nausea, vomiting, diarrhea, intermittent stomach pain, effects on blood components, and drowsiness or lack of ability to concentrate.

▼ Rare: Rare side effects can occur in almost any part of the body. Contact your doctor if you experience any side effect not listed above.

Drug Interactions

• Large doses of drugs that make your urine more acidic, like megadoses of vitamin C, may increase the risk of kidney stone formation.

• Alcohol, diazoxide, mecamylamine, or pyrazinamide can increase the amount of uric acid in your blood; an increase in your allopurinol dose may be required.

• Allopurinol may increase the action of azathioprine, mercaptopurine, or cyclophosphamide and other anticancer drugs, leading to possible bleeding or infection.

• Taking allopurinol with dacarbazine, probenecid, or sulfinpyrazone may cause excessive reduction of uric acid.

• Allopurinol may interact with anticoagulant (blood-thinning) medications, reducing the rate at which the anticoagulant is broken down in the body. Dosage reduction is necessary.

• People who are susceptible to ampicillin, amoxicillin, bacampicillin, or hetacillin rash are more likely to develop such a reaction while also taking allopurinol.

• Combining a thiazide diuretic or an ACE-inhibitor (for high blood pressure or heart failure) with allopurinol increases the risk of a drug-sensitivity reaction.

• Combining vidarabine with allopurinol may increase the risk of neurotoxic effects and anemia, nausea, pain, and itching.

• Large doses of allopurinol—more than 600 mg a day— may increase the effects of and risk of toxic reactions to theophylline by interfering with its clearance from the body.

Food Interactions

Take each dose with food or a full glass of water. Drink 10 to 12 glasses of water, juices, soda, or another liquid each day to avoid the formation of crystals in your urine or kidneys.

Usual Dose

Adult and Child (age 11 and over): 100–800 mg a day, depending on disease and response.

Child (age 6–10): 300–600 mg a day.

Child (under age 6): 150 mg a day.

The dose should be reviewed periodically by your doctor to be sure that it is producing the desired therapeutic effect.

Overdosage

The expected symptoms of overdose are exaggerated side effects. Allopurinol overdose victims should be taken to a hospital. ALWAYS bring the prescription bottle or container.

Special Information

Allopurinol can make you drowsy or make it difficult to concentrate: Take care while driving a car or operating hazardous equipment.

Call your doctor at once if you develop rash, hives, itching, chills, fever, nausea, muscle aches, unusual tiredness, fever, yellowing of the whites of the eyes or skin, painful urination, blood in the urine, irritation of the eyes, or swelling of the lips or mouth.

Avoid large doses of vitamin C, which can cause the formation of kidney stones during allopurinol treatment. Be sure to drink 10 to 12 8-oz. glasses of water a day while taking this medication.

If you forget to take a dose of allopurinol, take it as soon as possible. If it is almost time for your next regular dose, double this dose. For example, if your regular dose is 100 mg and you miss a dose, take 200 mg at the next usual dose time.

Special Populations

Pregnancy/Breast-feeding

Allopurinol may cause birth defects or interfere with fetal development. Check with your doctor before taking it if you are or might be pregnant.

Allopurinol passes into breast milk. Nursing mothers who must take allopurinol should consider bottle-feeding.

Seniors

No special precautions are required. Follow your doctor's directions and report any side effects at once.

Generic Name

Alprazolam (al-PRAY-zoe-lam) Ⓖ

Brand Name

Xanax

Type of Drug

Benzodiazepine tranquilizer.

Prescribed for

Anxiety, tension, fatigue, and agitation; also prescribed for irritable bowel syndrome, panic attacks, depression, and pre-menstrual syndrome (PMS).

General Information

Alprazolam is a member of a group of drugs known as benzodiazepines. Benzodiazepines directly affect the brain. They can relax you and make you more tranquil or sleepier, or they can slow nervous system transmissions in such a way as to act as an anticonvulsant. Many doctors prefer benzodiazepines to other drugs that can be used to similar effect because they tend to be safer, have fewer side effects, and are usually as effective, if not more so.

Cautions and Warnings

Do not take alprazolam if you know you are **sensitive** or **allergic** to it or to another benzodiazepine drug, including clonazepam.

Alprazolam can aggravate narrow-angle **glaucoma,** but you may take it if you have open-angle glaucoma.

Other conditions where alprazolam should be avoided are: severe **depression,** severe **lung disease, sleep apnea** (inter-mittent cessation of breathing during sleep), **liver disease, drunkenness,** and **kidney disease**. In each of these conditions, the depressive effects of alprazolam may be enhanced or could be detrimental to your overall condition.

Alprazolam should not be taken by **psychotic patients** because it is not effective for them and can trigger unusual excitement, stimulation, and rage.

Alprazolam is meant to be used for no more than 3 to 4 months in a row. Your condition should be reassessed before continuing your medicine beyond that time.

Alprazolam may be addictive. Drug withdrawal may develop if you stop taking it after only 4 weeks of regular use but is more likely after longer use. It may start with anxiety and progress to tingling in the hands or feet, sensitivity to bright light, sleep disturbances, cramps, tremors, muscle ten-sion or twitching, poor concentration, flu-like symptoms, fatigue, appetite loss, sweating, and changes in mental state.

Possible Side Effects

▼ Most common: mild drowsiness during the first few days of therapy. Weakness and confusion may occur, especially in seniors and in those who are sickly. If these effects persist, contact your doctor.

▼ Less common: depression, lethargy, disorientation, headache, inactivity, slurred speech, stupor, dizziness, tremors, constipation, dry mouth, nausea, inability to control urination, sexual difficulties, irregular menstrual cycle, changes in heart rhythm, low blood pressure, fluid retention, blurred or double vision, itching, rash, hiccups, nervousness, inability to fall asleep, and occasional liver dysfunction. If you experience any of these symptoms, stop taking the medicine and contact your doctor immediately.

▼ Rare: Rare side effects can occur in almost any part of the body. Contact your doctor if you experience any side effect not listed above.

Drug Interactions

• Alprazolam is a central-nervous-system depressant. Avoid alcohol, other tranquilizers, narcotics, barbiturates, monoamine oxidase inhibitors (MAOIs), antihistamines, and antidepressants. Taking alprazolam with these drugs may result in excessive depression, tiredness, sleepiness, breathing difficulties, or related symptoms.

• Smoking may reduce the effectiveness of alprazolam by increasing the rate at which it is broken down by the body.

• The effects of alprazolam may be prolonged when taken together with cimetidine, oral contraceptives, disulfiram, fluoxetine, isoniazid, itraconazole, ketoconazole, metoprolol, probenecid, propoxyphene, propranolol, rifampin, and valproic acid.

• Theophylline may reduce alprazolam's sedative effects.

• If you take antacids, separate them from your alprazolam dose by at least 1 hour to prevent them from interfering with the absorption of alprazolam into the bloodstream.

• Alprazolam may raise digoxin blood levels and the chances of digoxin toxicity.

• The effect of levodopa may be decreased if it is taken together with alprazolam.

• Combining alprazolam with phenytoin may increase phenytoin blood concentrations and the chances of phenytoin toxicity.

Food Interactions

Alprazolam is best taken on an empty stomach but may be taken with food if it upsets your stomach.

Usual Dose

Adult: 0.75–4 mg a day. Dosage must be tailored to your individual needs.

Child (under age 18): not recommended.

Overdosage

Symptoms of overdose are confusion, sleepiness, poor coordination, lack of response to pain such as a pinprick, loss of reflexes, shallow breathing, low blood pressure, and coma. The victim should be taken to a hospital emergency room. ALWAYS bring the prescription bottle or container.

Special Information

Alprazolam can cause tiredness, drowsiness, inability to concentrate, or related symptoms. Be careful if you are driving, operating machinery, or performing other activities that require concentration.

Anyone taking alprazolam for more than 3 or 4 months at a time may have a drug withdrawal reaction if the medicine is stopped suddenly (see "Cautions and Warnings").

If you forget a dose of alprazolam, take it as soon as you remember. If it is almost time for your next dose, skip the dose you forgot and return to your regular schedule. Do not take a double dose.

Special Populations

Pregnancy/Breast-feeding

Alprazolam may cause birth defects if taken during the first 3 months of pregnancy. You should avoid alprazolam while pregnant.

Alprazolam may pass into breast milk. Nursing mothers who must take alprazolam should bottle-feed.

Seniors

Seniors, especially those with liver or kidney disease, are more sensitive to the effects of alprazolam and generally require smaller doses to achieve the same effect.

Generic Name

Alprostadil (al-PROS-tuh-dil) Ⓖ

Brand Names

Caverject   Muse
Edex

Type of Drug

Anti-impotence agent.

Prescribed for

Erectile dysfunction; also prescribed for atherosclerosis (hardening of the arteries), gangrene, pain due to blood vessel disease, and congenital heart defects in newborns.

General Information

A male erection happens when blood flows into blood vessels and holding areas inside the penis. Problems occur when blood cannot move into the penis as it normally should. Alprostadil (prostaglandin E1 or PGE1) helps men get and keep an erection by dilating blood vessels that supply the penis and by relaxing muscles to help expand holding areas. Alprostadil also dilates other vessels and reduces platelet stickiness—which slows blood-clotting rates—and relaxes some muscle groups. Alprostadil must be injected into the tissue of the penis or inserted into the urethra.

Cautions and Warnings

Do not take alprostadil if you are **allergic** to it or to other prostaglandin drugs. Alprostadil can cause **priapism** (painful erection lasting more than 6 hours). People with diseases where priapism is a possibility—**sickle cell anemia or trait, multiple myeloma, leukemia**—those with **penile deformities,** or **penile implants, women, children,** or **those for whom sexual activity could be dangerous** should not use alprostadil.
  Penile pain is common after using either form of alprostadil, although it is usually mild or moderate.

Possible Side Effects

Injection

▼ Most common: penile pain.

▼ Less common: prolonged erection; penile fibrosis (deformity); blood blister or black-and-blue marks at the injection site, usually caused by poor injection technique; penis disorders, including yeast infection, numbness, irritation, sensitivity, itching, redness, and torn skin; penile rash or swelling; headache; dizziness; fainting; respiratory infection; flu symptoms; sinus inflammation; runny or stuffed nose; cough; blood pressure changes; local pain; prostate problems; back pain; and general pain.

▼ Rare: Rare side effects can affect the penis, kidney and urinary tract, heart and blood, skin, and eyes. Contact your doctor if you experience any side effect not listed above.

Pellets

▼ Most common: penile pain.

▼ Common: urethral pain, burning or bleeding, and testicular pain.

▼ Less common: headache, dizziness, respiratory infection, flu symptoms, runny nose, sinus inflammation, low blood pressure, back pain, pelvic pain, and general pain.

▼ Rare: Rare side effects can affect the kidney and urinary tract, heart and blood, skin, and eyes. Contact your doctor if you experience any side effect not listed above.

Drug Interactions

• Alprostadil can increase the effect of anticoagulant (blood-thinning) drugs. Your doctor may have to adjust the dose of your anticoagulant.

• Alprostadil may decrease the amount of cyclosporine in your blood.

• The safety of combining alprostadil with other drugs that affect blood vessels is not known. These combinations should be used with caution.

Food Interactions

None known.

Usual Dose

Dosage must be individualized to your need and response.

Overdosage

Alprostadil overdose can lead to an extended and painful erection, as well as other side effects. Overdose victims should seek medical attention.

Special Information

Patient information leaflets are included with each alprostadil prescription. Read this information before you use your prescription.

You must be trained in proper injection technique by your doctor. Self-injection should be permitted only after your doctor has made sure you know how to do it properly.

Alprostadil begins working within 5 to 10 minutes after taking it. Dosage should be set so that your erection lasts for about 30 to 60 minutes. Use the lowest dose that works.

Special Populations

Pregnancy/Breast-feeding

This product should not be used by women. Men using alprostadil must use a condom if they have intercourse with a pregnant woman. Alprostadil passes into semen and will affect the development of a fetal heart if a condom is not worn.

Seniors

Seniors may use alprostadil without special precaution.

Generic Name

Amantadine (uh-MAN-tuh-dene) Ⓖ

Brand Name

Symmetrel

Type of Drug

Antiviral and antiparkinsonian.

Prescribed for

Flu viruses, all varieties of Parkinson's disease, and uncontrolled muscle movements caused by phenothiazines and other psychoactive drugs; also used for fatigue associated with multiple sclerosis.

General Information

Although its action is not entirely understood, amantadine hydrochloride appears to prevent the release of the infectious part of some flu viruses into body cells; it may also interfere with the penetration of the virus into body cells. Amantadine is used to prevent and treat flu. It is 70% to 90% effective in preventing type A flu and will reduce symptoms of type A flu when taken within 2 days after they begin. Amantadine does not work for type B flu.

Cautions and Warnings

Do not take amantadine if you are **sensitive** or **allergic** to it. People with a history of **epilepsy** may experience increased seizure activity. People have developed **heart failure** while taking amantadine; those who already have heart failure should be carefully monitored for signs that the disease might be worsening. Amantadine is released unmetabolized from the body through the kidneys. People with **kidney disease** must receive reduced doses.

Amantadine should be used with caution by people with **liver disease,** a history of recurrent **eczema,** or **psychosis or severe psychoneurosis** that is not controlled by drug treatment.

Possible Side Effects

▼ Most common: nausea, dizziness, light-headedness, and sleeplessness.

▼ Common: depression; anxiety; irritability; hallucinations; confusion; appetite loss; dry mouth; constipation; weakness; blue or purple discoloration of the skin, which goes away 2 to 12 weeks after treatment is stopped; swelling in the arms, legs, or ankles; dizziness when rising suddenly from a sitting or lying position; low blood pressure; and headache.

▼ Less common: heart failure, psychotic reactions, urinary difficulties, breathing difficulties, fatigue, rash, vomiting, weakness, slurred speech, and visual disturbances.

▼ Rare: convulsions, increased white-blood-cell counts, eczema-type rash, and spasms of the eye muscles leading to uncontrollable eye movement and rolling.

Drug Interactions

• Combining amantadine with anticholinergic drugs like benztropine produces increased side effects. Altering the dose of either drug can solve this problem.

• Hydrochlorothiazide-triamterene (a diuretic combination) interferes with amantadine elimination through the kidneys.

• Alcohol may worsen some amantadine side effects, interfering with your ability to drive or concentrate.

Food Interactions

None known.

Usual Dose

Adult and Child (age 10 and over): 100–300 mg daily.
Senior (age 65 and over): 100 mg a day.
Child (age 1–9): 2–4 mg per lb. a day, up to 150 mg.

Overdosage

Symptoms of overdose include nausea, vomiting, appetite loss, and nervous system side effects—excitability, tremors, weakness, tiredness, blurred vision, slurred speech, and convulsions. Potentially fatal abnormal heart rhythms may also occur with large doses. Overdose victims should be taken to a hospital emergency room for treatment at once. ALWAYS bring the prescription bottle or container.

Special Information

Be careful while driving or operating any complex or hazardous equipment; avoid alcoholic beverages while taking amantadine.

Call your doctor immediately if you experience fainting; dizziness or light-headedness; visual difficulties; mood changes; swelling of the arms, legs, or ankles; or any other unusual or intolerable side effect.

A stool softener—for example, docusate—will usually relieve constipation. Dry mouth, nose, or throat can be easily relieved with candy or gum. Dry mouth also leads to tooth and gum disease. Maintain good oral hygiene to prevent cavities and gum disease while taking amantadine.

People taking amantadine for Parkinson's disease may not see any effect for at least 2 weeks.

It is important to take amantadine as your doctor has prescribed. If you are taking amantadine syrup, be sure to use the measuring spoon supplied with your prescription.

If you forget to take a dose of amantadine, take it as soon as possible. If it is almost time for your next dose, skip the dose you forgot and continue with your regular schedule. Do not take a double dose.

Special Populations

Pregnancy/Breast-feeding

In high doses, amantadine can be toxic and may cause malformations in animal fetuses. A cardiovascular malformation was reported in one infant exposed to amantadine in the first 3 months of pregnancy. Pregnant women should take this drug only if it is absolutely necessary and only after reviewing all of the possible risks with their doctors.

Amantadine passes into breast milk and may cause side effects in infants; nursing mothers should bottle-feed.

Seniors

Seniors require reduced doses of amantadine because of normal losses of kidney function.

Amaryl   see *Sulfonylurea Antidiabetes Drugs, page 957*

Ambien   see *Zolpidem, page 1108*

Generic Name

Aminolevulinic Acid (ah-MEE-noe-lev-ue-LIH-nic)

Brand Name

Levulan Kerastick

Type of Drug

Photodynamic therapy (PDT) sensitizer.

Prescribed for

Actinic keratoses.

General Information

Actinic keratoses are skin lesions that develop on sun-exposed areas of the face or hands in older adults with fair skin. Dermatologists consider them precancerous. Aminolevulinic acid solution is applied to the lesions in the doctor's office in preparation for PDT. By enhancing light sensitivity in treated skin, aminolevulinic acid increases the effectiveness of PDT, which is a form of light therapy. PDT is administered 1 day after application of this drug.

Cautions and Warnings

Aminolevulinic acid should not be applied around the **eyes** or inside the **nose** or **mouth**. Do not use this drug if you are **allergic** to it or porphyrins or have **porphyria**.

This drug causes **increased sensitivity to the sun and bright indoor lighting**. Skin reactions that may occur as a result of this sensitivity cannot be prevented by using sunscreen (see "Special Information").

Possible Side Effects

▼ Most common: scaling, crusting, itching, and changes in skin color. During PDT, which lasts for about 17 minutes, you will experience tingling, stinging, and a prickling or burning sensation in the treated lesions. These effects should begin to go away at the conclusion of PDT, though the lesions and surrounding skin will appear red. Swelling and scaling may also occur. These effects are temporary and should completely resolve within 4 weeks.

▼ Common: skin erosion and welts.

▼ Less common: pain, tenderness, swelling, skin ulcers, small blisters, oozing, loss of sensation in the area of application, scabs, and scratch marks.

Drug Interactions

• Other drugs that enhance your sensitivity to light may increase the effects of aminolevulinic acid. These drugs include griseofulvin, thiazide diuretics, sulfonylureas, phenothiazines, sulfonamides, and tetracycline medications.

Usual Dose

Aminolevulinic acid is applied to lesions in the doctor's office 14–18 hours prior to PDT.

Overdosage

Little is known about the effects of accidental ingestion, which is unlikely to occur because this drug is administered in a doctor's office.

Special Information

Only qualified medical personnel should administer this drug.

After application of the drug, avoid exposing the lesions to sunlight or bright indoor lighting for at least 40 hours. Wear a wide-brimmed hat and protective clothing during this period; sunscreen is not effective. Do not wash treated lesions until PDT has been administered.

If you experience a stinging or burning sensation, you may be able to alleviate these effects by shielding the lesions from light.

Special Populations

Pregnancy/Breast-feeding

The safety of using aminolevulinic acid during pregnancy is not known. When this drug is considered crucial by your doctor, its potential benefits must be carefully weighed against its risks.

It is not known if aminolevulinic acid passes into breast milk. Nursing mothers who must use it should consider bottle-feeding.

Seniors

Seniors may use this drug without special precaution.

Generic Name

Amiodarone (ah-mee-OE-duh-rone) [G]

Brand Name

Cordarone   Pacerone

Type of Drug

Antiarrhythmic.

Prescribed for

Abnormal heart rhythms.

General Information

Amiodarone should be prescribed only in situations where the abnormal rhythm is so severe as to be life-threatening and does not respond to other drug treatments. Amiodarone works by decreasing the sensitivity of heart tissue to nervous impulses within the heart. It has not been proven that people taking this drug will live longer than those with similar conditions who do not take it. Amiodarone may exert its effects 2 to 5 days after you start taking it, but often takes 1 to 3 weeks to affect your heart. Amiodarone's antiarrhythmic effects can last for weeks or months after you stop taking it.

Cautions and Warnings

Do not take amiodarone if you are **allergic** or **sensitive** to it or if you have **heart block**.

Amiodarone can cause **potentially fatal drug side effects**. At high doses, 10% or more of people taking this drug can develop potentially fatal **lung and respiratory effects,** beginning with cough and progressive breathing difficulties. **Liver damage** caused by amiodarone is usually mild. In rare cases, amiodarone has been associated with liver failure that resulted in death.

Amiodarone can cause **heart block,** a drastic slowing of electrical impulse movement between major areas of the heart, or extreme slowing of the heart rate. Amiodarone heart block occurs about as often as heart block caused by some other antiarrhythmic drugs, but its effects may last longer than those of the other drugs. Amiodarone can also **worsen existing abnormal heart rhythms** in 2% to 5% of people who take the drug. These effects can be fatal.

People taking amiodarone may develop optic nerve irritation, leading to **partial or complete loss of vision**. Most adults who take amiodarone for 6 months or more develop tiny deposits in the corneas of their eyes. These deposits may cause **blurred vision** or **halos** in up to 10% of people taking amiodarone. Some people develop dry eyes and sensitivity to bright light.

One in ten people taking amiodarone can experience **unusual sensitivity to the effects of the sun**. Use an appropriate sunscreen product and reapply it frequently.

Amiodarone can cause **thyroid abnormalities**. It may worsen an already sluggish thyroid gland in 2% to 10% of people taking the drug, and increase thyroid activity in 2% of people taking it.

Antiarrhythmic drugs are less effective and cause abnormal rhythms if blood potassium is low.

Possible Side Effects

About 75% of people taking 400 mg or more of amiodarone a day develop some drug side effects. As many as 18% have to stop taking the drug because of a side effect.

▼ Common: fatigue, not feeling well, tremors, unusual involuntary movements, loss of coordination, an unusual walk, muscle weakness, dizziness, tingling in the hands or feet, reduced sex drive, sleeplessness, headache, nervous system problems, nausea, vomiting, constipation, appetite loss, abdominal pain, dry eyes, unusual sensitivity to bright light, and seeing halos around bright lights. Unusual sun sensitivity is the most common skin reaction to amiodarone, but people taking this drug can develop a blue skin discoloration that may not go away completely when the drug is stopped. Other skin reactions are sun rashes, hair loss, and black-and-blue spots.

▼ Rare: inflammation of the lung or fibrous deposits in the lungs, changes in thyroid function, changes in taste or smell, bloating, unusual salivation, and changes in blood clotting. Amiodarone can cause heart failure, reduced heart rate, and abnormal rhythms. Up to 9% of people taking amiodarone develop abnormalities in liver function.

Drug Interactions

• Amiodarone increases the effects of metoprolol and other beta blockers, digoxin, flecainide, procainamide, quinidine, theophylline, and warfarin and other anticoagulants. These interactions can take from 2 or 3 days to several weeks to develop. The dosage of these drugs must be drastically reduced.

• When amiodarone and phenytoin are taken together, both drugs can be affected. Amiodarone can be antagonized by phenytoin and other hydantoin anticonvulsants, and the effect of phenytoin can be increased by amiodarone.

• Cholestyramine interferes with the absorption of amiodarone into the bloodstream.

• Cimetidine and ritonavir interfere with the breakdown of amiodarone, leading to high drug blood levels and the increased possibility of side effects.

Food Interactions

Amiodarone should be taken on an empty stomach, as food delays its absorption into your bloodstream. If amiodarone upsets your stomach, however, you may take it with food.

Usual Dose

Starting dose—800–1600 mg a day, taken in 1 or 2 doses. Maintenance dose—400 mg a day. You should take the lowest effective dose in order to minimize side effects.

Overdosage

Little is known about the effects of amiodarone overdose. Overdose victims should be taken to a hospital emergency room for treatment. ALWAYS bring the prescription bottle or container.

Special Information

Side effects are very common with amiodarone; 75% of people taking the drug will experience some drug-related problem.

Call your doctor if you develop chest pain, breathing difficulties or any other sign of changes in lung function, abnormal heartbeat, bloating in your feet or legs, tremors, fever, chills, sore throat, unusual bleeding or bruising, changes in skin color, unusual sunburn, or any other unusual side effect. See your doctor for an eye exam if your vision changes at all while taking amiodarone.

Amiodarone can make you dizzy or light-headed. Take care while driving a car or performing complex tasks.

If you take amiodarone once a day and forget to take a dose, but remember within 12 hours, take it as soon as possible. If you do not remember until later, skip the dose you forgot and continue with your regular schedule. If you take amiodarone twice a day and remember within 6 hours of your regular dose, take it as soon as you remember. Call your doctor if you forget to take 2 or more doses in a row. Do not take a double dose.

Special Populations

Pregnancy/Breast-feeding

In high doses, amiodarone has been found to be toxic to animal fetuses. Women of childbearing age should use an effective contraceptive while taking amiodarone. If you are or might be pregnant and this drug is considered crucial by your doctor, its potential benefits must be weighed against its risks.

Amiodarone passes into breast milk. Nursing mothers who must take this drug should bottle-feed.

Seniors

Dosage reduction may be needed in seniors with poor liver function.

Generic Name

Amlexanox (am-LEX-an-ox)

Brand Name

Aphthasol

Type of Drug

Skin-ulcer treatment.

Prescribed for

Mouth ulcers in people with normal immune systems.

General Information

Amlexanox slows the production or release of factors involved in the body's inflammatory response. It aids in the healing of mouth ulcers, but the exact way that it accelerates the healing process is not known.

Cautions and Warnings

Do not use amlexanox if you are **sensitive** or **allergic** to it or to any ingredient in the paste.

Possible Side Effects

▼ Less common: pain, stinging, or burning after application.

▼ Rare: mouth irritation, diarrhea, and nausea.

Drug Interactions

None known.

Food Interactions

Do not apply amlexanox while you have any food in your mouth.

Usual Dose

Apply a small amount (¼ in.) to each mouth ulcer after breakfast, lunch, and dinner, and at bedtime.

Overdosage

Swallowing even a whole tube of amlexanox would probably cause only upset stomach, nausea, diarrhea, and vomiting. Call your local poison control center or hospital emergency room for more information.

Special Information

Begin using amlexanox as soon as possible after noticing a mouth ulcer and use it until your ulcers heal. Call your doctor if the pain does not get better or the sores do not heal after 10 days of using amlexanox.

Make sure your teeth and mouth are clean before applying amlexanox paste. Squeeze ¼ in. of the paste onto your finger and apply it to each mouth ulcer using gentle pressure.

Wash your hands immediately after using amlexanox. If you get the paste into your eyes, wash it out at once using cool water.

If you forget a dose of amlexanox, use it as soon as you remember. If it is almost time for your next dose, skip the dose you forgot and continue with your regular schedule. Do not apply more than the recommended amount at any time.

Special Populations

Pregnancy/Breast-feeding

The effect of amlexanox on pregnancy is not known; use it only after discussing the possible risks and benefits with your doctor.

Amlexanox passes into the milk of nursing animals, but its effect in humans is not known. Nursing mothers should use this drug with caution.

Seniors

Seniors may use amlexanox without special precaution.

Generic Name

Amlodipine (am-LOE-dih-pene)

Brand Name

·Norvasc

Type of Drug

Calcium channel blocker.

Prescribed for

Angina pectoris, Prinzmetal's angina, and high blood pressure; has also been studied for heart failure.

General Information

Amlodipine is one of many calcium channel blockers available in the United States. These drugs block the passage of calcium, an essential factor in muscle contraction, into the heart and smooth muscles. Such blockage interferes with the contraction of these muscles, which in turn dilates (widens) the veins and vessels that supply blood to them. This dilating effect reduces blood pressure, the amount of oxygen used by the heart muscles, and the risk of blood vessel spasm. Amlodipine is therefore useful in treating not only high blood pressure but also angina pectoris (brief attacks of chest pain), a condition related to poor oxygen supply to the heart muscles.

Amlodipine affects the movement of calcium only into muscle cells; it has no effect on calcium in the blood.

Cautions and Warnings

Amlodipine may, in rare instances, cause unwanted **low blood pressure** in some people taking it for reasons other than hypertension. This is more of a problem with other calcium channel blockers.

Amlodipine may worsen **heart failure** in some people and should be used with caution if heart failure is present.

Calcium channel blockers, alone and with aspirin, have caused **bruises, black-and-blue marks,** and **bleeding** due to an anticoagulant effect. This is mostly a problem with nifedipine but should be considered for all members of the group.

Amlodipine may cause **angina** when treatment is first started, when dosage is increased, or if the drug is rapidly withdrawn. This can be avoided by gradually reducing dosage.

Studies have shown that people taking calcium channel blockers—usually those taken several times a day, not those taken only once daily—have a greater chance of having a **heart attack** than people taking beta blockers or another medicine for the same purposes. Discuss this with your doctor to be sure you are receiving the best possible treatment.

Do not take this drug if you have had an **allergic reaction** to it in the past.

People with severe **liver disease** may require reduced dosage.

Possible Side Effects

▼ Most common: headache, dizziness or light-headedness, anxiety, nausea, swelling in the arms or legs, heart palpitations, and flushing.

▼ Less common: sleepiness, muscle weakness, cramps or abdominal discomfort, itching, rash, sexual difficulties, wheezing or shortness of breath, muscle cramps, pain, and inflammation.

▼ Rare: Rare side effects can occur in almost any part of the body. Contact your doctor if you experience any side effect not listed above.

Drug Interactions

• Amlodipine may interact with beta-blocking drugs to cause heart failure, very low blood pressure, or an increased incidence of angina.

• Amlodipine may cause unexpected blood-pressure reduction when combined with other antihypertensive drugs; however, this interaction is more likely with other calcium channel blockers.

• The combination of quinidine (prescribed for abnormal heart rhythm) and amlodipine must be used with caution because it can produce low blood pressure, very slow heart rate, abnormal heart rhythms, and swelling in the arms or legs.

• Amlodipine can increase the effects of theophylline—prescribed for asthma and other respiratory problems—and related drugs.

• Patients taking amlodipine who are given fentanyl as a short-term surgical anesthetic may experience very low blood pressure.

Food Interactions

None known.

Usual Dose

5–10 mg once a day. Do not stop taking amlodipine abruptly. The dosage should be gradually reduced over a period of time.

Overdosage

Overdose of amlodipine can cause nausea, weakness, dizziness, confusion, and slurred speech. Take overdose victims to a hospital emergency room, or call your local poison control center for directions. You may be asked to make the patient vomit to remove the medication from the stomach. If you go to the emergency room, ALWAYS bring the prescription bottle or container.

Special Information

Call your doctor if you develop constipation, nausea, weakness or dizziness, swelling in the hands or feet, breathing difficulties, or increased heart pains, or if other side effects are bothersome or persistent.

If you are taking amlodipine for high blood pressure, be sure to continue taking your medication even if you feel well, and follow any instructions for diet restriction or other treatments.

It is important to maintain good dental hygiene while taking amlodipine and to use extra care when using your toothbrush or dental floss because of the chance that the drug will make you more susceptible to certain infections.

If you forget a dose of amlodipine, take it as soon as you remember. If it is almost time for your next dose, skip the dose you forgot and continue with your regular schedule. Do not take a double dose.

Special Populations

Pregnancy/Breast-feeding

Animal studies of amlodipine show that it may damage a fetus. Other calcium channel blockers can be used to treat severe high blood pressure associated with pregnancy, so there is no reason for women who are or might become pregnant to take amlodipine.

It is not known if amlodipine passes into breast milk. Nursing mothers who take amlodipine should consider bottle-feeding.

Seniors

Seniors, especially those with liver disease, are more sensitive to the effects of this drug and may require reduced dosage.

Amoxil   *see Penicillin Antibiotics, page 785*

Generic Name

Amprenavir   (am-PREN-ah-vire)

Brand Name

Agenerase

Type of Drug

Protease inhibitor.

Prescribed for

Human immunodeficiency virus (HIV) infection.

General Information

Protease inhibitors revolutionized the fight against acquired immunodeficiency syndrome (AIDS) because, when combined with other drugs, they reduce the amount of HIV virus in the bloodstream to levels that are often undetectable by current methods, CD_4 cell immune system counts and viral load measurements (amount of virus in the blood). Amprenavir is taken together with other anti-HIV medications in "drug cocktails" to take advantage of different avenues of attack against the HIV virus. Triple-drug cocktails were responsible for the reduction in the AIDS death rate that began in 1996. Protease inhibitors are always taken together with 1 or 2 nucleoside antiviral drugs, such as AZT, ddI, ddC, or 3TC. Multiple drug therapy has changed the current view of HIV from a fatal disease to a manageable chronic illness.

Protease inhibitors work in a unique way, but they are not a cure for HIV infection or AIDS. When the HIV virus attacks a cell, it must be converted into viral DNA. Other drugs, known as reverse transcriptase inhibitors, interfere with this step, but they need help in fighting HIV. Protease inhibitors work at the end of the HIV reproduction process, when proteins are "cut" by a protease enzyme into strands of exactly the right size to duplicate HIV. Protease inhibitors prevent the mature HIV virus from being formed by interfering with this cutting process. Proteins that are cut incorrectly or that remain uncut are inactive.

People taking a protease inhibitor may still develop secondary infections or conditions associated with HIV disease. Because of this, it is very important for you to remain under the care of a doctor or other health care provider. The long-term effects of amprenavir are not known. You may be able to pass the HIV virus to others even if you are on triple-drug therapy.

Cautions and Warnings

Do not take amprenavir if you are **sensitive** or **allergic** to it. People allergic to **sulfa drugs** may also be allergic to amprenavir.

People with **liver disease** may require reduced dosage.

Severe and **life-threatening skin reactions** can develop in people taking amprenavir.

Amprenavir may raise your blood sugar, worsen **diabetes,** or bring out latent diabetes. Treatment with insulin or an oral diabetes drug may be required in such cases.

The risk of bleeding may be increased in people with **hemophillia** who take protease inhibitors.

Protease inhibitors can cause the redistribution of body fat, leading to **buffalo hump, breast enlargement, abnormal thinness,** or a **round, moon-shaped face.**

Possible Side Effects

Amprenavir is always taken with other drugs, so the side effects listed here are associated with multiple drug therapy rather than amprenavir taken alone.

▼ Most common: nausea, vomiting, diarrhea, mild rash, itching, high blood sugar, and high blood-triglyceride levels.

▼ Common: changes in sense of taste, and tingling in or around the mouth or in the hands or feet.

▼ Less common: depression and high blood-cholesterol levels.

▼ Rare: life-threatening rash, diabetes, and buffalo hump.

Amprenavir has been studied in children age 4 to 12 and side effects are the same as in adults.

Drug Interactions

Amprenavir can interact with many drugs. Be sure to tell your doctor about all the medications you are taking.

• . Astemizole, bepridil, cisapride, dihydroergotamine, ergotamine, lidocaine injection, midazolam, triazolam, tricyclic antidepressants, and quinidine should never be combined with amprenavir because of the risk of severe, life-threatening reactions.

• You may require dosage adjustments of amiodarone, lidocaine injection, warfarin, and tricyclic antidepressants when you start taking amprenavir.

• Do not combine rifampin with amprenavir because it reduces drug levels by 90%. Rifabutin reduces the amount of amprenavir in the blood by 15%.

• Combining amprenavir and sildenafil drastically increases the risk of sildenafil side effects including low blood pressure, visual changes, and a persistent and painful erection.

• Amprenavir can reduce the effectiveness of birth control pills. Use another means of contraception while taking amprenavir.

• Amprenavir must be taken at least 1 hour before or after antacids.

• Combining amprenavir with statin cholesterol-lowering drugs increases the risk of drug toxicity.

• Carbamazepine, phenytoin, and phenobarbital reduce the effectiveness of amprenavir.

• Other drugs that could interact with amprenavir and should be used with caution are: dapsone, erythromycin, itraconazole, alprazolam, clorazepate, diazepam, flurazepam, calcium channel blockers, delavirdine, efavirenz, nevirapine, estrogens, progestogens, corticosteroids, clozapine, carbamazepine, loratidine, and pimozide.

Food Interactions

This drug can be taken without regard to food or meals, but high-fat foods may reduce the effectiveness of amprenavir.

Usual Dose

Capsules
   Adult and Child (age 13–16): 1200 mg (8 capsules) twice a day with other anti-HIV drugs. Adults with moderate-to-severe liver disease should take 300–450 mg twice a day.

Child (age 4–12): 9 mg per lb. 2 times a day or 6.8 mg per lb. 3 times a day with other anti-HIV drugs, up to 2400 mg a day. This dosage also applies to older children who weigh less than 110 lbs.

Child (under age 4): not recommended.

Oral Solution

Child (age 4–12): 10.2 mg per lb. 2 times a day or 7.7 mg per lb. 3 times a day with other anti-HIV drugs, up to 2800 mg a day. This dosage also applies to older children who weigh less than 110 lbs.

Child (under age 4): not recommended.

Overdosage

Overdose symptoms are likely to be exaggerated side effects. Overdose victims should be taken to a hospital emergency room. ALWAYS bring the prescription bottle or container.

Special Information

Amprenavir oral solution is absorbed less efficiently than the capsules. They cannot be interchanged for each other on a milligram for milligram basis.

Tell your doctor about all other prescription and over-the-counter drugs you are taking because of the risk of drug interactions.

It is very important to take amprenavir exactly as prescribed. If you forget a dose of amprenavir, take it as soon as you remember. If you miss a dose by more than 4 hours, skip the forgotten dose and continue with your regular schedule. Never take a double dose.

Call your doctor if you have a rash, nausea, diarrhea, or vomiting, or any intolerable drug side effect.

Amprenavir capsules contain large amounts of vitamin E. Do not take a vitamin E supplement while taking this drug.

Special Populations

Pregnancy/Breast-feeding

Amprenavir caused abortions and birth defects in pregnant animals. Its effect on pregnant women is not known and the drug should be taken only after risks and possible benefits have been discussed with your doctor.

Nursing mothers who must take amprenavir should bottle-feed.

Seniors

Amprenavir was not studied in seniors. Seniors taking this drug must use caution.

Generic Name

Anagrelide (ah-NAG-rel-ide)

Brand Name

Agrylin

Type of Drug

Antiplatelet.

Prescribed for

Essential thrombocythemia (ET), to reduce blood-platelet count and the risk of excess blood clotting associated with high blood-platelet levels.

General Information

Blood platelets play an important role in the body. They help to form blood clots that "seal off" minor cuts and wounds and prevent excessive bleeding. When platelet counts are too high, as in ET, unwanted clots may form almost anywhere in the body. These clots may obstruct blood vessels, leading to leg cramps, heart attack, stroke, or other medical problems. Exactly how anagrelide reduces blood-platelet count is not known, but it may interfere with the formation of new platelets. Anagrelide is not approved for general use by children under age 16, but it has been used without apparent harm by 8 children between the ages of 8 and 17, who took it in doses up to 4 mg a day.

Cautions and Warnings

This drug should be used with caution by people who have **heart disease**.

Unusually **low blood-platelet counts** can develop in people treated with anagrelide. Platelet counts should be periodically checked while you are taking this drug; they usually rise soon after the drug is stopped.

Anagrelide can cause **liver or kidney toxicity** and worsen diseases of those organs.

Possible Side Effects

▼ Most common: heart palpitations, diarrhea, abdominal pain, nausea, gas, headache, weakness, swelling, pain, dizziness, and difficulty breathing.

▼ Common: chest pain, rapid heartbeat, vomiting, upset stomach, appetite loss, rash or itching, tingling in the hands or feet, back pain, and not feeling well.

▼ Less common: fever, flu symptoms, chills, neck pain, sensitivity to bright light, abnormal heart rhythms, bleeding, heart disease, stroke, angina pain, heart failure, dizziness when rising from a sitting or lying position, flushing, migraine, fainting, depression, confusion, tiredness, high blood pressure, nervousness, memory loss, itching, skin disease, hair loss, stomach bleeding, blood in the stool, stomach irritation, vomiting, anemia, thrombocytopenia (low blood-platelet count), black-and-blue marks, swollen lymph glands, painful urination, blood in the urine, muscle and joint ache, leg cramps, runny nose, nosebleeds, lung disease, sinus inflammation, pneumonia, bronchitis, asthma, double vision, other visual difficulties, ringing or buzzing in the ears, liver inflammation, and dehydration.

Drug Interactions

• Sucralfate may interfere with the absorption of anagrelide. Do not combine these drugs.

Food Interactions

For optimal effectiveness, take anagrelide on an empty stomach.

Usual Dose

Adult: 0.5–4 mg a day, or 1 mg twice a day, to start. After at least a week, the lowest effective dose should be sought.

Child (under age 17): not recommended.

Overdosage

Little is known about the effects of anagrelide overdose, but symptoms are likely to include a sudden drop in blood-platelet count and heart or nervous system side effects. Overdose victims should be taken to a hospital emergency room at once. ALWAYS bring the prescription bottle or container.

Special Information

If you forget a dose, take it as soon as possible. If it is almost time for your next dose, skip the dose you forgot and continue with your regular schedule. Call your doctor if you forget 2 or more doses in a row. Do not take a double dose.

Special Populations

Pregnancy/Breast-feeding

At high doses, anagrelide caused birth defects in animal studies. When this drug is considered crucial by your doctor, its potential benefits must be carefully weighed against its risks.

It is not known if this drug passes into breast milk. Nursing mothers who must take anagrelide should bottle-feed.

Seniors

Seniors may take anagrelide without special precaution.

Generic Name

Anastrozole (ah-NAS-troe-zole)

Brand Name

Arimidex

The information in this profile also applies to the following drug:

Generic Ingredient: Letrozole
Femara

Type of Drug

Aromatase inhibitor.

Prescribed for

Advanced breast cancer in postmenopausal women.

General Information

Anastrozole is recommended for use in breast cancer that has advanced despite treatment with tamoxifen. Anastrozole reduces the amount of estradiol, an estrogenic hormone, in the blood. It does this by interfering with the action of the aromatase enzyme, an element involved in the manufacture of estradiol. Most of anastrozole is broken down in the liver.

Cautions and Warnings

Anastrozole **increases blood-cholesterol levels**.

Women with estrogen-receptor negative disease and those who did not respond at all to tamoxifen are **not likely to respond to anastrozole**.

Possible Side Effects

▼ Most common: weakness, nausea, headache, flushing, pain, and back pain.

▼ Less common: breathing difficulties; vomiting; cough; diarrhea; constipation; abdominal pain; appetite loss; bone pain; sore throat; dizziness; rash; dry mouth; swelling in the arms, legs, or feet; pelvic pain; depression; chest pain; and tingling in the hands or feet.

▼ Rare: Rare side effects can occur in almost any part of the body. Contact your doctor if you experience any side effect not listed above.

Drug Interactions

Usual doses of anastrozole do not affect other medications; however, high doses of anastrozole can reduce the ability of the liver to break down certain drugs.

Food Interactions

Food can reduce the amount of anastrozole absorbed into the blood. Take this drug either 1 hour before or 2 hours after a meal.

Usual Dose

Anastrozole
  Adult: 1 mg once a day.

Letrozole
  Adult: 2.5 mg once a day.

Overdosage

Symptoms of overdose can be exaggerated side effects. Overdose victims should be taken to a hospital emergency room. ALWAYS bring the prescription bottle or container.

Special Information

Call your doctor if your side effects become severe or intolerable.

Use a condom, diaphragm, or other non-hormonal contraceptive while taking anastrozole.

If you forget a dose of anastrozole, take it as soon as you remember. If it is almost time for your next dose, skip the dose you forgot and continue with your regular schedule. Call your doctor if you forget more than 2 doses in a row.

Special Populations

Pregnancy/Breast-feeding
Animal studies have shown that anastrozole can harm the fetus. Pregnant women who take anastrozole have a good chance of losing the pregnancy or harming the fetus. Conception should be prevented in women taking this drug by the use of a condom, diaphragm, or other non-hormonal contraceptive.

It is not known if anastrozole passes into breast milk. Nursing mothers who must take this drug should consider bottle-feeding.

Seniors
Seniors may take this drug without special precaution.

Type of Drug

Angiotensin II Blockers (AN-jee-oe-TEN-sin)

Brand Names

Generic Ingredient: Candesartan
Atacand

Generic Ingredient: Irbesartan
Avapro

Generic Ingredient: Losartan Potassium
Cozaar

*Generic Ingredients: Losartan Potassium
+ Hydrochlorothiazide*
Hyzaar

Generic Ingredient: Telmisartan
Micardis

Generic Ingredient: Valsartan
Diovan

Prescribed for

High blood pressure.

General Information

These drugs work by blocking the effects of angiotensin II, a hormone found in blood vessels and other tissue. Angiotensin II plays an important role in regulating blood pressure. Unlike angiotensin-converting enzyme (ACE) inhibitors—another group of blood-pressure-lowering medication—angiotensin II (AII) blockers do not cause chronic cough. AII blockers can be used alone or with a thiazide diuretic such as hydrochlorthiazide, as in Hyzaar. While Hyzaar is a single tablet, your doctor may prescribe an AII blocker and a diuretic as separate pills. Combining an AII blocker and a diuretic may reduce blood pressure twice as much as an AII blocker alone.

While approved by the FDA for high blood pressure, AII blockers may be useful in treating other conditions, such as heart failure. Irbesartan is being studied to slow the progression of kidney disease in people with diabetes and high blood pressure.

Cautions and Warnings

Do not take an AII blocker if you are **sensitive** or **allergic** to it. It is possible to be sensitive to one AII blocker and tolerant of another.

People being treated with diuretics may have insufficient fluid levels. This could lead to a sudden drop in blood pressure (symptoms include dizziness and fainting). Once your body has adjusted to a diuretic-AII blocker combination, this problem should subside.

Telmisartan is noticeably less effective in **African Americans**. Some studies indicate that losartan is less effective in African Americans, but recent research suggests that a higher drug dosage may compensate. Irbesartan and candesartan are also somewhat less effective in African Americans.

People with serious **liver disease** or **cirrhosis** should receive a lower starting dosage of losartan. Telmisartan should be used with caution by people with liver disease and related problems; alternate drug therapy should be considered. People with liver disease or cirrhosis should be cautious about taking valsartan, though no dosage adjustment is required.

Some people who take an AII blocker develop **kidney function changes** similar to those associated with ACE inhibitor drugs. Valsartan dosage may have to be modified in the presence of severe **kidney disease.** No adjustment is required for other AII blockers.

AII blockers have not been studied in **children under age 18**.

Possible Side Effects

AII blockers are generally very well tolerated. In clinical studies, the risk of side effects was about the same for an AII blocker as for a placebo (sugar pill).

Candesartan
▼ Common: respiratory infection.
▼ Less common: dizziness, headache, fatigue, diarrhea, nausea and vomiting, abdominal and other pain, joint pain, sinus problems, sore throat, runny nose, bronchitis, chest pain, and swollen arms or legs.
▼ Rare: Rare side effects can occur in almost any part of the body. Contact your doctor if you experience any side effect not listed above.

Irbesartan
▼ Common: respiratory infection.
▼ Less common: dizziness, headache, fatigue, anxiety, nervousness, diarrhea, upset stomach, heartburn, nausea and vomiting, abdominal and other pain, accidents, cough, sinus problems, sore throat, runny nose, flu-like symptoms, swelling, chest pain, rash, rapid heart beat, and urinary infection.

Possible Side Effects *(continued)*

▼ Rare: Rare side effects can occur in almost any part of the body. Contact your doctor if you experience any side effect not listed above.

Losartan
▼ Common: respiratory infection.
▼ Less common: dizziness, sleeplessness, diarrhea, upset stomach, heartburn, pain, muscle cramps, muscle aches, cough, stuffy nose, and sinus problems.
▼ Rare: rash, rapid heartbeat, and urinary infection. Other rare side effects can occur in almost any part of the body. Contact your doctor if you experience any side effect not listed above.

Telmisartan
▼ Common: respiratory infection.
▼ Less common: dizziness, headache, fatigue, anxiety or nervousness, diarrhea, upset stomach, heartburn, nausea and vomiting, abdominal pain, back and leg pain, muscle aches, cough, sinus irritation, sore throat, influenza, chest pain, urinary infection, swelling in the arms or legs, and high blood pressure.
▼ Rare: Rare side effects can occur in almost any part of the body. Contact your doctor if you experience any side effect not listed above.

Valsartan
▼ Less common: dizziness, sleeplessness, headache, fatigue, diarrhea, upset stomach, heartburn, abdominal pain, joint pain, respiratory infection, cough, sore throat, sinus problems, runny nose, virus infection, and swelling.
▼ Rare: Rare side effects can occur in almost any part of the body. Contact your doctor if you experience any side effect not listed above.

Drug Interactions

• Telmisartan may slightly reduce warfarin blood levels, but not enough to require a change in warfarin dosage.
• Combining telmisartan and digoxin can increase digoxin blood levels by up to 50%, leading to possible drug side effects. This combination should be used with caution.

• Combining an AII blocker and another blood-pressure-lowering drug, especially a diuretic, reduces blood pressure more efficiently than either drug used alone. People taking a diuretic who start an AII blocker may initially experience a rapid blood pressure drop and should start with a lower AII blocker dosage.

Food Interactions

For optimal effectiveness, take valsartan at least 1 hour before or 2 hours after meals. Other AII blockers can be taken with or without food.

Usual Dose

Candesartan
  Adult: 8–32 mg once a day. Usual starting dosage is 16 mg a day.
  Child: not recommended.

Irbesartan
  Adult: 150 mg once a day to start, increasing to 300 mg once a day if necessary. A lower dosage (75 mg) may be prescribed for people who are dehydrated or salt-depleted.
  Child: not recommended.

Losartan
  Adult: 25–50 mg once a day to start, increasing gradually up to 100 mg in 1 or 2 doses a day.
  Child: not recommended.

Telmisartan
  Adult: 20–80 mg a day. Usual starting dosage is 40 mg a day.
  Child: not recommended.

Valsartan
  Adult: 80–320 mg once a day.
  Child: not recommended.

Overdosage

Little is known about AII blocker overdose, though it could be fatal. The most likely overdose symptoms are very low blood pressure, dizziness, and rapid heart- beat. Overdose victims should be taken to a hospital emergency room. ALWAYS bring the prescription bottle or container.

Special Information

Avoid strenuous exercise and very hot weather because heavy sweating or dehydration can cause a rapid blood pressure drop.

People on dialysis who take telmisartan may become dizzy or faint when rising quickly from a sitting or lying position at the beginning of treatment.

Avoid over-the-counter diet pills, decongestants, and stimulants because they may contain ingredients that can raise blood pressure.

If you take an AII blocker once a day and forget a dose, take it as soon as you remember. If it is within 8 hours of your next dose, skip the one you forgot and continue with your regular schedule. If you take an AII blocker twice a day and forget a dose, take it as soon as you remember. If it is within 4 hours of your next dose, take 1 dose right away and another in 5 or 6 hours, then go back to your regular schedule. Never take a double dose.

Special Populations

Pregnancy/Breast-feeding

AII blockers should not be taken during the last 6 months of pregnancy because they can cause fetal injury or death. If necessary, you should take another drug for high blood pressure if you are or might be pregnant.

It is not known if AII blockers pass into breast milk, though they do in animal studies. Nursing mothers who must take an AII blocker should bottle-feed.

Seniors

Seniors may take AII blockers without special precautions.

Type of Drug

Antiemetics (5HT$_3$ Type)

Brand Names

Generic Ingredient: Dolasetron
Anzemet

Generic Ingredient: Granisetron
Kytril

Generic Ingredient: Ondansetron
Zofran   Zofran ODT

Prescribed for

Nausea and vomiting caused by chemotherapy, general anesthesia, and radiation therapy.

General Information

These drugs prevent nausea and vomiting by interfering with a form of the neurohormone serotonin (5HT) known as $5HT_3$. They block its effects in the part of the brain that controls vomiting and in the vagus nerve in the stomach and intestines. These drugs are very effective and often work in cases in which older antiemetics have failed. Another related medication alosetron (Lotronex) focuses on $5HT_3$ in the intestines and is effective against irritable bowel syndrome.

Cautions and Warnings

Do not take these drugs if you are **allergic** or **sensitive** to them.

People with **heart rhythm problems,** especially those taking diuretics and antiarrhythmic drugs, should be cautious about taking dolasetron.

People with **liver problems** should be cautious about taking ondansetron and should probably use another drug in this group.

These drugs should only be used when the risk of nausea and vomiting is relatively high.

Possible Side Effects

Dolasetron

▼ Common: diarrhea and headache.

▼ Less common: high or low blood pressure, abdominal pain, dizziness or light-headedness, fever or chills, and tiredness.

▼ Rare: blood in the urine; chest pain; kidney problems; painful urination or difficulty urinating; rapid heartbeat; pain; severe stomach pain with nausea or vomiting; rash; hives; itching; slow or irregular heartbeat; swollen face, feet, or lower legs; and breathing difficulties.

Possible Side Effects *(continued)*

Granisetron
▼ Most common: headache, constipation, weakness, and low white-blood-cell count.
▼ Common: abdominal pain, diarrhea, appetite loss, shivers, and anemia.
▼ Less common: stimulation, tiredness, sleeplessness, changes in sense of taste, hair loss, and low blood-platelet count.
▼ Rare: unusual muscle movements and drug sensitivity reactions.

Ondansetron
▼ Most common: headache, feeling unwell, and constipation.
▼ Common: anxiety, agitation, dizziness, drowsiness, sleepiness, diarrhea, gynecological problems, itching, urinary difficulties, abnormal heart rhythms, and low blood pressure.
▼ Less common: weakness, fever or chills, dry mouth, liver inflammation, diarrhea, abdominal pain, and rash.
▼ Rare: liver failure, drug allergy, bronchial spasm, unusual tiredness or weakness, dizziness or light-headedness, rapid heartbeat, angina pain, low blood potassium, and grand mal seizures.

Drug Interactions

No important drug interactions are known.

Food Interactions

These drugs may be taken with or without food.

Usual Dose

Dolasetron
  Adult and Child (age 17 and over): a single dose of 100 mg.
  Child (age 2–16): 0.8 mg per lb. of body weight, up to 100 mg.

Granisetron
  Adult and Child (age 17 and over): 1 mg 2 times a day.
  Child (age 2–16): 0.008 mg per lb. of body weight, up to 1 mg, 2 times a day.

Ondansetron
   Adult and Child (age 12 and over): 8 mg 3 times a day. Peo-
ple with liver failure should take no more than 8 mg a day.
   Child (age 4–11): 4 mg 3 times a day.
   Child (age 3 and under): not recommended.

Overdosage

Symptoms may include severe constipation, temporary
blindness, high blood pressure, fainting, and mild
headache. Call your local poison control center or a hospital emergency room for more information. If you go for
treatment, ALWAYS bring the prescription bottle or
container.

Special Information

Call your doctor if you develop chest tightness, wheezing,
breathing difficulties, chest pain, or any bothersome or persistent side effect.
   Maintain good dental hygiene while taking these drugs.
Chronic dry mouth can increase the risk of tooth decay and
gum disease.
   If you forget a dose, take it as soon as you remember. If it is
almost time for your next dose, skip the dose you forgot and
continue with your regular schedule. Missing more than 1
dose may increase the risk of vomiting.

Special Populations

Pregnancy/Breast-feeding
These drugs may be associated with a slight risk of birth
defects. When your doctor considers any of these drugs crucial, its potential benefits must be carefully weighed against
its risks.
   Ondansetron may pass into breast milk. Nursing mothers
who must take any of these drugs should consider bottle-
feeding.

Seniors
Seniors may take these drugs without special restriction.

Type of Drug

Antihistamine-Decongestant Combination Products

Brand Names

Generic Ingredients: Acrivastine + Pseudoephedrine
Semprex-D

Generic Ingredients: Azatadine + Pseudoephedrine
Trinalin Repetabs

Generic Ingredients: Brompheniramine + Phenylpropanolamine
E.N.T.

Generic Ingredients: Brompheniramine + Phenylephrine + Phenylpropanolamine
Bromophen T.D.   Tamine S.R.

Generic Ingredients: Brompheniramine + Pseudoephedrine

Allent	Respahist
Bromfed	Rondec
Dallergy-JR	Touro A & H
Endafed	ULTRAbrom
Lodrane LD	

Generic Ingredients: Dexbrompheniramine + Pseudoephedrine
Disobrom   Dexaphen-SA

Generic Ingredients: Carbinoxamine + Pseudoephedrine

Carbiset	Cardec-S
Carbiset TR	Rondec*
Carbodec	Rondec-TR
Carbodec TR	

Generic Ingredients: Chlorpheniramine + Pseudoephedrine

Anamine	Codimal L.A.
Anamine T.D.	Colfed-A
Anaplex A S	Cophene No.2
Atrohist Pediatric	Deconamine*
Brexin L.A.	Deconomed SR
Chlordrine SR	Duralex
Chlorphedrine SR	Dura-Tap/PD

Fedahist Gyrocaps
Fedahist Timecaps
Histalet Ⓐ
Klerist-D
Kronofed-A
Kronofed-A Jr.
ND Clear

Novafed A
Rescon
Rescon ED
Rescon JR
Rinade B.I.D.
Tanafed
Time-Hist

Generic Ingredients: Chlorpheniramine + Phenylephrine
Dallergy-D Ⓐ
Ed A-Hist
Histor-D

Prehist
Rolatuss Plain
Ru-Tuss

Generic Ingredients: Chlorpheniramine +
Phenylpropanolamine
A.R.M.
Drize
Dura-Vent/A
Ornade Spansules

Resaid
Rhinolar-EX
Vanex Forte-R

Generic Ingredients: Chlorpheniramine + Phenylephrine +
Phenylpropanolamine
Hista-Vadrin

Generic Ingredients: Chlorpheniramine + Phenindamine +
Phenylpropanolamine
Nolamine

Generic Ingredients: Chlorpheniramine + Phenyltoloxamine
+ Phenylephrine
Comhist

Generic Ingredients: Chlorpheniramine + Phenyltoloxamine
+ Phenylephrine + Phenylpropanolamine
Naldecon*
Naldecon Pediatric
Naldelate
Naldelate Pediatric
Nalgest*

Tri-Phen-Chlor
Tri-Phen-Mine SR
Tri-Phen-Mine Pediatric
Uni-Decon

Generic Ingredients: Chlorpheniramine + Pyrilamine +
Phenylephrine
Atrohist Pediatric

Rhinatate

R-Tannate   Triotann
R-Tannamine   Tritan
Rynatan   Tri-Tannate
Tanoral

Generic Ingredients: Chlorpheniramine + Pyrilamine + Phenylephrine + Phenylpropanolamine
Histalet Forte

Generic Ingredients: Fexofenadine + Pseudoephedrine
Allegra-D

Generic Ingredients: Loratadine + Pseudoephedrine
Claritin-D 12-Hour   Claritin-D 24-Hour

Generic Ingredients: Pheniramine + Pyrilamine + Phenyl-propanolamine [G]
Triaminic   Tri-P Oral Infant Drops

Generic Ingredients: Pheniramine + Phenyltoloxamine + Pyrilamine + Phenylpropanolamine
Iohist   Poly-Histine-D
Liqui-Histine-D   Poly-Histine-D Ped Caps

Generic Ingredients: Promethazine + Phenylephrine
Phenergan VC   Promethazine VC Plain
Promethazine VC   Prometh VC Plain

Some products in this brand-name group are alcohol- or sugar-free. Consult your pharmacist.

Prescribed for

Sneezing, watery eyes, runny nose, itchy or scratchy throat, nasal congestion, and other symptoms of the common cold, allergies, and upper respiratory conditions.

General Information

The basic formula for each of these antihistamine-decongestant combinations is the same: An antihistamine is used to relieve allergy symptoms and a decongestant to treat the symptoms of either a cold or allergy.

Most of these products are taken several times a day, while others are long-acting and are taken once or twice a day.

Since nothing can cure a cold or allergy, the best you can hope to achieve from a cold and allergy remedy is relief from symptoms.

Cautions and Warnings

Antihistamines in these products may cause **drowsiness**. Decongestants may cause **anxiety** and **nervousness** and may interfere with sleep.

People who are **allergic** to antihistamines or decongestants should use these products with caution.

People with narrow-angle **glaucoma, prostate disease,** certain **stomach ulcers,** and **bladder obstruction** should not use these products. People having **asthma attacks** and those taking a **monoamine oxidase inhibitor (MAOI)** for depression or high blood pressure should not take these products. People with serious **liver disease** and those taking **erythromycin, ketoconazole,** or **itraconazole** should not take terfenadine.

Possible Side Effects

▼ Most common: restlessness, nervousness, sleeplessness, drowsiness, sedation, excitation, dizziness, poor coordination, and upset stomach.

▼ Less common: low blood pressure, heart palpitations, rapid heartbeat and abnormal heart rhythms, chest pain, anemia, fatigue, confusion, tremors, headache, irritability, euphoria (feeling high), tingling or heaviness in the hands, tingling in the feet or legs, blurred or double vision, convulsions, hysterical reaction, ringing or buzzing in the ears, fainting, increase or decrease in appetite, nausea, vomiting, diarrhea or constipation, frequent urination, difficulty urinating, early menstrual periods, loss of sex drive, breathing difficulties, wheezing with chest tightness, stuffed nose, itching, rash, unusual sensitivity to the sun, chills, excessive perspiration, and dry mouth, nose, or throat.

Drug Interactions

• Combining these products with alcoholic beverages, antianxiety drugs, tranquilizers, or narcotic pain relievers may lead to excessive drowsiness or difficulty concentrating.

• Avoid these products if you are taking an MAOI for depression or high blood pressure because the MAOI may cause a very rapid rise in blood pressure or increase side effects such as dry mouth and nose, blurred vision, and abnormal heart rhythms.

• The decongestant component of these products may interfere with the normal effects of blood-pressure-lowering medications and can aggravate diabetes, heart disease, hyperthyroid disease, high blood pressure, prostate disease, stomach ulcer, and urinary blockage.

• If your doctor has prescribed one of these products, do not self-medicate with an additional over-the-counter drug for the relief of cold symptoms. This combination may aggravate high blood pressure, heart disease, diabetes, or thyroid disease.

Food Interactions

These drugs are best taken on an empty stomach but may be taken with food if they upset your stomach.

Usual Dose

Dosages vary. Generally, these products are taken every 4–12 hours.

Overdosage

Symptoms of overdose are drowsiness, chills, dry mouth, fever, nausea, nervousness, irritability, rapid or irregular heartbeat, chest pain, and urinary difficulties. Most cases should be treated by inducing vomiting as soon as possible with ipecac syrup—available at any pharmacy. Then call your local poison control center for more information or take the victim to a hospital emergency room. ALWAYS bring the prescription bottle or container.

Special Information

Use extra caution while doing anything that requires concentration, such as driving a car or operating hazardous machinery.

Call your doctor if your side effects are severe or become intolerable.

If you forget to take a dose of your medication, take it as soon as you remember. If it is almost time for your next dose, skip the dose you forgot and continue with your regular schedule. Do not take a double dose.

Special Populations

Pregnancy/Breast-feeding

Animal studies suggest that some older antihistamines cause birth defects but the antihistamines in these products have not been proven harmful. If you are or might be pregnant, do not take any of these products without your doctor's knowledge.

Small amounts of antihistamine or decongestant pass into breast milk. Nursing mothers who must use these products should bottle-feed.

Seniors

Seniors are more sensitive to the side effects of these medications.

Generic Name

Apraclonidine (ah-prah-KLON-ih-dene)

Brand Name

Iopidine

Type of Drug

Sympathomimetic.

Prescribed for

Post-surgical increases in eye pressure; also prescribed as additional short-term treatment in people who are using other glaucoma medicines.

General Information

Apraclonidine hydrochloride reduces both elevated and normal fluid pressure inside the eye and selectively blocks certain nerve endings without acting as a local anesthetic. The exact way it works is not known, but apraclonidine, like other drugs that reduce eye pressure, may work by decreasing the production of eye fluid. The drug starts to work within 1 hour after it is put into the eye and reaches its maximum effect in 3 to 5 hours.

Cautions and Warnings

Do not use apraclonidine if you are **allergic** to it or to clonidine. This drug can cause an allergic-like reaction, including

red eye, swelling of the lid and white of the eye, itching, burning, and the **feeling of something in your eye**. If this happens, stop using the drug and call your doctor. Taking this drug with a **monoamine oxidase inhibitor (MAOI)** may result in severe side effects—do not combine them.

Using this medicine with other eye-pressure-lowering drugs may not provide additional benefit: Other drugs work in the same way and a further effect may not be possible.

The ability of apraclonidine to lower eye pressure decreases over time. Most **people continuously benefit for less than 1 month**.

People with **kidney or liver disease** should be monitored by their doctors while taking this medicine.

Possible Side Effects

▼ Most common: eye redness, itching, tearing, eye discomfort, lid swelling, dry mouth, feeling of something in your eye, headache, and weakness.

▼ Less common: blanching of the eye; upper lid elevation; dilated pupils; blurred vision and other eye disorders; allergic reactions; lid crusting; abnormal vision; eye pain; abdominal pain; diarrhea; stomach discomfort; vomiting; dry mouth or nose; nasal burning; runny nose; sore throat; worsening asthma; constipation and nausea; slow heartbeat; heart palpitations; abnormal heart rhythms; chest pain; fainting; swelling; difficulty sleeping; irritability; reduced sex drive; pain, numbness, or tingling in the hands or feet; clammy or sweaty palms; taste changes; a feeling of having a head cold; and rash.

Drug Interactions

• Apraclonidine can reduce pulse and blood pressure. If you are also taking drugs to treat high blood pressure or other cardiovascular drugs, check your pulse and blood pressure.

• MAOI drugs can slow the breakdown of apraclonidine and increase the risk of drug side effects. This combination should be avoided.

Usual Dose

Adult: 1–2 drops in the affected eye 3 times a day.

Overdosage

Exaggerated side effects, especially those that affect the nervous system, are symptoms of overdose. Call your local poison control center for more information. ALWAYS take the prescription bottle or container with you if you go to the emergency room.

Special Information

Apraclonidine can cause dizziness and tiredness. Be careful doing anything that requires concentration, coordination, or alertness while taking this medication.

To prevent infection, do not touch the dropper tip to your finger or eyelid. Wait 5 minutes before using any other eyedrop or ointment.

If you forget a dose of apraclonidine, take it as soon as you remember. If it is almost time for your next dose, take one dose as soon as you remember and then go back to your regular schedule. Do not take a double dose.

Special Populations

Pregnancy/Breast-feeding

In animal studies, apraclonidine was toxic to embryos when given by mouth. It should be used with caution during pregnancy.

It is not known if this drug passes into breast milk, but nursing mothers should bottle-feed their babies while using it.

Seniors

Seniors may use this medicine without special precautions.

Generic Names

Aspirin, Buffered Aspirin (AS-prin) Ⓖ

Brand Names

Adprin-B	Aspergum
Alka-Seltzer with Aspirin	Asprimox
Arthritis Pain Formula	Bayer
Arthritis Foundation Pain Reliever	Bufferin
	Buffex
Ascriptin	Cama Arthritis Pain Reliever

Easprin
Ecotrin
Empirin
Genprin
Halfprin
Heartline

Magnaprin
Norwich
St. Joseph Adult Chewable
  Aspirin
ZORprin

Type of Drug

Analgesic and anti-inflammatory agent.

Prescribed for

Mild to moderate pain, fever, arthritis, and inflammation of bones, joints, or other body tissues. People who have had a stroke or transient ischemic attack (TIA)—oxygen shortage to the brain—may have aspirin prescribed to reduce the risk of having another such attack. Aspirin may also be prescribed as an anticoagulant (blood-thinning) drug in people with unstable angina and to protect against heart attack. Aspirin has a definite beneficial effect if it is taken as soon as possible after having a heart attack.

General Information

Aspirin may be the closest thing we have to a wonder drug. It has been used for more than a century for pain and fever relief and is now used for its effect on the blood as well.

Aspirin is the standard against which all other drugs are compared for relieving pain and for reducing inflammation. Chemically, aspirin is a member of the group of drugs called salicylates. Other salicylates include sodium salicylate, sodium thiosalicylate, choline salicylate, and magnesium salicylate (trilisate). These drugs are no more effective than regular aspirin, although two of them—choline salicylate and magnesium salicylate—may be a little less irritating to the stomach. They are all more expensive than aspirin.

Aspirin reduces fever by causing the blood vessels in the skin to open, allowing heat to leave the body more rapidly. Its effects on pain and inflammation are thought to be related to its ability to prevent the manufacture of complex body hormones called prostaglandins. Of all the salicylates, aspirin has the greatest effect on prostaglandin production.

Many people find that they can take buffered aspirin but not regular aspirin. The addition of antacids to aspirin can be important to people who must take large doses of aspirin for chronic arthritis or other conditions. In many cases, aspirin is the only effective drug and can be tolerated only with the antacids present.

Cautions and Warnings

People with **liver damage** should avoid aspirin. People who are **allergic** to aspirin may also be allergic to nonsteroidal anti-inflammatory drugs (NSAIDs) such as indomethacin, sulindac, ibuprofen, fenoprofen, naproxen, tolmetin, and meclofenamate sodium or to products containing tartrazine (a commonly used orange dye and food coloring). People with **asthma** and/or **nasal polyps** are more likely to be allergic to aspirin.

Alcoholic beverages may worsen the stomach irritation caused by aspirin. Alcohol increases the risk of aspirin-related ulcers.

Stop taking aspirin if you develop **dizziness, hearing loss, or ringing or buzzing in your ears.**

Reye's syndrome is a life-threatening condition characterized by vomiting and stupor or dullness and may develop in children with influenza (flu) or chickenpox that is treated with aspirin or other salicylates. Up to 30% of people who develop Reye's syndrome can die, and permanent brain damage is possible in those who survive. Because of this, authorities advise against giving children under age 16 aspirin or another salicylate, especially those with chickenpox or the flu; acetaminophen should be given instead.

Aspirin **interferes with normal blood clotting** and should therefore be avoided for 1 week **before surgery**. Ask for your surgeon or dentist's recommendation before taking aspirin for pain after surgery.

Possible Side Effects

▼ Most common: nausea, upset stomach, heartburn, loss of appetite, and loss of small amounts of blood in the stool.

▼ Less common: hives, rashes, liver damage, fever, thirst, and visual difficulties. Aspirin may contribute to the formation of stomach ulcers and bleeding. People who are allergic to aspirin and those with a history of nasal polyps, asthma, or rhinitis may experience breathing difficulty and a stuffed nose.

Drug Interactions

• People taking anticoagulant (blood-thinning) drugs should avoid aspirin because it increases the effect of the anticoagulant.

• Aspirin may increase the possibility of stomach ulcer when taken together with adrenal corticosteroids, phenylbutazone, or alcoholic beverages.

• Aspirin will counteract the uric-acid-eliminating effect of probenecid and sulfinpyrazone. Aspirin may counteract the blood-pressure-lowering effect of ACE inhibitor and beta-blocking drugs. Aspirin may also counteract the effects of some diuretics in people with severe liver disease.

• Aspirin may increase blood levels of methotrexate and of valproic acid when taken with either of these drugs, leading to increased chances of drug toxicity. Mixing aspirin and nitroglycerin tablets may lead to an unexpected drop in blood pressure.

• Do not take aspirin with an NSAID. There is no benefit to the combination, and the chance of side effects—especially stomach irritation—is vastly increased.

• Large aspirin doses (2000 mg a day or more) can lower blood sugar. This can be a problem in people with diabetes who take insulin or oral antidiabetes drugs to control their condition.

Food Interactions

Because aspirin can cause upset stomach and bleeding, take each dose with food, milk, or a glass of water.

Usual Dose

Adult: aches, pains, and fever—325–650 mg every 4 hours. Arthritis and rheumatic conditions—up to 5200 mg a day in divided doses. Rheumatic fever, up to 7800 mg a day in divided doses. To prevent heart attack, stroke, or TIA—325 mg every 2 days or 80–160 mg a day.

Child (under age 16): not recommended because of the risk of Reye's syndrome (see "Cautions and Warnings").

Overdosage

Aspirin may be lethal for adults in overdoses of 30 regular-strength tablets—325 mg each—or 20 maximum-strength tablets—500 mg. Aspirin may be lethal for children in overdoses of 12 regular-strength tablets or 8 maximum-strength tablets.

Symptoms of mild overdose are rapid and deep breathing, nausea, vomiting, dizziness, ringing or buzzing in the ears, flushing, sweating, thirst, headache, drowsiness, diarrhea, and rapid heartbeat.

Severe overdose may cause fever, excitement, confusion, convulsions, liver or kidney failure, coma, and bleeding.

The initial treatment of aspirin overdose involves inducing vomiting to remove any drug remaining in the stomach. Further treatment depends on how the situation develops and what must be done to maintain the patient. Do not induce vomiting until you have spoken with your doctor or poison control center. If in doubt, go to a hospital emergency room. ALWAYS bring the aspirin bottle or container.

Special Information

Contact your doctor if you develop continuous stomach pain or ringing or buzzing in the ears.

Do not use an aspirin product if it has a strong odor of vinegar. This is an indication that the product has started to break down in the bottle.

If you forget to take a dose of aspirin, take it as soon as you remember. If it is almost time for your next dose, skip the dose you forgot and continue with your regular schedule. Do not take a double dose.

Special Populations

Pregnancy/Breast-feeding

Check with your doctor before taking any aspirin-containing product during pregnancy. Aspirin may cause bleeding problems in the fetus during the last 2 weeks of pregnancy. Taking aspirin during the last 3 months of pregnancy may extend the length of pregnancy, prolong labor, and lead to a low-birth-weight infant. It can also cause bleeding in the mother before, during, or after delivery.

Aspirin passes into breast milk, but has not caused any problems in nursing babies. Nursing mothers should speak to their doctors before using aspirin.

Seniors

Aspirin, especially in the larger doses that an older adult may take to treat arthritis and rheumatic conditions, may be irritating to the stomach. Seniors with liver disease should not use aspirin.

Generic Name

Atenolol (ah-TEN-uh-lol) Ⓖ

Brand Name

Tenormin

Combination Products
Generic Ingredients: Atenolol + Chlorthalidone Ⓖ
Tenoretic 50   Tenoretic 100

Type of Drug

Beta-adrenergic blocking agent.

Prescribed for

High blood pressure, abnormal heart rhythms, angina pectoris, prevention of second heart attack and migraine, alcohol withdrawal, stage fright and other anxieties, and bleeding from the esophagus.

General Information

Atenolol is one of many beta-adrenergic blocking drugs, or beta blockers, that interfere with the action of a specific part of the nervous system. Beta receptors are found all over the body and affect many body functions. Each beta blocker has particular characteristics that may make it more suitable for certain conditions or people.

Cautions and Warnings

People with **angina** who take atenolol for high blood pressure risk aggravating their angina if they suddenly stop taking the drug. These people should have their drug dosage reduced gradually over 1 to 2 weeks.

Atenolol should be used with caution if you have **liver or kidney disease,** because your ability to eliminate this drug from your body may be impaired.

Atenolol reduces the amount of blood the heart pumps. This reduction in blood flow may aggravate the condition of people with **poor circulation** or **circulatory disease**.

If you are undergoing **major surgery,** your doctor may want you to stop taking atenolol at least 2 days before surgery.

Possible Side Effects

Side effects are relatively uncommon and usually mild; they usually develop early in the course of treatment and are rarely a reason to stop taking atenolol.

▼ Most common: impotence.

▼ Less common: unusual tiredness or weakness, slow heartbeat, heart failure (symptoms include swelling of the legs, ankles, or feet), dizziness, breathing difficulties, bronchospasm, depression, confusion, anxiety, nervousness, sleeplessness, disorientation, short-term memory loss, emotional instability, cold hands and feet, constipation, diarrhea, nausea, vomiting, upset stomach, increased sweating, urinary difficulties, cramps, blurred vision, rash, hair loss, stuffy nose, facial swelling, aggravation of lupus erythematosus (chronic condition affecting the body's connective tissue), itching, chest pain, back or joint pain, colitis, drug allergy (symptoms include fever and sore throat), and liver toxicity.

Drug Interactions

• Atenolol may interact with surgical anesthetics to increase the risk of heart problems during surgery. Some anesthesiologists recommend gradually stopping the drug by 2 days before surgery.

• Atenolol may interfere with the normal signs of low blood sugar and with oral antidiabetic drugs.

• Atenolol increases the blood-pressure-lowering effects of other blood-pressure-reducing agents, including clonidine, guanabenz, and reserpine; and calcium channel blockers, such as nifedipine.

• Aspirin-containing drugs, indomethacin, sulfinpyrazone, and estrogen drugs may interfere with the blood-pressure-lowering effect of atenolol.

• Cocaine may reduce the effectiveness of all beta blockers.

• Atenolol may worsen the problem of cold hands and feet associated with taking ergot alkaloids, used to treat migraine. Gangrene is a possibility in people taking both an ergot and atenolol.

• Atenolol will counteract thyroid hormone replacements.
• Calcium channel blockers, flecainide, hydralazine, oral contraceptives, propafenone, haloperidol, phenothiazine tranquilizers—molindone and others—quinolone antibacterials, and quinidine may increase the amount of atenolol in the bloodstream and lead to increased atenolol effects.
• Atenolol should not be taken within 2 weeks of taking a monoamine oxidase inhibitor (MAOI) antidepressant.
• Cimetidine increases the amount of atenolol absorbed into the bloodstream from oral tablets.
• Atenolol may interfere with the effectiveness of some antiasthma drugs, including theophylline and aminophylline, and especially ephedrine and isoproterenol.
• Combining atenolol with phenytoin or digitalis drugs may result in excessive slowing of the heart, possibly causing heart block (disruption of the electrical impulses that control heart rate).
• If you stop smoking while taking atenolol, your dose may have to be reduced because your liver will break down the drug more slowly.

Food Interactions

None known.

Usual Dose

Adult: starting dose—50 mg a day, increased gradually up to 200 mg. Maintenance dose—50–200 mg once a day. People with kidney disease may need only 50 mg every other day. Older adults should be treated more cautiously and may need a lower dose.

Overdosage

Symptoms of overdose include changes in heartbeat—unusually slow, unusually fast, or irregular—severe dizziness or fainting, breathing difficulties, bluish-colored fingernails or palms, and seizures. The victim should be taken to a hospital emergency room. ALWAYS bring the prescription bottle or container.

Special Information

Atenolol is meant to be taken continuously. When ending atenolol treatment, dosage should be reduced gradually over a period of about 2 weeks. Do not stop taking this drug unless directed to do so by your doctor: Abrupt withdrawal may cause chest pain, breathing difficulties, increased sweating, and unusually fast or irregular heartbeat.

Call your doctor at once if you develop back or joint pain, breathing difficulties, cold hands or feet, depression, rash, or changes in heartbeat. Atenolol may produce an undesirable lowering of blood pressure, leading to dizziness or fainting; call your doctor if this happens. Call your doctor if you experience persistent or bothersome anxiety, diarrhea, constipation, impotence, headache, itching, nausea or vomiting, nightmares or vivid dreams, upset stomach, insomnia, stuffy nose, frequent urination, unusual tiredness, or weakness.

Atenolol may cause drowsiness, light-headedness, dizziness, or blurred vision. Be careful when driving or performing complex tasks.

It is best to take atenolol at the same time each day. If you forget a dose, take it as soon as you remember. If you take atenolol once a day and it is within 8 hours of your next dose, skip the dose you forgot and continue with your regular schedule. If you take atenolol twice a day and it is within 4 hours of your next dose, skip the one you forgot and continue with your regular schedule. Never take a double dose.

Special Populations

Pregnancy/Breast-feeding

Infants born to women who took a beta blocker while pregnant had lower birth weights, low blood pressure, and reduced heart rates. Atenolol should be avoided by pregnant women and women who might become pregnant while taking it.

Atenolol passes into breast milk. Nursing mothers should avoid taking atenolol.

Seniors

Seniors taking atenolol may be more likely to suffer from cold hands and feet, reduced body temperature, chest pain, general feelings of ill health, sudden breathing difficulties, increased sweating, or changes in heartbeat.

Generic Name

Atovaquone (ah-TOE-vuh-quone)

Brand Name

Mepron [S]

Type of Drug

Anti-infective.

Prescribed for

Pneumocystis carinii pneumonia (PCP).

General Information

Atovaquone is an anti-infective with specific activity against PCP, an infection commonly associated with AIDS. It is used in people who cannot take trimethoprim and sulfamethoxazole. In studies comparing atovaquone with trimethoprim-sulfamethoxazole, approximately 60% of people with PCP improved on each drug. However, more people died of PCP and other infections while being treated with atovaquone. Of those who died, most had less atovaquone in their bloodstream than those who lived. In studies comparing oral atovaquone with intravenous pentamidine for treating PCP in people with AIDS, both drugs were equally effective, at 14%. Again, there was a direct correlation between the amount of atovaquone in the blood and survival. The drug stays in the body for several days and is eliminated through the liver.

Cautions and Warnings

Do not take atovaquone if you are or may be **allergic** to it or to any of the product's components.

This drug has not been studied for PCP prevention or for severe PCP, or in those who are failing on TMP-SMZ.

Atovaquone only works against PCP. People with PCP who have bacterial, viral, fungal, or other infections of the lung may continue to worsen despite atovaquone therapy. If this happens, it may be a sign that another kind of infecting organism is the cause. Additional medicine will be necessary.

Since atovaquone absorption is so strongly influenced by high-fat foods, **people who cannot eat enough** may not be able to absorb enough medicine, and may have to take intra-

venous treatments of other PCP anti-infectives while taking
atovaquone.

Possible Side Effects

Overall, only 4% to 7% of people stopped taking the drug
because of side effects, a much smaller percentage than
occurs with other PCP treatments.

▼ Most common: rash, nausea, diarrhea, headache,
vomiting, fever, sleeplessness, weakness, itching, oral fungal infections, abdominal pain, upset stomach, appetite
loss, constipation, cough, dizziness, pain, increased sweating, anxiety, sinus inflammation, and runny nose.

▼ Less common: changes in sense of taste, low blood
sugar, and low blood pressure.

Drug Interactions

• Atovaquone may increase blood levels of warfarin, oral
antidiabetes drugs, digoxin, and other drugs that bind
strongly to blood proteins.

• Rifampin and rifabutin may reduce blood levels of atovaquone, possibly diminishing its effectiveness.

• Taking atovaquone with TMP-SMZ has resulted in
reduced blood levels of TMP-SMZ. This should not reduce
TMP-SMZ's effectiveness.

• Taking atovaquone with zidovudine (AZT) drastically
reduces the rate at which zidovudine is eliminated from the
body. For most people, this is not a problem.

Food Interactions

Take atovaquone with food or meals to improve drug absorption. A high-fat meal can increase the amount absorbed by
300%.

Usual Dose

750 mg 2 times a day for 3 weeks, taken with food.

Overdosage

Little is known about the effects of atovaquone overdose;
symptoms are likely to be exaggerated drug side effects. Call
your local poison control center or hospital emergency room
for more information. If you go to the hospital, ALWAYS
bring the prescription bottle or container.

Special Information

Taking atovaquone regularly and with food is essential to the drug's effectiveness. If you cannot eat 2 meals a day, your doctor may have to prescribe another PCP treatment.

Call your doctor if you develop any persistent or bothersome side effects.

If you forget a dose, take it as soon as you remember. If it is almost time for your next dose, space your remaining doses equally throughout the rest of the day so that you can still take a total daily dose of 1500 mg, or 2 tsp.

Special Populations

Pregnancy/Breast-feeding

In animal studies, atovaquone has affected fetal development. If you are pregnant this drug should be used only if the potential risks and benefits have been carefully weighed by you and your doctor.

Atovaquone is likely to pass into breast milk because of its affinity for body fat. Nursing mothers should bottle-feed while taking atovaquone.

Seniors

This drug has not been tested systematically in people over age 65. Seniors, especially those with kidney, heart, or liver disease, may be more sensitive to atovaquone side effects.

Atrovent   see Ipratropium, page 524

Augmentin   see Penicillin Antibiotics, page 785

Brand Name

Auralgan Otic

Generic Ingredients

Antipyrine + Benzocaine + Glycerin

Other Brand Names
Allergen Ear Drops   Otocalm Ear
Auroto Otic

Type of Drug

Analgesic.

Prescribed for

Earache.

General Information

Auralgan contains benzocaine, a local anesthetic that deadens nerves inside the ear that transmit painful impulses; antipyrine, an analgesic that provides additional pain relief; and glycerin, which absorbs any water present in the ear. This drug is often used to treat painful conditions caused by water in the ear canal, such as "swimmer's ear."

Cautions and Warnings

Do not use the product if you are **allergic** to any of its ingredients.

Possible Side Effects

▼ Most common: local irritation.

Drug Interactions

• Do not use other ear medications at the same time as Auralgan.

Usual Dose

Place drops of Auralgan in the ear canal until the canal is filled. Saturate a piece of cotton with Auralgan, and put it in the ear canal to keep the drug from leaking out. Leave the drug in the ear for several minutes. Repeat 3–4 times a day.

Overdosage

Auralgan overdose is not likely to cause serious effects. In the case of overdose or accidental ingestion, call your local poison control center.

Special Information

Before using the product, warm the medicine bottle to body temperature by holding it in your hand for several minutes. Do not warm the bottle to a temperature above normal body temperature. Protect the bottle from light.

Call your doctor if you develop a burning or itching sensation or if the pain does not go away after 2 to 4 days of treatment.

If you forget a dose of Auralgan, take it as soon as you remember. If it is almost time for your next dose, skip the dose you forgot and continue with your regular schedule.

Special Populations

Pregnancy/Breast-feeding

Pregnant and breast-feeding women may use this product without special restriction.

Seniors

Seniors may use this product without restriction.

Generic Name

Azithromycin (uh-ZIH-throe-MYE-sin)

Brand Name

Zithromax

Type of Drug

Macrolide antibiotic.

Prescribed for

Upper and lower respiratory tract infections, skin infections, sexually transmitted diseases (STDs), middle ear infections, tonsillitis, and pharyngitis.

General Information

Azithromycin is an azalide antibiotic, a subgroup of the macrolides. Macrolide drugs are either bactericidal (bacteria-killing) or bacteriostatic (inhibiting bacterial growth) depending on the organism in question and amount of antibiotic present.

Cautions and Warnings

Do not take azithromycin if you are **allergic** to it or any macrolide antibiotic.

Azithromycin is excreted primarily through the liver. People with **liver disease or damage** should consult their doctors. Those on long-term therapy with this drug should have periodic blood tests.

Colitis (bowel inflammation) has been associated with all antibiotics (see "Possible Side Effects").

Azithromycin is considered appropriate only for the treatment of more mild forms of pneumonia in non-hospitalized patients. People with other underlying conditions, those who are **immune-compromised,** and those who contract pneumonia in a hospital or other institutional setting probably should be treated with other antibiotics.

Possible Side Effects

Most side effects are mild and go away once you stop taking azithromycin.

▼ Most common: nausea, vomiting, stomach cramps, stomach gas, and diarrhea. Colitis (symptoms include severe abdominal cramps and severe, persistent, and possibly bloody diarrhea) may develop.

▼ Less common: heart palpitations, chest pain, hairy tongue, vaginal irritation, kidney inflammation, dizziness, headache, fainting, tiredness, unusual sun sensitivity, rash, and swelling.

▼ Rare: serious abnormal heart rhythms.

Drug Interactions

• Pimozide should not be taken by anyone also taking a macrolide antibiotic. Two people died while taking this combination.

• Antacid products containing aluminum or magnesium may delay the absorption of azithromycin into the blood. Separate your antacid dose from azithromycin by at least 1 hour.

• All macrolide antibiotics increase blood levels of cyclosporin and may cause kidney damage.

• Mixing azithromycin with a statin cholesterol-lowering drug increases the risk of developing a potentially fatal condition involving severe muscle pain and destruction.

Food Interactions

It is important to take azithromycin on an empty stomach, 1 hour before or 2 hours after meals.

Usual Dose

Respiratory Tract Infections, Skin Infections, and STDs
   Adult (age 16 and over): 500 mg as a single dose on day 1, then 250 mg once a day on days 2–5 of treatment. Some STDs are treated with a single dose of 1000 mg.

Middle Ear Infections
   Child (age 6 months and over): 100–400 mg on day 1, then 50–200 mg on days 2–5 of treatment. Actual dose depends on body weight.

Tonsillitis and Sore Throat
   Child (age 2 and over): 100–500 mg a day for 5 days. Actual dose depends on body weight.

Overdosage

Overdose may cause severe side effects, especially nausea, vomiting, stomach cramps, and diarrhea. Call your local poison control center or hospital emergency room for more information.

Special Information

Call your doctor if you develop nausea, vomiting, diarrhea, stomach cramps, or severe abdominal pain.

It is crucial that you follow your doctor's directions on how to take the drug and how many days to take it—even if you feel well sooner. This drug's effectiveness may be severely reduced otherwise. Taking azithromycin at the same time each day may help you remember your medication.

If you forget a dose of azithromycin, take it as soon as you remember. If it is almost time for your next dose, skip the dose you forgot and go back to your regular schedule.

Special Populations

Pregnancy/Breast-feeding

It is not known if azithromycin passes into the fetal circulation. This medication should be taken by pregnant women only if it is clearly needed.

It is not known if azithromycin passes into breast milk, but other macrolide antibiotics do. Nursing mothers who must take this drug should bottle-feed.

Seniors

Seniors with liver disease should use caution. Seniors who have pneumonia or are especially sickly or debilitated probably should be treated with other medications.

Azmacort   see *Corticosteroids, Inhalers, page 270*

Generic Name

Baclofen (BAK-loe-fen) Ⓖ

Brand Name

Lioresal

Type of Drug

Skeletal muscle relaxant.

Prescribed for

Muscle spasms associated with multiple sclerosis (MS), spinal cord injury or disease, or other nervous system conditions; may also be used to treat trigeminal neuralgia (tic douloureux), and hiccups.

General Information

Baclofen may work by interfering with nervous system reflexes at the spinal cord, although it may also have some effect outside the spinal cord. Baclofen is chemically similar to a natural nerve transmitter known as GABA; baclofen's effect on muscle spasm may be related to its effect on GABA nerve receptors.

Cautions and Warnings

Do not take baclofen if you are **allergic** or sensitive to it. It should not be taken for muscle spasm resulting from **rheumatic disease, stroke, cerebral palsy,** or **Parkinson's dis-**

ease because its benefit in these situations has not been proven. The condition of people with **epilepsy** or **psychotic disorders** may worsen while taking baclofen.

About 4% of women with MS who take baclofen for less than 1 year develop **ovarian cysts** that usually disappear on their own. This is within the normal range for all women—1% to 5%—for developing ovarian cysts.

Abruptly stopping baclofen can lead to **hallucinations** and **seizure**. Dosage should always be gradually reduced, except in cases of severe side effects.

Possible Side Effects

Baclofen may affect lab tests for liver function and can raise blood sugar levels.

▼ Most common: drowsiness, low blood pressure, weakness, dizziness, light-headedness, nausea and vomiting, headache, and sleeplessness.

▼ Less common: frequent urination, fatigue or lethargy, confusion, euphoria, excitement, depression, hallucinations, tingling in the hands or feet, muscle pain, ringing or buzzing in the ears, coordination difficulties, tremors, rigidity, weakness, loss of muscle tone, unusual eye movement and other muscle-control problems, double vision, pinpoint or wide-open pupils, breathing difficulties, heart palpitations, dry mouth, appetite loss, changes in sense of taste, abdominal pain, diarrhea, bedwetting, difficulty urinating, painful urination, impotence, blood in the urine, rash, itching, swelling of the ankle, excessive sweating, weight gain, and stuffy nose.

▼ Rare: slurred speech, blurred vision, seizure, fainting, chest pain, and testing positive for blood in the stool.

Drug Interactions

• Avoid alcoholic beverages and other nervous system depressants while taking baclofen.

• Combining a monoamine oxidase inhibitor (MAOI) antidepressant with baclofen may cause drowsiness, nervous system depression, and low blood pressure.

• Combining a tricyclic antidepressant with baclofen may lead to severe muscle weakness.

• Baclofen may increase blood sugar. Diabetics may need to increase their dosage of antidiabetic drugs to account for this effect.

• Combining blood-pressure-lowering drugs with baclofen may lead to dizziness or fainting due to severe lowering of blood pressure.

Food Interactions

This drug may be taken without regard to food or meals.

Usual Dose

Adult and Child: 15 mg a day for 3 days, gradually increased until the desired effect is achieved, usually at 40–80 mg a day. People with kidney disease require lower doses.

Overdosage

Symptoms of baclofen overdose include vomiting, loss of muscle tone, twitching, convulsions, pinpoint or wide-open pupils, drowsiness, blurred or double vision, breathing difficulties, seizure, and coma. Overdose victims should be taken to a hospital emergency room for treatment. ALWAYS bring the prescription bottle or container.

Special Information

Baclofen is a nervous system depressant. Take care when driving or doing anything that requires concentration and physical coordination.

Call your doctor if you develop a frequent urge to urinate, painful urination, constipation, nausea, headache, sleeplessness, or persistent confusion.

Do not stop taking baclofen on your own. Abruptly stopping this drug may lead to hallucinations or seizure.

Your pharmacist may prepare a baclofen liquid. This mixture should be kept in the refrigerator and must be thrown away after 1 month.

If you forget a dose of baclofen and remember within 1 hour of your scheduled time, take it immediately. If you do not remember until more than 1 hour later or if you forget it completely, skip the dose you forgot and continue with your regular schedule. Do not take a double dose.

Special Populations

Pregnancy/Breast-feeding

Baclofen increases the chances of certain birth defects in lab animals. Pregnant women should only take baclofen after carefully weighing its possible benefits against its risks with their doctor.

Baclofen taken by mouth passes into breast milk. Nursing mothers who must take this drug should bottle-feed or receive the drug by injection directly into the spinal cord, because baclofen administered by injection does not pass into breast milk.

Seniors

Seniors may be more sensitive to nervous system side effects including hallucinations, depression, drowsiness, and confusion.

Bactroban   *see Mupirocin, page 691*

Generic Name

Becaplermin   (beh-CAP-ler-min)

Brand Name

Regranex

Type of Drug

Human growth factor.

Prescribed for

Diabetic foot and leg wounds.

General Information

Becaplermin is a type of human growth factor produced in a laboratory. While it is not a substitute for good wound care, becaplermin can stimulate wound tissue to heal faster. Studies of the drug have produced mixed results. In some studies, people using becaplermin were 1½ to 2 times more likely to have complete healing of their wounds. In another study, the results with becaplermin were the same as those with good wound care alone.

Cautions and Warnings

Do not use becaplermin if you are **sensitive** or **allergic** to it.

Becaplermin should not be used to **speed the healing** of wounds that are healing by themselves.

Becaplermin should not be applied to **exposed bones, joints, tendons, or ligaments** because its effect on these body structures is not known.

Possible Side Effects

People treated with becaplermin plus wound care had a slightly larger risk of developing a rash than those who received wound care alone.

Drug Interactions

None known.

Usual Dose

Adult and Child (age 16 and over): Apply a thin layer to the wound and leave in place for 12 hours. Then, remove the becaplermin bandage, rinse the wound, and cover it with a plain saline-soaked bandage for the rest of the day. Continue this process until the wound has healed completely.

Child (under age 16): not recommended.

Overdosage

Little is known about the effects of accidental ingestion. Call your local poison control center or a hospital emergency room for information.

Special Information

Call your doctor if your wound worsens or is irritated by becaplermin.

Wash your hands before applying becaplermin.

Do not allow the tip of the becaplermin tube to touch any surface, including the wound being treated.

Your doctor should reassess your treatment if the wound is not 30% smaller in 10 weeks and completely healed in 20 weeks.

Applying more becaplermin than recommended will not make your wound heal better or faster.

If you forget a dose, apply it as soon as you remember. If it is almost time for your next dose, skip the missed dose and continue with your regular schedule.

Special Populations

Pregnancy/Breast-feeding

The safety of using becaplermin during pregnancy is not known. The drug should only be used during pregnancy if it is absolutely necessary.

It is not known if becaplermin passes into breast milk. Nursing mothers who must take this drug should bottle-feed.

Seniors

Seniors may take this drug without special precautions.

Generic Name

Benazepril (ben-AY-zuh-pril)

Brand Name

Lotensin

Type of Drug

Angiotensin-converting enzyme (ACE) inhibitor.

Prescribed for

High blood pressure.

General Information

Benazepril hydrochloride and other ACE inhibitors prevent the conversion of a hormone called angiotensin I to another hormone called angiotensin II, a potent blood-vessel constrictor. Preventing this conversion relaxes blood vessels, thus reducing blood pressure and relieving symptoms of heart failure. Benazepril also affects the production of other hormones and enzymes that participate in the regulation of blood-vessel dilation. Benazepril starts working in 1 hour and continues to work for about 24 hours.

Some people who start taking benazepril after they are already on a diuretic (agent that increases urination) experience a rapid drop in blood pressure after their first dose or when their dosage is increased. To prevent this from happening, your doctor may tell you to stop taking your diuretic 2 or 3 days before starting benazepril or to increase your salt intake during that time. The diuretic may then be restarted gradually.

Cautions and Warnings

Do not take benazepril if you have had an **allergic reaction** to it in the past.

Benazepril occasionally causes **very low blood pressure**.

Benazepril may affect **kidney function**. Your doctor should check your urine for protein content during the first few months of treatment. Dosage adjustment is necessary if you have reduced kidney function.

Benazepril can affect white-blood-cell counts, possibly increasing your susceptibility to **infection**. Your doctor should monitor your blood counts periodically.

Possible Side Effects

▼ Most common: dizziness, tiredness, headache, nausea, and chronic cough. The cough usually goes away a few days after you stop taking the medication.

▼ Rare: Rare side effects can occur in almost any part of the body. Contact your doctor if you develop any side effect not listed above.

Drug Interactions

• The blood-pressure-lowering effect of benazepril is additive with diuretics and beta blockers. Any other drug that causes a rapid drop in blood pressure should be used with caution if you are taking benazepril.

• Benazepril may increase blood-potassium levels, especially if taken with Dyazide or other potassium-sparing diuretics.

• Benazepril may increase the effect of lithium; this combination should be used with caution.

• Antacids and benazepril should be taken at least 2 hours apart.

• Capsaicin may trigger or aggravate the cough associated with benazepril therapy.

• Indomethacin may reduce the blood-pressure-lowering effects of benazepril.

• Phenothiazine tranquilizers and antivomiting drugs may increase the effects of benazepril.

• Combining allopurinol and benazepril increases the risk of side effects.

• Benazepril increases blood levels of digoxin, which may increase the chance of digoxin-related side effects.

Food Interactions

You may take benazepril with food if it upsets your stomach.

Usual Dose

10–40 mg 1–2 times a day. People with poor kidney function may need less medication.

Overdosage

The principal effect of benazepril overdose is a rapid drop in blood pressure, as evidenced by dizziness or fainting. Take the overdose victim to a hospital emergency room immediately. ALWAYS bring the prescription bottle or container.

Special Information

Benazepril can cause swelling of the face, lips, hands, and feet. This swelling can also affect the larynx (throat) and tongue and interfere with breathing. If this happens, go to a hospital at once. Call your doctor if you develop a sore throat, mouth sores, abnormal heartbeat, sudden difficulty breathing, chest pain, persistent rash, or loss of taste perception.

You may get dizzy if you rise to your feet too quickly from a sitting or lying position.

Avoid strenuous exercise or very hot weather because heavy sweating or dehydration can cause a rapid drop in blood pressure.

While taking benazepril, avoid over-the-counter diet pills, decongestants, and other stimulants that can raise blood pressure.

If you take benazepril once a day and forget a dose, take it as soon as you remember. If it is within 8 hours of your next dose, skip the dose you forgot and continue with your regular schedule. If you take benazepril twice a day and miss a dose, take the missed dose right away. If it is within 4 hours of your next dose, take 1 dose immediately and another in 5 or 6 hours, and then go back to your regular schedule. Never take a double dose.

Special Populations

Pregnancy/Breast-feeding
ACE inhibitors can cause fetal injury or death. Women who are or might become pregnant should not take ACE inhibitors. If you become pregnant, stop taking the medication and call your doctor immediately.

Small amounts of benazepril pass into breast milk. Nursing mothers who must take this drug should consider bottle-feeding.

Seniors
Seniors may be more sensitive to the effects of this drug due to age-related losses in kidney or liver function.

Generic Name

Benztropine (BENZ-troe-pene) Ⓖ

Brand Name

Cogentin

The information in this profile also applies to the following drugs:

Generic Ingredient: Biperiden
Akineton

Generic Ingredient: Procyclidine
Kemadrin

Generic Ingredient: Trihexyphenidyl Ⓖ
Artane   Trihexy-2
Artane Sequels   Trihexy-5

Type of Drug

Anticholinergic.

Prescribed for

Parkinson's disease; also used to prevent and manage muscle spasms caused by phenothiazines and other psycho-active medicines.

General Information

Benztropine mesylate works like atropine sulfate, but its side effects are less frequent and less severe. Benztropine counteracts the effects of acetylcholine, one of the body's major transmitters of nerve impulses. Benztropine can reduce muscle spasms by about 20%. This property makes the drug useful in treating Parkinson's disease and other diseases associated with spasms of skeletal muscles. Benztropine also reduces other symptoms of Parkinson's disease, such as drooling.

Cautions and Warnings

Benztropine should be used with caution if you have narrow-angle **glaucoma, stomach ulcers, heart disease, obstructions in the gastrointestinal tract, prostatitis,** or **myasthenia gravis**.

Benztropine reduces the ability to perspire and can interfere with the body's heat-control mechanisms. When taken in hot weather—especially by seniors, chronically ill people, alcoholics, and people with nervous system disease—or by people who work in hot environments, this effect may lead to **heat exhaustion** or **heatstroke**. In severe instances, it can be fatal.

Possible Side Effects

▼ Most common: urinary difficulties including painful urination, constipation, blurred vision, and increased sensitivity to bright light.

▼ Less common: rash, disorientation, confusion, memory loss, hallucinations, psychosis, agitation, nervousness, delusions, delirium, paranoia, listlessness, depression, drowsiness, euphoria (feeling high), excitement, light-headedness, dizziness, headache, weakness, giddiness, heaviness or tingling in the hands or feet, rapid heartbeat, palpitations, mild reduction in heart rate, low blood pressure, dizziness when rising quickly from a sitting or lying position, dry mouth including extreme dryness, swollen glands, nausea, vomiting, upset stomach, interference with normal bowel function, duodenal ulcer, double vision, dilated pupils, glaucoma, muscle weakness or cramping, high temperature, flushing, decreased sweating, heatstroke, and impotence.

Drug Interactions

• Side effects may increase if benztropine is taken with antihistamines, phenothiazines, antidepressants, or other anticholinergic drugs.

• Benztropine should be used with caution by people taking barbiturates. Avoid alcoholic beverages.

• Benztropine may reduce the absorption and effect of some drugs, including levodopa, haloperidol, and phenothiazines.

• Combining amantadine with benztropine may result in excessive side effects.

Food Interactions

All of these drugs—except procyclidine—are best taken on an empty stomach, although they may be taken with food if they upset your stomach.

Usual Dose

Benztropine: 0.5–6 mg a day.

Biperiden: 2–8 mg a day.

Ethopropazine: 50–600 mg a day.

Procyclidine: 2.5–5 mg 3 times a day after meals.

Trihexyphenidyl: 1–2 mg to start, increased gradually to 6–10 mg daily. This drug may be taken in sustained-release form, a convenient way to take a high daily dosage once maintenance levels have been reached.

Overdosage

Overdose symptoms include clumsiness or unsteadiness; severe drowsiness; severe dryness of the mouth, nose, or throat; hallucinations; mood changes; breathing difficulties; rapid heartbeat; and unusually warm and dry skin. Victims should be taken to a hospital emergency room at once. ALWAYS bring the prescription bottle or container.

Special Information

Dry mouth can be relieved by chewing gum or sucking hard candy. Be aware that dry mouth may lead to cavities and gum disease. It is important that you maintain good oral hygiene to prevent dental problems while taking benztropine.

A stool softener, like docusate, will usually relieve constipation. Sunglasses will reduce the irritation brought on by bright lights.

Benztropine may cause drowsiness and blurred vision. Take care while driving or performing other tasks that require concentration and reliable vision. Avoid alcohol and nervous system depressants.

Call your doctor if you develop confusion, rash, eye pain, or a pounding heartbeat.

Limit your exposure to heat to reduce the chance of developing heat exhaustion or heatstroke.

If you take benztropine several times a day and you forget a dose, take it as soon as you remember. If it is within 2 hours of your next dose, skip the dose you forgot and continue with your regular schedule. Do not take a double dose. If you take your benztropine twice a day and forget a dose, take it as soon as you remember. If it is within 4 hours of your next dose, take 1 dose immediately and take the next 2 doses 8 hours apart. Then continue with your regular schedule.

Special Populations

Pregnancy/Breast-feeding

Women who are or may become pregnant while taking benztropine should discuss changing medication with their doctor because of the possibility of birth defects.

Benztropine may reduce the amount of breast milk produced. Infants are also particularly sensitive to benztropine; nursing mothers who must take this drug should bottle-feed.

Seniors

Seniors who take benztropine on a regular basis may be more sensitive to side effects, including a predisposition to developing glaucoma, confusion, disorientation, agitation, and hallucinations.

Generic Name

Bepridil (bep-RIH-dil)

Brand Name

Vascor

Type of Drug

Calcium channel blocker.

Prescribed for

Angina pectoris.

General Information

Bepridil hydrochloride is one of many calcium channel blockers available in the U.S. These drugs block the passage of calcium, an essential factor in muscle contraction, into the heart and smooth muscles. Such blockage of calcium interferes with the contraction of these muscles, which in turn dilates (widens) the veins and vessels that supply blood to them. This dilating effect reduces blood pressure, the amount of oxygen used by the heart muscles, and the risk of blood vessel spasm. Bepridil is therefore useful in treating not only high blood pressure but also angina pectoris (brief attacks of chest pain), a condition related to poor oxygen supply to the heart muscles.

Bepridil affects the movement of calcium only into muscle cells; it has no effect on calcium in the blood.

Cautions and Warnings

Do not take this drug if you have had an **allergic reaction** to it.

Bepridil should be used with extreme caution if you have a history of problems related to **heart rhythm**. It has caused serious derangement of heart rhythm and has affected white-blood-cell counts; therefore, it is usually reserved only for people who do not respond to other treatments.

Low blood pressure may occur, especially in people also taking a beta blocker.

Use bepridil with caution if you have **heart failure,** since the drug can worsen the condition. Bepridil may cause **angina** when treatment is first started, when the dosage is increased, or if the drug is rapidly withdrawn. This can be avoided by reducing the dosage gradually.

Studies have shown that people taking calcium channel blockers—usually those taken several times a day, not those taken only once daily—have a greater chance of having a **heart attack** than do people taking beta blockers or other medications for the same purposes. Discuss this with your doctor to be sure you are receiving the best possible treatment.

Calcium channel blockers can affect **blood platelets,** leading to possible bruising, black-and-blue marks, and bleeding.

People with **kidney problems** or serious **liver disorders** may require dosage adjustments.

Possible Side Effects

▼ Most common: diarrhea, nausea, and light-headedness.

▼ Less common: abnormal heart rhythms; very slow or very rapid heartbeat; breathing difficulties; coughing or wheezing, which may be signs of lung congestion or heart failure; constipation; headache; and unusual tiredness or weakness.

▼ Rare: low blood pressure, fainting, and swelling in the ankles, feet, or legs. Other rare side effects can occur in almost any part of the body. Contact your doctor if you experience any side effect not listed above.

Drug Interactions

• Bepridil may interact with beta-blocking drugs to cause heart failure, very low blood pressure, or an increased incidence of angina. However, many people have taken these drugs together with no problem.

• Bepridil may, in rare instances, increase the effects of anticoagulant (blood-thinning) drugs.

• Some calcium channel blockers may increase the amount of digoxin in the blood, but this interaction does not occur with bepridil.

Food Interactions

Taking bepridil with food has a minor effect on the absorption of the drug. You may take it with food if it upsets your stomach.

Usual Dose

200–400 mg a day in 2 doses. Do not stop taking this drug abruptly: The dosage should be gradually reduced over a period of time.

Overdosage

Bepridil overdose can cause nausea, dizziness, weakness, drowsiness, confusion, slurred speech, very low blood pressure, reduced heart efficiency, and unusual heart rhythms. Overdose victims should be taken to a hospital emergency room. ALWAYS bring the prescription bottle or container.

Special Information

Call your doctor if you develop swelling in the arms or legs, breathing difficulties, abnormal heartbeat, increased heart pain, dizziness, constipation, nausea, light-headedness, or very low blood pressure.

If you forget to take a dose of bepridil, take it as soon as you remember. If it is almost time for your next dose, skip the dose you forgot and continue with your regular schedule. Do not take a double dose.

Special Populations

Pregnancy/Breast-feeding

Very high doses of bepridil affect the development of animal fetuses. Women who are or might be pregnant should take it only with their doctor's approval. When this drug is considered crucial by your doctor, its potential benefits must be carefully weighed against its risks.

Bepridil passes into breast milk. If you must take bepridil, you should consider the potential effect on your infant before nursing.

Seniors

Older adults are likely to have reduction in kidney or liver function and may require dosage adjustments. Seniors require more frequent monitoring by their doctors after treatment has started.

Generic Name

Betaine (BEE-tane)

Brand Name

Cystadane

Type of Drug

Homocysteine antagonist.

Prescribed for

Homocysteinuria.

General Information

Homocysteinuria is a group of 3 disorders of the metabolism characterized by too much homocysteine in the blood and urine. People with this problem tend to have skeletal problems, problems with the lens of the eye, and blood-clotting problems that can cause chest pain or heart attack. Virtually all people treated with betaine experience a decrease of homocysteine in their blood. When used together with other homocysteinuria treatments, including folate and vitamins B_{12} and B_6, betaine's effect has been additive to those treatments. Betaine starts working in several days and has been used for several years with no loss of effect. Most patients treated with betaine have been children. The effects of homocysteinuria can be devastating in children and include developmental problems, lethargy, seizures, and eye problems.

Cautions and Warnings

None known.

Possible Side Effects

Side effects, which are uncommon, include nausea, upset stomach, diarrhea, choking if the powder is inhaled, and bad odors. Reported psychological changes from betaine are questionable.

Drug Interactions

None known. Betaine has been used successfully together with folate and vitamins B_{12} and B_6.

Food Interactions

None known.

Usual Dose

Adult and Child: 3 g twice a day. Dosage for children under age 3 may be started at about 50 mg per lb. a day and then increased in weekly 50-mg steps. Dosage should be increased in all patients until homocysteine is either undetectable in the blood or present in small amounts; doses up to 20 g a day have been required. Carefully measure all doses with the scoop provided. Each level scoopful is equal to 1 g of betaine.

Overdosage

Little is known about the effects of betaine overdose. People have been safely and successfully treated at doses up to 20 g a day. Call your poison control center or a hospital emergency room for more information.

Special Information

Shake the bottle lightly before removing the cap to loosen the powder. Protect the powder from moisture.

Mix each dose with 4 to 6 oz. of water until it dissolves completely, then drink it at once.

Do not use the product if the final solution is either not clear or colored, or if the powder does not completely dissolve.

If you forget a dose, take it as soon as you remember. If it is almost time for your next dose, skip the dose you forgot and continue with your regular schedule. Tell your doctor about any missed doses.

Special Populations

Pregnancy/Breast-feeding

The safety of using betaine during pregnancy is not known. This drug should only be used during pregnancy if it is absolutely necessary.

It is not known if betaine passes into breast milk. Nursing mothers who must take this drug should consider bottle-feeding.

Seniors

Seniors may use this drug without special precaution.

Generic Name

Betaxolol (bay-TAX-uh-lol) Ⓖ

Brand Names

Betoptic   Betoptic S   Kerlone

Type of Drug

Beta-adrenergic blocking agent.

Prescribed for

High blood pressure and glaucoma.

General Information

Betaxolol hydrochloride is one of many beta-adrenergic blocking drugs, or beta blockers, which interfere with the action of a specific part of the nervous system. Beta receptors are found all over the body and affect many body functions. Each beta blocker has particular characteristics that make it more suitable for certain conditions or people. Applied as eyedrops, betaxolol reduces ocular pressure (pressure inside the eye) by slowing the production of eye fluids and by slightly increasing the rate at which these fluids flow through and leave the eye.

Cautions and Warnings

You should be cautious about taking betaxolol if you have **asthma, severe heart failure,** a **very slow heart rate,** or **heart block** (disruption of the electrical impulses that control heart rate) because the drug may aggravate these conditions.

People with **angina** who take betaxolol for high blood pressure risk aggravating their angina if they suddenly stop taking the drug. These people should have their betaxolol dosage reduced gradually over 1 to 2 weeks.

Liver or kidney problems may reduce your ability to eliminate betaxolol from your body.

Betaxolol reduces the amount of blood your heart pumps with each beat. This reduction in blood flow may aggravate the condition of people with **poor circulation** or **circulatory disease**.

If you are undergoing **major surgery,** your doctor may want you to stop taking betaxolol at least 2 days before surgery.

Betaxolol eyedrops should be avoided by people who cannot take oral beta-blocking drugs such as propranolol.

Possible Side Effects

Side effects are relatively uncommon and usually mild.
▼ Most common: impotence.

Possible Side Effects *(continued)*

▼ Less common: unusual tiredness or weakness, slow heartbeat, heart failure, dizziness, breathing difficulties, bronchospasm, depression, confusion, anxiety, nervousness, sleeplessness, disorientation, short-term memory loss, emotional instability, cold hands and feet, constipation, diarrhea, nausea, vomiting, upset stomach, increased sweating, urinary difficulties, cramps, blurred vision, rash, hair loss, stuffy nose, facial swelling, aggravation of lupus erythematosus, itching, chest pain, back or joint pain, colitis, drug allergy (symptoms include fever and sore throat), and liver toxicity.

Drug Interactions

• Betaxolol may interact with surgical anesthetics to increase the risk of heart problems during surgery. Some anesthesiologists recommend gradually stopping the drug by 2 days before surgery.

• Betaxolol may interfere with the normal signs of low blood sugar and with the action of oral antidiabetes drugs.

• Betaxolol increases the blood-pressure-lowering effects of other blood-pressure-reducing agents, including clonidine, guanabenz, and reserpine, and calcium channel blockers, such as nifedipine.

• Aspirin-containing drugs, indomethacin, sulfinpyrazone, and estrogen drugs may interfere with the blood-pressure-lowering effect of betaxolol.

• Cocaine may reduce the effectiveness of all beta blockers.

• Betaxolol may worsen the problem of cold hands and feet associated with taking ergot alkaloids, used to treat migraine. Gangrene is a possibility in people taking both an ergot and betaxolol.

• Betaxolol will counteract thyroid hormone replacements.

• Calcium channel blockers, flecainide, hydralazine, oral contraceptives, propafenone, haloperidol, phenothiazine tranquilizers—molindone and others—quinolone antibacterials, and quinidine may increase the amount of betaxolol in the bloodstream and lead to increased betaxolol effects.

• Betaxolol should not be taken within 2 weeks of taking a monoamine oxidase inhibitor (MAOI) antidepressant.

• Cimetidine increases the amount of betaxolol absorbed into the bloodstream from oral tablets.

• Betaxolol may lessen the effectiveness of some anti-asthma drugs, including theophylline and aminophylline, and especially ephedrine and isoproterenol.

• Combining betaxolol with phenytoin or digitalis drugs can result in excessive slowing of the heart, possibly causing heart block.

• If you stop smoking while taking betaxolol, your dose may have to be reduced because your liver will break down the drug more slowly afterward.

• If you use other glaucoma eye medications, separate your doses to avoid physically combining them.

• Small amounts of betaxolol eyedrops are absorbed into the bloodstream and may interact with other drugs in the same way as oral beta blockers, although this is unlikely.

Food Interactions

None known.

Usual Dose

Tablets: 5–20 mg once a day. People with kidney failure should take 5 mg to start.

Eyedrops: 1 drop in the affected eye twice a day.

Overdosage

Symptoms of overdose are changes in heartbeat—unusually slow, unusually fast, or irregular—severe dizziness or faint-ing, breathing difficulties, bluish-colored fingernails or palms, and seizures. The victim should be taken to a hospital emergency room. ALWAYS bring the prescription bottle or container with you.

Special Information

Do not stop taking betaxolol unless directed to do so by your doctor. It is meant for continuing use. Abrupt withdrawal may cause chest pain, breathing difficulties, increased sweating, and unusually fast or irregular heartbeat. Dosage should be reduced gradually over a period of about 2 weeks when biso-prolol treatment is stopped.

Call your doctor at once if you develop back or joint pain, breathing difficulties, cold hands or feet, depression, rash, or changes in heartbeat. Betaxolol may produce an undesirable lowering of blood pressure, leading to dizziness or fainting; call your doctor if this happens to you. Also call your doctor if you experience persistent or bothersome anxiety, diarrhea, constipation, impotence, headache, itching, nausea or vomiting, nightmares or vivid dreams, upset stomach, trouble sleeping, stuffy nose, frequent urination, unusual tiredness, or weakness.

Betaxolol may cause drowsiness, light-headedness, dizziness, or blurred vision. Be careful when driving or performing complex tasks.

It is best to take betaxolol at the same time each day. If you forget a dose, take it as soon as you remember. If you take betaxolol once a day and it is within 8 hours of your next dose, skip the dose you forgot and continue with your regular schedule. If you take betaxolol twice a day and it is within 4 hours of your next dose, skip the one you forgot and continue with your regular schedule. Never take a double dose.

If you forget a dose of betaxolol eyedrops, administer it as soon as you remember. If it is almost time for your next dose, skip the dose you forgot and continue with your regular schedule. Do not take a double dose.

Special Populations

Pregnancy/Breast-feeding

Infants born to women who took a beta blocker while pregnant had lower birth weights, low blood pressure, and reduced heart rates. Betaxolol should be avoided by pregnant women and women who might become pregnant while taking it.

Beta blockers pass into breast milk. Nursing mothers taking betaxolol should bottle-feed.

Seniors

Seniors may require less of the drug to achieve results. Seniors taking betaxolol may be more likely to suffer from cold hands and feet, reduced body temperature, chest pain, general feelings of ill health, sudden breathing difficulties, increased sweating, or changes in heartbeat.

Biaxin *see Clarithromycin, page 217*

Generic Name

Bicalutamide (BYE-kal-UTE-uh-mide)

Brand Name

Casodex

The information in this profile also applies to the following drug:

Generic Ingredient: Nilutamide
Nilandron

Type of Drug

Antiandrogen.

Prescribed for

Prostate cancer.

General Information

Antiandrogens are prescribed together with another hormone product for prostate cancer. Bicalutamide competes with testosterone and other natural androgens (male hormones) by binding to the same places in body tissue where androgens normally bind. Prostate cancer is androgen sensitive and responds to treatments that counteract the effects of androgen or remove the sources of androgen.

Cautions and Warnings

Do not take bicalutamide if you are **allergic** to it or any ingredient in the product. Almost 40% of men taking this drug as single therapy for prostate cancer develop **breast pain and enlargement**. Bicalutamide may **reduce sperm count**.

Two of every 100 people taking the related drug nilutamide develop **interstitial pneumonitis** (symptoms include cough, chest pain, fever, and breathing difficulties). Report any symptoms to your doctor at once.

People taking nilutamide or flutamide may develop **liver inflammation.** Call your doctor if you experience any signs of liver damage (severe itching, dark-colored urine, flu, tiredness, appetite loss, yellowing of skin or whites of the eyes, abdominal pain, and stomach or intestinal problems).

Isolated cases of **aplastic anemia** (a potentially fatal blood disorder) have been reported in people taking nilutamide, but the relationship between the drug and the disease is not established.

Possible Side Effects

▼ Most common: Bicalutamide—hot flashes. Nilutamide—pain, headache, weakness, back or abdominal pain, nausea, constipation, flushing, sleeplessness, breathing difficulties, difficulty seeing in the dark, loss of testicle function, and breast swelling and tenderness.

▼ Common: diarrhea, constipation, nausea, pain, back pain, weakness, and pelvic pain.

▼ Less common: vomiting, abdominal pains, chest pain, flu symptoms, high blood pressure, swelling in the ankles or lower legs, high blood sugar, weight loss, dizziness, tingling in the hands or feet, sleeplessness, sweating, rash, nighttime urination, blood in the urine, urinary or other infection, impotence, breast swelling or pain, painful urination, anemia, difficulty breathing, bone pain, and headache.

▼ Rare: Rare side effects can occur in almost any part of the body. Contact your doctor if you experience any side effect not listed above.

Drug Interactions

• Bicalutamide increases the effect of oral anticoagulant (blood-thinning) drugs such as warfarin. Dosage adjustment may be necessary.

Food Interactions

None known.

Usual Dose

Bicalutamide
    Adult: 50 mg once a day, morning or night.

Nilutamide
    Adult: 300 mg a day, reduced to 150 mg a day after 30 days.

Overdosage

Symptoms of overdose include slow breathing, poor muscle

coordination, reduced activity, teariness, appetite loss, vomiting, and tiredness. Overdose victims should be taken to a hospital emergency room. ALWAYS bring the prescription bottle or container.

Special Information

Treatment with bicalutamide should always be started at the same time as a luteinizing hormone-releasing hormone agent such as leuprolide or goserelin. Do not stop taking either drug without your doctor's knowledge.

For maximum effect, nilutamide treatment should be started on the same day or day after surgical castration. Nilutamide can also be used together with leuprolide.

Up to half of people taking nilutamide can take from a few seconds to a few minutes to adapt to darkness. This can be a problem especially when driving at night or through tunnels. Wearing tinted glasses will minimize this effect.

Bicalutamide should be taken at the same time each day for best results. If you forget a dose of bicalutamide, take it as soon as you remember. If it is almost time for your next dose, skip the dose you forgot and continue with your regular schedule. Call your doctor if you forget to take more than 1 dose.

Special Populations

Pregnancy/Breast-feeding
Antiandrogens are not intended for use by women.

Seniors
Seniors may take this drug without special precautions.

Generic Name

Bisoprolol (bye-SOPE-roe-lol)

Brand Name

Zebeta

Combination Products

Generic Ingredients: Bisoprolol + Hydrochlorothiazide
Ziac

Type of Drug

Beta-adrenergic blocking agent.

Prescribed for

High blood pressure, angina pectoris, and abnormal heart rhythms.

General Information

Bisoprolol fumarate is one of many beta-adrenergic blocking drugs, or beta blockers, which interfere with the action of a specific part of the nervous system. Beta receptors are found all over the body and affect many body functions. Each beta blocker has particular characteristics that make it more suitable for certain conditions or people. Hydrochlorothiazide is a diuretic that lowers blood pressure.

Cautions and Warnings

People with **angina** who take bisoprolol for high blood pressure risk aggravating their angina if they suddenly stop taking the drug. These people should have their dosage reduced gradually over 1 to 2 weeks.

Bisoprolol should be used with caution if you have **liver or kidney disease,** because your ability to eliminate the drug from your body may be impaired.

Bisoprolol reduces the amount of blood pumped by the heart with each beat. This blood flow reduction may aggravate the condition of people with **poor circulation** or **circulatory disease**.

If you are undergoing **major surgery,** your doctor may want you to stop taking bisoprolol at least 2 days before surgery.

Possible Side Effects

Side effects are relatively uncommon and usually mild.

▼ Most common: impotence.

▼ Less common: unusual tiredness or weakness, slow heartbeat, heart failure, dizziness, breathing difficulties, bronchospasm, depression, confusion, anxiety, nervousness, sleeplessness, disorientation, short-term memory loss, emotional instability, cold hands and feet, constipation, diarrhea, nausea, vomiting, upset stomach, increased sweating, urinary difficulties, cramps, blurred vision, rash, hair loss, stuffy nose, facial swelling, aggravation of lupus erythematosus, itching, chest pain, back or joint pain, colitis, drug allergy (symptoms include fever and sore throat), and liver toxicity.

Drug Interactions

• Bisoprolol may interact with surgical anesthetics to increase the risk of heart problems during surgery. Some anesthesiologists recommend gradually stopping the drug by 2 days before surgery.

• Bisoprolol may interfere with the normal signs of low blood sugar and with the action of oral antidiabetes drugs.

• Bisoprolol increases the blood-pressure-lowering effects of other blood-pressure-reducing agents, including clonidine, guanabenz, and reserpine, and calcium channel blockers, such as nifedipine.

• Aspirin-containing drugs, indomethacin, sulfinpyrazone, and estrogen drugs may interfere with the blood-pressure-lowering effect of bisoprolol.

• Cocaine may reduce the effectiveness of all beta blockers.

• Bisoprolol may worsen the problem of cold hands and feet associated with taking ergot alkaloids, used to treat migraine. Gangrene is possible in people taking both an ergot and bisoprolol.

• Bisoprolol will counteract thyroid hormone replacements.

• Calcium channel blockers, flecainide, hydralazine, oral contraceptives, propafenone, haloperidol, phenothiazine tranquilizers—molindone and others—quinolone antibacterials, and quinidine may increase the amount of bisoprolol in the bloodstream and lead to increased bisoprolol effects.

• Bisoprolol should not be taken within 2 weeks of taking a monoamine oxidase inhibitor (MAOI) antidepressant.

• Cimetidine increases the amount of bisoprolol absorbed into the bloodstream from oral tablets.

• Bisoprolol may lessen the effectiveness of some anti-asthma drugs, including theophylline and aminophylline, and especially ephedrine and isoproterenol.

• Combining bisoprolol with phenytoin or digitalis drugs may result in excessive slowing of the heart, possibly causing heart block.

• Smoking makes the liver break this drug down more quickly. If you stop smoking while taking bisoprolol, your daily dose may have to be reduced.

Food Interactions

This drug may be taken without regard to food or meals.

Usual Dose

Adult: starting dose—5 mg once daily. The daily dose may
be gradually increased up to 20 mg. Maintenance dose—5–10
mg once daily. People with kidney or liver disease may need
only 2.5 mg a day to start. Seniors should be treated cautiously; they may respond to lower doses.

Overdosage

Symptoms of overdose include changes in heartbeat—
unusually slow, unusually fast, or irregular—severe dizziness
or fainting, breathing difficulties, bluish-colored fingernails or
palms, and seizures. The victim should be taken to a hospital
emergency room. ALWAYS bring the prescription bottle or
container.

Special Information

Do not stop taking bisoprolol unless directed to do so by your
doctor. It is meant for continuous use. Abrupt withdrawal
may cause chest pain, breathing difficulties, increased sweating, and unusually fast or irregular heart beat.

Call your doctor at once if you develop back or joint pain,
breathing difficulties, cold hands or feet, depression, rash, or
changes in heartbeat. Bisoprolol may produce an undesirable
lowering of blood pressure, leading to dizziness or fainting;
call your doctor if this happens to you. Also call your doctor if
you experience persistent or bothersome anxiety, diarrhea,
constipation, impotence, headache, itching, nausea or vomiting, nightmares or vivid dreams, upset stomach, trouble
sleeping, stuffed nose, frequent urination, unusual tiredness,
or weakness.

Bisoprolol may cause drowsiness, dizziness, blurred vision,
or light-headedness. Be careful when driving or performing
complex tasks.

It is best to take bisoprolol at the same time every day. If you
forget a dose, take it as soon as you remember. If it is within 8
hours of your next dose, skip the dose you forgot and continue
with your regular schedule. Do not take a double dose.

Special Populations

Pregnancy/Breast-feeding

Infants born to women who took a beta blocker while pregnant had lower birth weights, low blood pressure, and

reduced heart rates. Bisoprolol should be avoided by pregnant women and women who might become pregnant while taking it.

It is not known if bisoprolol passes into breast milk. Nursing mothers taking bisoprolol should bottle-feed.

Seniors
Seniors taking bisoprolol may be more likely to suffer from cold hands and feet, reduced body temperature, chest pain, general feelings of ill health, sudden breathing difficulties, increased sweating, or changes in heartbeat.

Type of Drug

Bisphosphonates (bis-FOS-fuh-nates)

Brand Names

Generic Ingredient: Alendronate
Fosamax

Generic Ingredient: Etidronate
Didronel

Generic Ingredient: Risedronate
Actonel

Generic Ingredient: Tiludronate
Skelid

Prescribed for

Osteoporosis (a condition characterized by loss of bone mass due to depletion of minerals, especially calcium) in post-menopausal women, Paget's disease of bone, and high blood calcium associated with cancer.

General Information

Bisphosphonates have been used for many years to treat a variety of conditions associated with low bone mass due to calcium depletion. In osteoporosis, bones become weak and brittle, increasing the risk of fractures. Bisphosphonates help prevent loss of bone mass and can make bones stronger. Exactly how they work is not well understood. Etidronate has been used occasionally in children, but these drugs generally are not considered safe for use in children.

Cautions and Warnings

Do not use a bisphosphonate if you are **sensitive** or **allergic** to it. Do not use a bisphosphonate if you have severe **kidney disease** or active **stomach or intestinal disease** such as difficulty swallowing, ulcers, or stomach irritation because the drug may worsen your condition.

It is not known if **men with osteoporosis** benefit from taking a bisphosphonate.

Alendronate and risedronate can cause **low blood calcium**.

Possible Side Effects

Side effects are generally mild.

Alendronate
▼ Most common: pain.
▼ Common: abdominal pain and discomfort, gas, stomach ulcers, and back pain.
▼ Less common: upset stomach, constipation, diarrhea, nausea, difficulty swallowing, muscle pain, headache, flu-like symptoms, accidents, and swelling in the arms or legs.
▼ Rare: vomiting and changes in taste.

Etidronate
▼ Most common: fever.
▼ Common: nausea and flu-like symptoms.
▼ Less common: convulsions, constipation, inflammation of the lining of the mouth, changes in liver function, low blood levels of magnesium or phosphate, breathing difficulties, and changes in sense of taste.
▼ Rare: allergic reactions including itching, rash, itchy sores, and sudden swelling that goes away on its own.

Risedronate
▼ Most common: headache, diarrhea, abdominal pain, and severe joint pain.
▼ Common: chest pain, dizziness, swelling in the arms or legs, constipation, nausea, sinus irritation, and bone pain.

Possible Side Effects (continued)

▼ Less common: leg cramps, weakness, bronchitis, poor vision in one eye, dry eyes, ringing or buzzing in the ears, parathyroid gland problems, infection, rash and other skin problems, tooth problems, and vitamin D deficiency.

▼ Rare: fatigue.

Tiludronate

▼ Most common: diarrhea and nausea.

▼ Common: headache, upset stomach, respiratory infection, runny nose, fluid in the lungs, and sinus irritation.

▼ Less common: vomiting, dizziness, tingling in the hands or feet, coughing, sore throat, gas, aches and pains, cataracts, eye redness, glaucoma, rash, skin disorders, tooth problems, swelling, infection, vitamin D deficiency, and muscle aches.

▼ Rare: fatigue, high blood pressure, fainting, appetite loss, constipation, abdominal pain, tiredness, and sleeplessness.

Drug Interactions

• Antacids and calcium supplements can interfere with the absorption of bisphosphonates. Separate doses of these drugs and a bisphosphonate by at least 30 minutes.

• Separate doses of tiludonate and aluminum-containing antacids by 1 hour.

• Combining alendronate and aspirin or other nonsteroidal anti-inflammatory drugs (NSAIDs) or other anti-inflammatory drugs can increase the risk of developing stomach or intestinal side effects.

• Aspirin can interfere with the absorption of tiludronate.

• Indomethacin can increase the amount of tiludronate absorbed into the blood by 2 to 4 times.

Food Interactions

Take these medicines only with plain water. Food and drink—even mineral water, orange juice, or coffee—interfere with the absorption of these drugs. Take alendronate or risedronate every morning at least 30 minutes before eating, drinking, or taking other medications. Etidronate should be taken on an empty stomach 2 hours before a meal. Tiludronate should be taken when you first get up; wait 4 hours before eating breakfast.

Usual Dose

Alendronate
    Adult: 10–40 mg a day.
    Child: not recommended.

Etidronate
    Adult: up to 4.5 mg per lb. a day to start, gradually increasing to no more than 9 mg per lb. per day.
    Child: not recommended.

Risedronate
    Adult: 30 mg a day.
    Child: not recommended.

Tiludronate
    Adult: 480 mg (2 tablets) a day.
    Child: not recommended.

Overdosage

Little is known about the effects of bisphosphonate overdose. Very low blood-calcium is the most serious symptom and requires emergency treatment. Other symptoms include upset stomach, heartburn, ulcer and irritation of the esophagus. Milk or antacids may reverse these effects. Overdose victims should be taken to a hospital emergency room. ALWAYS bring the prescription bottle or container.

Special Information

Food interferes with the effectiveness of these drugs. Carefully follow the directions in "Food Interactions" above.

To reduce the risk of stomach and throat irritation, do not lie down for at least 30 minutes after taking alendronate or risedronate.

Separate doses of calcium and vitamin D supplements from those of a bisphosphonate by at least 2 hours.

If you forget a dose, take it as soon as you remember. If it is almost time for your next dose, skip the dose you forgot and continue with your regular schedule. If you forget a morning dose and take it later in the day, you must still follow the instructions in "Food Interactions" about avoiding food.

Special Populations

Pregnancy/Breast-feeding

Bisphosphonates cause abnormal bone development in animal fetuses and are toxic to pregnant animals. When any of these drugs is considered crucial by your doctor, its potential benefits must be carefully weighed against its risks.

It is not known if bisphosphonates pass into breast milk. Since these drugs affect bone formation, nursing mothers who must take a bisphosphonate should bottle-feed.

Seniors

Seniors may use these drugs without special restriction.

Generic Name

Bitolterol (bye-TOL-ter-ol)

Brand Name

Tornalate

Type of Drug

Bronchodilator.

Prescribed for

Asthma and bronchospasm.

General Information

Bitolterol mesylate is currently available only as an inhalant, but may be taken with other medications to control your asthma. The drug starts working 3 to 4 minutes after it is taken and continues to work for 5 to 8 hours. It can be used as necessary to treat asthma attacks or on a regular basis to prevent them.

Cautions and Warnings

Bitolterol should be used with caution by people with a history of **angina pectoris** (a condition characterized by brief attacks of chest pain), **heart disease, high blood pressure, stroke, seizures, diabetes, prostate disease,** or **glaucoma.**

Using excessive amounts of bitolterol can lead to increased breathing difficulties, rather than relief. In the most extreme cases, people have had heart attacks after using excessive amounts of inhalant.

Possible Side Effects

▼ Most common: tremors, cough, and dry or sore throat.

▼ Common: restlessness, weakness, anxiety, shakiness and nervousness, tension, sleeplessness, dizziness and fainting, headache, pallor, sweating, nausea, vomiting, and muscle cramps.

▼ Less common: light-headedness, angina, abnormal heart rhythm, heart palpitations, breathing difficulties, bronchospasm, and flushing.

▼ Rare: abnormalities in liver tests, white-blood-cell counts, and tests for urine protein. The importance of these reactions is not known.

Drug Interactions

• Bitolterol's effects may be enhanced by monoamine oxidase inhibitor (MAOI) antidepressants, thyroid drugs, other bronchodilators, and some antihistamines.

• Bitolterol is antagonized by beta-blocking drugs, such as propranolol.

• Bitolterol may antagonize the effects of blood-pressure-lowering drugs, especially reserpine, methyldopa, and guanethidine.

• The risk of heart damage may be increased in people taking both bitolterol and theophylline.

Food Interactions

None known.

Usual Dose

Adult and Child (age 12 and over): to treat an attack—2 inhalations at an interval of at least 1–3 minutes, followed by a third inhalation, if needed. To prevent an attack—2 inhalations every 8 hours. Do not take more than 3 puffs in 6 hours or 2 every 4 hours.

Overdosage

Bitolterol overdose can result in exaggerated side effects, including chest pain and high blood pressure, although the pressure can drop to a low level after a short period of elevation. People who inhale too much bitolterol should see a doctor or go to a hospital emergency room.

Special Information

The drug should be inhaled during the second half of your inward breath. This will allow the medication to reach more deeply into your lungs.

Be sure to follow your doctor's directions for the use of bitolterol. Using more than you need can lead to drug tolerance and actually worsen your symptoms. If your condition worsens after taking bitolterol, stop taking it and call your doctor at once.

Call your doctor at once if you develop chest pains, rapid heartbeat, palpitations, muscle tremors, dizziness, headache, or facial flushing, or if you still have trouble breathing after using the medication.

If a dose of bitolterol is forgotten, take it as soon as you remember. If it is almost time for your next dose, skip the dose you forgot and continue with your regular schedule. Do not take a double dose.

Special Populations

Pregnancy/Breast-feeding

Bitolterol should be used by a pregnant or breast-feeding woman only when it is absolutely necessary. The potential benefit of using this medication must be carefully weighed against its risks.

It is not known if bitolterol passes into breast milk. Nursing mothers who take this may want to consider bottle-feeding.

Seniors

Seniors are more sensitive to the effects of this drug. Follow your doctor's directions and report any side effects at once.

Generic Name

Brimonidine (brim-ON-ih-dene)

Brand Name

Alphagan

Type of Drug

Alpha agonist.

Prescribed for

Glaucoma and ocular hypertension (high pressure inside the eye).

General Information

Brimonidine tartrate stimulates alpha-2 receptors in the eye and lowers pressure there. The maximum effect occurs 2 hours after the drops are administered. Brimonidine reduces the amount of aqueous humor (liquid) produced inside the eye and increases the rate at which fluid flows out of the eyeball. That portion of brimonidine that finds its way into the bloodstream is broken down by the liver.

Cautions and Warnings

Do not use this drug if you are **sensitive** or **allergic** to it.

People with **kidney or liver disease** should use this drug with caution. People with **cardiovascular disease** should exercise caution with this medication because it can affect blood pressure. It should be used with caution in people with **depression, cerebral or coronary insufficiency, Raynaud's disease,** and **dizziness or fainting** when rising from a sitting or lying position.

Brimonidine's effectiveness may decrease over time. Your doctor should check your eye pressure periodically to make sure the drug is still working.

Possible Side Effects

▼ Most common: dry mouth; redness, burning, and stinging of the eye; headache; blurred vision; sensation of something in the eye; drowsiness; and eye allergy and itching.

▼ Common: staining or erosion of the cornea, unusual sensitivity to bright light, eyelid redness or swelling, eye pain or ache, dry eye, respiratory symptoms, dizziness, eye irritation, upset stomach, weakness, abnormal vision, and muscle pain.

▼ Less common: crusty deposit on the eyelid, eye bleeding, abnormal taste sensation, sleeplessness, eye discharge, high blood pressure, anxiety, heart palpitations, dry nose, and fainting.

Drug Interactions

• Brimonidine may enhance the effects of alcohol, barbiturates, sedatives, anesthetics, beta-blocking drugs, blood-pressure-lowering drugs, and cardiac glycosides.

• Tricyclic antidepressants can increase the breakdown of brimonidine.

Usual Dose

Adult: 1 drop in the affected eye every 8 hours, 3 times a day.

Overdosage

Little is known about the effects of accidental ingestion. Victims should be taken to a hospital emergency room for treatment. ALWAYS bring the prescription bottle or container.

Special Information

If you wear soft contact lenses, wait at least 15 minutes between the time you put the drops in your eye and when you put your lenses in.

To prevent possible infection, do not allow the dropper to touch your fingers, eyelids, or any surface. Wait at least 5 minutes before using any other eyedrops.

Brimonidine may make you drowsy. Be careful while driving or doing anything else that requires concentration while you are taking this drug.

It is important that brimonidine be used according to your doctor's directions. If you forget to administer a dose of brimonidine, do so as soon as you remember. If it is almost time for your next dose, skip the dose you forgot and continue with your regular schedule. Do not take a double dose.

Special Populations

Pregnancy/Breast-feeding

A small amount of brimonidine may pass into the circulation of the fetus. Pregnant women should use this drug with care.

It is not known if this drug passes into breast milk. Nursing mothers who must use this drug should consider bottle-feeding.

Seniors

Seniors may use brimonidine without special precaution.

Generic Name

Bupropion (bue-PROE-pee-on) Ⓖ

Brand Names

Wellbutrin   Zyban
Wellbutrin SR

Type of Drug

Antidepressant and smoking deterrent.

Prescribed for

Depression and nicotine addiction.

General Information

Bupropion hydrochloride is usually used for severe or major depression only after other drugs have failed because of the risk of seizure with bupropion. It is chemically different from other antidepressants and is similar to diethylpropion, an appetite suppressant. Bupropion may work as a smoking deterrent by acting on key hormone systems in the brain. Studies of bupropion in smoking cessation found that people taking 150 to 300 mg a day of the drug were able to stop smoking for 4 weeks of the 7-week study. The people in these studies were not depressed. Bupropion is not likely to work until you have taken it for 3 to 4 weeks. The drug clears your system about 2 weeks after you stop taking it.

Cautions and Warnings

People with **seizure disorders,** people who have had a seizure in the past, and people with **bulimia** or **anorexia nervosa** should be very careful about taking bupropion because they are at a higher risk of having a seizure. About 4 in 1,000 people taking bupropion in dosages up to 450 mg a day develop a seizure. This is about 4 times the seizure rate associated with other antidepressants. The risk of developing a seizure increases by about 10 times with dosages between 450 and 600 mg a day. About half of the people who developed a seizure on bupropion had a risk factor such as a history of head injury, a previous seizure, or a nervous system tumor, or were taking another drug associated with increased seizure risk.

People with unstable **heart disease** or those who have had a recent **heart attack** should take this drug with caution because of possible side effects. Many people taking bupropion experience some restlessness, agitation, anxiety, and sleeplessness, especially soon after they start taking the drug. Some even require sleeping pills to counter this effect, and others find the stimulation so severe that they have to stop taking bupropion.

People taking bupropion may experience **hallucinations, delusions,** or **psychotic episodes.** Dosage reduction or drug withdrawal is usually necessary to manage these reactions.

One-quarter of those who take bupropion **lose their appetite** and 5 or more lbs. of body weight. People who have lost weight due to their depression should be cautious about taking bupropion.

People switching from bupropion to a **monoamine oxidase inhibitor (MAOI) antidepressant,** or vice versa, should allow at least 2 weeks to pass between stopping one drug and starting the other.

People with **kidney or liver disease** require less bupropion at the beginning of treatment. Dosage should be increased cautiously.

An antidepressant other than bupropion should be seriously considered for people with a history of drug abuse because of the mild stimulation bupropion causes. These people may require larger-than-usual dosages, but they are still susceptible to seizures at these higher dosages.

Suicide is always a risk in severely depressed people, who should only have minimal quantities of medication in their possession.

Possible Side Effects

About 10% of people stop taking bupropion due to side effects.

▼ Most common: dry mouth; dizziness; rapid heartbeat; headache, including migraine; excessive sweating; nausea; vomiting; constipation; appetite loss; weight changes; sedation; agitation; sleeplessness; and tremors.

▼ Less common: upset stomach, diarrhea, increased appetite, menstrual complaints, impotence, urinary difficulties, slowness of movement, salivation, muscle spasms, warmth, uncontrolled muscle movement, compulsion to move around or change positions, abnormal heart rhythms, blood-pressure changes, heart palpitations, fainting, itching, redness and rash, confusion, hostility, loss of concentration, reduced sex drive, anxiety, delusions, euphoria (feeling high), fatigue, joint pain, fever or chills, respiratory infection, and visual, taste, and hearing disturbances.

Many other side effects have been reported with bupropion, but their link to the drug is not well established.

Drug Interactions

• Carbamazepine may reduce blood concentrations of bupropion.

• People taking both bupropion and levodopa experience increased side effects. People taking levodopa should have their bupropion dosage increased gradually.

• Ritonavir may significantly increase bupropion blood levels and the risk of side effects.

• Phenelzine (an MAOI) increases the risk of bupropion side effects. Allow at least 2 weeks to pass between stopping an MAOI and starting bupropion.

• Don't mix bupropion with other drugs that increase the risk of seizures—including tricyclic antidepressants, haloperidol, lithium, loxapine, molindone, phenothiazine tranquilizers, and thioxanthene tranquilizers.

Food Interactions

Bupropion may be taken with food if it upsets your stomach.

Usual Dose

Depression
   Adult: 200–450 mg a day divided into 3 or 4 daily doses; normal daily dosage is 300 mg.
   Child (under age 18): not recommended.

Smoking Cessation
   Adult: 150 mg twice a day. Begin treatment while you are still smoking.
   Child (under age 18): not recommended.

Overdosage

Symptoms of overdose are likely to include severe side effects, such as seizures—present in ⅓ of overdoses—hallucinations, loss of consciousness, and abnormal heart rhythms. Overdose victims should be taken to a hospital emergency room at once. ALWAYS bring the prescription bottle or container.

Special Information

Do not stop taking bupropion without your doctor's knowledge. Suddenly stopping the drug may cause withdrawal reactions and side effects.

Call your doctor if you experience agitation or excitement, restlessness, confusion, difficulty sleeping, fast or abnormal heart rhythm, severe headache, seizure, rash, fainting, or any unusual or persistent side effect.

To reduce the risk of a seizure, take bupropion in 3 or 4 equal doses each day. Total daily dosage should not exceed 450 mg; single doses should not exceed 150 mg.

Bupropion may make you tired, dizzy, or light-headed. Be careful when driving or doing any task that requires concentration.

Alcohol, tranquilizers, and other nervous-system depressants increase the depressant effects of this drug. Alcohol also increases the risk of a seizure.

If you forget a dose, take it as soon as you remember. If it is almost time for your next dose, take 1 dose as soon as you remember and another in 3 or 4 hours, then go back to your regular schedule. Do not take a double dose.

Special Populations

Pregnancy/Breast-feeding

The safety of using bupropion during pregnancy is not known. When your doctor considers this drug crucial, its potential benefits must be carefully weighed against its risks. Pregnant women trying to quit smoking should use non-drug methods until their pregnancy is completed.

Bupropion passes into breast milk. Nursing mothers who must use bupropion should bottle-feed.

Seniors

Seniors with reduced kidney or liver function may require reduced dosage.

BuSpar   *see Buspirone, below*

Generic Name

Buspirone (bue-SPYE-rone)

Brand Name

BuSpar

Type of Drug

Minor tranquilizer and antianxiety drug.

Prescribed for

Anxiety; also prescribed for the aches, pains, fatigue, and cramps of premenstrual syndrome (PMS).

General Information

Buspirone hydrochloride has a potent antianxiety effect. It is approved by the Food and Drug Administration (FDA) for short-term relief of anxiety, but it may apparently be used safely for more than 4 weeks. The exact way in which buspirone works is not known, but it seems to lack the addiction dangers associated with other antianxiety drugs, including benzodiazepines. It neither severely depresses the nervous system nor acts as an anticonvulsant or muscle relaxant, as other antianxiety drugs do. Minor improvement will be apparent after only 7 to 10 days of drug treatment, but the maximum effect does not occur for 3 or 4 weeks.

Cautions and Warnings

Do not take buspirone if you are **allergic** to it.

Buspirone should be used cautiously by people with **liver or kidney disease**.

Buspirone does not have any antipsychotic effect and should not be taken for symptoms of **psychosis**.

Although buspirone has not shown a potential for **drug abuse,** you should be aware of this possibility.

Possible Side Effects

▼ Most common: dizziness, nausea, headache, fatigue, nervousness, light-headedness, and excitement.

▼ Common: heart palpitations, muscle aches and pains, tremors, rash, sweating, and clamminess.

▼ Less common: sleeplessness, chest pain, rapid heartbeat, low blood pressure, fainting, stroke, heart attack, heart failure, dream disturbances, difficulty concentrating, euphoria (feeling high), anger or hostility, depression, depersonalization or disassociation, fearfulness, loss of interest, hallucinations, suicidal tendencies, claustrophobia, stupor, slurred speech, intolerance to noise, and intolerance to cold temperatures.

▼ Rare: Rare side effects can occur in almost any part of the body. Contact your doctor if you experience any side effect not listed above.

Drug Interactions

• Combining buspirone with a monoamine oxidase inhibitor (MAOI) antidepressant may produce severe hypertension and may be dangerous.

• The effects of combining buspirone with other drugs that work in the central nervous system (CNS) are not known. Do not take other tranquilizers or antianxiety or psychoactive drugs with buspirone unless prescribed by a doctor familiar with your complete medical history.

• Buspirone may increase the side effects of haloperidol.

• Studies show that buspirone is not affected by alcohol, but this combination should still be used with caution because buspirone causes drowsiness and dizziness.

• The combination of buspirone and trazodone may cause liver inflammation.

Food Interactions

This drug may be taken either with or without food, but for the most consistent results, always take your dose at the same time of day in the same way—that is, with or without food.

Usual Dose

Starting dosage—15 mg a day in 3 divided doses. Dosage may be increased gradually to 60 mg a day.

Overdosage

Symptoms of overdose are nausea, vomiting, dizziness, drowsiness, pinpointed pupils, and upset stomach. The overdose victim should be taken to a hospital emergency room. ALWAYS bring the prescription bottle or container.

Special Information

Buspirone may cause nervous-system depression, drowsiness, and dizziness. Be careful while driving or operating hazardous equipment. Avoid other CNS drugs and alcoholic beverages because they will enhance buspirone's effects.

Contact your doctor if you become restless, develop uncontrolled or repeated movements of the head, face, or neck, or have any intolerable side effects. About 1 in 10 people stop taking buspirone because of side effects.

If you forget a dose, take it as soon as you remember. If it is almost time for your next dose, skip the dose you forgot and go back to your regular schedule. Do not take a double dose.

Special Populations

Pregnancy/Breast-feeding

Though buspirone has not been found to cause birth defects, be sure to inform your doctor if you are or might be pregnant while taking this drug. When this drug is considered crucial by your doctor, its potential benefits must be carefully weighed against its risks.

It is not known how much buspirone passes into breast milk. Nursing mothers who must take this drug should consider bottle-feeding.

Seniors

Several hundred seniors participated in drug evaluation studies without any unusual problems. However, the effect of this drug in seniors is not well known, and special problems may surface, particularly in those with kidney or liver disease.

Generic Name

Butenafine (bue-TEN-uh-fene)

Brand Name

Mentax

Type of Drug

Antifungal.

Prescribed for

Athlete's foot.

General Information

Butenafine hydrochloride works by blocking the natural syn-
thesis of a chemical—ergosterol—essential to the cell membrane (outer skin) of the fungus cell. Butenafine may actually
kill the fungus if enough of it is present. Some butenafine is
absorbed into the bloodstream.

Cautions and Warnings

Do not use butenafine if you are **sensitive** or **allergic** to it.

Possible Side Effects

▼ Common: rash, burning, stinging, worsening of the
infection, swelling, irritation, and itching.

Drug Interactions

When you apply butenafine to the skin, do not combine it
with any other medication.

Usual Dose

Adult and Child (age 12 and over): Apply enough to cover
the affected area and surrounding skin once a day for 4
weeks. Wash your hands after each application.

Child (under age 12): not recommended.

Overdosage

Little is known about the effects of accidental ingestion. Call
your local poison control center or hospital emergency room
for more information.

Special Information

This drug may irritate sensitive skin. Call your doctor if this
happens—another medication may be more appropriate.
Also call your doctor if you experience redness, itching, burning, blistering, swelling, or oozing.

Athlete's foot is relatively common and may be caused by a number of different kinds of fungi. Do not use this drug without your doctor's knowledge.

Butenafine is to be applied only to your skin. It should not be applied to other areas, including the eyes, nose, mouth, or vagina.

If you apply the cream after bathing, be sure that your feet are completely dry, especially the areas between your toes.

As is often the case when using an anti-infective, your symptoms may begin to improve before you have completed the full course of treatment. Be sure to use all of the medication as directed. Also, follow your doctor's instructions about the kind of bandage or dressing to use.

Call your doctor if the condition does not improve after 4 weeks of using the cream.

Special Populations

Pregnancy/Breast-feeding
Butenafine should only be used during pregnancy if absolutely necessary.

It is not known if this drug passes into breast milk. Nursing mothers who must use this drug should consider bottle-feeding.

Seniors
Seniors may use this medication without special precaution.

Generic Name

Calcitonin (kal-sih-TONE-in)

Brand Names

Calcimar   Osteocalcin
Miacalcin   Salmonine

Type of Drug

Peptide hormone.

Prescribed for

Osteoporosis (condition characterized by loss of bone mass due to depletion of minerals, especially calcium) in postmenopausal women; also prescribed for Paget's disease of bone.

General Information

Calcitonin helps to strengthen bone by adding more calcium to it and slowing the natural process by which bone is broken down. The calcitonin used in this drug is essentially identical to human calcitonin except that it is more potent. It is a synthetic version of the natural calcitonin found in salmon. Calcitonin can increase bone density and reduce the risk of fractures of the vertebrae (bones that comprise the spinal column), which are associated with back pain and loss of height. Calcitonin has been available for years as an injection, but the development of the nasal spray makes the drug easier to use.

Cautions and Warnings

Do not use this drug if you are **sensitive** or **allergic** to it. Although **serious allergic reactions** were reported with the injectable form, none have occurred with the nasal spray.

Changes in the **tissues lining your nose** are possible with long-term use of this product. Periodic nasal examinations are recommended.

Possible Side Effects

▼ Most common: stuffy nose, runny nose, and other nasal symptoms; and back pain.

▼ Less common: flu-like symptoms, rash, muscle ache, joint problems, sinus irritation, upper respiratory infection, bronchial spasm, high blood pressure, angina, upset stomach, constipation, abdominal pain, nausea, diarrhea, cystitis, dizziness, tingling in the hands or feet, eye tearing, swollen lymph glands, and infections.

▼ Rare: Rare side effects can occur in almost any part of the body. Contact your doctor if you experience any side effect not listed above.

Food and Drug Interactions

None known.

Usual Dose

Adult: 1 spray (200 IU) a day.

Child: Information is lacking on the use of this drug in children.

Overdosage

Little is known about the effects of calcitonin overdose or accidental ingestion. No adverse effects have been reported after high doses. Call your local poison control center for more information. Overdose victims should be taken to a hospital emergency room. ALWAYS bring the prescription bottle or container.

Special Information

Alternate nostrils daily when using the nasal spray.

Before you take your first dose, you must activate the pump. Hold the bottle upright and press the two white arms toward the bottle 6 times until a faint spray is emitted. Once this occurs, the pump is activated and ready for use. It is not necessary to reactivate the pump every day.

If you forget to administer a dose of the nasal spray, do so as soon as you remember. If it is almost time for the next dose, skip the dose you forgot and continue with your regular schedule. Call your doctor if you forget 2 or more doses or if you develop severe nose irritation or any unusual or intolerable symptom.

Special Populations

Pregnancy/Breast-feeding

Calcitonin does not cross into the fetal circulation, though animal studies have associated the injectable form of the drug with low birth weight. This drug is recommended for use during pregnancy only if its possible benefits outweigh its risks.

It is not known if calcitonin passes into breast milk, though animal studies have shown that it reduces the amount of milk produced. Nursing mothers who must use calcitonin should consider bottle-feeding.

Seniors

Seniors may use this product without special precaution.

Generic Name

Capecitabine (cape-SE-tah-been)

Brand Name

Xeloda

Type of Drug

Antimetabolite.

Prescribed for

Breast cancer that has metastasized (spread) to other parts of the body.

General Information

Capecitabine is prescribed for women whose breast cancer has metastasized despite previous cancer treatment. This drug is converted in the body to 5-FU, a widely used anticancer agent. Unlike some anticancer medications, capecitabine can be taken by mouth and has relatively few serious side effects.

Cautions and Warnings

People who are **allergic** or **sensitive** to 5-FU should not take capecitabine.

People with **liver or kidney disease** should be carefully monitored by their doctors because capecitabine's effect on these conditions is not known.

Capecitabine can **reduce fertility**.

Capecitabine use is associated with **heart and blood vessel disease**.

Possible Side Effects

▼ Most common: diarrhea, constipation, nausea, vomiting, mouth sores, abdominal pain, hand-and-foot syndrome (see "Special Information"), inflammation of the skin, tingling or pain in the hands or feet, fatigue, loss of appetite, low blood-cell counts, eye irritation, and fever.

▼ Common: upset stomach, nail problems, headache, dizziness, sleeplessness, dehydration, swelling, muscle aches, and pain in the arms or legs.

Possible Side Effects *(continued)*

Less common and rare side effects can affect the stomach and intestines, skin, nervous system, lungs and respiratory system, heart and blood vessels, blood, urinary and reproductive tracts, liver, and other organs.

Other side effects can occur in almost any part of the body. Contact your doctor if you experience any side effect not listed above.

Drug Interactions

• Combining antacids and capecitabine can increase the amount of drug absorbed by about 20%. Separate doses of antacids and capecitabine by 2 hours.

• Leucovorin (a drug used in cancer treatment) increases the side effects of 5-FU. This combination has caused death in several seniors.

Food Interactions

Capecitabine should be taken within 30 minutes of a meal to avoid stomach problems.

Usual Dose

Adult: 1500–2800 mg a day, depending on height and weight.

Child: not recommended.

Overdosage

Symptoms include nausea, vomiting, diarrhea, bleeding and reduced blood-cell counts, and stomach irritation. Overdose victims should be taken to a hospital emergency room. ALWAYS bring the prescription bottle or container.

Special Information

Stop taking capecitabine and call your doctor if you have 4 to 6 more bowel movements a day than normal, vomit 2 to 5 times in 1 day, or become very nauseous. Depending on the severity of your symptoms, your doctor may reduce your dosage.

Capecitabine has caused hand-and-foot syndrome. Symptoms of this condition include numbness, tingling, pain, swelling, redness, skin loss and blistering of the hands or feet. Stop taking the drug and call your doctor if you experience any of these symptoms.

People who develop stomatitis (symptoms include swelling, pain, or sores in the area of the mouth or tongue) should stop taking the drug and call their doctors at once.

Call your doctor, but do not stop taking the drug, if you develop a fever of 100.5°F or higher or other signs of infection.

If you forget a dose, take it as soon as you remember. If it is almost time for your next dose, take 1 dose right away and space the remaining daily dosage evenly throughout the day. Go back to your regular schedule the next morning. Call your doctor if you miss more than 2 doses in a row.

Special Populations

Pregnancy/Breast-feeding
Capecitabine can harm the fetus. Its potential benefits must be carefully weighed against its risks when capecitabine is considered crucial by your doctor. Effective contraception is absolutely necessary while taking this drug.

It is not known if capecitabine passes into breast milk. Nursing mothers who must take this drug should bottle-feed.

Seniors
Seniors may be more sensitive to side effects, especially diarrhea and other stomach problems.

Generic Name

Captopril (KAP-toe-pril) G

Brand Name

Capoten

Combination Products

Generic Ingredients: Captopril + Hydrochlorothiazide G
Capozide

Type of Drug

Angiotensin-converting enzyme (ACE) inhibitor; antihypertensive.

Prescribed for

High blood pressure and congestive heart failure; also used to treat and prevent diabetic kidney disease and high blood pressure associated with other medical conditions, such as scleroderma and Takayasu's disease. Captopril combined with the diuretic hydrochlorothiazide is used to treat high blood pressure.

General Information

Captopril and other ACE inhibitors work by preventing the conversion of a hormone called angiotensin I to another hormone called angiotensin II, a potent blood-vessel constrictor. Preventing this conversion relaxes blood vessels, helps to reduce blood pressure, and relieves the symptoms of heart failure. Captopril also affects the production of other hormones and enzymes that participate in the regulation of blood-vessel dilation. Captopril usually begins working about 1 hour after it is taken.

People who are already taking a diuretic (an agent that increases urination) may experience a rapid blood-pressure drop after their first dose of captopril or when their captopril dose is increased. To prevent this, your doctor may tell you to stop taking your diuretic or to increase your salt intake 2 or 3 days before starting captopril. The diuretic may then be restarted gradually.

In addition to its labeled uses, captopril has been studied in the diagnosis of certain kidney diseases and of primary aldosteronism, and in the treatment of rheumatoid arthritis, swelling and fluid accumulation, Bartter's syndrome, Raynaud's disease, and post-heart-attack treatment when the function of the left ventricle is affected.

Cautions and Warnings

Do not take captopril if you are **allergic** to it.

Although not common, captopril may cause **very low blood pressure**. It may also affect your **kidneys,** especially if you have congestive **heart failure.** Your doctor should check your urine for protein content during the first few months of captopril treatment. Captopril may cause a decline in kidney function. Dosage adjustment of captopril is necessary if you have reduced kidney function because the drug is generally eliminated from the body via the kidneys.

Captopril may affect white-blood-cell counts, possibly increasing your susceptibility to **infection**. Your doctor should monitor your blood counts periodically.

Possible Side Effects

▼ Most common: rash, itching, and cough that usually goes away a few days after you stop taking the drug.

▼ Less common: dizziness, tiredness, sleep disturbances, headache, tingling in hands or feet, chest pain, heart palpitations, feeling unwell, abdominal pain, nausea, vomiting, diarrhea, constipation, appetite loss, dry mouth, breathing difficulties, and hair loss.

▼ Rare: Rare side effects can occur in almost any part of the body. Contact your doctor if you experience any side effect not listed above.

Drug Interactions

• The blood-pressure-lowering effect of captopril is additive with diuretic drugs and beta blockers. Any other drug that causes a rapid blood-pressure drop should be used with caution if you are taking captopril.

• Captopril may increase blood-potassium levels, especially when taken with Dyazide or other potassium-sparing diuretics.

• Captopril may increase the effects of lithium; this combination should be used with caution.

• Antacids and captopril should be taken at least 2 hours apart.

• Capsaicin may trigger or aggravate the cough associated with captopril.

• Indomethacin may reduce the blood-pressure-lowering effect of captopril.

• Phenothiazine tranquilizers and antivomiting agents may increase the effects of captopril.

• Probenecid increases this drug's effect as well as the chance of side effects.

• The combination of allopurinol and captopril increases the chance of an adverse drug reaction.

• Captopril may increase blood levels of digoxin, which may increase the chance of digoxin-related side effects.

Food Interactions

Captopril should be taken on an empty stomach, at least 1 hour before or 2 hours after a meal.

Usual Dose

Adult: 75 mg a day to start. Dosage may be increased to 450 mg a day in divided doses, if needed. Dosage must be tailored to your needs. People with poor kidney function must take lower doses.

Child: approximately 0.15 mg per lb. of body weight, 3 times a day.

Overdosage

The principal effect of captopril overdose is a rapid drop in blood pressure, which may lead to dizziness or fainting. Take the overdose victim to a hospital emergency room immediately. ALWAYS bring the prescription bottle or container.

Special Information

Captopril may cause swelling of the face, lips, hands, and feet. This swelling may also affect the larynx (throat) and tongue and interfere with breathing. If this happens, go to a hospital emergency room at once. Call your doctor if you develop a sore throat, mouth sores, abnormal heartbeat, chest pain, a persistent rash, or losses in the sense of taste.

You may get dizzy if you rise to your feet too quickly from a sitting or lying position.

Avoid strenuous exercise or very hot weather because heavy sweating or dehydration may lead to a rapid drop in blood pressure.

Avoid over-the-counter stimulants that can raise blood pressure while taking captopril, including diet pills and decongestants.

If you forget to take a dose of captopril, take it as soon as you remember. If it is within 4 hours of your next dose, take 1 dose immediately and another in 5 or 6 hours, then go back to your regular schedule. Do not take a double dose.

Special Populations

Pregnancy/Breast-feeding

ACE inhibitors can cause fetal injury or death. Women who are or might be pregnant should not take ACE inhibitors. If you become pregnant, stop taking captopril and call your doctor immediately.

Small amounts of captopril pass into breast milk. Nursing mothers who must take this drug should consider bottle-feeding.

Seniors

Seniors may be more sensitive to the effects of captopril due to age-related declines in kidney or liver function.

Generic Name

Carbamazepine (car-bam-A-zuh-pene) Ⓖ

Brand Names

Atretol	Tegretol
Carbatrol	Tegretol-XR
Epitrol	

Type of Drug

Anticonvulsant.

Prescribed for

Seizure disorders as well as trigeminal and other neuralgias; also used to treat severe pain; psychiatric disorders including depression, bipolar disorder, intermittent explosive disorder, post-traumatic stress disorder, psychotic disorders, and schizophrenia; withdrawal from alcohol, cocaine, or benzodiazepine-type drugs; restless leg syndrome; non-hereditary chorea in children; and diabetes insipidus.

General Information

Carbamazepine was first approved for relief of the severe pain of trigeminal neuralgia. Over the years, it has gained wide use in seizure control, especially in people whose seizures are uncontrolled with phenytoin, phenobarbital, or primidone, or who have suffered severe side effects from these drugs. Carbamazepine is not a simple pain reliever and should not be taken for everyday aches and pains. It is associated with potentially fatal side effects.

Cautions and Warnings

Carbamazepine should not be used if you have had **bone marrow depression** or if you are **sensitive** or **allergic** to this drug or any tricyclic antidepressant.

Monoamine oxidase inhibitor (MAOI) antidepressants should be discontinued 2 weeks before starting carbamazepine.

Carbamazepine may cause severe, **possibly life-threatening blood reactions.** People who have had blood reactions to other drugs are at particular risk for another reaction with carbamazepine. Your doctor should have a complete blood count done before you start taking this drug and repeat these tests weekly during the first 3 months of treatment, and then every month for the next 2 to 3 years. Unexplained fever or infection may be a sign of a blood reaction.

Severe, **possibly fatal skin reactions** have developed in a few people taking carbamazepine.

Carbamazepine may aggravate **glaucoma** and should be used with caution by people with this condition. This drug may activate underlying **psychosis,** confusion, or agitation, especially in older adults.

Possible Side Effects

▼ Most common: dizziness, drowsiness, unsteadiness, nausea, and vomiting. Other common side effects are blurred or double vision, confusion, hostility, headache, and severe water retention.

▼ Less common: mood and behavioral changes, especially in children. Hives, itching, rash, and other allergic reactions may also occur.

▼ Rare: Rare side effects can affect your breathing, speech, emotions, liver function, urinary function, and many other parts of the body. Contact your doctor if you experience any side effect not listed above.

Drug Interactions

• Carbamazepine blood levels may be increased by cimetidine, danazol, diltiazem, isoniazid, propoxyphene, erythromycin-type antibiotics (except azithromycin), fluoxetine, fluvoxamine, mexiletine, nicotinamide, troleandomycin, or verapamil, leading to possible carbamazepine toxicity.

• Carbamazepine may reduce the effectiveness of oral contraceptives and cause breakthrough bleeding.

• Charcoal tablets or powder, phenobarbital and other barbiturates, phenytoin, and primidone may decrease the absorption of carbamazepine. Levels of phenobarbital, a breakdown product of primidone, may be increased by combining primidone and carbamazepine.

• Carbamazepine reduces the effects of acetaminophen, the anticoagulant (blood thinner) warfarin, and theophylline (prescribed for asthma). Increased dosage of these drugs may be necessary. Other drugs counteracted by carbamazepine are cyclosporine, dacarbazine, digitalis drugs, disopyramide, doxycycline, haloperidol, levothyroxine, and quinidine.

• Combining carbamazepine and other antiseizure drugs, including felbamate, hydantoins, succinimides, and valproic acid, may cause unpredictable results. Combination treatments to control seizures must be customized to each person.

• Combining carbamazepine and lithium may increase nervous system side effects.

Food Interactions

Take carbamazepine with food if it causes stomach upset.

Usual Dose

Adult and Child (age 13 and over): 400–1200 mg a day, depending on the condition. Usual maintenance dose is 400–800 mg a day in 2 divided doses.

Child (age 6–12): 200–1000 mg a day, or 10–15 mg per lb. of body weight a day, divided into 3–4 equal doses.

Dosage varies according to form. Liquid carbamazepine must be taken 3 times a day, regular carbamazepine tablets twice a day, and sustained-release tablets once daily. Never change your dosage schedule without first checking with your doctor.

Overdosage

Carbamazepine is a potentially lethal drug. Overdose symptoms appear in 1 to 3 hours. These include irregularity or difficulty in breathing, rapid heartbeat, changes in blood pressure, shock, loss of consciousness or coma, convulsions, muscle twitching, restlessness, uncontrolled body movements, drooping eyelids, psychotic mood changes, nausea, vomiting, and reduced urination. Induce vomiting right away with ipecac syrup—available at any pharmacy. Then take the victim to a hospital emergency room. ALWAYS bring the prescription bottle or container.

Special Information

Carbamazepine may cause dizziness and drowsiness. Take care while driving or doing any task that requires concentration.

Call your doctor at once if you experience yellowing of the skin or whites of the eyes, unusual bleeding or bruising, abdominal pain, pale stools, dark urine, impotence, mood changes, nervous system symptoms, swelling, fever, chills, sore throat, or mouth sores. These may be signs of a potentially fatal drug reaction.

If you forget a dose, skip it and go back to your regular schedule. If you miss more than 1 dose in a day, call your doctor. Do not stop taking this drug without first consulting your doctor.

Special Populations

Pregnancy/Breast-feeding

Carbamazepine caused birth defects in animal studies. Seizure disorder itself also increases the risk of birth defects. Pregnant women should take carbamazepine only after discussing with their doctors its potential benefits and risks.

Carbamazepine passes into breast milk. Nursing mothers who must take carbamazepine should bottle-feed.

Seniors

Seniors taking this drug are more likely to develop heart problems, psychosis, confusion, or agitation.

Type of Drug

Carbonic-Anhydrase Inhibitors, Eyedrops (kar-BON-ik an-HYE-drase)

Brand Names

Generic Ingredient: Dorzolamide
Trusopt

Generic Ingredient: Brinzolamide
Azopt

Prescribed for

Glaucoma.

General Information

These drugs are similar to acetazolamide, a carbonic-anhydrase inhibitor taken by mouth. Carbonic anhydrase is an enzyme found in many parts of the body, including the eyes. By blocking the effects of this enzyme, dorzolamide and brinzolamide slow the production of fluid inside the eye, reducing pressure there. This effect is useful in treating glaucoma because the disease is characterized by elevated eye pressure.

Cautions and Warnings

Do not use these drugs if you are **sensitive** or **allergic** to it or to other sulfa drugs. Small amounts of these drugs enter the bloodstream. Rarely, people using them experience **side effects or allergies associated with sulfa drugs**.

These drugs have not been studied in people with very **poor kidney or liver function**. Since these drugs are eliminated via the kidneys, people with impaired kidney function should use an alternate glaucoma medication.

Possible Side Effects

Dorzolamide

▼ Most common: eye burning, stinging, or discomfort and a bitter taste in the mouth immediately after administering the eyedrops.

▼ Less common: allergic reactions, blurred vision, tearing, dry eye, and increased sensitivity to bright light.

▼ Rare: headache, nausea, weakness, tiredness, rash, and kidney stones. Dorzolamide can cause the same types of side effects as other sulfa drugs, but this is very unlikely. Report any unusual symptoms to your doctor.

Possible Side Effects *(continued)*

Brinzolamide

▼ Common: blurred vision and a bitter, sour, or unusual taste in the mouth.

▼ Less common: eyelid inflammation; rash; dry eye; sensation of something in the eye; headache; eye redness, itching, discharge, or pain; and runny nose.

▼ Rare: allergic reactions, hair loss, chest pain, pinkeye, diarrhea, nausea, sore throat, tearing, itchy rash, double vision, dizziness, dry mouth, breathing difficulties, upset stomach, tired eyes, kidney pain, cornea problems, and formation of a crust or sticky sensation around the eyelid. Brinzolamide can cause the same types of side effects as other sulfa drugs, but this is very unlikely. Report any unusual symptoms to your doctor.

Drug Interactions

• If you are using more than 1 eyedrop product, separate doses of these drugs by at least 10 minutes.

Usual Dose

Adult: 1 drop in the affected eye 3 times a day.

Overdosage

Accidental ingestion of a bottle of dorzolamide or brinzolamide may affect blood levels of potassium and other electrolytes. The victim should be taken to a hospital emergency room. ALWAYS bring the prescription bottle or container.

Special Information

Call your doctor and stop using your eyedrops if you develop any unusual eye reaction or condition, including swollen eyelids and pinkeye.

If you wear soft contact lenses, take them out before using the eyedrops and put them back in 15 minutes after a dose.

To prevent infection, do not allow the eyedropper tip to touch your fingers, eyelids, or any surface. Wait at least 10 minutes before using any other eyedrops.

If you forget to administer a dose, do so as soon as you remember. If it is almost time for your next dose, skip the one you forgot and continue with your regular schedule. Do not take a double dose.

Special Populations

Pregnancy/Breast-feeding
Very high dosages of dorzolamide or brinzolamide caused birth defects in animal studies. While the risks of using these drugs during pregnancy are small in people, pregnant women should use dorzolamide or brinzolamide only after discussing its potential benefits and risks with their doctors.

It is not known if these drugs pass into breast milk. Nursing mothers who must use either drug should bottle-feed.

Seniors
Seniors may be more sensitive to side effects.

Cardizem CD   *see Diltiazem, page 330*

Cardura   *see Doxazosin, page 352*

Generic Name

Carisoprodol (kar-ih-SOP-roe-dol) Ⓖ

Brand Name
Soma

Type of Drug
Skeletal muscle relaxant.

Prescribed for
Pain and discomfort associated with sprain, strain, and back problems.

General Information
Carisoprodol is prescribed as part of a coordinated program of rest, physical therapy, and other treatments. The drug may relieve pain by interfering with central nerves that cause the

muscles to go into spasm. This drug begins working within 30 minutes after it is taken and lasts for 4 to 6 hours.

Cautions and Warnings

Do not take carisoprodol if you are sensitive or **allergic** to it or to meprobamate, or if you have **acute intermittent porphyria**. A few people experience unusual side effects within a few minutes or hours of taking their first dose of carisoprodol. They may include extreme weakness, temporary loss of use of the arms and legs, dizziness, muscle weakness, temporary loss of vision, double vision, dilated pupils, agitation, joint pain, euphoria (feeling high), confusion, and disorientation.

People can become **dependent** on this drug and may experience withdrawal (symptoms include abdominal cramps, sleeplessness, chills, headache, and nausea) after taking it for an extended period of time.

People with **kidney or liver disease** should use carisoprodol with care.

Possible Side Effects

▼ Common: drowsiness.

▼ Less common: rapid heartbeat; dizziness or lightheadedness; fainting; depression; large hive-like swellings on the face, eyelids, mouth, lips, or tongue; breathing difficulties; chest tightness or wheezing; allergic fever; stinging or burning eyes; headache; unusual stimulation; trembling; upset stomach or abdominal cramps; hiccups; and nausea or vomiting.

▼ Rare: Rare side effects can affect your vision, breathing, blood, skin, and other body parts. Contact your doctor if you experience any side effect not listed above.

Drug Interactions

• Avoid alcoholic beverages, sleeping pills, tranquilizers, and other nervous system depressants while taking carisoprodol.

Food Interactions

You may take carisoprodol with food if it upsets your stomach.

Usual Dose

Adult: 350 mg 3–4 times a day and at bedtime.
Child (under age 12): not recommended.

Overdosage

Symptoms of carisoprodol overdose include slurred speech, stupor, coma, shock, and breathing difficulties. In rare cases, carisoprodol overdose is fatal. The effects of a carisoprodol overdose are amplified by alcohol and other nervous system depressants. Victims should be taken to a hospital emergency room for treatment at once. ALWAYS bring the prescription bottle or container.

Special Information

Carisoprodol may adversely affect your ability to concentrate and slow your physical reactions. Be careful when driving a car or doing anything else that requires concentration and alertness.

Avoid alcohol and other nervous system depressants while taking carisoprodol.

Call your doctor if you become dizzy or faint while taking carisoprodol, or if you develop a rapid or pounding heartbeat.

If you forget a dose of carisoprodol, take it immediately if you remember within 1 hour of your scheduled time. If you do not remember until more than 1 hour later or you forget it completely, skip the dose you forgot and continue with your regular schedule. Do not take a double dose.

Special Populations

Pregnancy/Breast-feeding

Pregnant women should not use this drug unless they have thoroughly discussed its risks and benefits with their doctor.

Carisoprodol passes into breast milk in large amounts. Nursing mothers should avoid this drug because it may affect their babies.

Seniors

Seniors with kidney or liver disease should be careful about taking carisoprodol; it may cause sleepiness or affect the ability to concentrate.

Generic Name

Carteolol (car-TEE-uh-lol)

Brand Names

Cartrol   Ocupress

Type of Drug

Beta-adrenergic blocking agent.

Prescribed for

High blood pressure, angina pectoris, and glaucoma.

General Information

Carteolol hydrochloride is one of many beta-adrenergic blocking drugs, or beta blockers, that interfere with the action of a specific part of the nervous system. Beta receptors are found all over the body and affect many body functions. Each beta blocker has particular characteristics that make it more suitable for certain conditions or people. When applied as eyedrops, carteolol reduces ocular pressure (pressure inside the eye) by slowing the production of eye fluids and by slightly increasing the rate at which these fluids flow through and leave the eye.

Cautions and Warnings

You should be cautious about taking carteolol if you have **asthma, severe heart failure,** a **very slow heart rate,** or **heart block** (disruption of the electrical impulses that control heart rate) because the drug may aggravate these conditions.

People with **angina** who take carteolol for high blood pressure risk aggravating their angina if they suddenly stop taking the drug. These people should have their drug dosage reduced gradually over 1 to 2 weeks.

Carteolol should be used with caution if you have **liver or kidney disease** because the ability to eliminate the drug from your body may be impaired.

Carteolol reduces the amount of blood pumped by the heart with each beat. This reduction in blood flow may aggravate the condition of people with **poor circulation** or **circulatory disease**.

If you are undergoing **major surgery,** your doctor may want you to stop taking carteolol at least 2 days before surgery.

Carteolol eyedrops should be avoided by people who cannot take oral beta-blocking drugs such as propranolol.

Possible Side Effects

Side effects are relatively uncommon and usually mild.

▼ Most common: impotence.

▼ Less common: unusual tiredness or weakness, slow heartbeat, heart failure, dizziness, breathing difficulties, bronchospasm, depression, anxiety, nervousness, sleeplessness, disorientation, short-term memory loss, emotional instability, cold hands and feet, constipation, diarrhea, nausea, vomiting, upset stomach, increased sweating, urinary difficulties, cramps, blurred vision, rash, hair loss, stuffy nose, facial swelling, aggravation of lupus erythematosus, itching, chest pain, back or joint pain, colitis, and drug allergy (symptoms include fever and sore throat).

Drug Interactions

• Carteolol may interact with surgical anesthetics to increase the risk of heart problems during surgery. Some anesthesiologists recommend gradually stopping the drug by 2 days before surgery.

• Carteolol may interfere with the normal signs of low blood sugar and with the action of oral antidiabetes drugs.

• Carteolol increases the blood-pressure-lowering effects of other blood-pressure-reducing agents, including clonidine, guanabenz, and reserpine, as well as calcium channel blockers, such as nifedipine.

• Aspirin-containing drugs, indomethacin, sulfinpyrazone, and estrogen drugs may interfere with the blood-pressure-lowering effect of carteolol.

• Cocaine may reduce the effectiveness of all beta blockers.

• Carteolol may worsen the problem of cold hands and feet associated with ergot alkaloids, used to treat migraine. Gangrene is a possibility in people taking both an ergot and carteolol.

• Carteolol will counteract thyroid hormone replacements.

• Calcium channel blockers, flecainide, hydralazine, oral contraceptives, propafenone, haloperidol, phenothiazine tranquilizers—molindone and others—quinolone antibacterials, and quinidine may increase the amount of carteolol in the bloodstream and lead to increased carteolol effects.

• Carteolol should not be taken within 2 weeks of taking a monoamine oxidase inhibitor (MAOI) antidepressant.

• Cimetidine increases the amount of carteolol absorbed into the bloodstream from oral tablets.

• Carteolol may reduce the effect of some antiasthma drugs, including theophylline and aminophylline, and especially ephedrine and isoproterenol.

• Combining carteolol with phenytoin or digitalis drugs may result in excessive slowing of the heart, possibly causing heart block.

• If you stop smoking while taking carteolol, your dose may have to be reduced because your liver will break down the drug more slowly afterward.

• If you use other glaucoma eye medications, separate your dose to avoid physically combining them.

• Small amounts of carteolol eyedrops are absorbed into the bloodstream and may interact with other drugs in the same way as oral beta blockers, although it is unlikely.

Food Interactions

None known.

Usual Dose

Tablets: 2.5–10 mg once a day. People with poor kidney function may need to take their dose as infrequently as once every 72 hours.

Eyedrops: 1 drop in the affected eye 1–2 times a day.

Overdosage

Symptoms of overdose include changes in heartbeat—unusually slow, unusually fast, or irregular—severe dizziness or fainting, breathing difficulties, bluish-colored fingernails or palms, and seizures. The victim should be taken to a hospital emergency room. ALWAYS bring the prescription bottle or container.

Special Information

Carteolol should be taken continuously. When ending carteolol treatment, dosage should be lowered gradually over a period of about 2 weeks. Do not stop taking this drug unless directed to do so by your doctor. Abrupt withdrawal may cause chest pain, breathing difficulties, increased sweating, and unusually fast or irregular heartbeat.

Call your doctor at once if you develop back or joint pain, breathing difficulties, cold hands or feet, depression, rash, or changes in heartbeat. This drug may produce an undesirable lowering of blood pressure, leading to dizziness or fainting; call your doctor if this happens to you. Call your doctor if you experience persistent or bothersome anxiety, diarrhea, constipation, impotence, headache, itching, nausea or vomiting, nightmares or vivid dreams, upset stomach, trouble sleeping, stuffy nose, frequent urination, unusual tiredness, or weakness.

Carteolol can cause drowsiness, light-headedness, dizziness, or blurred vision. Be careful when driving or performing complex tasks.

It is best to take carteolol at the same time each day. If you forget a dose of carteolol tablets, take it as soon as you remember. If you take carteolol once a day and it is within 8 hours of your next dose, skip the dose you forgot and continue with your regular schedule. If you take carteolol twice a day and it is within 4 hours of your next dose, skip the one you forgot and continue with your regular schedule. Never take a double dose.

To prevent possible infection, do not allow the dropper to touch your fingers, eyelids, or any surface. Wait at least 5 minutes before using any other eyedrops.

If you forget a dose of carteolol eyedrops, administer it as soon as you remember. If it is almost time for your next dose, skip the one you forgot and continue with your regular schedule. Do not take a double dose.

Special Populations

Pregnancy/Breast-feeding

Infants born to women who took a beta blocker while pregnant had lower birth weights, low blood pressure, and reduced heart rates. Carteolol should be avoided by pregnant women and women who might become pregnant while taking it.

It is not known if carteolol passes into breast milk. Nursing mothers taking carteolol should bottle-feed.

Seniors

Seniors may require less of the drug to achieve results. Seniors taking carteolol may be more likely to suffer from cold hands and feet, reduced body temperature, chest pain, general feelings of ill health, sudden breathing difficulties, increased sweating, or changes in heartbeat.

Generic Name

Carvedilol (car-VAY-dih-lol)

Brand Name

Coreg

Type of Drug

Alpha-beta-adrenergic blocker.

Prescribed for

Heart failure, high blood pressure, angina pain, and cardiomyopathy.

General Information

Carvedilol was the first beta blocker approved for heart failure. Carvedilol blocks both the alpha- and beta-adrenergic portions of the central nervous system. This dual action reduces the amount of blood pumped with each heartbeat and also decreases the risk of tachycardia (very rapid heartbeat). Carvedilol's beta-blocking effects begin within an hour of taking the first dose; maximum blood pressure lowering occurs after 1 or 2 weeks. The drug also causes blood vessels to dilate (widen), allowing the heart to pump blood more efficiently.

Cautions and Warnings

Carvedilol causes **liver injury** in about 1 of every 100 people who take it. Those with severe liver disease should not take this medication. Call your doctor at once if you develop signs of liver damage (symptoms include severe itching, dark-colored urine, flu-like symptoms, appetite loss, and yellowing of the skin or whites of the eyes).

Check with your doctor about continuing carvedilol if you are to receive **general anesthesia**; heart function that is depressed by anesthetics can worsen if carvedilol is used at the same time.

Carvedilol can mask signs of **low blood sugar** and may increase the effects of insulin or oral antidiabetes drugs, making it more difficult to recover from the effects of low blood sugar.

Carvedilol can mask symptoms of an **overactive thyroid gland.** Abruptly stopping carvedilol can trigger an attack of hyperthyroidism.

Possible Side Effects

Most side effects are considered mild or moderate.

▼ Most common: dizziness, sleepiness or sleeplessness, diarrhea, abdominal pain, slow heartbeat, dizziness when rising from a sitting or lying position, swelling of the hands or feet, sore throat, breathing difficulties, tiredness, back pain, urinary infection, viral infection, high blood-triglyceride levels, and low blood-platelet counts.

▼ Less common: extra heartbeats; palpitations; blood-pressure changes; fainting; reduced blood supply to the arms and legs (symptoms include aches, cramps, pain, or tiredness on walking, or pain in the foot, thigh, hip, or buttocks); tingling in the hands or feet; reduced sensation; depression; nervousness; constipation; gas; liver irritation; cough; impotence and reduced sex drive in men; itching; rash; visual difficulties; ringing or buzzing in the ears; high blood cholesterol, sugar, or uric acid; anemia; weakness; hot flushes; leg cramps; dry mouth; not feeling well; sweating; and muscle ache.

▼ Rare: Rare side effects can affect the heart, mental status, the respiratory tract, the urinary tract, and the kidney. It can also cause hair loss, weight gain, and sugar in the urine.

Drug Interactions

• Carvedilol increases the effects of insulin and oral antidiabetes drugs. People taking this combination must monitor their blood sugar levels regularly. Call your doctor if there is any change from your normal pattern.

• Carvedilol increases the effects of verapamil, diltiazem, and similar calcium-channel blocking drugs.

• Carvedilol increases the blood-pressure-lowering effect of clonidine. People taking this combination may need less clonidine to control their pressure.

• Carvedilol increases the amount of digoxin in the blood by about 15%. Your digoxin dosage may have to be adjusted.

• Cimetidine increases the amount of carvedilol absorbed into the blood by about 30%, but the importance of this interaction is not clear.

• Rifampin reduces the amount of carvedilol in the blood by about 70%. Dosage adjustment is necessary.

Food Interactions

Take carvedilol with food to reduce the risk of dizziness or fainting.

Usual Dose

Heart Failure
  Adult: 3.125 mg 2 times a day for 2 weeks. Dose may be doubled every 2 weeks to the highest level tolerated. Maximum daily dosage is 25 mg 2 times a day in people weighing less than 187 lbs., and 50 mg twice a day in people who weigh more.

High Blood Pressure and Cardiomyopathy
  Adult: 6.25 mg twice a day to start, increased to 25 mg twice a day if needed.
  Senior: Seniors may require smaller doses than younger adults.
  Child: not recommended.

Overdosage

Overdose may lead to very low blood pressure (symptoms include dizziness and fainting), slow heartbeat and other cardiac symptoms including shock and heart attack, breathing difficulties, bronchial spasm, vomiting, periods of unconsciousness, and seizures. Overdose victims must be taken to a hospital emergency room. ALWAYS bring the prescription bottle or container.

Special Information

Carvedilol should be taken continuously. Do not stop taking it without your doctor's knowledge, because abrupt withdrawal may cause chest pain, breathing difficulties, increased sweating, and unusually fast or irregular heartbeat. The dose should be gradually reduced over a period of about 2 weeks.

People taking carvedilol may become dizzy or faint when rising quickly from a sitting or lying position. If this happens to you, sit or lie down until you feel better. Carvedilol can also cause drowsiness, light-headedness, or blurred vision. Be careful when driving or doing any task that requires concentration.

Contact lens wearers are more likely to experience dry eyes with carvedilol.

It is best to take carvedilol at the same time each day. If you forget a dose, take it as soon as you remember. If it is within 4 hours of your next dose, skip the dose you forgot and continue with your regular schedule. Do not take a double dose.

Special Populations

Pregnancy/Breast-feeding

Animal studies indicate that carvedilol passes into the fetal bloodstream and may interfere with pregnancy. When this drug is considered crucial by your doctor, its potential benefits must be carefully weighed against its risks.

It is not known if carvedilol passes into human breast milk, though it passes into rat breast milk. Beta-blocking drugs like carvedilol may affect babies' hearts. Nursing mothers who must take this drug should bottle-feed.

Seniors

Seniors are more likely to develop side effects, especially dizziness, and may require reduced dosage.

Ceftin   *see Cephalosporin Antibiotics, page 178*

Cefzil   *see Cephalosporin Antibiotics, page 178*

Celebrex   *see Celecoxib, page 174*

Generic Name

Celecoxib (sel-EH-sox-ib)

Brand Name

Celebrex

Type of Drug

Cyclooxygenase-2 (COX-2) inhibitor NSAID (non-steroidal anti-inflammatory drug).

Prescribed for

Osteoarthritis and rheumatoid arthritis; familial adenomatous polyposis (FAP).

General Information

Traditional NSAIDs work primarily by blocking the effects of COX-2, a body enzyme that plays an important role in regulating pain and inflammation. But these NSAIDs also have an unwanted effect: They interfere with cyclooxygenase-1 (COX-1), a related enzyme that helps to maintain the stomach's protective lining. NSAIDs that block the effects of this enzyme may produce side effects such as stomach irritation, gas, and stomach ulcers.

COX-2 inhibitors, such as celecoxib are a new class of NSAIDs that work about as well as the older NSAIDs. In fact, both 200 mg a day and 400 mg a day of celecoxib work as well as naproxen 500 mg twice a day. They interfere only with COX-2, leaving the stomach-protecting COX-1 unaffected. This means that COX-2 inhibitor NSAIDs can relieve pain and inflammation just like traditional NSAIDs but are less likely to cause gastrointestinal (GI) side effects. Another advantage of celecoxib is that it does not cause thinning of the blood or affect blood platelets as can happen with older NSAIDs. Celecoxib is broken down in the liver. African Americans absorb about 40% more celecoxib than Caucasians. Celecoxib is the first drug proven effective in reducing the number of intestinal polyps in people with the rare genetic disorder FAP.

Cautions and Warnings

Do not take celecoxib if you are **sensitive** or **allergic** to it or to sulfa drugs. NSAIDs should not be taken by people with

asthma or **itchy sores** or by those who have had an **allergic reaction to aspirin**. They can develop a group of symptoms (runny nose with or without nasal polyps and a severe, potentially fatal bronchial spasm) known as the aspirin triad. People with these symptoms must seek emergency treatment at once.

Early studies indicate that 1 in 2,500 people who take celecoxib develop serious **stomach and intestinal problems**. By contrast, 1 in 100 people who take a traditional NSAID for 3 to 6 months and 2 to 4 of 100 people who take a traditional NSAID for 1 year develop upper GI ulcers, gross bleeding, or perforation.

NSAIDs can cause **GI bleeding and ulcers** and **stomach perforation**. This can occur at any time, with or without warning, in people who take NSAIDs regularly. Minor upper GI problems, such as upset stomach, are common and may occur at any time during NSAID therapy. People who develop bleeding or ulcers and continue NSAID treatment should be aware of the risk of developing more serious side effects.

Celecoxib should be used with caution by people who have had **ulcers,** or stomach or intestinal bleeding.

People with **kidney problems** usually have about 40% less celecoxib in their blood than normal. Celecoxib has not been studied in people with severe kidney disease. They should not use this drug unless their doctors closely monitor their kidney function.

Celecoxib can cause **liver irritation** and should be used with caution by people with **hepatitis** or **cirrhosis**.

People with moderate liver disease can have twice as much celecoxib in their blood and require a reduced dosage. The effect of celecoxib in people with severe liver failure is not known.

Possible Side Effects

Side effects are similar to those of traditional NSAIDs. Stomach and intestinal side effects are about half as common.

▼ Most common: headache.

▼ Common: diarrhea, upset stomach, sinus irritation, and respiratory infection.

Possible Side Effects *(continued)*

▼ Less common: abdominal pain, gas, nausea, back pain, swelling in the legs or arms, accidental injuries, sleeplessness, dizziness, sore throat, runny nose, and rash.

▼ Rare: Rare side effects can occur in almost any part of the body. Contact your doctor if you experience any side effect not listed above.

Drug Interactions

• Combining celecoxib with an aluminum and magnesium antacid slightly reduces the amount of drug absorbed. Separate doses of these antacids and celecoxib by 1 to 2 hours.

• Fluconazole and lithium may raise celecoxib blood levels and increase the risk of side effects.

• While celecoxib may be combined with low dosages of aspirin, taking these drugs together can increase the risk of stomach or intestinal ulcers or other complications. The ulcer risk associated with this combination is less than that posed by single-drug therapy with a traditional NSAID.

• Celecoxib can reduce the blood-pressure-lowering effect of angiotensin-converting enzyme (ACE) inhibitors and diuretic drugs. This combination can also increase the risk of kidney damage after chronic celecoxib use.

Food Interactions

Celecoxib can be taken without regard to food or meals. For optimal effectiveness, avoid taking this drug with high-fat meals.

Usual Dose

Adult (age 18 and over): 100–200 mg twice a day.
Child (under age 18): not recommended.

Overdosage

Symptoms include lethargy, drowsiness, nausea, vomiting, and stomach pain. Stomach or intestinal bleeding or severe allergic reactions can occur. High blood pressure, kidney failure, breathing difficulties, and coma are rare. You may be asked to make the victim vomit with syrup of Ipecac—available at any pharmacy—to remove any remaining medication from the stomach. The victim should be taken to a hospital emergency room. ALWAYS bring the prescription bottle or container.

Special Information

Call your doctor if you develop rash, itching, unexplained weight gain, nausea, fatigue, yellowing of the skin or whites of the eyes, flu-like symptoms, lethargy, swelling, black stools, severe stomach pain, persistent headache, or any bothersome or persistent side effect.

If you forget a dose and remember within 1 or 2 hours of your scheduled time, take it right away. If you do not remember until later, skip the forgotten dose and continue with your regular schedule.

Special Populations

Pregnancy/Breast-feeding
Celecoxib has caused birth defects in animal studies. Any NSAID may affect fetal heart development during the second half of pregnancy. Pregnant women should not take celecoxib without their doctor's approval. When this drug is considered crucial by your doctor, its potential benefits must be carefully weighed against its risks.

NSAIDs may pass into breast milk. There is a possibility that a nursing mother taking celecoxib could affect her baby's heart or cardiovascular system. Nursing mothers who must take this drug should bottle-feed.

Seniors
Generally, seniors can take this drug without special precaution. Those who weigh less than 110 lbs. should begin with the lowest possible dosage.

Celexa *see Citalopram, page 213*

Type of Drug

Cephalosporin Antibiotics

(CEF-uh-loe-SPOR-in)

Brand Names

Generic Ingredient: Cefaclor G
Ceclor   Ceclor Pulvules
Ceclor CD

Generic Ingredient: Cefadroxil G
Duricef

Generic Ingredient: Cefdinir
Omnicef

Generic Ingredient: Cefixime
Suprax

Generic Ingredient: Cefpodoxime Proxetil
Vantin

Generic Ingredient: Cefprozil
Cefzil

Generic Ingredient: Ceftibuten
Cedax

Generic Ingredient: Cefuroxime Axetil
Ceftin

Generic Ingredient: Cephalexin G
Keflex

Generic Ingredient: Cephalexin Hydrochloride
Keftab

Generic Ingredient: Cephradine G
Velosef

Generic Ingredient: Loracarbef
Lorabid

Prescribed for

Bacterial infections.

General Information

These antibiotics are related to cephalosporin C, which is similar to penicillin and is isolated from the *Cephalosporium acremonium* fungus. Of the more than 20 different antibiotic drugs derived from cephalosporin C, only those that are taken by mouth are included in *The Pill Book.* Injectable drugs are not discussed. Most common infections can be treated with these antibiotics, but they are not interchangeable. Your doctor must select the appropriate antibiotic for a particular infection.

Cautions and Warnings

Up to 15% of people **allergic** to penicillin may also be allergic to cephalosporins. The most common cephalosporin allergic reaction is a hive-like condition with redness over large areas of the body. Other sensitivity reactions include rash, fever, and joint aches or pain. Such reactions generally begin after a few days of taking the antibiotic and resolve within a few days after the antibiotic is stopped.

Prolonged or repeated use of a cephalosporin may lead to a **secondary infection** not susceptible to the antibiotic.

Occasionally, people taking a cephalosporin develop **colitis**. Call your doctor if you develop severe diarrhea while taking one of these drugs.

People with **poor kidney function** may require less medicine to treat their infections. Rarely, people taking a cephalosporin have had a **seizure,** especially those with kidney disease where the dose was not reduced.

Some injectable cephalosporins have caused **blood-clotting problems**. This has not occurred in people taking an oral drug.

Rarely, severe **anemia** occurs in people taking cephalosporin antibiotics. Report any signs of anemia (such as pale skin color, weakness, tiredness, difficulty breathing, and abnormal heart rhythms) to your doctor.

Cefprozil oral suspension contains phenylalanine and cannot be taken by people with **phenylketonuria (PKU disease)**.

Possible Side Effects

Most side effects are mild.

▼ Most common: abdominal pain and gas, upset stomach, nausea, vomiting, diarrhea, itching, and rash.

Possible Side Effects *(continued)*

▼ Less common: headache, dizziness, tiredness, tingling in the hands or feet, seizure, confusion, drug allergy, fever, joint pain, chest tightness, redness, muscle aches and swelling, appetite loss, and changes in taste perception. Colitis may develop.

Cefaclor may cause serum sickness (symptoms include fever, joint pain, and rash).

Cephalosporins may cause changes in blood cells, kidney problems, liver inflammation, and jaundice, but these side effects are rarely a problem with oral cephalosporins.

Drug Interactions

• Antacids can reduce the amounts of cefaclor, cefdinir, and cefpodoxime in the blood. Do not take antacids within 2 hours of these antibiotics

• Cimetidine, famotidine, ranitidine, or nizatidine can reduce the effectiveness of cefpodoxime and cefuroxime—do not combine these drugs.

• Iron and iron-fortified foods may interfere with the absorption of cefdinir. Separate your iron dose from the antibiotic by at least 2 hours. Iron-fortified infant formula does not produce this effect.

• Probenecid may increase blood levels of some cephalosporins.

• Potent (loop-type) diuretics can lead to kidney damage if mixed with a cephalosporin antibiotic.

• Cephalosporins may cause a false-positive test result for sugar in the urine with Clinitest tablets or similar products. They do not affect Clinistix or Tes-Tape.

• Cefuroxime may cause a false-positive test result for blood sugar.

• Drinking alcohol with or within 72 hours of some injectable cephalosporins can lead to a severe reaction. This reaction has not occurred with oral cephalosporins.

• Mixing warfarin with some injectable cephalosporins can lead to unexpected bleeding. This reaction has not occurred with oral cephalosporins.

Food Interactions

Generally, cephalosporins may be taken with food or milk if they upset your stomach. Food increases the absorption of cefpodoxime and cefuroxime.

Usual Dose

Cefaclor
   Adult: 250 mg every 8 hours, or 375–500 mg every 12 hours.
   Child: 9 mg per lb. of body weight a day, in 2–3 equal doses.

Cefadroxil
   Adult: 1–2 g a day, in 1–2 doses.
   Child: 13 mg per lb. of body weight a day, in 1–2 doses.

Cefdinir
   Adult and Child (age 13 and over): 300 to 600 mg a day.
   Child: 3–6½ mg per lb. of body weight per day for 5–10 days.

Cefixime
   Adult: 400 mg a day, in 1–2 doses.
   Child: 3.5 mg per lb. of body weight a day, in 1–2 doses.

Cefpodoxime Proxetil
   Adult and Child (age 13 and over): 200–400 mg a day, in 1–2 doses.
   Child (age 5 months–12 years): 2.5–5 mg per lb. of body weight a day. Maximum daily dose for middle-ear infections is 400 mg; 200 mg for sore throat or tonsillitis.

Cefprozil
   Adult: 250–1000 mg a day.
   Child (age 6 months–12 years): 13 mg per lb. of body weight every 12 hours.

Ceftibuten
   Adult and Child (age 12 and over): 400 mg once a day for 10 days.
   Child: 4 mg per lb. of body weight, up to 400 mg, once a day for 10 days.

Cefuroxime
   Adult and Child (age 12 and over): 125–500 mg every 12 hours.
   Child (under age 12): 125–250 mg every 12 hours.

Cephalexin
    Adult: 250–1000 mg every 6 hours. Some urinary infections may be treated with 500 mg every 12 hours.
    Child: 11–23 mg per lb. of body weight a day. The dose may be increased to 46 mg per lb. of body weight for middle-ear infections.

Cephradine
    Adult: 250–500 mg every 6–12 hours.
    Child (age 9 months and over): 11–45 mg per lb. of body weight a day, in 2–4 doses.

Loracarbef
    Adult and Child (age 13 and over): 200–400 mg every 12 hours.
    Child (age 6 months–12 years): 6.5–13 mg per lb. of body weight a day.

Overdosage

Common symptoms of overdose are nausea, vomiting, and upset stomach. These can often be treated with milk or antacid. Cephalosporin overdoses are generally not serious; contact a hospital emergency room or local poison control center for more information.

Special Information

You must take the full course of treatment prescribed—even if you feel better in 2 or 3 days—to obtain the maximum benefit from any antibiotic.

Proper diagnosis is key to the effectiveness of an antibiotic: Do not take any antibiotic without consulting your doctor.

If you miss a dose that you take once a day, take it as soon as you remember. If it is almost time for your next dose, take the dose you forgot right away and your next one 10 to 12 hours later. Then go back to your regular schedule. If you take the medication 2 times a day, take the dose you forgot right away and the next dose 5 to 6 hours later. Then go back to your regular schedule. If you take the medication 3 or more times a day, take the dose you missed right away and your next dose 2 to 4 hours later. Then go back to your regular schedule.

Diabetics taking cephradine should not change their diet or diabetes medication without consulting their doctor.

Most cephalosporin liquids must be kept in the refrigerator to maintain their strength. Only cefixime liquid does not require refrigeration. All of the liquid cephalosporins have a very limited shelf life. Do not keep any of these liquids beyond the 10 days to 2 weeks specified on the label. Follow your pharmacist's storage instructions.

Special Populations

Pregnancy/Breast-feeding
These drugs are considered relatively safe during pregnancy, though small amounts pass into the fetus. Little information is available about the newer members of the group. Also, cephalosporins pass more quickly out of the bodies of pregnant women. Cephalosporins should be taken during pregnancy only if the benefit outweighs the risk.

Small amounts of most cephalosporin antibiotics pass into breast milk. Nursing mothers who must take a cephalosporin should bottle-feed.

Seniors
Seniors may require a lower dosage because of reduced kidney function.

Generic Name

Cetirizine (seh-TERE-ih-zene)

Brand Name

Zyrtec

The information in this profile also applies to the following drug:

Generic Ingredient: Fexofenadine
Allegra

Type of Drug

Antihistamine.

Prescribed for

Cetirizine: stuffy and runny nose, itchy eyes, and scratchy throat caused by seasonal and year-round allergy, and for other symptoms of allergy such as rash, itching, and hives; also prescribed for chronic itching and for asthma. Fexofenadine:

sneezing, stuffy and runny nose, scratchy throat and mouth, and itchy, watery, and red eyes caused by seasonal allergies.

General Information

Antihistamines generally work by blocking the release of histamine (a chemical released by body tissue during an allergic reaction) from the cell at the H_1 histamine receptor site, drying up secretions of the nose, throat, and eyes. Cetirizine causes less sedation than older antihistamines and appears to be just as effective.

Cautions and Warnings

Do not take cetirizine if you are **allergic** or **sensitive** to it.

People with **kidney disease** should receive reduced dosage of cetirizine.

Possible Side Effects

Occasional side effects include headache, nervousness, weakness, upset stomach, nausea, vomiting, sore throat, nosebleeds, cough, stuffy nose, changes in bowel habits, and dry mouth, nose, or throat.

Drug Interactions

Cetirizine is less likely than other antihistamines to interact with drugs.

Food Interactions

Take cetirizine on an empty stomach, 1 hour before or 2 hours after meals; it may be taken with food or milk if it upsets your stomach.

Usual Dose

Cetirizine
  Adult (age 12 and over): 5–10 mg once a day. Reduced dosage is necessary in people with kidney disease.
    Child (age 6–11): 10 mg a day.
    Child (age 2–5): 5 mg a day.

Fexofenadine
  Adult (age 12 and over): 60 mg twice a day. People with kidney disease should take 60 mg a day.
    Child: not recommended.

Overdosage

Drug overdose is likely to cause severe side effects. Overdose victims should be given ipecac syrup—available at any pharmacy—to make them vomit and be taken to a hospital emergency room. ALWAYS bring the prescription bottle or container.

Special Information

Report sore throat, unusual bleeding, bruising, tiredness, weakness, or any other unusual side effect to your doctor. Do not combine this drug with alcohol or other nervous system depressants.

If you forget to take a dose of cetirizine, take it as soon as you remember. If it is almost time for your next dose, skip the one you forgot and continue with your regular schedule. Do not take a double dose.

Special Populations

Pregnancy/Breast-feeding

Antihistamines are generally considered safe for use during pregnancy. But, do not take any antihistamine without your doctor's knowledge if you are or might become pregnant—especially during the last 3 months of pregnancy, because newborns may have severe reactions to antihistamines.

Small amounts of antihistamine pass into breast milk. Nursing mothers who must take cetirizine should bottle-feed.

Seniors

Seniors may take cetirizine without special precaution.

Generic Name

Chlordiazepoxide (klor-dye-az-uh-POX-ide) Ⓖ

Brand Names

Libritabs   Librium

Type of Drug

Benzodiazepine tranquilizer.

Prescribed for

Anxiety, tension, fatigue, and agitation; also prescribed for irritable bowel syndrome and panic attacks.

General Information

Chlordiazepoxide is a member of the group of drugs known as benzodiazepines.

Benzodiazepines work by a direct effect on the brain. They can relax you and make you more tranquil or sleepier, or they can slow nervous system transmissions in such a way as to act as an anticonvulsant. Many doctors prefer benzodiazepines to other drugs that can be used to similar effect because they tend to be safer, have fewer side effects, and are usually as effective, if not more so.

Cautions and Warnings

Do not take chlordiazepoxide if you know you are **sensitive** or **allergic** to it or another member of the group, including clonazepam.

Chlordiazepoxide can aggravate narrow-angle **glaucoma,** but you may take it if you have open-angle glaucoma.

Other conditions in which chlordiazepoxide should be avoided are severe **depression,** severe **lung disease, sleep apnea** (intermittent cessation of breathing during sleep), **liver disease, drunkenness,** and **kidney disease.** In each of these conditions, the depressive effects of chlordiazepoxide may be enhanced or could be detrimental to your overall situation.

Chlordiazepoxide should not be taken by **psychotic patients** because it is not effective for them and can trigger unusual excitement, stimulation, and rage.

Chlordiazepoxide is not intended for more than 3 to 4 months of continuous use. Your condition should be reassessed before continuing chlordiazepoxide beyond that time.

Chlordiazepoxide may be **addictive**. Drug withdrawal may develop if you stop taking it after only 4 weeks of regular use, but is more likely after longer use. It may start with anxiety and progress to tingling in the hands or feet, sensitivity to bright light, sleep disturbances, cramps, tremors, muscle tension or twitching, poor concentration, flu symptoms, fatigue, appetite loss, sweating, and changes in mental state.

Possible Side Effects

Weakness and confusion may occur, especially in seniors and in those who are sickly.

▼ Most common: mild drowsiness during the first few days of therapy.

▼ Less common: depression, lethargy, disorientation, headache, inactivity, slurred speech, stupor, dizziness, tremor, constipation, dry mouth, nausea, inability to control urination, sexual difficulties, irregular menstrual cycle, changes in heart rhythm, low blood pressure, fluid retention, blurred or double vision, itching, rash, hiccups, nervousness, inability to fall asleep, and occasional liver dysfunction. If you experience any of these symptoms, stop taking the medicine and contact your doctor immediately.

▼ Rare: Rare side effects can occur in almost any part of the body. Contact your doctor if you experience any side effect not listed above.

Drug Interactions

• Chlordiazepoxide is a central-nervous-system depressant. Avoid alcohol, other tranquilizers, narcotics, barbiturates, monoamine oxidase inhibitors (MAOIs), antihistamines, and antidepressants. Taking chlordiazepoxide with these drugs may result in excessive depression, tiredness, sleepiness, breathing difficulties, or related symptoms.

• Smoking may reduce the effectiveness of chlordiazepoxide by increasing the rate at which it is broken down by the body.

• The effects of chlordiazepoxide may be prolonged when it is taken with cimetidine, oral contraceptives, disulfiram, fluoxetine, isoniazid, ketoconazole, metoprolol, probenecid, propoxyphene, propranolol, rifampin, or valproic acid.

• Theophylline may reduce chlordiazepoxide's sedative effects.

• If you take antacids, separate them by at least 1 hour from your chlordiazepoxide dose to prevent them from interfering with the passage of chlordiazepoxide into the bloodstream.

• Chlordiazepoxide may increase blood levels of digoxin and the chances for digoxin toxicity.

• Levodopa's effectiveness may be reduced by chlordiazepoxide.

• Phenytoin blood concentrations may be increased when taken with chlordiazepoxide, resulting in possible phenytoin toxicity.

Food Interactions

Chlordiazepoxide is best taken on an empty stomach but may be taken with food if it upsets your stomach.

Usual Dose

Adult: 5–100 mg a day. This range is due to individual response related to age, weight, disease severity, and other characteristics.

Child (age 6 and over): may be given if deemed appropriate by a doctor. Starting dose—5 mg 2–4 times a day. Maintenance dose—up to 30–40 mg a day for some children, but must be individualized to obtain maximum benefit.

Child (under age 6): not recommended.

Overdosage

Symptoms of overdose are confusion, sleepiness, poor coordination, lack of response to pain such as a pin prick, loss of reflexes, shallow breathing, low blood pressure, and coma. The victim should be taken to a hospital emergency room. ALWAYS bring the prescription bottle or container.

Special Information

Chlordiazepoxide can cause tiredness, drowsiness, inability to concentrate, or similar symptoms. Be careful if you are driving, operating machinery, or performing other activities that require concentration.

If you forget a dose of chlordiazepoxide, take it as soon as you remember. If it is almost time for your next dose, skip the dose you forgot and continue with your regular schedule. Do not take a double dose.

Special Populations

Pregnancy/Breast-feeding

Chlordiazepoxide may cause birth defects if taken during the first 3 months of pregnancy. Avoid chlordiazepoxide while pregnant.

Chlordiazepoxide may pass into breast milk. Nursing mothers who must take chlordiazepoxide should bottle-feed.

Seniors

Seniors, especially those with liver or kidney disease, are more sensitive to the effects of chlordiazepoxide and generally require smaller doses to achieve the same effect.

Generic Name

Chlorpheniramine Maleate

(KLOR-fen-ERE-uh-mene MAL-ee-ate) G

Brand Names

Chlorpheniramine E.R.   Pro-Hist-8
Chlor-Phen

The information in this profile also applies to the following drugs:

Generic Ingredient: Azatadine Maleate
Optimine

Generic Ingredient: Brompheniramine Maleate G
Colhist   ND-Stat
Nasahist B

Generic Ingredient: Cyproheptadine Hydrochloride G
Periactin

Generic Ingredient: Dexchlorpheniramine Maleate G
Polaramine   Polarmine Repetabs

Generic Ingredient: Tripelennamine Hydrochloride G
PBZ   PBZ-SR

Type of Drug

Antihistamine.

Prescribed for

Stuffy and runny nose, itchy eyes, and scratchy throat caused by seasonal allergy, and other symptoms of allergy such as rash, itching, and hives.

General Information

Antihistamines generally work by blocking the release of histamine (a chemical released by body tissue during an allergic reaction) from body cells at the H_1 histamine receptor site, drying up secretions of the nose, throat, and eyes.

Cautions and Warnings

Do not use this drug if you are **allergic** to it.

Use chlorpheniramine maleate with care if you have a history of **thyroid disease, heart disease, high blood pressure,** or **diabetes**. This drug should be avoided or used with extreme care if you have narrow-angle **glaucoma, stomach ulcer** or other **stomach problems, enlarged prostate,** or **problems passing urine**. It should not be used by people who have **deep-breathing problems** such as asthma.

Possible Side Effects

▼ Less common: rash or itching, sensitivity to bright light, increased sweating, chills, lowered blood pressure, headache, rapid heartbeat, sleeplessness, dizziness, disturbed coordination, confusion, restlessness, nervousness, irritability, euphoria (feeling "high"), tingling in the hands or feet, blurred or double vision, ringing in the ears, upset stomach, appetite loss, nausea, vomiting, constipation, diarrhea, urinary difficulties, chest tightness, wheezing, stuffy nose, and dryness of the mouth, nose, or throat. Young children may also develop nervousness, irritability, tension, and anxiety.

Drug Interactions

• Chlorpheniramine maleate should not be taken with a monoamine oxidase inhibitor (MAOI) antidepressant, because the combination may cause severe side effects.

• The effects of tranquilizers, benzodiazepines, sedatives, and sleeping medications will be increased when any of these drugs is combined with chlorpheniramine maleate. It is extremely important for your doctor to know if you are taking any other medication with chlorpheniramine maleate so that the dosage of that medication can be properly adjusted.

• Be extremely cautious when drinking alcoholic beverages while taking this drug, which enhances the intoxicating and sedating effects of alcohol.

Food Interactions

You may take this drug with food if it upsets your stomach.

Usual Dose

Azatadine
1–2 mg twice a day.

Brompheniramine
 Adult and Child (age 13 and over): 4 mg 3–4 times a day.
 Child (age 6–12): 2–4 mg 3–4 times a day; do not take more than 12 mg a day.
 Child (under age 6): 0.25 mg per lb. of body weight a day, in divided doses.

Chlorpheniramine
 Adult and Child (age 13 and over): 4-mg tablet every 4–6 hours; do not take more than 24 mg a day.
 Child (age 6–12): 2-mg tablet every 4–6 hours; do not take more than 8 mg a day.
 Child (age 2–5): 1 mg every 4–6 hours; do not take more than 4 mg a day.

Chlorpheniramine, Sustained-Release
 Adult and Child (age 13 and over): 8–12 mg at bedtime, or every 8–12 hours during the day.
 Child (age 6–12): 8 mg during the day or at bedtime.
 Child (under age 6): not recommended.

Cyproheptadine
 Adult and Child (age 15 and over): do not exceed 32 mg a day.
 Child (age 7–14): 4 mg 2–3 times a day; do not exceed 16 mg a day.
 Child (age 2–6): 2 mg 2–3 times a day; do not exceed 12 mg a day.

Dexchlorpheniramine
 Adult and Child (age 12 and over): 2 mg every 4–6 hours.
 Child (age 6–11): 1 mg every 4–6 hours.
 Child (age 2–5): 0.5 mg every 4–6 hours.

Dexchlorpheniramine, Sustained-Release

   Adult and Child (age 12 and over): 4–6 mg every 8–10 hours and at bedtime.

   Child (age 6–11): 4 mg once a day and at bedtime.

   Child (under age 6): not recommended.

Tripelennamine

   Adult and Child (age 12 and over): 25–50 mg every 4–6 hours; do not take more than 600 mg a day. Adults may take up to 3 100-mg, sustained-release tablets a day, although this much is not usually needed.

   Child (under age 12): 2 mg per lb. of body weight a day in divided doses; no more than 300 mg should be given a day.

Overdosage

Symptoms of overdose include depression or stimulation, especially in children; dry mouth; fixed or dilated pupils; flushing of the skin; and upset stomach. Overdose victims should be made to vomit as soon as possible with ipecac syrup—available at any pharmacy—to remove excess drug from the stomach. Take the victim to a hospital emergency room immediately if the victim is unconscious or if you cannot induce vomiting. ALWAYS bring the prescription bottle or container.

Special Information

This drug may cause tiredness or loss of concentration: Be extremely cautious when driving or doing anything that requires close attention.

   If you forget a dose of this drug, take it as soon as you remember. If it is almost time for your next dose, skip the one you forgot and continue with your regular schedule. Do not take a double dose.

Special Populations

Pregnancy/Breast-feeding

Animal studies have shown that some antihistamines may cause birth defects. Do not take any antihistamine without your doctor's knowledge if you are or might be pregnant—especially during the last 3 months of pregnancy, because newborns may have severe reactions to antihistamines.

Small amounts of some antihistamines pass into breast milk. Nursing mothers who must take chlorpheniramine maleate should bottle-feed.

Seniors
Seniors are more sensitive to antihistamine side effects.

Generic Name

Chlorpromazine (klor-PROE-muh-zene) Ⓖ

Brand Name

Thorazine*

The information in this profile also applies to the following drugs:

Generic Ingredient: Fluphenazine Hydrochloride Ⓖ
Permitil   Prolixin

Generic Ingredient: Mesoridazine Besylate
Serentil Ⓢ

Generic Ingredient: Thioridazine Hydrochloride Ⓖ
Mellaril   Mellaril-S

Generic Ingredient: Trifluoperazine Hydrochloride Ⓖ
Stelazine

Some products in this brand-name group are alcohol- or sugar-free. Consult your pharmacist.

Type of Drug

Phenothiazine antipsychotic.

Prescribed for

Psychotic disorders, moderate to severe depression with anxiety, agitation or aggressiveness in disturbed children, alcohol withdrawal, intractable pain, and senility; may also be used to relieve nausea, vomiting, hiccups, restlessness, and apprehension before surgery or other procedures.

General Information

Chlorpromazine and other phenothiazines act upon a portion of the brain called the hypothalamus. Phenothiazines affect parts of the hypothalamus that control metabolism, body temperature, alertness, muscle tone, hormone balance, and vomiting. Chlorpromazine is available in suppositories and as liquid for those who have trouble swallowing tablets.

Cautions and Warnings

Chlorpromazine may depress the **cough reflex**. People have accidentally choked to death because the cough reflex failed to protect them. Because of its effect in reducing vomiting, chlorpromazine may obscure symptoms of disease or toxicity due to overdose of another drug.

Do not take chlorpromazine if you are **allergic** to it or any phenothiazine drug. Do not take it if you have very **low blood pressure, Parkinson's disease,** or **blood, liver, kidney, or heart disease**.

Use chlorpromazine under your doctor's strict supervision if you have **glaucoma, epilepsy, ulcers,** or **urinary difficulties**.

Avoid exposure to **extreme heat,** because this drug may upset your body's temperature-control mechanism. Do not allow the liquid forms of this drug to come in contact with your skin, because they are highly irritating.

Possible Side Effects

▼ Most common: drowsiness, especially during the first or second week of therapy. If drowsiness becomes troublesome, contact your doctor.

▼ Less common: changes in blood components including anemias, raised or lowered blood pressure, abnormal heart rate, heart attack, and faintness or dizziness.

▼ Rare: Rare side effects can occur in almost any part of the body. Contact your doctor if you experience any side effect not listed in this section.

Jaundice (symptoms include yellowing of the whites of the eyes or skin) may appear; when it does it is usually within the first 2 to 4 weeks of treatment. Normally it goes away when the drug is discontinued, but there have been cases when it has not.

Possible Side Effects *(continued)*

Phenothiazines may produce extrapyramidal side effects, including spasm of the neck muscles, rolling back of the eyes, convulsions, difficulty swallowing, and symptoms associated with Parkinson's disease. These side effects seem very serious but usually disappear after the drug has been withdrawn; however, symptoms affecting the face, tongue, or jaw may persist for as long as several years, especially in older adults with a history of brain damage.

Chlorpromazine may cause an unusual increase in psychotic symptoms or may cause paranoid reactions, tiredness, lethargy, restlessness, hyperactivity, confusion at night, bizarre dreams, sleeplessness, depression, and euphoria (feeling high).

Drug Interactions

• Be cautious about taking chlorpromazine with barbiturates, alcohol, sleeping pills, narcotics or other tranquilizers, or any other drug that may produce a depressive effect.

• Aluminum antacids may reduce the effectiveness of phenothiazine drugs.

• Chlorpromazine may reduce the effectiveness of bromocriptine and appetite suppressants.

• Anticholinergic drugs may reduce the effectiveness of chlorpromazine and increase the chance of side effects.

• Phenothiazine drugs may counter the blood-pressure-lowering effect of guanethidine.

• Taking lithium together with a phenothiazine drug may lead to disorientation, loss of consciousness, or uncontrolled muscle movements.

• Combining propranolol and a phenothiazine drug may lead to unusually low blood pressure.

• Combining tricyclic antidepressants with a phenothiazine drug can lead to antidepressant side effects.

Food Interactions

Take liquid chlorpromazine with fruit juice or other liquids, you may also take it with food if it upsets your stomach.

Usual Dose

Adult: 30–1000 mg or more a day, individualized according to your disease and response.

Child (age 6 months and over): 0.25 mg per lb. of body weight every 4–6 hours, up to 200 mg or more a day, depending on disease, age, and response.

Overdosage

Overdose symptoms include depression, extreme weakness, tiredness, lowered blood pressure, agitation, restlessness, uncontrolled muscle spasms, convulsions, fever, dry mouth, abnormal heart rhythms, and coma. The victim should be taken to a hospital emergency room immediately. ALWAYS bring the prescription bottle or container.

Special Information

Call your doctor at once if you develop sore throat, fever, rash, weakness, visual problems, tremors, muscle movements or twitching, yellowing of the skin or whites of the eyes, or darkening of the urine.

This drug may cause drowsiness. Use caution when driving or operating hazardous equipment. Avoid alcoholic beverages.

Chlorpromazine may cause unusual sensitivity to the sun and may turn your urine reddish-brown to pink.

If dizziness occurs, avoid rising quickly from a sitting or lying position and avoid climbing stairs. Use caution in hot weather, because this drug may make you more prone to heat stroke.

If you are using sustained-release capsules, do not chew them or break them: Swallow them whole. Liquid forms of phenothiazines must be protected from light. Do not take them out of their opaque bottles.

If you take chlorpromazine more than once a day and forget to take a dose, take it right away if you remember within an hour. If you do not remember within an hour, skip the dose you forgot and continue with your regular schedule. If you take 1 dose a day and forget a dose, skip the dose you forgot and continue your regular schedule the next day. Never take a double dose.

Special Populations

Pregnancy/Breast-feeding

Infants born to women taking this drug have experienced side effects—including jaundice and nervous system effects.

Check with your doctor about taking chlorpromazine if you are or might be pregnant.

This drug may pass into breast milk. Consider bottle-feeding if you must take chlorpromazine.

Seniors

Seniors are more sensitive to the effects of this drug and usually achieve desired results with lower dosages. Some experts feel that seniors should receive ½ to ¼ the usual adult dose.

Generic Name

Chlorzoxazone (klor-ZOX-uh-zone) Ⓖ

Brand Names

Paraflex   Remular-S
Parafon Forte DSC

Type of Drug

Skeletal muscle relaxant.

Prescribed for

Pain and spasm of muscular conditions, including strain, sprain, bruising, and lower back problems.

General Information

Chlorzoxazone works primarily on the spinal cord level and on the brain, acting as a mild sedative. This results in fewer spasms, less pain, and greater mobility. Chlorzoxazone provides only temporary relief and is not a substitute for other types of therapy, such as rest, surgery, and physical therapy.

Cautions and Warnings

Do not take chlorzoxazone if you are **allergic** to it or if you have a condition known as **porphyria**.

People with **poor liver or kidney function** should take this drug with caution because it is broken down by the liver and passes out of the body in the urine.

Chlorzoxazone may worsen **depression** or interact with other drugs that cause nervous system depression (see "Drug Interactions").

Because it is possible to become **dependent** on this drug, people with a history of substance abuse should take chlorzoxazone with caution.

Possible Side Effects

▼ Most common: dizziness, drowsiness, and light-headedness.

▼ Less common: headache, stimulation, stomach cramps or pain, diarrhea, constipation, heartburn, nausea, and vomiting.

▼ Rare: internal bleeding, liver problems, severe allergic reactions and breathing problems. Contact your doctor if you experience any unlisted side effect.

Drug Interactions

• The depressive effects of chlorzoxazone may be enhanced by taking it with alcohol, tranquilizers, sleeping pills, or other nervous system depressants. Avoid these combinations.

Food Interactions

Take this drug with food if it upsets your stomach. The tablets may be crushed and mixed with food.

Usual Dose

Adult: 250–750 mg 3–4 times a day.
Child: 125–500 mg 3–4 times a day.

Do not take more medication than is prescribed.

Overdosage

Early signs of chlorzoxazone overdose may include nausea, vomiting, diarrhea, drowsiness, dizziness, light-headedness, and headache. Victims may also feel sluggish or sickly and lose the ability to move their muscles. Breathing may become slow or irregular, and blood pressure may drop. Contact a doctor immediately or go to a hospital emergency room for treatment. ALWAYS bring the prescription bottle or container.

Special Information

Chlorzoxazone may make you drowsy or reduce your ability to concentrate. Be extremely careful while driving or operating hazardous equipment. Avoid alcoholic beverages.

Chlorzoxazone may turn your urine orange to purple-red; this is not dangerous.

Call your doctor if you develop drowsiness, weakness, an allergic reaction, breathing difficulties, black or tarry stools, vomiting of material that resembles coffee grounds, liver problems, or any other severe or bothersome side effect.

If you miss a dose of chlorzoxazone by more than an hour, skip the dose you forgot and continue with your regular schedule. Do not take a double dose.

Special Populations

Pregnancy / Breast-feeding

As with all drugs, chlorzoxazone should not be used by pregnant women and women who might become pregnant without their doctor's approval.

It is not known if chlorzoxazone passes into breast milk. Nursing mothers should consider bottle-feeding.

Seniors

Seniors, especially those with severe liver disease, are more sensitive to the effects of chlorzoxazone.

Generic Name

Cholestyramine (kol-es-TYE-rah-meen) G

Brand Names

LoCHOLEST Prevalite   Questran
LoCHOLEST Light   Questran Light

The information in this profile also applies to the following drug:

Generic Ingredient: Colestipol
Colestid

Type of Drug

Anti-hyperlipidemic (blood-fat reducer).

Prescribed for

High blood-cholesterol levels; generalized itching associated with bile duct obstruction—cholestyramine only; colitis; digitalis or thyroid overdose; and pesticide poisoning.

General Information

Cholestyramine resin lowers blood-cholesterol levels by absorbing bile acids in the bowel. Since the body uses cholesterol to make the bile acids—needed to digest fat—fat digestion can only continue by making more bile acid from blood cholesterol. This results in lower blood-cholesterol levels 4 to 7 days after starting cholestyramine.

Cholestyramine works entirely within the bowel and is never absorbed into the bloodstream. Though usually given 3 to 4 times a day, there appears to be no advantage to taking it more often than 2 times a day. The cholesterol-lowering effect of cholestyramine may be increased when it is taken with an HMG-CoA inhibitor or nicotinic acid. In some kinds of hyperlipidemia, colestipol may be more effective in lowering total blood cholesterol than clofibrate.

Cautions and Warnings

Do not use cholestyramine if you are **sensitive** to it or if your **bile duct is blocked**. The powder form should not be taken dry; doing so may result in the inhalation of powder into your lungs or a clogged esophagus.

Cholestyramine may cause or worsen **constipation** and **hemorrhoids**. Most constipation is mild but some people may need to stop the medication or take less of it.

Possible Side Effects

▼ Most common: constipation, which may be severe and result in bowel impaction. Hemorrhoids may be worsened.

▼ Less common: abdominal pain and bloating, and bleeding disorders or black-and-blue marks due to interference with the absorption of vitamin K, a necessary factor in the blood clotting process. One person developed night-blindness because the medication interfered with vitamin A absorption into the blood. Other side effects include belching, gas, nausea, vomiting, diarrhea, heartburn, and appetite loss. Your stool may have an unusual appearance because of a high fat level.

Possible Side Effects *(continued)*
▼ Rare: Rare side effects can affect your mouth, stomach and intestines, muscles and joints, mental status, urinary tract, and breathing. Contact your doctor if you experience any side effect not listed above.

Drug Interactions

• Cholestyramine interferes with the absorption of virtually all oral drugs, including acetaminophen, amiodarone, aspirin, cephalexin, chenodiol, clindamycin, clofibrate, corticosteroids, diclofenac, iron, digitalis drugs, furosemide, gemfibrozil, glipizide, hydrocortisone, imipramine (an antidepressant), methyldopa, mycophenolate, nicotinic acid, penicillin, phenobarbital, phenytoin, piroxicam, propranolol, tetracycline, thiazide diuretics, thyroid drugs, tolbutamide, trimethoprim, warfarin and other anticoagulant (blood-thinning) drugs, and vitamins A, D, E, and K. Take other medications at least 1 hour before or 4 to 6 hours after taking cholestyramine.

Food Interactions

Take this medication before meals. It may be mixed with soda, water, juice, cereal, or pulpy fruits, such as applesauce or crushed pineapple. Cholestyramine bars should be thoroughly chewed and taken with plenty of fluids.

Usual Dose

Cholestyramine: 4 g (1 packet) taken 1–6 times a day.

Colestipol: 5–30 g (1–6 packets) a day in 2–4 divided doses.

Overdosage

The most severe effect of overdose is bowel impaction. Take the overdose victim to a hospital emergency room. ALWAYS bring the prescription bottle or container.

Special Information

Do not swallow the granules or powder in their dry form. Prepare each packet of powder by mixing it with soup, cereal, or pulpy fruit or by adding the powder to a 6-oz. glass of liquid, such as a carbonated beverage. If some of the drug sticks to the sides of the glass, rinse it with liquid and drink the remainder.

. Constipation, gas, nausea, and heartburn may occur and then disappear with continued use of this medication. Call your doctor if these side effects persist or if you develop unusual problems such as bleeding from the gums or rectum.

If you miss a dose of cholestyramine, skip it and continue with your regular schedule. Do not take a double dose.

Special Populations

Pregnancy/Breast-feeding
While cholestyramine does not affect the fetus directly, it may prevent the absorption of vitamins A, D, and E and other nutrients essential to the fetus' proper development—even when you take a prenatal vitamin supplement. When this drug is considered crucial by your doctor, its potential benefits must be carefully weighed against its risks.

Cholestyramine is not absorbed into the body. However, reduced absorption of vitamins A, D, and E and other nutrients may make your milk less nutritious. Nursing mothers who must take cholestyramine should bottle-feed.

Seniors
Seniors are more likely to experience side effects, especially those relating to the bowel.

Generic Name

Ciclopirox (sye-kloe-PERE-ox)

Brand Names

Loprox   Penlac Nail Lacquer

Type of Drug

Antifungal.

Prescribed for

Fungus and yeast infections of the nails and skin, including athlete's foot and candida.

General Information

Ciclopirox slows the growth of a variety of fungus organisms and yeasts and kills many others. The drug penetrates the skin, hair, hair follicles, and sweat glands. Cicloprox nail lacquer is used for toenail and fingernail fungus infections.

Cautions and Warnings

Do not use this product if you are **allergic** to it.

Possible Side Effects

▼ Common: burning, itching, and stinging at the application site.

Drug Interactions

None known.

Usual Dose

Cream/Lotion: Apply enough to cover affected areas and massage it into the skin twice a day.

Nail Lacquer: Apply to infected nails once a day.

Overdosage

Accidental ingestion may cause nausea and upset stomach. Call your local poison control center or hospital for more information.

Special Information

Clean the affected areas before applying ciclopirox, unless otherwise directed by your doctor.

This product can be expected to relieve symptoms within the first week of use. Follow your doctor's directions for the complete 2- to 4-week course of treatment with the cream or lotion to gain maximum benefit. The nail lacquer may be used for up to 48 weeks. Stopping the medication too soon can lead to a relapse.

When using ciclopirox nail lacquer, do not apply it to any skin other than that which surrounds the infected nails because of possible irritation. Do not apply nail polish or any other nail lacquer to infected nails while you are using this product.

Avoid using cicloprox nail lacquer near an open flame since the product is flammable.

Call your doctor if the affected area burns, stings, or becomes red after you use this product, or if your symptoms do not clear up after 4 weeks of treatment; by then it is unlikely that the cream will be effective.

If you forget a dose of ciclopirox, apply it as soon as you remember. Do not apply more than prescribed to make up for the missed dose.

Special Populations

Pregnancy/Breast-feeding

Ciclopirox may pass to the fetus in very small amounts. In animal studies, high doses of ciclopirox given by mouth did not harm the fetus. As with all drugs, caution should be exercised when using ciclopirox during pregnancy.

It is unknown if ciclopirox passes into breast milk. Nursing mothers who must use this drug should consider bottle-feeding.

Seniors

Seniors may use this drug without special restriction.

Generic Name

Cilostazol (sil-oe-STAY-zol)

Brand Name

Pletal

Type of Drug

Antiplatelet.

Prescribed for

Intermittent claudication.

General Information

In intermittent claudication, leg muscles go into spasm due to reduced blood flow. This occurs when plaque buildup narrows blood vessels leading to the calf or other leg muscles. People with this condition often develop leg pain after walking only a short distance. Cilostazol prevents blood platelets from "clumping together" to begin the process of forming a blood clot, which can further obstruct arteries and worsen intermittent claudication. This drug is broken down in the liver.

Cautions and Warnings

Do not take this drug if you are **sensitive** or **allergic** to it.
    People with **heart failure** should not take cilostazol.

Possible Side Effects

The risk of side effects increases with dosage.
    ▼ Most common: headache, infection, muscle aches, abnormal bowel movements, and diarrhea.
    ▼ Common: palpitations, rapid heartbeat, dizziness, fainting, upset stomach, nausea, sore throat, runny nose, back pain, and swelling in the arms or legs.
    ▼ Less common: gas, cough, and abdominal pain.
    ▼ Rare: Rare side effects can occur in almost any part of the body. Contact your doctor if you experience any side effect not listed above.

Drug Interactions

• Avoid mixing cilostazol with ketoconazole, itraconazole, fluconazole, miconazole, fluvoxamine, fluoxetine, nefazodone, or sertraline because this interaction may slow the breakdown of cilostazol, prolonging its effects. Take half the regular dose of cilostazol when combining it with any of these drugs.

• Aspirin can increase the anticoagulant (blood-thinning) effect of cilostazol, but this combination has not caused serious bleeding problems. There is no information on the effect of combining cilostazol and other antiplatelet or anticoagulant drugs. Take half the regular dose of cilostazol when combining it with any of these drugs.

• Diltiazem increases cilostazol blood levels by about 50%. Take half the regular dose of cilostazol when combining it with diltiazem.

• Erythromycin and similar antibiotics increase cilostazol blood levels. Take half the regular dose of cilostazol when combining it with any of these drugs.

* Smoking reduces the effectiveness of cilostazol by causing the liver to break it down faster.

Food Interactions

Take this drug on an empty stomach at least 1 hour before or 2 hours after meals. Do not drink grapefruit juice at any time while taking cilostazol because it can interfere with the breakdown of the drug.

Usual Dose

Adult: 100 mg twice a day. Take 50 mg twice a day if you are taking other drugs that may increase the effect of cilostazol.
Child: not recommended.

Overdosage

Symptoms of overdose are likely to be the most common side effects. Overdose victims should be taken to a hospital emergency room. ALWAYS bring the prescription bottle or container.

Special Information

Several weeks of cilostazol treatment may be necessary before you notice any improvement in symptoms. Maximum benefit usually occurs after 12 weeks.

If you forget a dose, take it as soon as you remember. If it is almost time for your next dose, skip the forgotten dose and continue with your regular schedule. Do not take a double dose.

Special Populations

Pregnancy/Breast-feeding

Animal studies suggest that cilostazol may harm the fetus, but there is no information on the effect of cilostazol in pregnant women. When this drug is considered crucial by your doctor, its potential benefits must be carefully weighed against its risks.

Cilostazol may pass into breast milk. Nursing mothers who must take this drug should consider bottle-feeding.

Seniors

Seniors can take this drug without special precaution.

Generic Name

Cimetidine (sih-MET-ih-dene) Ⓖ

Brand Names

Tagamet   Tagamet HB Ⓢ

Type of Drug

Histamine H_2 antagonist.

Prescribed for

Ulcers of the stomach and duodenum (upper intestine); also used for upset stomach, gastroesophageal reflux disease (GERD), benign stomach ulcer, bleeding in the stomach and duodenum, colorectal cancer, prevention of stress ulcer, hyperparathyroidism, fungal infections of the hair and scalp, herpes virus infection, excessive hairiness in women, chronic itching of unknown cause, skin reactions, warts, acetaminophen overdose, and other conditions characterized by the production of large amounts of gastric fluids. Cimetidine may be prescribed to stop the production of stomach acid during surgery. The non-prescription version is recommended for heartburn and stomach gas.

General Information

Histamine H_2 antagonists work by turning off the system that produces stomach acid and other secretions. Cimetidine is effective in treating the symptoms of ulcer and preventing complications of the disease, although an ulcer that does not respond to another histamine H_2 antagonist will probably not respond to cimetidine. Histamine H_2 antagonists differ only in their potency. Cimetidine is the least potent; 1000 mg are roughly equal to 300 mg of either nizatidine or ranitidine, or 40 mg of famotidine. These drugs are roughly equal in their ability to treat ulcer disease and their risk of side effects.

Cautions and Warnings

Do not take cimetidine if you have had an **allergic reaction** to it or any histamine H_2 antagonist. Cimetidine has a mild antiandrogen effect, which probably causes the painful, swollen breasts that some people experience after taking this drug for a month or more.

People with **kidney or liver disease** should take cimetidine with caution because it is broken down in the liver and passes out of the body through the kidneys.

The fact that symptoms are alleviated by cimetidine does not preclude the possibility of **stomach cancer**, which can have symptoms similar to other gastrointestinal (GI) disorders. Make sure your doctor screens for possible malignancy.

Some people—mostly the very ill—experience confusion, agitation, psychosis, hallucinations, depression, anxiety, or disorientation, usually within 2 or 3 days of starting cimetidine. Normally these symptoms stop 3 to 4 days after discontinuing the drug. Call your doctor if this happens to you.

Possible Side Effects

Serious side effects are uncommon.

▼ Most common: mild diarrhea, dizziness, rash, painful breast swelling, nausea and vomiting, headache, confusion, drowsiness, hallucinations, and impotence.

▼ Less common: liver inflammation, peeling or red and swollen rash, breathing difficulties, tingling in the hands or feet, delirious feelings, and oozing from the nipples.

▼ Rare: Cimetidine may affect white blood cells or blood platelets. Some symptoms of these effects are unusual bleeding or bruising, unusual tiredness, and weakness. Other rare side effects are inflammation of the pancreas, hair loss (reversible), abnormal heart rhythms, heart attack, reversible muscle or joint pains, and reversible drug reactions.

Drug Interactions

• Separate cimetidine from antacid doses by about 3 hours to avoid reducing cimetidine's effectiveness. Other drugs that may reduce the absorption of cimetidine are metoclopramide and anticholinergic drugs, including trihexyphenidyl hydrochloride, oxybutynin, and benztropine mesylate.

• Cigarette smoking reverses the healing effect cimetidine has on ulcers.

• Cimetidine may increase the side effects of a variety of drugs, possibly leading to drug toxicity. These drugs include alcohol; aminophylline; oral antidiabetes drugs; benzodiazepine tranquilizers and sleeping pills, except lorazepam, oxazepam, and temazepam; caffeine; calcium channel blockers; carbamazepine; carmustine; chloroquine; flecainide; fluorouracil; labetalol; lidocaine; metoprolol; metronidazole; moricizine; mexiletine; narcotic pain relievers; ondansetron; pentoxifylline; phenytoin; procainamide; propafenone; propranolol; quinine; quinidine; tacrine; theophylline drugs, except dyphylline; triamterene; tricyclic antidepressants; valproic acid; and warfarin (a blood-thinner).

• Drugs whose absorption may be decreased by cimetidine are iron, indomethacin, fluconazole, ketoconazole, and tetracycline antibiotics.

• Enteric-coated tablets should not be taken with cimetidine. The change in stomach acidity causes the tablets to disintegrate prematurely in the stomach.

• Cimetidine may decrease the effects of digoxin and tocainide.

Food Interactions

None known.

Usual Dose

Adult: 400–800 mg at bedtime; 300 mg 4 times a day with meals and at bedtime, or 400 mg 2 times a day. To treat GERD—400 mg 4 times a day. Do not exceed 2400 mg a day. Smaller doses may be as effective for seniors or those with impaired kidney function.

Overdosage

Little is known about the effects of cimetidine overdose, but victims may experience exaggerated side effects. Two deaths have occurred. Your local poison control center may advise giving ipecac syrup—available at any pharmacy—to induce vomiting and remove any drug remaining in the stomach. Victims who have definite symptoms should be taken to a hospital emergency room. ALWAYS bring the prescription bottle or container.

Special Information

Take cimetidine exactly as directed and follow your doctor's instructions regarding diet and other treatment in order to get the maximum benefit from the drug.

Cigarettes are associated with stomach ulcers and reduce cimetidine's effectiveness.

Call your doctor at once if you develop any unusual side effects such as bleeding or bruising, tiredness, diarrhea, dizziness, rash, or hallucinations. Black, tarry stools or vomiting material that resembles coffee grounds may indicate your ulcer is bleeding.

If you miss a dose of cimetidine, take it as soon as possible. If it is almost time for your next dose, skip the dose you forgot and continue with your regular schedule. Do not take a double dose.

Special Populations

Pregnancy/Breast-feeding
Animal studies reveal no damage to the fetus, although cimetidine does pass into the fetal blood. When this drug is considered crucial by your doctor, its potential benefits must be carefully weighed against its risks.

Large amounts of cimetidine pass into breast milk. Nursing mothers who must take this drug should bottle-feed.

Seniors
Seniors may need less medication due to loss of kidney function and be more susceptible to side effects, especially confusion and other nervous system effects (see "Cautions and Warnings").

Cipro *see Fluoroquinoline Anti-Infectives, page 442*

Generic Name
Cisapride (SIS-uh-pride)

Brand Name
Propulsid

Type of Drug
Gastrointestinal (GI) stimulant.

Prescribed for
Nighttime heartburn caused by gastroesophageal reflux disease (GERD).

General Information

Cisapride stimulates the release of the hormone acetylcholine at key nerve endings in the GI tract. This stimulation causes the stomach and intestines to move food through the GI tract faster. It also increases pressure in the lower esophagus, which in turn helps to draw food that has refluxed (risen into the lower esophagus) back into the stomach. These effects are useful in treating nighttime heartburn caused by GERD. People with GERD have reduced lower-esophageal pressure; cisapride restores that pressure to normal levels. Cisapride has no consistent effect on daytime heartburn or other GI problems. Its safety and effectiveness in children have not been established. Children taking this drug may suffer severe side effects.

Cautions and Warnings

Cisapride should be avoided by people with **stomach or intestinal bleeding, bowel obstruction or perforation,** or other conditions in which stimulation of the GI tract may be harmful. Rarely, serious **abnormal heart rhythms, heart attack,** or **sudden death** occur in people taking cisapride who have a condition that predisposes them to abnormal rhythms. People who have **kidney failure,** or **heart failure** or other forms of heart disease, should not take cisapride. Cisapride **drug interactions may be fatal** (see "Drug Interactions").

Possible Side Effects

▼ Most common: headache, diarrhea, abdominal pain, nausea, constipation, and runny nose.

▼ Less common: upset stomach, gas, sinus inflammation, upper respiratory infection, coughing, pain, fever, urinary infection, frequent urination, sleeplessness, anxiety, nervousness, rash, itching, viral infection, joint pain, changes in vision, and vaginal irritation.

▼ Rare: dizziness, vomiting, sore throat, chest pain, back pain, depression, dehydration, muscle aches, dry mouth, tiredness, heart palpitations, migraine, tremors, swelling in the feet or legs, seizure, uncontrollable muscle movements, rapid heartbeat, liver inflammation, hepatitis, and low white-blood-cell and blood-platelet counts.

Drug Interactions

• Combining cisapride and ketoconazole (an antifungal) leads to serious abnormal heart rhythms due to high blood levels of cisapride. Itraconazole, miconazole administered intravenously, fluconazole, clarithromycin, erythromycin, nefazodone, indinavir, ritonavir, and troleandomycin can interact with cisapride in this way.

• Do not combine cisapride and drugs that can cause abnormal heart rhythms, such as disopyramide, moricizine, procainamide, maprotiline, quinidine, amiodarone, sotalol, tricyclic antidepressants, sertindole, chlorpromazine and similar phenothiazine-type antipsychotic drugs, astemizole, bepridil, sparfloxacin, and terodiline.

• Cisapride's stimulating effect on the GI tract interferes with the absorption of most oral drugs into the bloodstream. Your doctor should determine if dosage adjustments are necessary.

• Combining cimetidine and cisapride increases blood levels of both drugs. Cisapride increases the amount of ranitidine absorbed. Your doctor must adjust these drug dosages to fit your needs.

• Cisapride may increase the effects of anticoagulant (blood-thinning) drugs. Your anticoagulant dosage may need to be adjusted or you may have to stop taking cisapride.

• Anticholinergic drugs including atropine, benztropine, donnatal, oxybutynin, and trihexyphenidyl interfere with the effects of cisapride.

Food Interactions

Take cisapride at least 15 minutes before meals and at bedtime.

Usual Dose

40–80 mg a day.

Overdosage

Symptoms include stomach rumbling, gas, and frequent stools and urination. Other possible symptoms are droopy eyelids, tremors, convulsions, breathing difficulties, catatonic reaction, loss of muscle tone, and diarrhea. Overdose victims should be taken to a hospital emergency room. ALWAYS bring the prescription bottle or container.

Special Information

Use cisapride with care if you take a benzodiazepine tranquilizer or sleeping medication; avoid alcohol.

Call your doctor if you develop any bothersome or persistent side effect.

If you forget a dose, take it as soon as you remember, as long as it is before a meal. If it is almost time for your next dose, skip the one you forgot and continue with your regular schedule. Do not take a double dose.

Special Populations

Pregnancy/Breast-feeding

Animal studies indicate that cisapride may harm the fetus. When this drug is considered crucial by your doctor, its potential benefits must be carefully weighed against its risks.

Cisapride passes into breast milk. Nursing mothers who must take this drug should bottle-feed.

Seniors

Seniors may use this drug without special restriction.

Generic Name

Citalopram (sih-TAL-oe-pram)

Brand Name

Celexa

Type of Drug

Selective serotonin reuptake inhibitor (SSRI).

Prescribed for

Depression.

General Information

Citalopram and other SSRIs, which are unrelated to the older tricyclic and tetracyclic antidepressant drugs, work by preventing the movement of the neurohormone serotonin into nerve endings. This forces serotonin to remain in the spaces surrounding nerve endings, where it works. The drug is effective in treating common symptoms of depression. It can help improve mood and mental alertness, increase physical activity, and improve sleep patterns. The drug takes about 4 weeks to work and stays in the body for several weeks after you stop taking it. This fact may be important when your doctor starts or stops treatment.

Cautions and Warnings

Do not take citalopram if you are **allergic** to it.

Serious, **potentially fatal reactions** may occur if citalopram and a **monoamine oxidase inhibitor (MAOI)** antidepressant are taken together (see "Drug Interactions").

Citalopram is broken down by your liver; people with severe **liver disease** should use caution with this drug and be treated with lower doses. People with **reduced kidney function** should take citalopram with caution.

A few people with **mania** or **hypomania** may experience an activation of their condition while taking citalopram.

Citalopram should be used with caution by people who suffer from **seizure** disorders.

SSRIs can affect **blood platelets**, but their exact effect is not known. Some people have had abnormal bleeding while taking these drugs.

Citalopram causes low blood levels of **uric acid**, but has not caused kidney failure.

The possibility of **suicide** exists in severe depression and may be present until the condition is significantly improved. Severely depressed patients only carry small quantities of citalopram with them to reduce the risk of overdose.

Possible Side Effects

▼ Most common: dry mouth, headache, dizziness, tremors, nausea, diarrhea or loose stools, sleeplessness, tiredness or fatigue, sexual dysfunction (15% of men and 1.7% of women) or abnormal ejaculation and not feeling well.

▼ Common: excessive sweating, constipation, upset stomach, and agitation.

Possible Side Effects *(continued)*

▼ Less common: heart palpitations, chest pain, nervousness, anxiety, tingling or numbness in the hands or feet, twitching, muscle spasms, confusion, rash, muscle and joint aches, gas, appetite increase or decrease, menstrual disorders, sore throat, runny nose, yawning, changes in vision, frequent urination, fever, back pain, chills, confusion, reduced skin sensation, nightmares, depersonalization, weight gain, vomiting, changes in sense of taste, and ringing or buzzing in the ears.

▼ Rare: Rare side effects can affect your urinary tract, dreaming or thinking, stomach and intestines, skin, muscles and joints, and menstruation. Other rare side effects can affect virtually every body system. Contact your doctor if you experience any side effect not listed above.

Drug Interactions

• At least 5 weeks should elapse between stopping citalopram and starting an MAOI antidepressant. Two weeks should elapse between stopping an MAOI and starting citalopram. Taking these 2 drugs too close together or at the same time may cause serious, life-threatening reactions.

• Citalopram doubles the amount of metoprolol (a beta-blocker drug), in the blood. This interaction produced no important effect on blood pressure or heart rate.

• People taking warfarin may experience a slight increase in that drug's effect when taking citalopram. The importance of this effect is not known.

• People combining lithium and citalopram may experience increased amounts of either drug in the blood. Your doctor should check your blood lithium levels.

• Combining alcohol with citalopram is not recommended.

• Combining citalopram with azithromycin, clarithromycin, dirithromycin, erythromycin, troleandomycin, fluconazole, or itraconazole may increase citalopram levels.

• Mixing citalopram and imipramine can increase the amount of imipramine's active breakdown product in the blood. The importance of this effect is not known.

• Cimetidine increases levels of citalopram, but the importance of this effect is not known.

Food Interactions

For consistent blood levels, citalopram should be taken on an empty stomach at least 1 hour before or 2 hours after meals.

Usual Dose

40 mg once a day, morning or night. Seniors and people with liver disease should receive 20 mg a day.

Overdosage

Overdose symptoms are tiredness, nausea, vomiting, rapid heartbeat, anxiety, dilated pupils, and changes in electrocardiogram results. Overdose victims should be taken to a hospital emergency room at once. ALWAYS bring the prescription bottle or container.

Special Information

Citalopram may make you dizzy or drowsy. Take care when driving or doing tasks that require alertness and concentration.

Do not drink alcoholic beverages while taking citalopram.

Be sure your doctor knows if you are pregnant, breast-feeding, or taking other prescription or over-the-counter medications while taking citalopram. Notify your doctor if you experience any unusual side effect.

If you forget a dose, take it as soon as you remember. If it is almost time for your next dose, skip the forgotten dose and continue with your regular schedule. Do not take a double dose.

Special Populations

Pregnancy/Breast-feeding

Do not take citalopram if you are or might be pregnant without first weighing its potential benefits against its risks with your doctor.

It is not known if citalopram passes into breast milk. Nursing mothers who must take this drug should consider bottle-feeding.

Seniors

Seniors should begin at half the usual dose.

Claritin   *see **Loratadine**, page 600*

*see **Loratadine**, page 600*

Claritin-D   *see **Antihistamine-Decongestant** **Combination Products**, page 81*

*see **Antihistamine-Decongestant** **Combination Products**, page 81*

Generic Name

Clarithromycin   (klah-rith-roe-MYE-sin)

Brand Name

Biaxin

Type of Drug

Macrolide antibiotic.

Prescribed for

Mild to moderate infections of the upper and lower respiratory tract and for duodenal ulcers; also used for skin and other infections including membrane attack complex (MAC).

General Information

Clarithromycin and other macrolide antibiotics are either bactericidal (bacteria-killing) or bacteriostatic (inhibiting bacterial growth), depending on the organism in question and amount of antibiotic present. In ulcer disease, clarithromycin is used to fight *Helicobacter pylori* infection, which is present in almost all ulcers and most cases of stomach inflammation.

Cautions and Warnings

Do not take clarithromycin if you are **allergic** to it or any macrolide antibiotic.

Clarithromycin is primarily eliminated from the body through the liver and kidneys. People with severe **kidney disease** may require dose adjustments. Liver disease generally does not call for an adjustment.

Colitis (bowel inflammation) has been associated with all antibiotics (see "Possible Side Effects").

Possible Side Effects

Most side effects are mild and go away once you stop taking clarithromycin.

▼ Most common: nausea, vomiting, upset stomach, changes in sense of taste, stomach cramps, stomach gas, and headache. Colitis (symptoms include severe abdominal cramps and severe, persistent, and possibly bloody diarrhea) may develop.

Drug Interactions

• Clarithromycin may increase the anticoagulant (blood-thinning) effects of warfarin in people who take it regularly, especially older adults. This combination requires careful monitoring by your doctor.

• Mixing clarithromycin and omeprazole raises the amount of both drugs in the blood.

• Mixing clarithromycin with rifabutin or rifampin can interfere with the antibiotic's effect and increase the risk of intestinal side effects.

• Mixing clarithromycin with ranitidine bismuth-sulfate (for ulcers) can raise the amount of both drugs in the blood, but these effects are not considered important.

• Clarithromycin can prolong the effect of alprazolam, diazepam, midazolam, and triazolam, causing excessive nervous system depression.

• Clarithromycin increases the effects of buspirone and can lead to buspirone side effects.

• Clarithromycin can raise blood levels of carbamazepine. People mixing these drugs should be checked by their doctors for changes in blood-carbamazepine levels.

• Two deaths have been reported in people combining clarithromycin and pimozide. Pimozide should not be used by people taking a macrolide antibiotic.

• Clarithromycin may raise blood levels of theophylline, possibly leading to a theophylline overdose. It can also increase the effects of caffeine.

• Combining clarithromycin and digoxin, cyclosporine, ergot drugs, tacrolimus, or triazolam may lead to drug side effects.

• Mixing clarithromycin with a statin cholesterol lowering drug increases the risk of developing a potentially fatal condition involving severe muscle pain and destruction.

• Do not mix clarithromycin and cisapride; serious abnormal heart rhythms, some fatal, can result.

• Fluconazole increases the amount of clarithromycin in the blood.

• Mixing zidovudine (an AIDS drug—also known as AZT) with clarithromycin may affect the amount of zidovudine in the bloodstream.

Food Interactions

Clarithromycin can be taken without regard to food or meals. It may be taken with milk.

Usual Dose

Adult: infections—250–500 mg every 12 hours for 1–2 weeks. Dosage must be reduced in people with severe kidney disease. Ulcer—500 mg 3 times a day plus 40 mg omeprazole in the morning or ranitidine bismuth citrate 400 mg twice a day for 14 days, then omeprazole 20 mg every morning or ranitidine bismuth citrate 400 mg twice a day for 2 weeks.

Child: infections—6.8 mg per lb. of body weight every 12 hours, up to 250–500 mg a dose, depending on the offending organism.

Overdosage

Overdose may cause severe side effects, especially nausea, vomiting, stomach cramps, and diarrhea. Call your local poison control center or hospital emergency room for more information.

Special Information

Call your doctor if you develop nausea, vomiting, diarrhea, stomach cramps, or severe abdominal pain.

Clarithromycin suspension must be shaken well before each dose. Do not store it in the refrigerator.

Clarithromycin may be gentler on the digestive tract than erythromycin.

Remember to complete the full course of treatment exactly as prescribed, even if you feel well sooner. Clarithromycin's effectiveness may be severely reduced otherwise.

Take clarithromycin at the same time each day. If you forget a dose, take it as soon as you remember. If it is within 4 hours of your next dose, skip the one you forgot and go back to your regular schedule.

Special Populations

Pregnancy/Breast-feeding
Clarithromycin has affected animal fetuses. Pregnant women should take clarithromycin only if no alternative is available.

It is not known if clarithromycin passes into breast milk, but other macrolide antibiotics do. Nursing mothers who must take this drug should bottle-feed.

Seniors
Seniors with severe kidney disease require a dosage adjustment.

Generic Name

Clemastine (KLEH-mas-tene) Ⓖ

Brand Name
Tavist

Type of Drug
Antihistamine.

Prescribed for
Stuffy and runny nose, itchy eyes, and scratchy throat caused by seasonal allergy and for other symptoms of allergy such as rash, itching, and hives.

General Information
Antihistamines generally work by blocking the release of histamine (a chemical released by body tissue during an allergic reaction) from cells at the H_1 histamine receptor site, drying up secretions of the nose, throat, and eyes. Clemastine fumarate is less sedating than most antihistamines, but not less sedating than astemizole, cetirizine, or loratadine.

Cautions and Warnings
Clemastine should not be taken if you are **allergic** to it. People with **asthma** or other **deep-breathing problems, glaucoma,** or **stomach ulcers** or other **stomach problems** should avoid clemastine because its side effects can aggravate these problems.

Possible Side Effects

▼ Most common: headache, weakness, nervousness, stomach upset, nausea, vomiting, cough, stuffy nose, changes in bowel habits, sore throat, nosebleeds, and dry mouth, nose, or throat.

▼ Less common: drowsiness, hair loss, allergic reaction (symptoms include rash, itching, hives, and breathing difficulties), depression, sleeplessness, menstrual irregularities, muscle aches, sweating, tingling in the hands or feet, frequent urination, and visual disturbances.

Drug Interactions

• Combining clemastine with alcohol, tranquilizers, sleeping pills, or other nervous system depressants may increase the depressant effects of clemastine. Do not combine these drugs.

• The effects of oral anticoagulant (blood-thinning) drugs may be decreased by clemastine. Do not take this combination without your doctor's knowledge.

• Monoamine oxidase inhibitor (MAOI) antidepressants may increase the drying and other effects of clemastine. This combination can also worsen urinary difficulties.

Food Interactions

Clemastine is best taken on an empty stomach at least 1 hour before or 2 hours after eating; it may be taken with food if it upsets your stomach.

Usual Dose

Adult and Child (age 12 and over): 1.34 mg 2 times a day or 2.68 mg up to 3 times a day. Do not take more than 8.04 mg— 7 tablets of Tavist-1 or 3½ tablets of Tavist—daily.

Child (under age 12): not recommended.

Overdosage

Overdose is likely to cause severe side effects. Overdose victims should be given ipecac syrup—available at any pharmacy—to induce vomiting and should then be taken to a hospital emergency room for treatment. ALWAYS bring the prescription bottle or container.

Special Information

Clemastine may make it difficult for you to concentrate or perform complex tasks such as driving a car. Be sure to report any unusual side effects to your doctor.

If you forget to take a dose of clemastine, take it as soon as you remember. If it is almost time for your next dose, skip the one you forgot and continue with your regular schedule. Do not take a double dose.

Special Populations

Pregnancy/Breast-feeding

Do not take any antihistamines without your doctor's knowledge if you are or might be pregnant—especially during the last 3 months of pregnancy, because newborns may have severe reactions to antihistamines.

Small amounts of clemastine pass into breast milk. Nursing mothers who must take clemastine should bottle-feed.

Seniors

Seniors are more sensitive to side effects.

Generic Name

Clindamycin (klin-duh-MYE-sin) Ⓖ

Brand Name

Cleocin

Type of Drug

Antibiotic.

Prescribed for

Bacterial infections. The vaginal cream is used to treat bacterial vaginosis. Topical clindamycin is used to treat acne and rosacea.

General Information

Clindamycin is one of the few oral drugs that is effective against anaerobic bacteria, which grow only in the absence of oxygen and are often found in infected wounds, lung abscesses, abdominal infections, and infections of the female genital tract. It also works against bacteria usually treated by penicillin or erythromycin. Clindamycin may be useful for treating certain skin or soft tissue infections. It kills the bacteria that frequently cause acne.

Cautions and Warnings

Do not take clindamycin if you are **allergic** to it or lincomycin, another antibiotic.

Clindamycin can cause a severe intestinal irritation called **colitis**, which can be fatal. Signs of colitis are diarrhea, blood in the stool, and abdominal cramps. Any form of this drug, including products applied to the skin and the vaginal cream, can provoke colitis. Because of this, clindamycin should be reserved for serious infections or those that cannot be treated with other drugs.

Clindamycin should be used with caution if you have kidney or liver disease.

Possible Side Effects

Capsules
▼ Most common: stomach pain; nausea; vomiting; diarrhea, in up to 30 percent of people; and pain when swallowing.
▼ Less common: itching; rash; signs of serious drug sensitivity, such as difficulty in breathing and yellowing of the skin or the whites of the eyes; colitis (see "Cautions and Warnings"); effects on blood components; and joint pain.

Topical Lotion
▼ Most common: dry skin, redness, burning, or peeling; oily skin, and itching.
▼ Less common: diarrhea, abdominal pain, colitis, and gastrointestinal upset.

Vaginal Cream
▼ Most common: cervicitis, vaginitis, and irritation.
▼ Less common: nausea, vomiting, diarrhea, constipation, abdominal pain, dizziness, headache, and fainting.

Drug Interactions

• Do not mix clindamycin and erythromycin.

• The absorption of clindamycin capsules into the blood-stream is delayed by Kaolin-Pectin Suspension (prescribed for diarrhea). Separate these drugs by at least 1 hour.

Food Interactions

Take the oral medication with a full glass of water or with food to prevent irritation of the stomach and intestine.

Usual Dose

Capsules
   Adult: 150–450 mg every 6 hours.
   Child: 4–11 mg per lb. of body weight a day in divided doses. No child should be given less than 37.5 mg 3 times a day, regardless of weight.

Topical Lotion
Apply enough to cover the affected area(s) with a thin coat twice a day.

Vaginal Cream
Insert 1 applicator's worth at bedtime for 7 consecutive days.

Overdosage

Clindamycin overdose may lead to severe diarrhea and other drug side effects. Do not treat this diarrhea on your own. Call your local poison center for information. ALWAYS take the medicine bottle with you if you go to an emergency room for treatment.

Special Information

Unsupervised use of clindamycin can lead to secondary infections from susceptible organisms, such as fungi. Take this drug for the full course of therapy as indicated by your physician.

If you develop severe diarrhea or abdominal pain, call your doctor at once.

Women using the vaginal cream should not have vaginal intercourse until treatment is complete.

If you miss a dose of oral clindamycin, take it as soon as possible. If it is almost time for your next dose, double that dose and go back to your regular dosage schedule.

Special Populations

Pregnancy/Breast-feeding

This drug crosses into fetal blood circulation. When the drug is considered crucial by your doctor, its potential benefits must be carefully weighed against its risks.

Clindamycin passes into breast milk. Nursing mothers who must take oral clindamycin should consider bottle-feeding.

Seniors

Seniors with other illnesses may be unable to tolerate diarrhea and other clindamycin side effects.

Generic Name

Clofibrate (cloe-FIH-brate) Ⓖ

Brand Name

Atromid-S

Type of Drug

Anti-hyperlipidemic (blood-fat reducer).

Prescribed for

High blood levels of triglycerides; also prescribed for high cholesterol and low-density lipoprotein (LDL) cholesterol levels and for diabetes insipidus.

General Information

Clofibrate reduces cholesterol and triglyceride levels by interfering with the body's production of these blood fats and increasing the rate at which they are broken down. Less predictable and effective than other cholesterol-lowering medications, it is usually prescribed for people whose blood fats remain high despite changes in diet, weight control, and exercise. People with high cholesterol and low triglycerides should not take clofibrate because it is most effective in lowering triglycerides.

Cautions and Warnings

Clofibrate should be used with caution if you are **allergic** to it or have **cirrhosis of the liver, heart disease, gallstones** (clofibrate users have twice the risk of developing gallstones), **liver disease,** an **underactive thyroid,** or stomach **ulcer**.

People with **kidney disease** require dosage adjustments.

Clofibrate does not reduce the risk of a fatal heart attack. A 1978 study suggests that taking clofibrate regularly for many years increases the risk of dying from noncardiac causes, but this has not been confirmed by more recent research. Another clofibrate study shows an increase in side effects, including abnormal heart rhythms and intermittent leg pains due to blood-vessel spasm. Clofibrate should be used only by people whose other efforts to reduce their triglyceride or cholesterol levels have failed.

Possible Side Effects

▼ Most common: nausea.

▼ Less common: vomiting; loose stools; upset stomach; gas; abdominal pain; liver enlargement; gastric irritation; mouth sores; headache; dizziness; tiredness; cramped muscles; aching and weakness; rash; itching; brittle hair or hair loss; abnormal heart rhythms; blood clots in the lungs or veins; gallstones, especially in people who have taken clofibrate for a long time; decreased sex drive; and impotence.

If you suffer from angina pectoris (a condition characterized by brief attacks of chest pain), clofibrate may increase or decrease this pain. It may cause you to produce smaller quantities of urine and has been associated with blood in the urine, tiredness, weakness, drowsiness, and mildly increased appetite and weight gain. Some experts claim that clofibrate causes stomach ulcer, stomach bleeding, arthritis-like symptoms, uncontrollable muscle spasm, increased perspiration, blurred vision, breast enlargement, and effects on the blood.

Drug Interactions

• Your anticoagulant (blood thinner) dosage may have to be reduced by up to 50% if you start taking clofibrate. It is essential that your doctor know that you are taking both drugs so that the proper dosage adjustments can be made.

• Combining clofibrate and a statin cholesterol-lowering drug may lead to skeletal muscle destruction.

- Clofibrate may reduce the effect of chenodiol.
- Clofibrate may increase the effects of oral antidiabetics and any drug used to treat diabetes insipidus including carbamazepine, chlorpropamide, desmopressin, diuretics, and hormone replacement products.
- Contraceptive drugs may interfere with the effectiveness of clofibrate.
- Probenecid may increase the effectiveness and side effects of clofibrate.
- Rifampin may reduce clofibrate's effectiveness.
- Clofibrate may interfere with a number of blood tests. Make sure your doctor knows that you are taking the drug before any blood tests are done.

Food Interactions

Take this drug with food or milk to prevent upset stomach.

Usual Dose

2000 mg a day.

Overdosage

Symptoms are most likely to be severe side effects. Take the overdose victim to a hospital emergency room. ALWAYS bring the prescription bottle or container.

Special Information

Call your doctor if you develop chest pain, breathing difficulties, abnormal heart rates, severe stomach pain with nausea and vomiting, fever and chills, sore throat, swelling of the legs, weight gain, blood in the urine, changes in urinary habits, or any bothersome or persistent side effect.

Follow the diet recommended by your doctor. Limit alcohol consumption.

Clofibrate should be stored at room temperature in a dry place—not in a bathroom medicine cabinet—to protect this drug's gelatin covering.

Regular doctor visits are necessary to be sure that clofibrate is still working. It is also important to be screened with blood counts and liver function tests, which may uncover possible side effects.

If you forget a dose, take it as soon as possible. If it is almost time for your next dose, skip the one you forgot and continue with your regular schedule. Do not take a double dose.

Special Populations

Pregnancy/Breast-feeding

Pregnant women should not take clofibrate because large amounts of this drug pass into the bloodstream of the fetus. If you are planning to become pregnant, stop taking clofibrate several months before trying to conceive.

Clofibrate passes into breast milk. Nursing mothers who must take clofibrate should bottle-feed.

Seniors

Seniors with loss of kidney function may require dosage adjustments.

Generic Name

Clonazepam (klon-A-zeh-pam) Ⓖ

Brand Name

Klonopin

Type of Drug

Anticonvulsant.

Prescribed for

Petit mal and other seizure; also prescribed for panic attacks, periodic leg movements during sleep, speaking difficulty associated with Parkinson's disease, acute manic episodes, nerve pain, and schizophrenia.

General Information

Clonazepam is a benzodiazepine drug. Clonazepam is not used as a sedative or hypnotic. It is used only for the uses described above in people who have not responded to other drug treatments. Tolerance to the effects of clonazepam commonly develops within about 3 months of use. Your doctor may raise your clonazepam dosage periodically to maintain the drug's effect.

Cautions and Warnings

Do not take clonazepam if you are **sensitive** or **allergic** to it or any other benzodiazepine.

When stopping clonazepam treatments, the drug must be discontinued gradually. Abrupt discontinuance of clonazepam may lead to drug **withdrawal symptoms** including severe seizures, tremors, abdominal or muscle cramps, vomiting, and increased sweating.

Use clonazepam with caution if you have a chronic **respiratory illness**, since the drug tends to increase salivation and other respiratory secretions and can make breathing more labored. Avoid using clonazepam if you have severe **depression**, severe **lung disease**, **sleep apnea** (intermittent cessation of breathing during sleep), **liver disease**, **alcoholism**, or **kidney disease**. These conditions may exacerbate the depressive effects of benzodiazepines, and such effects may be detrimental to your overall condition.

Clonazepam can aggravate **narrow-angle glaucoma**, but if you have open-angle glaucoma, you may take it.

Possible Side Effects

▼ Most common: drowsiness, poor muscle control, and behavioral changes.

▼ Rare: Rare side effects can occur in almost any part of the body but are most likely to affect mental function, stomach and intestines, urinary function, blood, and liver. Contact your doctor if you experience any side effect not listed above.

Drug Interactions

• The depressant effects of clonazepam are increased by tranquilizers, sleeping pills, narcotic pain relievers, antihistamines, alcohol, monoamine oxidase inhibitors (MAOIs), tricyclic antidepressants, and other anticonvulsants.

• Mixing valproic acid and clonazepam may produce severe petit mal seizures.

• Smoking, phenobarbital and phenytoin may reduce clonazepam's effectiveness.

• Clonazepam may increase the requirement for other anticonvulsant drugs in people who suffer from multiple types of seizures.

• The effects of clonazepam may be prolonged when it is taken with cimetidine, oral contraceptives, disulfiram, fluoxetine, isoniazid, ketoconazole, metoprolol, probenecid, propoxyphene, propranolol, rifampin, or valproic acid.

• Theophylline may reduce clonazepam's sedative effects.

• Separate antacids from your clonazepam dose by at least 1 hour to prevent them from interfering with clonazepam being absorbed into the bloodstream.

• Clonazepam may increase blood levels of digoxin and the risk of digoxin toxicity.

• Clonazepam may decrease the effect of levodopa.

Food Interactions

Clonazepam is best taken on an empty stomach but may be taken with food if it upsets your stomach.

Usual Dose

Adult and Child (age 10 and over): starting dose—0.5 mg 3 times a day. The dose is increased by 0.5–1 mg every 3 days until seizures are controlled or side effects develop. The maximum daily dose is 20 mg. Other uses for clonazepam involve doses from 0.5–16 mg a day, depending on the condition and its severity.

Child (under age 10, or below 66 lbs.): starting dose— 0.004–0.013 mg per lb. of body weight a day. Dosage can be increased gradually to a maximum of 0.045–0.09 mg per lb. of body weight.

Clonazepam dosage must be reduced in people with impaired kidney function.

Overdosage

Overdose may cause confusion, coma, poor reflexes, sleepiness, low blood pressure, labored breathing, and other depressive effects. If the overdose is discovered within a few minutes and the victim is still conscious, it may be helpful to induce vomiting with ipecac syrup—available at any pharmacy. Overdose victims must be taken to a hospital emergency room. ALWAYS bring the prescription bottle or container.

Special Information

Clonazepam may interfere with your ability to drive or perform other complex tasks because it can cause drowsiness and difficulty in concentrating.

Your doctor should perform periodic blood counts and liver function tests while you are taking this drug to check for possible side effects.

Do not suddenly stop taking clonazepam—severe seizures may result. The dosage must be discontinued gradually by your doctor.

If you miss a dose by 1 hour or less, take it right away. Otherwise, skip the dose you forgot and go back to your regular schedule. Do not take a double dose.

Carry identification or wear a bracelet indicating that you have a seizure disorder for which you take clonazepam.

Special Populations

Pregnancy/Breast-feeding

Clonazepam crosses into the fetal circulation and can affect the fetus. Women who are or might be pregnant should avoid it. When the drug is considered crucial by your doctor, its potential benefits must be carefully weighed against its risks.

Some reports suggest a strong link between anticonvulsant drugs and birth defects, though most of the information pertains to phenytoin and phenobarbital, not clonazepam. It is also possible that the epileptic condition itself or genetic factors common to people with seizure disorders may figure in the higher incidence of birth defects.

Clonazepam may pass into breast milk. Nursing mothers who must take this drug should bottle-feed.

Seniors

Seniors, especially those with liver or kidney disease, are more sensitive to the effects of this drug—especially dizziness and drowsiness—and may require smaller doses.

Generic Name

Clonidine (KLAH-nih-dene) G

Brand Names

Catapres	Catapres-TTS-2
Catapres-TTS-1	Catapres-TTS-3

Type of Drug

Alpha receptor stimulant.

Prescribed for

High blood pressure, including hypertensive emergency (diastolic blood pressure over 120); also used for excess sweating, childhood growth delay, attention-deficit hyperactivity disorder (ADHD), Tourette's syndrome, migraine, ulcerative colitis, painful or difficult menstruation, flushing related to menopause, diagnosis of pheochromocytoma (adrenal gland tumor), diabetic diarrhea, smoking cessation, methadone and opiate detoxification, withdrawal from alcohol and benzodiazepines such as Valium, nerve pain following herpes attack, and allergic reactions in the presence of asthma triggered by external sources. Clonidine by epidural injection has been used to treat cancer pain.

General Information

Clonidine stimulates nerve endings in the brain called alpha-adrenergic receptors. It reduces blood pressure by dilating (widening) blood vessels. Clonidine works quickly, decreasing blood pressure within 1 hour. The other uses of clonidine relate to its stimulation of alpha receptors throughout the body.

Cautions and Warnings

Do not take clonidine if you are **allergic** to it. People who have had a recent **heart attack** or have chronic **kidney failure, cardiac insufficiency**, or **disease of blood vessels in the brain** should avoid clonidine.

Some people develop a **tolerance** of their clonidine dosage. If this happens, your blood pressure may increase and your doctor may prescribe a higher dose.

Never stop taking clonidine without your doctor's knowledge. If you **abruptly stop taking clonidine**, you may experience an unusual **increase in blood pressure** accompanied by **agitation, headache, nervousness** and severe reactions, possibly **death**. Restarting clonidine therapy or taking another antihypertensive can reverse these effects.

If you require **surgery**, your doctor will continue your clonidine therapy until about 4 hours before surgery and resume it as soon as possible afterward.

People who develop **skin sensitivity** (symptoms include rash, itching, and swelling) to Catapres-TTS, the transdermal patch form of clonidine, may experience the same reactions with oral clonidine.

Possible Side Effects

Tablets

▼ Most common: dry mouth, drowsiness, constipation, and sedation.

▼ Common: dizziness, headache, and fatigue. These effects tend to diminish within 4 to 6 weeks.

▼ Less common: appetite loss, swelling or pain in the glands of the throat, nausea, vomiting, weight gain, blood-sugar elevation, breast pain or enlargement, worsening of congestive heart failure, heart palpitations, rapid heartbeat, dizziness when rising quickly from a sitting or lying position, painful blood-vessel spasm, abnormal heart rhythms, electrocardiogram changes, feeling unwell, changes in dream patterns, nightmares, difficulty sleeping, hallucinations, delirium, anxiety, depression, nervousness, restlessness, headache, rash, hives, thinning or loss of scalp hair, difficult or painful urination, nighttime urination, retaining urine, decrease or loss of sex drive, weakness, muscle or joint pain, leg cramps, increased alcohol sensitivity, dryness and burning of the eyes, dry nose, loss of color, and fever.

Transdermal Patch

▼ Most common: dry mouth and drowsiness.

▼ Less common: constipation, nausea, changes in sense of taste, dry throat, fatigue, headache, lethargy, changes in sleep patterns, nervousness, dizziness, impotence, sexual difficulties, and mild skin reactions including itching, swelling, contact dermatitis, discoloration, burning, peeling, throbbing, white patches, and generalized rash. Rashes of the face and tongue have also occurred but cannot be specifically tied to transdermal clonidine.

Drug Interactions

• Avoid alcohol, barbiturates, sedatives, and tranquilizers because they increase the depressive effects of clonidine.

• Tricyclic and other antidepressants, appetite suppressants, estrogens, stimulants, indomethacin and other non-steroidal anti-inflammatory drugs (NSAIDs), and prazosin may counteract the effects of clonidine.

• Combining clonidine and a beta blocker may increase the severity of a drug-withdrawal reaction and rebound high blood pressure and may cause blood pressure to rise.

• Combining verapamil and clonidine may lead to very low blood pressure and atrioventricular (AV) block (abnormality in heartbeat patterns).

Food Interactions

The tablets are best taken on an empty stomach but may be taken with food if they upset your stomach.

Usual Dose

Tablets
   Adult: high blood pressure—100 mcg twice a day to start; may be raised by 100–200 mcg a day until maximum control is achieved. Take no more than 2400 mcg a day. Other uses— 100–900 mcg a day, or up to 0.8 mcg per lb. of body weight in divided doses. Seniors should start with a lower dose and increase more slowly.
   Child: 5–25 mcg a day for every 2.2 lbs. of body weight, divided into 4 doses given every 6 hours.

Transdermal Patch
   Adult: 100 mcg delivered daily from a patch applied once every 7 days. Up to two 300-mcg patches may be needed to control blood pressure. Transdermal dosage exceeding 600 mcg a day has not been shown to increase effectiveness.
   Child: not recommended.

Overdosage

Symptoms of overdose are slow heartbeat, nervous system depression, very slow breathing or no breathing, low body temperature, pinpoint pupils, seizures, lethargy, agitation, irritability, nausea, vomiting, abnormal heart rhythms, mild increases in blood pressure followed by a rapid drop in blood pressure, dizziness, weakness, loss of reflexes, and vomiting. Victims should be taken to a hospital emergency room immediately. ALWAYS bring the prescription bottle or container.

Special Information

Clonidine causes drowsiness in about a third of people who take it. Be extremely careful while driving or performing any task that requires concentration. This effect is prominent during the first few weeks of clonidine therapy and then tends to decrease.

Do not take over-the-counter cough and cold medications unless directed by your doctor.

Call your doctor if you become depressed or have vivid dreams or nightmares while taking clonidine, or if you develop swelling in your feet or legs, paleness or coldness in your fingertips or toes, or any persistent or bothersome side effect.

Apply the transdermal patch to a hairless area of skin such as the upper arm or torso. Use a different skin site each time. If the patch becomes loose, apply the supplied adhesive directly over it. If the patch falls off before 7 days are up, apply a new one. Do not remove the patch while bathing.

If you forget a dose of oral clonidine, take it as soon as possible and then go back to your regular schedule. If you miss 2 or more consecutive doses, consult your doctor; missed doses may cause blood pressure increases and severe adverse effects. Do not take a double dose.

Special Populations

Pregnancy/Breast-feeding
Clonidine passes into the fetal bloodstream. Animal studies show that clonidine may damage the fetus in doses as low as 1/3 the maximum dose. Women who are or might be pregnant should only take clonidine after talking with their doctor about its risks and possible benefits.

Clonidine passes into breast milk. Nursing mothers who must take this drug should bottle-feed.

Seniors
Seniors are more susceptible to the effects of this drug and should begin with lower doses.

Generic Name

Clopidogrel (kloe-PID-oe-grel)

Brand Name
Plavix

Type of Drug
Antiplatelet.

Prescribed for

Heart attack and stroke prevention; to thin the blood after placement of a vascular stent.

General Information

Artery-clogging blood clots are often the cause of heart attacks and strokes. Clopidogrel reduces the risk of both by helping prevent blood-clot formation. This drug thins the blood by making platelets—the cells that aggregate to form clots—less "sticky." It starts working in as little as 2 hours after taking a single tablet. The drug's blood-thinning effect lasts until inactivated platelets are replaced by the body. Studies suggest that clopidogrel is more effective than aspirin in preventing heart attack and stroke in people at risk. People taking clopidogrel after stent surgery usually take it for a relatively short period. Those taking it to prevent a heart attack or stroke must take it for life.

Cautions and Warnings

Do not take this drug if you are **sensitive** or **allergic** to it or ticlopidine, a related antiplatelet. Ticlopidine can cause a rapid drop in white-blood-cell count, but this has not occurred with clopidogrel.

People with **bleeding ulcers, brain hemorrhages,** or **other bleeding problems** should use clopidogrel with caution.

People with **liver problems** should use clopidogrel with caution.

Possible Side Effects

▼ Most common: rash and other skin problems.

▼ Common: chest pain, accidents, flu-like symptoms, pain, headache, dizziness, abdominal pain, upset stomach, joint pain, back pain, black-and-blue marks, and respiratory infection.

▼ Less common: tiredness, swollen arms or legs, high blood pressure, diarrhea, nausea, bleeding, nosebleeds, breathing difficulties, runny nose, coughing, bronchitis, high blood cholesterol, urinary infection, and depression.

▼ Rare: bleeding in the brain and stomach ulcer.

Drug Interactions

• Clopidogrel may interfere with the body's ability to break down fluvastatin, nonsteroidal anti-inflammatory drugs (NSAIDs), phenytoin, tamoxifen, tolbutamide, torsamide, and warfarin.

• Combining clopidogrel and NSAIDs may increase blood loss and bleeding in the stomach and intestines.

• Do not combine clopidogrel and other antiplatelet drugs or the anticoagulant (blood thinner) warfarin unless you are under your doctor's direct supervision. This interaction may prevent normal blood clotting and lead to severe bleeding problems.

Food Interactions

Clopidogrel may be taken without regard to food or meals.

Usual Dose

Adult: 75 mg a day.

Overdosage

Little is known about the effects of clopidogrel overdose aside from reduced blood clotting. Overdose victims should be taken to a hospital emergency room. ALWAYS bring the prescription bottle or container.

Special Information

Minor cuts may take longer to stop bleeding during treatment with clopidogrel. If you forget a dose, take it as soon as you remember. If it is almost time for your next dose, skip the forgotten dose and continue with your regular schedule.

Special Populations

Pregnancy/Breast-feeding

The safety of using clopidogrel during pregnancy is not known. Other antiplatelet drugs, like aspirin, are not used during pregnancy due to their possible effects on mother and fetus.

Clopidogrel may pass into breast milk. Nursing mothers who must take this drug should bottle-feed.

Seniors

Seniors may take this drug without special precaution.

Generic Name

Clorazepate (klor-AZ-uh-pate) Ⓖ

Brand Names

Gen-Xene   Tranxene-SD
Tranxene

Type of Drug

Benzodiazepine tranquilizer.

Prescribed for

Anxiety, tension, fatigue, and agitation; also prescribed for irritable bowel syndrome and panic attacks.

General Information

Clorazepate dipotassium is a benzodiazepine. Benzodiazepines directly affect the brain. They can relax you and make you more tranquil or sleepier, or they can slow nervous system transmissions in such a way as to act as an anticonvulsant. Many doctors prefer benzodiazepines to other drugs that can be used to similar effect because they tend to be safer, have fewer side effects, and usually work as well, if not better.

Cautions and Warnings

Do not take clorazepate if you know you are **sensitive** or **allergic** to it or to another benzodiazepine drug, including clonazepam.

Clorazepate can aggravate narrow-angle **glaucoma**, but you may take it if you have open-angle glaucoma.

Other conditions in which clorazepate should be avoided are: severe **depression**, severe **lung disease**, **sleep apnea** (intermittent cessation of breathing during sleep), **liver disease**, **drunkenness**, and **kidney disease**. In each of these conditions, the depressive effects of clorazepate may be enhanced or could be detrimental to your overall condition.

Clorazepate should not be taken by **psychotic patients** because it is not effective for them and can trigger unusual excitement, stimulation, and rage.

Clorazepate is not intended to be used for more than 3 to 4 months at a time. Your doctor should reassess your condition before continuing your prescription beyond that time.

Clorazepate may be **addictive**. Drug withdrawal may develop if you stop taking it after only 4 weeks of regular use but is more likely after longer use. It may start with anxiety and progress to tingling in the hands or feet, sensitivity to bright light, sleep disturbances, cramps, tremors, muscle tension or twitching, poor concentration, flu symptoms, fatigue, appetite loss, sweating, and changes in mental state.

Possible Side Effects

Weakness and confusion may occur, especially in seniors and in those who are more sickly.

▼ Most common: mild drowsiness during the first few days of therapy.

▼ Less common: confusion, depression, lethargy, disorientation, headache, inactivity, slurred speech, stupor, dizziness, tremors, constipation, dry mouth, nausea, inability to control urination, sexual difficulties, irregular menstrual cycle, changes in heart rhythm, low blood pressure, fluid retention, blurred or double vision, itching, rash, hiccups, nervousness, inability to fall asleep, and occasional liver dysfunction. If you have any of these symptoms, stop taking the medicine and contact your doctor immediately.

▼ Rare: Rare side effects can affect your heart, stomach and intestines, urinary tract, blood, muscles and joints. Contact your doctor if you experience any side effects not listed above.

Drug Interactions

• Clorazepate is a central-nervous-system depressant. Don't mix it with alcohol, other tranquilizers, narcotics, barbiturates, monoamine oxidase inhibitors (MAOIs), antihistamines, and antidepressants. Taking clorazepate with these drugs may result in excessive depression, tiredness, sleepiness, breathing difficulties, or related symptoms.

• Smoking may reduce clorazepate's effectiveness by increasing the rate at which it is broken down by the body.

• Clorazepate's effects may be prolonged when it is mixed with cimetidine, oral contraceptives, disulfiram, fluoxetine, isoniazid, ketoconazole, metoprolol, probenecid, propoxyphene, propranolol, rifampin, or valproic acid. Theo-phylline may reduce clorazepate's sedative effects.

• If you take antacids, separate them from your clorazepate dose by at least 1 hour to prevent them from interfering with the absorption of clorazepate into the bloodstream.

• Clorazepate may increase blood levels of digoxin and the chances of digoxin toxicity.

• The effect of levodopa may be decreased if it is taken together with clorazepate.

• Combining clorazepate with phenytoin may increase phenytoin blood concentrations and the chances of pheny-toin toxicity.

Food Interactions

Clorazepate is best taken on an empty stomach, but it may be taken with food if it upsets your stomach.

Usual Dose

Immediate-Release
   Adult and Child (age 9 and over): 15–60 mg daily. The aver-age dose is 30 mg in divided quantities, but dosage must be adjusted to individual response for maximum effect.
   Child (under age 9): not recommended.

Sustained-Release
   Adult: The sustained-release form of clorazepate may be given as a single dose, either 11.25 or 22.5 mg, once every 24 hours.
   Child: not recommended.

Overdosage

Symptoms of overdose are confusion, sleepiness, poor coor-dination, lack of response to pain such as a pin prick, loss of reflexes, shallow breathing, low blood pressure, and coma. The victim should be taken to a hospital emergency room. ALWAYS bring the prescription bottle or container.

Special Information

Clorazepate can cause tiredness, drowsiness, inability to con-centrate, or similar symptoms. Be careful if you are driving, operating machinery, or performing other activities that require concentration.

People taking clorazepate for more than 3 or 4 months at a time may develop drug withdrawal reactions if the medication is stopped suddenly (see "Cautions and Warnings").

If you forget a dose of clorazepate, take it as soon as you remember. If it is almost time for your next dose, skip the dose you forgot and continue with your regular schedule. Do not take a double dose.

Special Populations

Pregnancy/Breast-feeding
Clorazepate may cause birth defects if taken during the first 3 months of pregnancy. Avoid this drug if you are or might be pregnant.

Clorazepate may pass into breast milk. Nursing mothers who must take clorazepate should bottle-feed.

Seniors
Seniors, especially those with liver or kidney disease, are more sensitive to the effects of clorazepate and generally require smaller doses to achieve the same effect.

Generic Name

Clotrimazole (kloe-TRIM-uh-zole) Ⓖ

Brand Names

Lotrimin   Mycelex-G
Mycelex

Type of Drug

Antifungal.

Prescribed for

Fungus infections of the mouth, skin, and vaginal tract.

General Information

Clotrimazole is useful against a variety of fungus organisms that other drugs do not affect. The exact way in which clotrimazole works is unknown.

Cautions and Warnings

If clotrimazole causes local **itching** or **irritation,** stop using it. Do not use clotrimazole in your **eyes.** Proper diagnosis is essential for effective treatment. Do not use this product without first consulting your doctor.

Possible Side Effects

Side effects are infrequent and usually mild.

Cream and Solution
▼ Most common: redness, stinging, blistering, peeling, itching, and swelling of local areas.

Vaginal Tablets
▼ Most common: mild burning, rash, mild cramps, frequent urination, and burning or itching in a sexual partner.

Lozenges
▼ Most common: stomach cramps or pain, diarrhea, nausea, and vomiting.

Drug Interactions

None known.

Food Interactions

The oral form of clotrimazole is best taken on an empty stomach, at least 1 hour before or 2 hours after meals. However, you may take it with food as long as you allow the lozenge to dissolve in your mouth.

Usual Dose

Topical Cream and Solution: Apply to affected areas morning and night.

Vaginal Cream: 1 applicator's worth at bedtime for 7–14 days.

Vaginal Tablet: 1 tablet inserted into the vagina at bedtime for 7 days, or 2 tablets a day for 3 days.

Lozenge: 1 lozenge 5 times a day for 2 weeks or more.

Overdosage

Little is known about the effects of clotrimazole overdose or accidental ingestion. Call your local poison control center for more information.

Special Information

If treating a vaginal infection, you should refrain from sexual activity or be sure that your partner wears a condom until treatment is finished. Call your doctor if burning or itching develops or if the condition does not improve within 7 days.

If you are using the vaginal cream, you may want to wear a sanitary napkin to avoid staining your clothing.

Dissolve the lozenge slowly in the mouth.

This medicine must be taken on consecutive days. If you forget a dose of oral clotrimazole, take it as soon as you remember. Do not double your dose.

Special Populations

Pregnancy/Breast-feeding

Women who are or might be pregnant should talk to their doctors about the medication's risks and benefits. Women who are in the first 3 months of pregnancy should use this drug only if directed to do so by their doctors. If you are pregnant, your doctor may want you to insert vaginal tablets by hand rather than use a vaginal applicator.

This drug is not likely to pass into breast milk. Nursing mothers need not worry about adverse effects on their infants while taking clotrimazole.

Seniors

Seniors may use this medication without special restriction.

Generic Name

Clozapine (KLOE-zuh-pene) G

Brand Name

Clozaril

Type of Drug

Antipsychotic.

Prescribed for

Severe schizophrenia.

General Information

Clozapine is a unique antipsychotic that has the capacity to treat people who do not respond to or cannot tolerate other drugs. It works by a mechanism that differs from those of other antipsychotic drugs.

A very small number of people who take clozapine develop a rapid drop in their white-blood-cell count, a condition called agranulocytosis. This effect usually reverses itself when the drug is stopped, but the drug must be stopped AS SOON AS IT IS DISCOVERED. An unusually large number of people who have developed clozapine agranulocytosis in the U.S. are of Eastern European Jewish descent, but the association is not very strong. Most cases of agranulocytosis occur between week 4 and week 10 of treatment. It is essential that blood samples be taken approximately every week and for 4 weeks after the drug is stopped to watch for this effect. Because of the risk of agranulocytosis, clozapine should not be tried until at least 2 other antipsychotic medicines have failed.

Some people taking antipsychotic drugs develop tardive dyskinesia, a potentially irreversible condition marked by uncontrollable movements. Tardive dyskinesia has not been seen in patients taking clozapine, a major advantage of this drug over other antipsychotic medicines. However, there is still a risk that this set of symptoms could occur with clozapine.

Cautions and Warnings

Women, seniors, people with **serious illnesses,** those who are **emaciated,** those with a history of **diseases affecting the white blood cells,** or those who are taking **other medication that could affect white blood cells** may be more susceptible to clozapine agranulocytosis.

About 5% of people taking the drug experience a **seizure** in the first year of treatment. Seizure is most likely to occur at higher drug doses.

People with **heart disease** should be carefully monitored while on clozapine because of possible cardiac risks.

A serious set of side effects, known as **neuroleptic malignant syndrome (NMS),** includes a high fever and has been associated with clozapine when it is used together with lithium or other drugs. The symptoms that constitute NMS include muscle rigidity, mental changes, irregular pulse or blood pressure, increased sweating, and abnormal heart rhythm. NMS is potentially fatal and requires immediate medical attention.

Use this drug with caution if you have **glaucoma, prostate problems,** or **liver, kidney, or heart disease**.

Clozapine may interfere with mental or physical abilities because of the **sedation** it usually causes during the first few weeks of treatment.

Possible Side Effects

▼ Most common: rapid heartbeat, low blood pressure, dizziness, fainting, drowsiness or sedation, salivation, and constipation.

▼ Less common: headache, tremor, sleep disturbance, restlessness, slow muscle motions, absence of movement, agitation, convulsions, rigidity, restlessness, confusion, sweating, dry mouth, visual disturbances, high blood pressure, nausea, vomiting, heartburn or abdominal discomfort, fever, and weight gain.

▼ Rare: agranulocytosis (symptoms include fever with or without chills, sore throat, and sores or white spots on the lips or mouth, tardive dyskinesia (symptoms include lip smacking or puckering, puffing of the cheeks, rapid or wormlike tongue movement, uncontrolled chewing motions, and uncontrolled arm and leg movements), and NMS (see "Cautions and Warnings"). Other rare side effects can occur in almost any part of the body. Contact your doctor if you experience any side effect not listed above.

Drug Interactions

• Clozapine's anticholinergic effects—blurred vision, dry mouth, and confusion—may be enhanced by interaction with other anticholinergics, such as tricyclic antidepressants like amitriptyline.

• Drugs that reduce blood pressure may enhance the blood-pressure-lowering effects of clozapine.

• Alcohol and other nervous system depressants, including benzodiazepines and other antianxiety drugs, may enhance clozapine's sedative action. At least 1 person has died as a result of combining diazepam and clozapine.

• Clozapine may increase blood levels of digoxin, warfarin, heparin, and phenytoin.
• The combination of lithium and clozapine may cause seizures, confusion, and NMS (see "Cautions and Warnings").
• Cigarette smoking may alter dosage requirements.

Food Interactions

None known.

Usual Dose

Starting dose—25 mg 2 times a day. Maintenance dose—generally, 300–450 mg a day. Dosage may be increased gradually to a daily maximum of 900 mg if required.

Overdosage

Symptoms of overdose are delirium, drowsiness, changes in heart rhythm, unusual excitement, nervousness, restlessness, hallucinations, excessive salivation, dizziness or fainting, slow or irregular breathing, and coma. Overdose victims must be taken to a hospital emergency room immediately. ALWAYS bring the prescription bottle or container.

Special Information

Clozapine may cause a fever during the first few weeks of treatment. Generally, the fever is not important, but it may occasionally be necessary to stop treatment due to persistent fever, a decision that would be made by your doctor.

Regular blood tests are necessary to monitor blood composition for any changes that might be caused by clozapine.

Call your doctor at once if you develop lethargy or weakness, a flu-like infection, sore throat, feelings of ill health, sweating, muscle rigidity, mental changes, irregular pulse or blood pressure, mouth ulcers, or dry mouth that lasts for more than 2 weeks. Dry mouth, a common side effect of clozapine, may be countered by using gum, candy, ice, or a saliva substitute such as Orex or Moi-Stir.

Do not stop taking clozapine without your doctor's knowledge and approval, because a gradual dosage reduction may be necessary to prevent side effects.

Avoid alcohol or any other nervous system depressant while taking clozapine.

Some of the side effects of clozapine—drowsiness, blurred vision, or seizures—may interfere with the performance of complex tasks like driving or operating hazardous equipment.

While taking clozapine, rapidly rising from a sitting or lying position may cause you to become dizzy or faint.

If you take clozapine twice a day and forget a dose, take it as soon as you remember. If it is almost time for your next dose, take 1 dose as soon as you remember and another in 5 or 6 hours, then go back to your regular schedule. If you take clozapine 3 times a day and forget a dose, take it as soon as you remember. If it is almost time for your next dose, take 1 dose as soon as you remember and another in 3 or 4 hours, then go back to your regular schedule. Never take a double dose.

Special Populations

Pregnancy/Breast-feeding
This drug should be used during pregnancy only if your doctor determines that it is absolutely necessary.

Clozapine may pass into breast milk. Nursing mothers who must take this drug should bottle-feed.

Seniors
Seniors may be more sensitive to the side effects of clozapine, such as dizziness on rapidly rising from a sitting or lying position, confusion, and excitability. Older men are also more likely to have prostate problems, a reason to be cautious with clozapine.

Generic Name

Codeine (KOE-deen) G

Brand Name
Only available in generic form.

The information in this profile also applies to the following drugs:

Generic Ingredient: Fentanyl
Actiq Lozenge on a Stick   Fentanyl Oralet (Lozenge)
Duragesic (Patch)

Generic Ingredient: Oxycodone

Oxycontin Controlled	OxyFAST Concentrate
Release Tablets	Percolone
Oxy/R	Roxicodone Solution

Type of Drug

Narcotic.

Prescribed for

Mild to moderate pain, and cough.

General Information

Codeine relieves pain and suppresses cough. The pain-relieving effect of 30 to 60 mg of codeine is equal to approximately 650 mg, or 2 tablets, of aspirin. Codeine may be less effective than aspirin for pain associated with inflammation because aspirin reduces inflammation and codeine does not. Codeine suppresses the cough reflex but does not cure the underlying cause of the cough. Other narcotic cough suppressants are stronger pain relievers, but codeine remains the best cough medication available.

Fentanyl is a potent pain reliever that can be substituted for other narcotic drugs. The patch form, which must be replaced about every 3 days, delivers fentanyl to the bloodstream at a steady rate. The lozenge has a shorter length of action than any other narcotic pain reliever, which make them useful when given to children before surgery because it provides doctors with the flexibility to obtain maximum benefit with minimal side effects. The lozenge on a stick is used for breakthrough cancer pain as a booster for people already taking narcotic pain relievers. These forms should only be used under controlled circumstances because of the risk of side effects or overdose. Low dosages of fentanyl relieve pain— larger amounts cause loss of consciousness and breathing difficulties.

Oxycodone is a narcotic used to control moderate to severe pain. Most people take it together with aspirin (Percodan) or acetaminophen (Percocet), but it can be used by itself. This is a potent pain reliever that carries a risk of addiction with continued use.

Cautions and Warnings

Do not take narcotics if you are **allergic** or **sensitive** to them. Use narcotics with extreme caution if you suffer from **asthma**

or other breathing problems. Long-term use of narcotics may cause drug dependence or **addiction.** Narcotics may make it difficult to monitor the progress of people who have suffered **head injuries.**

Possible Side Effects

▼ Most common: light-headedness, dizziness, sleepiness, nausea, vomiting, appetite loss, and sweating. If these occur, ask your doctor about lowering your dosage. Most of these side effects disappear if you lie down.

▼ Less common: euphoria (feeling "high"), headache, agitation, uncoordinated muscle movement, minor hallucinations, disorientation and visual disturbances, dry mouth, constipation, flushing of the face, rapid heartbeat, palpitations, faintness, urinary difficulties or hesitancy, reduced sex drive or impotence, itching, rash, anemia, lowered blood sugar, and yellowing of the skin or whites of the eyes. Narcotic analgesics may aggravate convulsions in those who have had them.

More serious side effects of codeine are shallow breathing or breathing difficulties.

Drug Interactions

• Avoid combining narcotics with alcohol, sleeping medications, tranquilizers, or other depressant drugs.

• Combining a narcotic pain reliever with any other medication that lowers blood pressure can lead to excessive blood-pressure lowering. Avoid this combination.

• Combining cimetidine with a narcotic pain reliever may cause confusion, disorientation, breathing difficulties, and seizure.

Food Interactions

Codeine may be taken with food to reduce upset stomach. The fentanyl patch may be used without regard to food.

Usual Dose

Codeine

Adult: 15–60 mg 4 times a day for relief of pain; 10–20 mg every few hours as needed to suppress cough.

Child: 1–2 mg per lb. of body weight in divided doses for relief of pain; 0.5–0.75 mg per lb. of body weight in divided doses to suppress cough.

Fentanyl Lozenge and Lozenge on a Stick
  Adult and Child: 100–400 mg. Dosage may be repeated up to 4 times daily. Allow the lozenge to dissolve in your mouth. DO NOT CHEW.

Fentanyl Patch
Apply to a clean and non-irritated patch of skin as directed, usually once every 3 days.

Overdosage

Symptoms include breathing difficulties or slowing of respiration, extreme tiredness progressing to stupor and then coma, pinpointed pupils, no response to pain stimulation, cold and clammy skin, slowing of heartbeat, lowering of blood pressure, convulsions, and cardiac arrest. The victim should be taken to a hospital emergency room immediately. ALWAYS bring the prescription bottle or container.

Special Information

Codeine is a respiratory depressant and affects the central nervous system (CNS), producing sleepiness, tiredness, or inability to concentrate. Be careful when driving or doing any task that requires concentration. Avoid alcohol.

Call your doctor if you develop breathing difficulties, constipation, dry mouth, or any bothersome or persistent side effect.

Apply the fentanyl patch only to non-irritated skin on a flat surface of the upper body. Hair at the application site should be clipped or cut, not shaved, before applying the patch. Do not use oils, soaps, lotions, alcohol, or anything else that might irritate the skin before applying the patch.

If you forget a dose of codeine, take it as soon as you remember. If it is almost time for your next dose, skip the one you forgot and continue with your regular schedule. Never take a double dose.

Special Populations

Pregnancy/Breast-feeding
Narcotics pass into the fetal circulation. Excessive use of them during pregnancy may cause drug dependence in new-

borns. Narcotics may also cause breathing difficulties in infants during delivery. Animal studies show that codeine may cause fetal harm. If given to a pregnant woman before cesarean section, fentanyl may cause drowsiness in newborns. When either of these drugs is considered crucial by your doctor, its potential benefits must be carefully weighed against its risks.

Narcotics pass into breast milk. Nursing mothers who must take codeine should bottle-feed.

Seniors

Seniors are more likely to be sensitive to side effects and should be treated with the smallest effective dosage.

Generic Name

Colchicine (KOLE-chih-sene) G

Brand Name

Only available in generic form.

Type of Drug

Antigout.

Prescribed for

Gouty arthritis; also prescribed for Mediterranean fever; chronic progressive multiple sclerosis; cirrhosis of the liver; biliary cirrhosis; Behçet's disease; pseudogout (a condition caused by calcium deposits); amyloidosis; very low blood-platelet count (also known as ITP); skin reactions, including scleroderma, psoriasis, and other conditions; and nerve disability associated with chronic progressive multiple sclerosis.

General Information

While no one knows exactly how colchicine works, it appears to help people with gout by reducing the inflammatory response to uric acid crystals that form inside joints and by interfering with the body's mechanism for making uric acid. Unlike drugs that affect uric acid levels, colchicine does not block the progression of gout to chronic gouty arthritis; it will, however, relieve the pain of acute attacks and lessen the frequency and severity of attacks. It has no effect on other kinds of pain.

Cautions and Warnings

Do not use colchicine if you suffer from any serious **blood, kidney, liver, stomach,** or **cardiac condition**.

Vomiting, abdominal pain, diarrhea, nausea, kidney damage, and **blood in the urine** may occur with colchicine, especially at maximum doses. This can worsen existing gastrointestinal (GI) or other conditions. Stop taking the medication and call your doctor if you develop one of these symptoms.

The **weakness** that people develop while taking colchicine is frequently related to high levels of colchicine in the blood caused by poor kidney function and improves without treatment 3 to 4 weeks after the drug is stopped. This reaction is often mistaken for other conditions.

Periodic **blood counts** should be done if you are taking colchicine for long periods of time.

Colchicine interferes with the absorption of vitamin B_{12} by affecting the lining of the GI tract.

Colchicine may affect the process of **sperm** generation in men.

The safety and effectiveness for **use by children** have not been established.

Possible Side Effects

▼ Common: vomiting, diarrhea, and abdominal pain may occur if you take maximum doses of colchicine for an acute gout attack. You may also experience severe diarrhea, kidney and blood-vessel damage, blood in the urine, and reduced urination.

▼ Less common: hair loss, rash, appetite loss, and muscle and nerve weakness.

Rare: with long-term colchicine therapy—reduced white-blood-cell and platelet counts, nerve inflammation, blood-clotting problems, rash, and other reactions. Colchicine may interfere with sperm formation.

Drug Interactions

• Colchicine interferes with the absorption of vitamin B_{12}.
• Colchicine may increase sensitivity to central-nervous-system depressants, such as tranquilizers and alcohol.

• The following drugs may reduce colchicine's effectiveness: anticancer drugs, bumetanide, diazoxide, thiazide diuretics, ethacrynic acid, furosemide, mecamylamine, pyrazinamide, and triamterene.

• Taking phenylbutazone with colchicine increases the risk of side effects.

Food Interactions

None known.

Usual Dose

Acute Gout Attack: 1–1.2 mg. This dose may be followed by 0.5–1.2 mg every 1–2 hours until pain is relieved or nausea, vomiting, or diarrhea occurs. The total dose needed to control pain and inflammation during an attack varies from 4–8 mg.

Gout Prevention: 0.5–1.8 mg daily. In mild cases, 0.5 mg or 0.6 mg may be taken 3–4 days a week.

Familial Mediterranean Fever: 1–3 mg a day.

Cirrhosis of the Liver: 1 mg a day for 5 days each week.

Biliary Cirrhosis: 0.6 mg 2 times a day.

Amyloidosis: 0.5 mg 1–2 times a day.

Behçet's Disease: 0.5–1.5 mg a day.

Pseudogout: 0.6 mg 2 times a day.

ITP: 1.2–1.8 mg a day for 2 weeks or more.

Scleroderma: 1 mg a day.

Other Skin Disorders: up to 1.8 mg a day, depending on the specific condition.

Overdosage

The lethal dose is estimated at 65 mg, although people have died after taking as little as 7 mg at once. Usually 1 to 3 days pass between the time that an overdose is taken and symptoms begin. Overdose symptoms start with nausea, vomiting, stomach pain, diarrhea—which may be severe and bloody—and burning sensations in the throat or stomach or on the skin. If you think you are experiencing overdose symptoms, contact your doctor immediately, or go to a hospital emergency room. ALWAYS bring the prescription bottle or container.

Special Information

Call your doctor if you develop rash, sore throat, fever, unusual bleeding or bruising, tiredness, or numbness or tingling. Seniors are more likely to develop drug side effects and should use this drug with caution.

Stop taking maximum doses of colchicine as soon as gout pain is relieved and reduce your dose to a maintenance level if your doctor has prescribed it for gout prevention. Stop taking the drug entirely and contact your doctor at the first sign of nausea, vomiting, stomach pain, or diarrhea.

If you forget a dose of colchicine, take it as soon as possible. If it is almost time for your next dose, skip the dose you forgot and continue with your regular schedule. Do not take a double dose.

Special Populations

Pregnancy/Breast-feeding
Colchicine can harm the fetus. Pregnant women should not take it unless the potential benefits clearly outweigh the risks.

It is not known if colchicine passes into breast milk. No problems with nursing infants are known, but nursing mothers who must take colchicine should consider bottle-feeding.

Seniors
Seniors are more likely to develop side effects and should use colchicine with caution.

Combivent see Ipratropium, page 524

Type of Drug
Contraceptives

Brand Names

Generic Ingredients: Low-Dose Estrogen + Low-Dose Progestin (Single-Phase Combination)

Alesse-21	Genora 1/50
Alesse-28	Levlite 21
Brevicon	Levlite 28
Genora 0.5/35	Loestrin 21 1/20
Genora 1/35	Loestrin 21 1.5/30

Loestrin Fe 1/20   Nelova 0.5/35E
Loestrin Fe 1.5/30   Nelova 1/35E
Modicon   Nelova 1/50M
Necon 0.5/35-21   Norethin 1/35E
Necon 0.5/35-28   Norethin 1/50M
Necon 1/35-21   Norinyl 1+35
Necon 1/35-28   Norinyl 1+50
Necon 1/50-21   Ortho-Novum 1/35
Necon 1/50-28   Ortho-Novum 1/50

Generic Ingredients: Low-Dose Estrogen + Intermediate Dose Progestin
Demulen 1/35   Lo-Ovral
Desogen   Lovlen
Levora 0.15/30-21   Nordette
Levora 0.15/30-28   Ortho-Cept
Loestrin 21 1.5/30   Ortho-Cyclen
Loestrin Fe 1.5/30   Zovia 1/35E

Generic Ingredients: Intermediate-Dose Estrogen + Low-Dose Progestin (Single-Phase Combination)
Ovcon-35   Ovcon-50   Ovral

Generic Ingredients: Intermediate-Dose Estrogen + Intermediate-Dose Progestin (Single-Phase Combination)
Demulen 1/50   Zovia 1/50

Generic Ingredients: Intermediate-Dose Estrogen + Low-Dose Progestin (2-Phase Combination)
Janest-28   Necon 10/11–21
Mircette   Necon 10/11–28
Nelova 10/11   Ortho-Novum 10/11

Generic Ingredients: Low-Dose Estrogen + Low-Dose Progestin (3-Phase Combination)
Ortho-Novum 7/7/7   Tri-Norinyl
Tri-Levlen   Triphasil
Tri-Levlen 28   Trivora-28

Generic Ingredients: Intermediate Dose Estrogen + Low Dose Progestin (3-Phase Combination)
Ortho Tri-Cyclen

Generic Ingredients: Intermediate Dose Estrogen + Intermediate Dose Progestin
Estrostep 21   Estrostep Fe

Generic Ingredient: Low-Dose Progestin (Mini-Pill)
Ovrette

Generic Ingredient: High-Dose Progestin (Mini-Pill)
Micronor   Nor-Q.D.

Generic Ingredient: Progestin (Implant)
Norplant System

Generic Ingredient: Progestin (Intrauterine Insert)
Progestasert

Generic Ingredient: High-Dose Progestin (Emergency Contraceptive)
Plan B

Generic Ingredient: High-Dose Progestin + Ethinyl Estradiol (Emergency Contraceptive)
Preven

Prescribed for

Prevention of pregnancy, endometriosis, excessive menstruation, cyclic withdrawal bleeding, and acne.

General Information

Oral contraceptives ("the pill") are synthetic hormones containing either progestin or a progestin-estrogen combination. These drugs are similar to natural female hormones, which cannot be used as contraceptives because very large dosages would be required. Synthetic hormones are more potent and are effective at smaller dosages. Oral contraceptives work by preventing sperm from reaching the unfertilized egg, preventing the implantation of a fertilized egg in the uterus, or preventing ovulation (the release of an unfertilized egg from the ovaries). They prevent acne by balancing hormone levels.

When properly used, oral contraceptives can be 97% to 99% effective at preventing pregnancy. These products vary in their effectiveness and in the amount and type of estrogen or progestin used. The side effects of these drugs tend to increase with the amount of hormone they contain. While low hormone dosages are preferred, contraceptives with the smallest amounts of estrogen may be less effective in some women than others.

Single-phase products provide constant levels of estrogen and progestin throughout the entire month-long pill cycle. In 2-phase combinations, the amount of estrogen remains at a steady low level throughout the cycle, while progestin levels increase and then decrease. This variation in progestin allows normal changes to take place in the uterus. Three-phase products are the newest estrogen-progestin combinations. Throughout the cycle, estrogen levels remain the same while those of progestin change to create a 3-part wave pattern. This 3-part pattern is meant to simulate the normal hormone cycle and reduce breakthrough bleeding. Breakthrough bleeding may occur with the older combination products from day 8 through 16 of the cycle. The amount of estrogen in 3-phase products is considered low.

The mini-pill, a progestin-only product, may cause irregular menstrual cycles and may be less effective than estrogen-progestin combinations. Mini-pills may be recommended to older women or women who should avoid estrogens (see "Cautions and Warnings").

Levonorgestrel, a progestin, is used in implants that provide effective contraception for up to 5 years after surgical implantation under the skin of the upper arm. Levonorgestrel implants should be replaced at least once every 5 years. They can be removed at any time, reversing the contraceptive effect. The intrauterine insert provides a continuous flow of progestin, and effective contraception, for about 1 year. The implant and intrauterine systems contain the same hormone found in the mini-pill and are associated with many of the same side effects and precautions as oral contraceptives.

Emergency contraceptives contain high doses of estrogen and progestin. They are intended for use after contraceptive failure or unprotected intercourse. They should never be taken by a pregnant woman.

Oral contraceptives in any form are associated with risks. These risks are greatest in women over age 35 who smoke and have high blood pressure.

Cautions and Warnings

You should not use contraceptive drugs if you are or might be **pregnant,** have had **blood clots** in veins or arteries, **stroke,** any **blood-coagulation disorder,** known or suspected **cancer** of the breast or sex organs, **liver cancer,** or **irregular or very light menstrual periods**. Contraceptive drugs may cause **eye problems**. Call your doctor at once if you develop visual difficulties of any kind.

The risks of using contraceptive drugs increase if you are **physically immobile** or have **asthma; cardiac insufficiency; epilepsy; migraine; kidney problems;** a strong **family history of breast cancer;** benign **breast disease; diabetes; endometriosis; gallbladder disease** or **gallstones; liver problems,** including jaundice; **high blood cholesterol; high blood pressure; estrogen or progestin intolerance; depression; tuberculosis;** or **varicose veins.**

There is an increased risk of **heart attack** in women who have taken oral contraceptives for more than 10 years, or who are between age 40 and 49 and have other coronary risk factors such as smoking, obesity, high blood pressure, diabetes, and high blood cholesterol. This risk remains even after the medication is stopped. Smokers who use oral contraceptives are 5 times more likely to have a heart attack than nonsmokers taking contraceptives, and 10 to 12 times more likely to have a heart attack than nonsmokers who do not use the pill.

Women with a history of **headaches, high blood pressure,** or **varicose veins** should avoid estrogen-containing products, as should older women and those who have experienced estrogen side effects.

Oral contraceptives may mask the onset of **menopause.**

Progestin-only products are associated with an increased risk of **blood-clotting problems.**

Possible Side Effects

▼ Common: Common side effects often result from using a product that is poorly suited to your body chemistry. Determining the right amount and type of hormone often minimizes these effects. If you are taking too much estrogen, you may experience nausea, bloating, high blood pressure, migraine, or breast tenderness. Too little estrogen may cause early or mid-cycle breakthrough bleeding, spotting, or reduced periodic flow. Too much progestin is associated with weight gain and increased appetite, tiredness or weakness, low periodic flow, acne, depression, breast regression, and oily scalp. Too little progestin may cause late breakthrough bleeding, excessive periodic bleeding, or missed periods.

Possible Side Effects *(continued)*

▼ Less common: abdominal cramps, infertility after discontinuance of the drug, breast tenderness, weight change, headache, rash, vaginal itching and burning, general vaginal infection, nervousness, dizziness, depression, cataract, changes in sex drive, hair loss, and increased sensitivity to the sun.

▼ Rare: Women who take oral contraceptives are more likely to develop several serious conditions, including blood clots in the deep veins, stroke, heart attack, liver cancer, gallbladder disease, and high blood pressure. Women who smoke cigarettes are at much higher risk for some of these adverse effects.

Drug Interactions

• Rifampin, barbiturates, phenylbutazone, phenytoin, ampicillin, neomycin, penicillin, tetracycline, chloramphenicol, sulfa drugs, griseofulvin, nitrofurantoin, protease inhibitor drugs for AIDS, tranquilizers, and antimigraine drugs make oral contraceptives less effective. Use backup birth control while taking these medications together.

• Oral contraceptives may elevate blood levels of benzodiazepine tranquilizers and sleeping pills, caffeine, metoprolol, corticosteroids, theophylline drugs, and tricyclic antidepressants, increasing the risk of side effects.

• Oral contraceptives may increase the toxic liver effects of acetaminophen and reduce the drug's effectiveness. Oral contraceptives may increase or decrease the effect of anticoagulant (blood-thinning) drugs. Discuss the risks of this combination with your doctor.

• Oral contraceptives may decrease the effects of salicylate pain relievers including aspirin, clofibrate, lorazepam, oxazepam, and temazepam.

• Oral contraceptives may increase blood-cholesterol levels and interfere with blood tests for thyroid function and blood sugar.

Food Interactions

None known.

Usual Dose

Single-Phase, 2-Phase, and 3-Phase Combinations: The first day of bleeding is day 1 of the menstrual cycle. Beginning on the 5th day of the cycle, take 1 pill a day for 20–21 days according to the number of pills supplied by the manufacturer. If menstrual flow has not begun 7 days after taking the last pill, begin the next month's cycle of pills. Some manufacturers recommend starting the pills on a Sunday to make it easy to remember to take them. In this case, start taking your pills on the first Sunday after your period begins. If menstruation begins on a Sunday, take the first pill that day.

Progestin-Only Mini Pill: Take 1 pill every day.

Emergency Contraception: Emergency contraceptive kits have only a few pills. Take half the pills (1 or 2 depending on the brand you use) within 72 hours of unprotected sex. Take the rest of the pills 12 hours after the first dose.

Overdosage

An overdose may cause nausea and withdrawal bleeding in adult women. Overdose victims should be taken to a hospital emergency room. ALWAYS bring the prescription package.

Special Information

Use backup birth control to prevent pregnancy in the first 3 weeks after you begin taking oral contraceptives.

Take your pill at the same time each day to establish a routine and ensure maximum contraceptive protection.

Call your doctor immediately if you experience severe abdominal pain; severe or sudden headache; pain in the chest, groin, or leg, especially the calf; sudden slurring of speech; changes in vision; weakness, numbness, or pain in the arms or legs; coughing up of blood; loss of coordination; or shortness of breath. These symptoms may require emergency treatment.

Other problems that may require medical attention are bulging eyes; changes in vaginal bleeding; fainting; frequent or painful urination; a gradual increase in blood pressure; breast lumps or secretions; depression; yellowing of the skin or whites of the eyes; rash; redness or irritation; upper abdominal swelling, pain, or tenderness; an unusual or dark-colored mole; thick, white vaginal discharge; or vaginal itching or tenderness.

See your doctor for a check-up every 6 to 12 months.

Some manufacturers include 7 inert or iron pills in their packaging to be taken on days when the drug is not taken. This makes it easier for women to stay on schedule with their pills. The 7 pills bridge the gap between contraceptive cycles and allow women to take 1 pill every day without stopping.

For single- or 2-phase combinations: If you forget to take a pill for 1 day, take 2 pills the following day. If you miss 2 consecutive days, take 2 pills for the next 2 days. Then return to your schedule of 1 pill a day. If you miss 3 consecutive days, do not take any pills for the next 7 days and use another form of contraception; then start a new cycle.

For 3-phase combinations: If you forget to take a pill for 1 day, take 2 pills the following day. If you miss 2 consecutive days, take 2 pills for the next 2 days. Then return to your schedule of 1 pill a day. If you forget to take a pill for 3 days in a row, stop taking the drug and use an alternate means of contraception until your period starts. ALWAYS use a backup contraceptive method for the remainder of your cycle if you forget even 1 pill of a 3-phase combination.

Missing a pill reduces your protection. If you keep forgetting to take your pills, you must use another birth control method.

If you take drugs that reduce the effectiveness of oral contraceptives (see "Drug Interactions"), use a backup contraceptive method during that cycle to prevent accidental pregnancy.

Good dental hygiene is essential while taking contraceptive drugs. See your dentist regularly and brush and floss carefully because contraceptives may increase the risk of an oral infection.

Oral contraceptives may increase your sensitivity to the sun.

Wearing contact lenses may be uncomfortable while taking an oral contraceptive because the pills can cause minor changes in the shape of your eyes.

All oral contraceptive prescriptions come with a "patient package insert." It gives detailed information about the drug and is required by federal law.

Special Populations

Pregnancy/Breast-feeding

Oral contraceptives cause birth defects and may interfere with fetal development. They are not safe for use during pregnancy.

Oral contraceptives pass into breast milk and reduce the amount of milk produced. Nursing mothers who must use any of these drugs should bottle-feed.

Seniors

These products are not intended for women who have completed menopause.

Type of Drug

Corticosteroids (kor-tih-koe-STER-oids)

━━━━━━━━━━━━━━━━━━━━━━━━━━━━━━━━━━━━━━━

Brand Names

Generic Ingredient: Betamethasone
Celestone

Generic Ingredient: Cortisone Acetate 🄶
Cortone Acetate

Generic Ingredient: Dexamethasone 🄶
Decadron   Dexone
Dexameth   Hexadrol

Generic Ingredient: Hydrocortisone 🄶
Cortef   Cortifoam
Cortenema   Hydrocortone

Generic Ingredient: Methylprednisolone 🄶
Medrol

Generic Ingredient: Prednisolone 🄶
Delta-Cortef   Prelone
Pediapred 🅂 🄰

Generic Ingredient: Prednisone 🄶
Deltasone   Prednicen-M
Liquid Pred   Prednisone Intensol
Meticorten   Sterapred
Orasone   Sterapred DS
Panasol-S

Generic Ingredient: Triamcinolone 🄶
Aristocort   Kenacort
Atolone

Prescribed for

A wide variety of disorders from rash to cancer, including adrenal disease, adrenal hormone replacement, bursitis, arthritis, severe skin reactions including psoriasis and other rashes, severe or disabling allergies, asthma, drug or serum sickness, severe respiratory diseases including pneumonitis, blood disorders, gastrointestinal (GI) disease including ulcerative colitis, and inflammation of the nerves, heart, or other organs. Dexamethasone is also used to treat mountain sickness, vomiting, bronchial disease in premature babies, excessive hairiness, and hearing loss associated with bacterial meningitis. Dexamethasone has been used to detect and manage depression, but its value is unproven.

General Information

Produced by the adrenal gland, natural corticosteroids are hormones that affect almost every body system. The major differences among corticosteroid drugs are potency and variation in secondary effects. Doctor preference and past experience with a corticosteroid usually determine which drug to prescribe for a specific disease.

Cautions and Warnings

If you are **allergic** to one corticosteroid, you are probably allergic to all corticosteroids and should avoid using them.

Corticosteroids may mask symptoms of an **infection**. Because these drugs compromise the immune system, new infections may occur during corticosteroid treatment; when this happens, a relatively minor infection that would respond to ordinary treatment can turn serious. Corticosteroids may impair immune response to **hepatitis B,** prolonging recovery. They may reactivate dormant **amebiasis** (an amoebic infection usually acquired in the tropics). Corticosteroids should not be taken if you have a **fungal blood infection,** because they can allow the infection to spread more easily. They should be used with caution by people with **tuberculosis**.

Long-term use of any corticosteroid may increase the risk of developing **cataracts, glaucoma,** or **eye infections**, especially viral or fungal.

When stopping a corticosteroid, dosage must be reduced gradually under a doctor's supervision—otherwise you may experience **adrenal gland failure**.

If you are taking large corticosteroid doses, you should not receive any **live virus vaccine** because corticosteroids interfere with the body's reaction to the vaccine.

Hydrocortisone and cortisone may lead to **high blood pressure**. Other corticosteroids are less likely to affect blood pressure.

Corticosteroids should be used with caution if you have severe **kidney disease**.

High-dose or long-term corticosteroid therapy may aggravate or worsen **stomach ulcers**. This may occur when total dosage reaches 1000 mg of prednisone, 150 mg of betamethasone or dexamethasone, 5000 mg of cortisone, 4000 mg of hydrocortisone, 1000 mg of prednisolone, or 800 mg of triamcinolone or methylprednisolone.

People who have recently stopped taking a corticosteroid and are going through a period of **stress** may need small doses of a rapid-acting corticosteroid, such as hydrocortisone to get them through this period. Call your doctor if you think you might be experiencing this kind of stress reaction.

Use corticosteroids with caution if you have had a recent **heart attack** or have **ulcerative colitis, heart failure, high blood pressure, blood-clotting tendencies, thrombophlebitis, osteoporosis, antibiotic-resistant infections, Cushing's disease, myasthenia gravis, metastatic cancer, diabetes, underactive thyroid disease, cirrhosis of the liver,** or **seizure disorders.**

Corticosteroid psychosis (symptoms include euphoria or feeling "high," delirium, sleeplessness, mood swings, personality changes, and severe depression) may develop in people taking dosages greater than 40 mg a day of prednisone. These symptoms may also develop with other corticosteroids taken in equivalent doses (see "Usual Dose" for relative equivalencies). Symptoms of corticosteroid psychosis usually develop within 15 to 30 days of beginning treatment. These symptoms may also be linked to other factors—women and those with a family history of psychosis are more at risk.

Corticosteroids can cause **loss of calcium,** which may result in bone fractures and aseptic necrosis of the femoral and humoral heads (a condition in which the large bones in the hip degenerate from loss of calcium).

Prednisone may aggravate **emotional instability**.

Corticosteroids do not cure multiple sclerosis (MS) or slow its progression, though they may speed recovery from attacks of the disease.

Corticosteroid products often contain **tartrazine dyes** and **sulfite preservatives**. Many people are allergic to these chemicals.

Possible Side Effects

▼ Most common: upset stomach, possibly leading to stomach or duodenal ulcer.

▼ Common: water retention, heart failure, potassium loss, muscle weakness, loss of muscle mass, slowed healing of wounds, black-and-blue marks, increased sweating, allergic rash, itching, convulsions, dizziness, and headache.

▼ Less common: irregular menstruation; slowed growth in children, particularly after lengthy periods of corticosteroid treatment; adrenal or pituitary gland suppression; diabetes; drug sensitivity or allergic reactions; blood clots; insomnia; weight gain; increased appetite; nausea; feeling unwell; euphoria; mood swings; personality changes; and severe depression.

Drug Interactions

• Tell your doctor if you are taking any oral anticoagulant (blood-thinning) drug. If you begin taking a corticosteroid, your anticoagulant dosage may have to be adjusted.

• Combining a corticosteroid and a diuretic such as hydrochlorothiazide may cause loss of blood potassium. Low blood potassium may increase the side effects of digitalis drugs.

• Oral contraceptives (the "pill"), estrogen, erythromycin, azithromycin, clarithromycin, and ketoconazole may increase the risk of corticosteroid side effects.

• Barbiturates, aminoglutethimide, phenytoin and other hydantoin anticonvulsants, rifampin, ephedrine, colestipol, and cholestyramine may reduce the effectiveness of corticosteroids.

• Corticosteroids may decrease the effects of aspirin and other salicylates, growth hormones, and isoniazid.

• Combining a corticosteroid and a theophylline drug may require a dosage adjustment of either or both drugs.

• Corticosteroids may interfere with laboratory tests. Tell your doctor if you are taking any of these drugs so that tests are properly analyzed.

Food Interactions

Take corticosteroids with food or a small amount of antacid to avoid stomach upset. If stomach upset continues, notify your doctor.

Usual Dose

Betamethasone: starting dosage—0.6–7.2 mg a day. Maintenance dosage—0.6–7.2 mg a day.

Cortisone: starting dosage—25–300 mg a day. Maintenance dosage—25–300 mg a day.

Dexamethasone: 0.75–9 mg a day. Daily dosage sometimes exceeds 9 mg. A temporary dosage increase may be necessary if you are experiencing emotional stress. In alternate-day therapy, twice the usual daily dose is taken every other day.

Hydrocortisone: 20–240 mg a day.

Methylprednisolone: starting dosage—4–48 mg or more a day. Maintenance dosage varies. A temporary dosage increase may be necessary if you are experiencing emotional stress. In alternate-day therapy, twice the usual daily dose is taken every other day.

Prednisone and Prednisolone: 5–60 mg a day. Daily dosage sometimes exceeds 60 mg. A temporary dosage increase may be necessary if you are experiencing emotional stress. In alternate-day therapy, twice the usual daily dose is taken every other day.

Equivalent doses: Using 5 mg of prednisone as the basis for comparison, equivalent doses of other corticosteroids are 0.6 mg–0.75 mg of betamethasone, 25 mg of cortisone, 0.75 mg of dexamethasone, 20 mg of hydrocortisone, 4 mg of methylprednisolone, 5 mg of prednisolone, and 4 mg of triamcinolone.

Overdosage

Symptoms of overdose are anxiety, depression or stimulation, stomach bleeding, increased blood sugar, high blood pressure, and water retention. The victim should be taken to a hospital emergency room immediately. ALWAYS bring the prescription bottle or container.

Special Information

Do not stop taking this medication without your doctor's knowledge. Suddenly stopping any corticosteroid drug may have severe consequences; the dosage must be gradually reduced by your doctor.

Call your doctor if you develop unusual weight gain, black or tarry stools, swelling of the feet or legs, muscle weakness, vomiting of blood, menstrual irregularity, prolonged sore throat, fever, cold or infection, appetite loss, nausea and vomiting, diarrhea, weight loss, weakness, dizziness, or low blood sugar.

If you take several doses a day and forget a dose, take the dose you forgot as soon as possible. If it is almost time for your next dose, skip the one you forgot and double the next dose. If you take 1 dose a day and forget a dose, skip the dose you forgot and continue with your regular schedule. Do not take a double dose.

If you take a corticosteroid every other day and forget a dose, take it immediately if you remember it in the morning of your regularly scheduled day. If it is much later in the day, skip the dose you forgot and take it the following morning, then go back to your regular schedule. Do not take a double dose.

Special Populations

Pregnancy/Breast-feeding

Studies have shown that long-term corticosteroid therapy at high dosages may cause birth defects, as may chronic corticosteroid use during the first 3 months of pregnancy. When this drug is considered crucial by your doctor, its potential benefits must be carefully weighed against its risks.

Corticosteroids taken by mouth may pass into breast milk. Most nursing mothers who must take a corticosteroid should bottle-feed, though low dosages of some of these drugs may be taken for short periods while breast-feeding. Consult your doctor.

Seniors

Seniors are more likely to develop high blood pressure while taking an oral corticosteroid. Older women are more susceptible to osteoporosis (a condition characterized by loss of bone mass due to depletion of minerals, especially calcium) associated with high dosages. Lower dosages are just as effective in seniors and cause fewer side effects.

Type of Drug

Corticosteroids, Eye Products

(kor-tih-koe-STER-oids)

Brand Names

Generic Ingredient: Dexamethasone G
AK-Dex   Maxidex
Decadron Phosphate

Generic Ingredient: Fluorometholone G
Flarex   FML Forte
Fluor-Op   FML S.O.P.
FML

Generic Ingredient: Loteprednol Etabonate
Alrex   Lotemax

Generic Ingredient: Medrysone
HMS

Generic Ingredient: Prednisolone
AK-Pred   Inflamase Mild
Econopred   Pred Mild
Econopred Plus   Pred Forte
Inflamase Forte

Generic Ingredient: Rimexolone
Vexol

Prescribed for

Allergic and inflammatory eye conditions and to speed healing after eye surgery or injury.

General Information

Corticosteroid eye products are prescribed for general relief of inflammation due to allergy and other causes. They are also used after eye surgery or serious eye injury to aid the healing process by reducing the natural inflammatory process. Very severe eye conditions that do not respond to these products may require treatment with corticosteroid drugs taken by mouth. Fluorometholone, medrysone, and prednisolone (up to 0.125%) are preferred for long-term treatment because they are least likely to raise the fluid pressure inside the eye. Corticosteroid eye products have not been widely studied in children, though fluorometholone has been proven safe for use in children age 2 and over.

Cautions and Warnings

Do not use any of these products if you are **allergic** or **sensitive** to corticosteroids. These products should be used with caution if you have a **fungal, herpes, tuberculosis, or viral infection of the eye,** or have **cataracts, glaucoma,** or **diabetes**. Do not use any of these products without your doctor's knowledge.

Long-term use of these products can lead to **eye damage,** including glaucoma, infection, and nerve damage.

Do not use any of these products in **children** without consulting a doctor.

Possible Side Effects

▼ Rare: watery eyes; glaucoma; optic nerve damage; gradual blurring, reduction, or loss of vision; eye pain; nausea; vomiting; eye infections; and eye burning, stinging, or redness.

Drug Interactions

• Corticosteroids applied to the eye may interfere with the effect of antiglaucoma drugs.

• The risk of raising fluid pressure inside the eye is increased when corticosteroid eye products are taken with anticholinergic drugs, especially atropine, over a long period of time.

Food Interactions

None known.

Usual Dose

Eyedrops: 1–2 drops several times a day.

Eye Ointment: Place a thin strip of ointment into the affected eye several times a day.

Overdosage

Swallowing a container of corticosteroid eyedrops or ointment usually does not produce serious effects. Call your local poison center or a hospital emergency room for more information.

Special Information

If you forget to administer a dose, do so as soon as you remember. If it is almost time for your next dose, skip the one you forgot and continue with your regular schedule.

To prevent infection, keep the eyedropper from touching your fingers, eyelids, or any surface. Wait at least 5 minutes before using any other eyedrops.

Special Populations

Pregnancy/Breast-feeding

Using large amounts of corticosteroid eyedrops during pregnancy may affect the adrenal gland of the fetus. When your doctor considers one of these products crucial, its potential benefits must be carefully weighed against its risks.

Oral corticosteroids pass into breast milk, but it is not known if this is also true of corticosteroid eyedrops. Nursing mothers who must use one of these medications should consider bottle-feeding.

Seniors

Seniors may use these products without special precaution.

Type of Drug

Corticosteroids, Inhalers
(kor-tih-koe-STER-oids)

Brand Names

Generic Ingredient: Beclomethasone Dipropionate
Beclovent
Vanceril
Vanceril Double Strength

Generic Ingredient: Budesonide
Pulmicort Turbohaler

Generic Ingredient: Flunisolide
AeroBid   AeroBid-M

Generic Ingredient: Fluticasone Propionate
Flovent   Flovent Rotadisk

Generic Ingredient: Triamcinolone Acetonide
Azmacort   Nasacort

Prescribed for

Chronic asthma and bronchial disease.

General Information

Corticosteroid inhalers relieve the symptoms associated with asthma and bronchial disease by reducing inflammation of bronchial mucous membranes, making it easier to breathe. Corticosteroid inhalers produce the same treatment effect as oral corticosteroids, with some important differences. Because inhalers deliver the drug directly to the lungs, smaller dosages can be used. They also have fewer side effects because little of the drug reaches the bloodstream. Corticosteroid inhalers can prevent asthma attacks if used regularly but do not relieve them once they start.

Cautions and Warnings

Do not use any of these drugs if you are **allergic** to corticosteroids.

Corticosteroid inhalers should not be used as the primary treatment of **severe asthma**. They are recommended only for people who take prednisone or another oral corticosteroid, or for people who do not respond to other asthma drugs.

Combining an oral corticosteroid with a corticosteroid inhaler may cause **pituitary gland suppression**.

During a period of severe **stress,** you may have to switch to an oral corticosteroid if the inhaler does not control your asthma. During periods of stress or a severe asthmatic attack, people who have stopped using an inhaler should ask their doctors about taking an oral corticosteroid.

In people with asthma, death from **adrenal gland failure** has occurred during and after switching from an oral corticosteroid to an inhaler. Adrenal function is impaired for several months after the switch.

Corticosteroid inhalers may be associated with immediate or delayed **drug reactions,** including breathing difficulties, rash, and bronchospasm.

Corticosteroid inhalers are not recommended for **children under age 6.**

Possible Side Effects

▼ Most common: dry mouth, hoarseness, rash, and bronchospasm.

▼ Rare: cough, wheezing, and facial swelling. Cough and wheezing are probably caused by an ingredient in the inhaler other than the corticosteroid itself. Newer administration systems that omit this ingredient may minimize the problem.

Food and Drug Interactions

None known.

Usual Dose

Beclomethasone
Adult and Child (age 13 and over): 2 inhalations (84 mcg) 3–4 times a day, or 4 inhalations twice a day. People with severe asthma may take up to 16 inhalations a day.
Child (age 6–12): 1–2 inhalations 3–4 times a day.

Budesonide
Adult: starting dose—200–400 mcg twice a day. Do not exceed 800 mcg twice a day.
Child (age 6 and over): 200 mcg twice a day. Do not exceed 400 mcg twice a day.

Flunisolide
Adult and Child (age 16 and over): 2 inhalations (500 mcg) morning and evening. Do not exceed 8 inhalations a day.
Child (age 6–15): 2 inhalations (500 mcg) morning and evening. Do not exceed 4 inhalations a day.

Fluticasone Inhalation
Adult and Child (age 12 and over): 88–880 mcg twice a day.

Fluticasone Rotadisk
Adult and Child (age 12 and over): 100–1000 mcg twice a day.
Child (age 4–11): 50–100 mcg twice a day.

Triamcinolone

Adult and Child (age 13 and over): 2 inhalations (200 mcg) 3–4 times a day. Do not exceed 16 inhalations a day without your doctor's knowledge.

Child (age 6–12): 1–2 inhalations (100–200 mcg) 3–4 times a day. Do not exceed 12 inhalations a day.

Overdosage

Serious adverse effects are unlikely. Excessive use of large amounts of an inhaled corticosteroid may cause overdose symptoms and require gradually stopping the drug. Call your local poison control center or a hospital emergency room for more information.

Special Information

People using both a corticosteroid inhaler and a bronchodilator, such as albuterol, should use the bronchodilator first, wait a few minutes, and then use the corticosteroid inhaler. This allows more corticosteroid to be absorbed.

These drugs are for preventive therapy only and will not affect an asthma attack. Inhaled corticosteroids must be taken regularly, as directed. Wait at least 1 minute between inhalations.

To properly take this medication, thoroughly shake the inhaler if it is one that must be shaken. Take a drink of water to moisten your throat. Place the inhaler 2 finger-widths away from your mouth and tilt your head back slightly. While activating the inhaler, take a slow, deep breath for 3 to 5 seconds, then hold your breath for about 10 seconds, and finally breathe out slowly. Allow at least 1 minute between puffs. Rinse your mouth after each use to reduce dry mouth and hoarseness.

If you forget to administer a dose, do so as soon as you remember. If it is almost time for your next dose, skip the dose you forgot and continue with your regular schedule. Do not take a double dose.

Special Populations

Pregnancy/Breast-feeding

Corticosteroids may cause birth defects or interfere with fetal development. When any of these drugs is considered crucial by your doctor, its potential benefits must be carefully weighed against its risks.

It is not known if inhaled corticosteroids pass into breast milk, though oral corticosteroids do. Nursing mothers who must take an inhaled corticosteroid should consider bottle-feeding.

Seniors

Seniors may use corticosteroid inhalers without special restriction. Tell your doctor if you have bone or bowel disease, colitis, diabetes, glaucoma, fungal or herpes infections, high blood pressure, high blood cholesterol, an underactive thyroid, or heart, kidney, or liver disease.

Type of Drug

Corticosteroids, Nasal
(kor-tih-koe-STER-oids)

Brand Names

Generic Ingredient: Beclomethasone Dipropionate

Beconase	Vancenase AQ
Beconase AQ	Vancenase Pockethaler
Vancenase	

Generic Ingredient: Budesonide
Rhinocort

Generic Ingredient: Flunisolide

Nasalide	Nasarel

Generic Ingredient: Fluticasone Propionate
Flonase

Generic Ingredient: Mometasone Furoate Monohydrate
Nasonex

Generic Ingredient: Triamcinolone Acetonide

Nasacort	Nasacort AQ

Prescribed for

Rhinitis (nasal inflammation) associated with seasonal or chronic allergy and other causes; also used to prevent recurrence of nasal polyps.

General Information

Nasal corticosteroids are used to treat severe symptoms of seasonal allergy that have not responded to other drugs such as decongestants. They work by reducing inflammation of the mucous membranes that line the nasal passages, making it easier to breathe. These drugs may take several days to produce an effect. Fluticasone and triamcinolone are approved only for allergic rhinitis; other nasal corticosteroids are approved for both allergic and non-allergic rhinitis.

Cautions and Warnings

Do not use a nasal corticosteroid if you are **allergic** to any of its ingredients. Rarely, serious and life-threatening drug-sensitivity reactions have occurred.

Combining prednisone or another oral corticosteroid with a nasal corticosteroid may cause **pituitary gland suppression,** although nasal corticosteroids alone rarely cause this problem.

Rarely, *Candida* (yeast) infections of the nose and throat develop.

During a period of severe **stress,** you may have to switch to an oral corticosteroid drug if the nasal form does not control your symptoms.

Possible Side Effects

▼ Most common: mild irritation of the nose, nasal passages, and throat; burning; stinging; dryness; and headache.

▼ Less common: light-headedness, nausea, nosebleed or bloody mucus, unusual nasal congestion, bronchial asthma, sneezing attacks, runny nose, throat discomfort, and loss of the sense of taste.

▼ Rare: ulcers of the nasal passages, watery eyes, sore throat, vomiting, hypersensitivity reactions (symptoms include itching, rash, swelling, bronchospasms, and breathing difficulties), nasal infection, wheezing, perforation of the wall between the nostrils, and increased eye pressure.

Possible Side Effects *(continued)*

Very rarely, deaths caused by failure of the adrenal gland have occurred in people taking adrenal corticosteroid tablets or syrup who were switched to a nasal corticosteroid. This is a rare complication and usually results from stopping the liquid or tablets suddenly instead of gradually.

Food and Drug Interactions

None known.

Usual Dose

Beclomethasone
   Adult and Child (age 13 and over): 1 spray (42 mcg) in each nostril 2–4 times a day.
   Child (age 6–12): 1 spray (42 mcg) in each nostril 3 times a day.

Budesonide
   Adult and Child (age 6 and over): 2 sprays (64 mcg) in each nostril morning and evening, or 4 sprays in the morning.
   Child (under age 6): not recommended.

Flunisolide
   Adult and Child (age 15 and over): 2 sprays (50 mcg) in each nostril 2 times a day to start; may be increased up to 8 sprays a day in each nostril.
   Child (age 6–14): 1 spray (25 mcg) in each nostril 3 times a day, or 2 sprays in each nostril 2 times a day.

Fluticasone
   Adult: 2 sprays (100 mcg) in each nostril once a day or divided in 2 doses, to start. Dosage may be reduced in half in a few days, if tolerated.
   Child (age 4 and over): 1 spray (50 mcg) in each nostril once a day; may be increased to 2 sprays a day in each nostril, if needed.
   Child (under age 4): not recommended.

Mometasone
   Adult and Child (age 12 and over): 2 sprays (100 mcg) in

each nostril once a day; may be increased to 4 sprays a day in each nostril.

Triamcinolone

Adult and Child (age 13 and over): 2 sprays (220 mcg) in each nostril once a day; may be increased to 4 sprays a day in each nostril.

Child (age 6–12): 1 (Nasacort AQ) or 2 (Nasacort) sprays in each nostril once a day; may be increased to 2 sprays a day in each nostril, if needed.

Child (under age 6): not recommended.

Overdosage

Serious adverse effects are unlikely after accidental ingestion. Excessive use of large amounts of nasal corticosteroids may cause overdose symptoms and require gradual discontinuation of the drug. Call your local poison control center or a hospital emergency room for more information.

Special Information

It may be necessary to clear your nasal passages with a nasal decongestant before using a nasal corticosteroid to allow it to reach the mucous membranes.

Some of these drugs take 10 to 14 days to start working. Beclomethasone, budesonide, and triamcinolone work faster, in 3 to 7 days; in some cases, triamcinolone provides relief in 12 hours. Flunisolide may take up to 3 weeks. Do not use any of these drugs continuously for more than 3 weeks unless you have experienced a definite benefit.

If you are using more than one spray at a time, wait at least 1 minute between sprays.

Nasal corticosteroids may cause irritation and drying of mucous membranes in the nose. Call your doctor if this effect persists or if symptoms get worse.

Rarely, nasal *Candida* infections develop in people using a nasal corticosteroid. These infections may require treatment with an antifungal drug, as well as the discontinuance of the nasal corticosteroid.

People using a nasal corticosteroid to prevent the return of nasal polyps after surgery may experience nosebleeds because the drug can slow healing of the wound.

If you forget to administer a dose, do so as soon as you remember. If it is almost time for your next dose, skip the dose you forgot and continue with your regular schedule. Do not take a double dose.

Special Populations

Pregnancy/Breast-feeding

Taking large amounts of corticosteroids during pregnancy may slow fetal growth. While the small amount of drug absorbed into the blood after nasal application is unlikely to have any effect, consult your doctor before taking any corticosteroid if you are or might be pregnant.

Dexamethasone passes into breast milk. Nursing mothers who must use this drug should bottle-feed. It is not known if other nasal corticosteroids pass into breast milk, though oral corticosteroids do. Nursing mothers should be cautious about using any of these drugs.

Seniors

Seniors may use nasal corticosteroids without special restriction. Tell your doctor if you have bone or bowel disease, colitis, diabetes, glaucoma, fungal or herpes infections, high blood pressure, high blood cholesterol, an underactive thyroid, or heart, kidney, or liver disease.

Type of Drug

Corticosteroids, Topical

(kor-tih-koe-STER-oids)

Brand Names

Generic Ingredient: Alclometasone Dipropionate
Aclovate

Generic Ingredient: Amcinonide
Cyclocort

Generic Ingredient: Augmented Betamethasone Dipropionate [G]
Diprolene   Diprolene AF

Generic Ingredient: Betamethasone [G]

Alphatrex	Diprosone
Betatrex	Luxiq
Beta-Val	Maxivate

Psorion Cream
Teladar

Valisone
Valisone Reduced Strength

Generic Ingredient: Clobetasol Propionate [G]
Cormak
Embeline
Embeline E

Temorate
Temorate E

Generic Ingredient: Clocortolone Pivalate
Cloderm

Generic Ingredient: Desonide [G]
DesOwen

Tridesilon

Generic Ingredient: Desoximetasone [G]
Topicort

Topicort LP

Generic Ingredient: Dexamethasone [G]
Aeroseb-Dex
Decadron

Decaspray

Generic Ingredient: Diflorasone Diacetate [G]
Florone
Florone E

Maxiflor
Psorcon

Generic Ingredient: Fluocinolone Acetonide [G]
Fluonid
Flurosyn
FS Shampoo

Synalar
Synalar-HP

Generic Ingredient: Fluocinonide [G]
Fluonex
Lidex

Lidex-E

Generic Ingredient: Flurandrenolide [G]
Cordran

Cordran SP

Generic Ingredient: Fluticasone Propionate
Cutivate

Generic Ingredient: Halcinonide
Halog

Halog-E

Generic Ingredient: Halobetasol Propionate
Ultravate

Generic Ingredient: Hydrocortisone [G]
1% HC

Acticort 100

Ala-Cort
Ala-Scalp
Analpram-HC
Anucort-HC
Anumed HC
Anusol-HC
Bactinė Hydrocortisone
Cetacort
CortaGel
Cortaid with Aloe
Cortaid Intensive Therapy
Cort-Dome
Cortenema
Cortifoam
Cortizone-5
Cortizone-10
Delcort
Dermacort
Dermol HC
Dermolate
Dermtex HC with Aloe
Eldecort
Gynecort
Hemril HC Uniserts
Hi-Cor 1.0
Hi-Cor 2.5
Hycort
Hydrocort
HydroTex
Hytone
LactiCare-HC
Lanacort-5
Lanacort-10
Locoid
Maximum Strength Cortaid
Maximum Strength Cortaid-Faststick
Maximum Strength KeriCort-10
Nutracort
Pandel
Penecort
Pramoxine HC
Procort
Proctocort
Proctocream-HC
Proctofoam-HC
Scalpicin
S-T Cort
Synacort
Tegrin-HC
Texacort
T Scalp
Westcort

Generic Ingredient: Mometasone Furoate
Elocon

Generic Ingredient: Prednicarbate
Dermatop

Generic Ingredient: Triamcinolone Acetonide G
Aristocort
Aristocort A
Delta-Tritex
Flutex
Kenalog
Kenalog-H
Kenonel
Triacet
Triderm

Prescribed for

Inflammation, itching, or other local skin problems; may also be used to treat psoriasis and severe diaper rash.

General Information

Topical corticosteroids do not cure the underlying cause of skin problems, but they can relieve symptoms of rash, itching, or inflammation by interfering with the body mechanisms that produce them. You should never use a topical corticosteroid without your doctor's knowledge because it could mask a symptom important in diagnosing your condition. Some generic versions of topical corticosteroids vary in potency from related brand-name forms. Ask your doctor or pharmacist which products are interchangeable.

Cautions and Warnings

Do not use a topical corticosteroid as the sole treatment for **viral skin diseases** such as herpes, **fungal skin infections** such as athlete's foot, or **tuberculosis** of the skin. These drugs should not be used in the **ear** if the eardrum is perforated. Do not use these drugs if you are **allergic** to any component of the aerosol, cream, gel, lotion, ointment, or solution.

Rectal corticosteroid products should not be used if you have any serious **bowel condition,** including bowel perforation, obstruction, abscess, and systemic fungal infection.

The **rectal foam** is not expelled after it has been applied and may result in higher drug blood levels than those associated with rectal enema products. The risk of systemic (whole-body) side effects is greater when more of the drug enters the blood. If there is no improvement after 2 or 3 weeks of using a rectal corticosteroid, contact your doctor.

Using a topical corticosteroid around the eyes for prolonged periods may cause **cataracts** or **glaucoma.**

Children may be more susceptible to serious side effects from topical corticosteroids, especially if they are applied to large areas over long periods. Augmented betamethasone propionate, clobetasol, desoximetasone, fluticasone, and halobetasol are not recommended for use on children's skin.

Possible Side Effects

▼ Most common: burning, itching, irritation, acne, dry and cracking skin, skin tightening, secondary infection, and skin discoloration. These effects are more likely when the treated area is covered with an occlusive bandage (one that prevents contact with water and air).

Possible Side Effects *(continued)*

Significant quantities of corticosteroids may be absorbed into the bloodstream if large amounts are used for long periods. This can result in systemic effects and may cause serious problems, particularly in people with liver disease.

Drug Interactions

None known.

Usual Dose

Cream, Ointment, Solution, and Aerosol: Apply a thin film to the skin 2–4 times a day.

Rectal Enema: 100 mg nightly for 21 days.

Rectal Foam: 1 applicator's worth, 1–2 times a day for 2–3 weeks.

Overdosage

Serious adverse effects are unlikely after accidental ingestion. Excessive use of large amounts of topical corticosteroids may cause overdose symptoms and require gradual discontinuation of the drug. Call your local poison control center or a hospital emergency room for more information.

Special Information

To prevent secondary infection, clean the skin before applying the drug. Apply a very thin film and rub in gently—effectiveness depends on contact area, not the thickness of the layer applied.

Do not wash, rub, or put clothing on the area until the medication has dried.

Flurandrenolide tape comes with specific directions for use; follow them carefully.

If your doctor instructs you to apply plastic wrap or any other occlusive dressing, follow directions carefully. These dressings can increase the penetration of the drug into your skin by as much as 10 times, which may be a crucial element in the medication's effectiveness. Occlusive dressings should not be used with augmented betamethasone, betamethasone propionate, clobetasol, halobetasol, or mometasone.

If you are using one of these products for diaper rash, do not use tight-fitting diapers or plastic pants, which can cause too much drug to be absorbed into the blood.

Your doctor may prescribe a specific form of the product with good reason. Do not change forms without your doctor's knowledge; a different form may not be as effective.

If you forget to administer a dose, do so as soon as you remember. If it is almost time for your next dose, skip the one you forgot and continue with your regular schedule. Do not administer a double dose.

Special Populations

Pregnancy/Breast-feeding

Corticosteroids applied to the skin in large amounts or for long periods of time may cause birth defects. When any of these drugs is considered crucial by your doctor, its potential benefits must be carefully weighed against its risks. Over-the-counter hydrocortisone products should not be used for more than a few days without your doctor's knowledge.

It is not known if topical corticosteroids pass into breast milk, though oral corticosteroids do. Nursing mothers who must use a topical corticosteroid should consider bottle-feeding. If you apply a corticosteroid to the nipple area, be sure to completely clean the area prior to nursing. Nursing mothers should never use clobetasol.

Seniors

Seniors are more susceptible to high blood pressure and osteoporosis (a condition characterized by loss of bone mass due to depletion of minerals, especially calcium) associated with large dosages. These effects are unlikely with topical corticosteroids unless a high-potency medication is used over a large area for an extended period.

Brand Name

Cortisporin Otic

Generic Ingredients

Hydrocortisone + Neomycin Sulfate + Polymyxin B Sulfate Ⓖ

Other Brand Names

AK-Spore H.C. Otic	Octicair
AntibiOtic	Otic-Care
Cortatrigen Ear Drops	Otocort
Drotic	Otomycin-HPN Otic
Ear-Eze	Pediotic
LazerSporin-C	UAD

Type of Drug

Antibiotic-corticosteroid combination.

Prescribed for

Superficial ear infection, ear inflammation or itching, and other outer ear problems.

General Information

Cortisporin Otic contains a corticosteroid to reduce inflammation and 2 antibiotics to treat local ear infections. This combination can be quite useful for local ear problems because of its dual method of action and its relatively broad applicability.

Cautions and Warnings

Do not use this product if you are **sensitive** or **allergic** to any of its ingredients.

Cortisporin Otic is designed for use in the ear. It can be **very damaging if placed into the eye**.

Possible Side Effects

Local irritation, such as itching or burning, may occur as a drug sensitivity or allergic reaction.

Drug Interactions

None known.

Usual Dose

2–4 drops in the affected ear 3–4 times a day.

Overdosage

The amount of drug contained in each bottle is too small to cause serious problems. Call a hospital emergency room or your local poison control center for more information.

Special Information

Use only when prescribed by a physician. Overuse of this or similar products can result in the growth of new organisms, such as fungi. If new infections or problems appear, stop using the drug and contact your doctor.

Wash your hands, then hold the closed bottle in your hand for a few minutes to warm it to body temperature. Shake well for 10 seconds. For best results, drops should not be self-administered, but given by another person. The person receiving the drops should lie on his or her side with the affected ear facing upward. Fill the dropper and instill the required number of drops directly in the ear canal.

If the drops are being given to an infant, hold the earlobe down and back to allow the drops to run in. If the drops are being given to an older child or adult, hold the earlobe up and back to allow them to run in. Do not put the dropper into the ear or allow it to touch any part of the ear or bottle. Keep the ear tilted for about 2 minutes after the drops have been put in or insert a soft cotton plug, whichever is recommended by your doctor.

If you forget to administer a dose of Cortisporin Otic, dose as soon as you remember. If it is almost time for your next dose, skip the dose you forgot and continue with your regular schedule. Do not apply a double dose.

Special Populations

Pregnancy/Breast-feeding
Pregnant and breast-feeding women may use this product.

Seniors
Seniors may use this product without special restriction.

Brand Name

Cosopt

Generic Ingredients

Dorzolamide + Timolol

Type of Drug

Carbonic-anhydrase inhibitor and beta blocker combination.

Prescribed for

Open-angle glaucoma.

General Information

Cosopt contains 2 glaucoma drugs that work in different ways. It is intended for people whose glaucoma does not respond to either drug used alone. Small amounts of dorzolamide and timolol—the active ingredients in Cosopt—enter the bloodstream.

Cautions and Warnings

Do not use Cosopt if you are **sensitive** or **allergic** to either of its ingredients or cannot take sulfa drugs or beta blockers. Cosopt should not be used by people with bronchial **asthma,** severe **chronic obstructive pulmonary disease, slow heart rate** or **heart block, heart failure,** or who are in **shock.**

People with **diabetes** or an **overactive thyroid** should use Cosopt with caution since beta blockers can mask the signs of low blood sugar or hyperthyroidism.

Small amounts of both ingredients enter the bloodstream and can produce the same kinds of **systemic (whole-body) reactions** associated with larger dosages of either a sulfa drug or beta blocker. Stop using the drug at once and call your doctor if a serious reaction develops.

Beta blockers may have to be discontinued prior to **major surgery** because they can affect the heart's ability to respond normally. Some people taking a beta blocker experience severe reductions while undergoing general anesthesia.

Dorzolamide should not be used by people with **kidney disease** and has not been studied in people with **liver disease**.

People with a history of **severe allergic reactions** who take a beta blocker may be at increased risk of experiencing a reaction because the drug blocks part of the body's natural allergic response.

Timolol can worsen the muscle weakness that accompanies **myasthenia gravis**.

Possible Side Effects

▼ Most common: changes in sense of taste, especially bitterness or sourness; and a burning or stinging sensation in the eye.

Possible Side Effects *(continued)*

▼ Common: eye redness, blurred vision, and eye irritation or itching.

▼ Less common: abdominal pain, back pain, eyelid inflammation, bronchitis, cloudy vision, eye discharge or swelling, conjunctivitis (pinkeye), corneal erosion, corneal staining, lens cloudiness, cough, dizziness, dry eye, upset stomach, drug particles in the eye, eye pain, tearing, eyelid scaling, eyelid pain or discomfort, sensation of something in the eye, headache, high blood pressure, influenza, lens discoloration, nausea, sore throat, cataracts, sinus irritation, respiratory infection, urinary infection, visual problems, and retinal detachment.

▼ Rare: slow heartbeat, heart failure, chest pain, stroke, depression, diarrhea, dry mouth, breathing difficulties, low blood pressure, heart attack, stuffy nose, rash, tingling in the hands or feet, increased sensitivity to the sun, kidney stones, and vomiting. Other rare side effects associated with oral dorzolamide or timolol may occur.

Drug Interactions

• If you use more than 1 eyedrop medication, separate doses of these drugs by at least 10 minutes.

• Cosopt can increase the effect of other carbonic-anhydrase inhibitors.

• Combining Cosopt with an oral beta blocker or another calcium antagonist may increase the risk of side effects, especially changes in heart rhythm and low blood pressure.

• Do not combine Cosopt and another beta-blocking eyedrop.

• Combining Cosopt and reserpine can lead to low blood pressure, slowing of heartbeat, and dizziness or fainting.

• Combining Cosopt with digitalis and a calcium antagonist, or with quinidine, can slow heartbeat.

Usual Dose

Adult: 1 drop in the affected eye 2 times daily.

Overdosage

Little is known about the effects of Cosopt overdose or accidental ingestion. Possible overdose symptoms include dizzi-.

ness, headache, shortness of breath, slow heartbeat, breathing difficulties, heart attack, and nervous system effects. Call your local poison control center or a hospital emergency room for more information. If you seek treatment, ALWAYS bring the prescription bottle or container.

Special Information

Conjunctivitis and eyelid reactions can occur due to an allergic reaction or as the result of local irritation. If you experience either of these problems, stop using the drug and call your doctor so that your condition can be evaluated.

To prevent infection, do not allow the eyedropper to touch your fingers, eyelids, or any surface. Wait at least 10 minutes before using any other eyedrops.

Cosopt contains benzalkonium chloride (a preservative), which may be absorbed by soft contact lenses. Remove your soft contact lenses before using the eyedrops; you may put them back in 15 minutes after a dose.

If you forget a dose of Cosopt, take it as soon as you remember. If it is almost time for your next dose, skip the forgotten dose and continue with your regular schedule.

Special Populations

Pregnancy/Breast-feeding
The safety of using Cosopt is not known. When this drug is considered crucial by your doctor, its potential benefits must be carefully weighed against its risks.

It is not known if dorzolamide passes into breast milk, though timolol does. Nursing mothers who must use Cosopt should bottle-feed.

Seniors
Seniors may use Cosopt without precaution.

Coumadin   see Warfarin, page 1084

Cozaar   see Angiotensin II Blockers, page 72

Generic Name

Cromolyn (KROE-muh-lin) G

Brand Names

Crolom
Cromoptic Gastrocrom
Intal

Nasalcrom
Opticrom

The information in this profile also applies to the following drug:

Generic Ingredient: Nedocromil
Tilade

Type of Drug

Allergy preventive and antiasthmatic.

Prescribed for

Prevention of severe allergy reactions, including asthma, runny nose, and mastocytosis; also prescribed for food allergies, eczema, dermatitis, chronic itching, and hay fever. It may be used to treat and prevent chronic inflammatory bowel disease. The eyedrops are used to treat conjunctivitis (pinkeye) and other eye irritations.

General Information

Unlike antihistamines, which work against histamine that has been released into the system, cromolyn sodium prevents allergy, asthma, and other conditions by stabilizing mast cells, a key component in any allergic reaction because they release histamine. Cromolyn prevents the release of histamine and other chemicals from mast cells. The drug works only in the areas to which it is applied; only 7% to 8% of an inhaled dose and 1% of a swallowed capsule is absorbed into the blood. Even the oral capsules, which one would normally expect to be absorbed into the blood, treat only gastrointestinal-tract allergies. Cromolyn products must be used on a regular basis to be effective in reducing the frequency and intensity of allergic reactions.

Cautions and Warnings

Cromolyn should never be used to treat an acute allergy attack. It is intended only to prevent or reduce the number of allergic attacks and their intensity. Once the proper dosage level has been established for you, reducing that level may result in a recurrence of attacks.

Rarely, people have experienced **severe allergic attacks** after taking cromolyn. People allergic to cromolyn should not take any product containing it.

People with **kidney or liver disease** require reduced dosage.

Cough or **bronchial spasm** may occasionally occur after the inhalation of a cromolyn dose. Severe bronchospasm is rare.

Cromolyn aerosol should be used with caution in people with **abnormal heart rhythm** or **diseased coronary blood vessels** because of a possible reaction to the propellants used in the product.

Possible Side Effects

▼ Most common: rash and itching. Capsules— headache and diarrhea. Most capsule side effects are minor and may be attributable to the underlying condition; a variety have been reported but cannot be tied conclusively to the drug.

▼ Less common: local irritation, including nasal stinging, sneezing, tearing, cough, and stuffy nose; urinary difficulty; dizziness; headache; joint swelling; a bad taste in the mouth; nosebleeds; abdominal pain; and nausea.

▼ Rare: severe drug reactions, consisting of coughing, difficulty in swallowing, hives, itching, breathing difficulties, or swelling of the eyelids, lips, or face.

Drug Interactions

None known.

Food Interactions

Inhaled or swallowed cromolyn products should not be mixed with any food, juice, or milk. The nasal and eye products may be taken without regard to food or meals.

Usual Dose

Inhaled Capsules or Solution

Adult and Child (age 2 and over): starting dose—20 mg 4 times a day. Children under age 5 may inhale cromolyn powder if their allergies are severe. The solution must be given with a power-operated nebulizer and face mask. Handheld nebulizers are not adequate. To prevent exercise asthma, 20 mg may be inhaled up to 1 hour before exercise.

Aerosol
   Adult and Child (age 5 and over): up to 2 sprays 4 times a day, spaced equally throughout the day. To prevent exercise asthma, 2 puffs may be inhaled up to 1 hour before exercise.

Nasal Solution
   Adult and Child (age 6 and over): 1 spray in each nostril 3–6 times a day at regular intervals. First blow your nose, and then inhale the spray.

Oral Capsules
   Adult: 2 capsules a half hour before meals and at bedtime.
   Child (age 2–12): 1 capsule (100 mg) 4 times a day a half hour before meals and at bedtime. Dosage may be increased to about 13–18 mg per lb. of body weight in 4 equal doses.
   Child (under age 2): about 10 mg per lb. of body weight a day divided into 4 equal doses. This product is recommended in infants and young children only if absolutely necessary.

Eyedrops
   Adult and Child (age 4 and over): 1–2 drops in each eye 4–6 times a day at regular intervals.

Overdosage

No action is necessary other than medical observation. Call your local poison control center or a hospital emergency room for more information.

Special Information

Cromolyn is taken to prevent or minimize severe allergic reactions. It is imperative that you take cromolyn products on a regular basis to provide equal protection throughout the day.

If you are taking cromolyn to prevent seasonal allergies, it is essential that you start taking the medication before you come into contact with the cause of the allergy and that you continue treatment while you are exposed to it.

Cromolyn oral capsules should be opened and their contents mixed with about 4 oz. of hot water. Stir until the powder completely dissolves and the solution is completely clear; then fill the rest of the glass with cold water. Drink the entire contents of the glass. Do not mix the solution with food, juice, or milk.

Do not wear soft contact lenses while using cromolyn eye-drops. The lenses may be replaced a few hours after you stop taking the drug.

Call your doctor if you develop wheezing, coughing, a severe drug reaction (see "Possible Side Effects"), rash, or any bothersome or persistent side effect.

Call your doctor if your symptoms do not improve or if they worsen.

If you forget to administer a dose, do so as soon as you remember and space the remaining daily dosage evenly throughout the day. Do not take a double dose.

Special Populations

Pregnancy/Breast-feeding
In animal studies, very large dosages of cromolyn adminis-tered by vein have affected the fetus, though no birth defects were reported. When this drug is considered crucial by your doctor, its potential benefits must be carefully weighed against its risks.

It is not known if cromolyn passes into breast milk. Nursing mothers who must use cromolyn should consider bottle-feeding.

Seniors
Older adults with reduced kidney or liver function may require lower dosages.

Generic Name

Cyclobenzaprine (sye-cloe-BEN-zuh-prene) Ⓖ

Brand Name
Flexeril

Type of Drug
Skeletal muscle relaxant.

Prescribed for
Serious muscle spasm and acute muscle pain; also used to treat fibrositis (muscular rheumatism).

General Information

Cyclobenzoprine hydrochloride is used to treat severe muscle spasms; it is prescribed as part of a coordinated program of rest, physical therapy, and other measures.

Cautions and Warnings

Do not take cyclobenzaprine if you are **allergic** to it. This drug should not be taken for several weeks following a **heart attack** or by people with **abnormal heart rhythms, heart failure, heart block** (disruption of the electrical impulses that control heart rate), or **hyperthyroidism** (overactive thyroid gland).

Cyclobenzaprine should be avoided by people with **urinary retention, glaucoma,** or **increased eye pressure**. This drug may increase the chances of **cavities** or **gum disease**.

Cyclobenzaprine is intended only for **short-term use** of 2 to 3 weeks.

Cyclobenzaprine is chemically similar to tricyclic antidepressants and may produce some of the more serious side effects associated with those drugs. Abruptly stopping cyclobenzaprine may cause **nausea, headache,** and **feelings of ill health;** this is not a sign of addiction.

Possible Side Effects

▼ Most common: dry mouth, drowsiness, and dizziness.

▼ Less common: muscle weakness, fatigue, nausea, constipation, upset stomach, unpleasant taste, blurred vision, headache, nervousness, and confusion.

▼ Rare: Rare side effects can occur in almost any part of the body. Contact your doctor if you experience any unlisted side effect not listed above.

Many other side effects have been reported by people taking cyclobenzaprine, but their relationship to the drug has not been established.

Drug Interactions

• The effects of alcohol, sedatives, or other nervous system depressants may be increased by cyclobenzaprine.

• Cyclobenzaprine may increase some side effects of atropine, ipratropium, and other anticholinergic drugs. These include blurred vision, constipation, urinary difficulties, dry mouth, confusion, and drowsiness.

• The combination of cyclobenzaprine and a monoamine oxidase inhibitor (MAOI) antidepressant may produce very high fever, convulsions, and possibly death. Do not take these drugs within 14 days of each other.

• Cyclobenzaprine may increase the effects of haloperidol, loxapine, molindone, pimozide, anticoagulant (blood-thinning) drugs, anticonvulsants, thyroid hormones, antithyroid drugs, phenothiazines, thioxanthenes, and nasal decongestants such as naphazoline, oxymetazoline, phenylephrine, and xylometazoline.

• Barbiturates and carbamazepine may counteract the effects of cyclobenzaprine.

• Fluoxetine, ranitidine, cimetidine, methylphenidate, estramustine, estrogens, and oral contraceptives may increase the effects and side effects of cyclobenzaprine.

• Cyclobenzaprine may counteract the effects of clonidine, guanadrel, and guanethidine.

Food Interactions

None known.

Usual Dose

Adult and Child (age 15 and over): 10 mg 3 times a day; may be increased up to 60 mg a day.

Child (under age 15): not recommended.

Overdosage

Cyclobenzaprine overdose may cause confusion, loss of concentration, hallucinations, agitation, overactive reflexes, fever or vomiting, rigid muscles, and other side effects of the drug. It may also cause drowsiness, low body temperature, rapid or irregular heartbeat and other kinds of abnormal heart rhythms, heart failure, dilated pupils, convulsions, very low blood pressure, stupor, coma, and sweating. Overdose victims must be taken to a hospital emergency room. ALWAYS bring the prescription bottle or container.

Special Information

Cyclobenzaprine causes drowsiness, dizziness, or blurred vision in more than 40% of people who take it, which may interfere with the ability to perform complex tasks like driving or operating equipment. Avoid alcohol, sedatives, and other nervous system depressants because they can enhance sedative effects of cyclobenzaprine.

Call your doctor if you develop rash; hives; itching; urinary difficulties; clumsiness; confusion; depression; convulsions; yellowing of the skin or whites of the eyes; swelling of the face, lips, or tongue; or any other persistent or bothersome side effect.

If you forget a dose of cyclobenzaprine, take it as soon as you remember. If you take cyclobenzaprine once a day and it is almost time for your next dose, skip the one you forgot and continue with your regular schedule. If you take cyclobenzaprine twice a day and it is almost time for your next dose, take 1 dose as soon as you remember, another in 5 or 6 hours, and then go back to your regular schedule. If you take cyclobenzaprine 3 times a day and it is almost time for your next dose, take 1 dose as soon as you remember, another in 3 or 4 hours, and then go back to your regular schedule. Never take a double dose.

Special Populations

Pregnancy/Breast-feeding
As with all drugs, cyclobenzaprine should be avoided by pregnant women unless the potential benefits clearly outweigh the risks.

It is not known if cyclobenzaprine passes into breast milk, but antidepressants with a similar chemical structure do pass into breast milk. Nursing mothers who must take this drug should consider bottle-feeding.

Seniors
Seniors are more likely to be sensitive to the effects of cyclobenzaprine.

Generic Name

Cyclosporine (sye-kloe-SPOR-in)

Brand Names

Neoral   Sangcya
Sandimmune

Type of Drug

Immunosuppressant.

Prescribed for

Kidney, heart, or liver transplantation; also used for bone-marrow, heart-lung, and pancreas transplants; also prescribed for patchy hair loss, rheumatoid arthritis, aplastic anemia, atopic dermatitis, Behçet's disease, cirrhosis of the liver, ulcerative colitis, dermatomyositis, eye symptoms of Graves' disease, insulin-dependent diabetes, kidney inflammation, multiple sclerosis (MS), severe psoriasis and psoriasis-related arthritis, myasthenia gravis, pemphigus, sarcoidosis of the lung, and pyoderma gangrenosum.

General Information

Cyclosporine is used to prevent rejection of transplanted organs. A product of fungus metabolism, cyclosporine was proven to be a potent immunosuppressant in 1972 and was first given to human kidney and bone marrow transplant patients in 1978. It works by blocking the activity of T-cells, which protect the body against invading microorganisms or foreign substances. Cyclosporine also prevents the production of a substance known as interleukin-II that activates T-cells. In 1995, a new form of cyclosporine called Neoral, a microemulsion, was introduced by its manufacturer. This form is as safe and effective as the original product but is better absorbed into the bloodstream and requires less medication to achieve the same effect.

Cautions and Warnings

Cyclosporine should be prescribed only by doctors experienced in immunosuppressive therapy and the care of organ-transplant patients. Sandimmune is always used with corticosteroid drugs like prednisone. Neoral has been used with a corticosteroid and azathioprine, an immune suppressant. When combined with other immune suppressants, cyclosporine must be used with great care because oversuppression of the immune system may lead to **lymphoma** or extreme susceptibility to **infection.**

Sandimmune, the original oral form of cyclosporine, is poorly absorbed into the bloodstream; it must be taken in a dosage that is 3 times greater than the injectable dosage. People taking this drug by mouth for a long period of time should have their blood checked for **cyclosporine levels** so that the dosage may be adjusted if necessary. Since more Neoral is absorbed into the blood you will probably need less of it. When you first start taking Neoral, your dosage will be about the same as that of the older oral liquid but then will be reduced according to the amount of cyclosporine in your blood. Follow your doctor's directions about drug dosage. Do not substitute Neoral for Sandimmune; they are not equivalent to each other.

Cyclosporine causes **kidney toxicosis** (kidney poisoning)—different from transplant rejection—in 25% to 35% of people taking it to prevent organ rejection. Mild symptoms usually start after about 2 or 3 months of treatment. Reducing drug dosage may control this effect. In one study, clonidine skin patches used before and after surgery decreased toxic risks to the kidney.

Liver toxicosis is seen in about 5% of transplant patients taking cyclosporine. It usually appears in the first month and may be controlled by reducing dosage.

Convulsions may develop, especially in people also taking high dosages of corticosteroids. Other nervous system side effects are listed below (see "Possible Side Effects").

Cyclosporine may cause **high blood-potassium or uric-acid levels**.

In one study, cyclosporine increased **cholesterol** and other blood-fat levels. It is not known how this affects people who take the drug on a long-term basis.

There is conflicting information on how cyclosporine affects blood sugar. Kidney-transplant patients taking the drug have developed **insulin-dependent diabetes,** which is related to the dosage of cyclosporine and reverses itself when you stop taking the drug. On the other hand, cyclosporine preserves the function of insulin-producing cells in the pancreas and has allowed many insulin-dependent diabetics to live without taking insulin.

Possible Side Effects

▼ Most common: Cyclosporine is known to be toxic to the kidneys. Your doctor will carefully monitor your kidney function while you are taking it. Other side effects are high blood pressure, increased hair growth, and enlargement of the gums. Lymphoma may develop in people whose immune systems are excessively suppressed. Almost 85% of people treated with cyclosporine develop an infection, compared with 94% of people on other immune-system suppressants.

Possible Side Effects (continued)

▼ Less common: tremors, cramps, acne, brittle hair or fingernails, convulsions, headache, confusion, diarrhea, nausea or vomiting, tingling in the hands or feet, facial flushing, reduced white-blood-cell and platelet counts, sinus inflammation, swollen and painful male breasts, drug allergy (symptoms include rash, itching, hives, and breathing difficulties), conjunctivitis (pinkeye), fluid retention and swelling, ringing or buzzing in the ears, hearing loss, high blood sugar, and muscle pain.

▼ Rare: blood in the urine, heart attack, itching, anxiety, depression, lethargy, weakness, mouth sores, difficulty swallowing, intestinal bleeding, constipation, pancreas inflammation, night sweats, chest pain, joint pain, visual disturbances, and weight loss.

Drug Interactions

• Cyclosporine should be used carefully with other kidney-toxic drugs including nonsteroidal anti-inflammatory drugs (NSAIDs) such as ibuprofen, naproxen, and others; gentamicin; tobramycin; vancomycin; trimethoprim-sulfamethoxazole; melphalan; amphotericin B; ketoconazole; azapropazon; diclofenac; cimetidine; ranitidine; and tacrolimus.

• Drugs that may increase blood levels of cyclosporine include amiodarone; diltiazem; nicardipine; verapamil; fluconazole; itraconazole; clarithromycin; danazol; erythromycin; methyltestosterone; methylprednisolone—this combination also causes convulsions; allopurinol; bromocriptine; danazol; and metoclopramide. With ketoconazole, your doctor may use this drug interaction to reduce your cyclosporine dosage.

• Drugs that decrease cyclosporine levels and may lead to organ rejection include nafcillin, rifabutin, rifampin, carbamazepine, probucol, phenobarbital, and phenytoin.

• Cyclosporine interferes with the body's ability to clear digoxin, prednisolone, and lovastatin. People taking any of these drugs who start on cyclosporine must have their drug dosage reduced.

• Combining colchicine and cyclosporine may lead to liver, kidney, stomach, and other side effects. Avoid this combination.

• Combining cyclosporine and nifedipine may lead to gum overgrowth.

• Cyclosporine increases blood potassium. Excessive blood-potassium levels may be reached if cyclosporine is taken with enalapril, lisinopril, a potassium-sparing diuretic such as spironolactone, salt substitutes, potassium supplements, or high potassium—low sodium—food.

• Cyclosporine prevents the normal body response to live vaccines. People taking cyclosporine should be vaccinated only after specific discussions with their doctors. You must wait for a period of several months to several years after stopping the medication before vaccination may be considered again.

Food Interactions

Cyclosporine may be taken with food if it upsets your stomach. For optimal effectiveness, avoid eating a fatty meal within half an hour of taking Neoral.

You may mix Neoral in a glass—not a paper or plastic cup—with room-temperature orange or apple juice or chocolate milk to make it taste better. DO NOT DRINK GRAPEFRUIT JUICE BECAUSE IT SPEEDS THE BREAKDOWN OF CYCLOSPORINE. Drink immediately after mixing, then put more juice or chocolate milk in the glass and drink it to be sure that the entire dose has been taken. Neoral should not be taken with unflavored milk because it may be unpalatable.

Usual Dose

In general, the usual dosage of Neoral is lower than Sandimmune, but dosage must be individualized for you by your doctor. Do not substitute one brand for the other.

Sandimmune

Adult: The usual oral dosage of cyclosporine is 6–8 mg per lb. of body weight a day. The first dose is given 4–12 hours before the transplant operation or immediately after surgery. This dosage is continued after the operation for 1–2 weeks and then slowly reduced to 2.25–4.5 mg per lb. of body weight.

Child: Similar dosages are usually prescribed, but because children tend to release the drug from their bodies faster than adults, larger and more frequent doses may be needed.

Neoral

Adult: The usual oral dosage of Neoral is 3–4 mg per lb. of body weight a day divided into 2 doses. The first dose is given 4–12 hours before the transplant operation or immediately after surgery. This dosage is continued after the operation for 1 -2 weeks and then slowly reduced to maintain a target amount of cyclosporine in the body.

Child: Similar dosages are usually prescribed but, because children tend to release the drug from their bodies faster than adults, larger and more frequent doses may be needed.

Overdosage

Overdose victims may be expected to develop side effects and symptoms of extreme immunosuppression. Induce vomiting with ipecac syrup—available at any pharmacy—which is recommended up to 2 hours after the overdose was taken. Call your doctor or local poison control center before inducing vomiting. If you must go to a hospital emergency room, ALWAYS bring the prescription bottle or container.

Special Information

Call your doctor at the first sign of fever; sore throat; tiredness; weakness; nervousness; unusual bleeding or bruising; tender or swollen gums; convulsions; irregular heartbeat; confusion; numbness or tingling of your hands, feet, or lips; breathing difficulties; severe stomach pain with nausea; or blood in the urine. Other side effects such as shaking or trembling of the hands, increased hair growth, acne, headache, leg cramps, nausea, or vomiting are less serious but should be brought to your doctor's attention, particularly if they are bothersome or persistent.

Maintain good dental hygiene while taking cyclosporine and use extra care when brushing and flossing because the drug increases your risk of oral infection. Cyclosporine may also cause swollen gums. See your dentist regularly.

Continue taking your medication as long as your doctor prescribes it. Do not stop taking it without your doctor's knowledge. If you cannot take one of the oral forms, cyclosporine can be given by injection.

Do not keep either brand of the oral liquid in the refrigerator. After the bottle is opened, use the medication within 2 months. At temperatures below 68°F, Neoral can form a gel and a light sediment can form in Sandimmune. These do not affect the potency of either product. They can still be used and are effective.

If you forget a dose, take it as soon as you remember if it is within 12 hours of your regular dose. If not, skip the dose you forgot and continue with your regular schedule. Do not take a double dose.

Special Populations

Pregnancy/Breast-feeding
In animal studies cyclosporine damages the fetus. Though a small number of pregnant women have taken cyclosporine without major problems, it is recommended that pregnant women avoid cyclosporine. When this drug is considered crucial by your doctor, its potential benefits must be carefully weighed against its risks.

Cyclosporine passes into breast milk. Nursing mothers who must take cyclosporine should bottle-feed.

Seniors
Due to decreased kidney function, seniors are more susceptible to kidney toxicosis.

Cycrin *see Medroxyprogesterone Acetate, page 616*

Daypro *see Oxaprozin, page 766*

Generic Name

Delavirdine (deh-LAV-er-dene)

Brand Name
Rescriptor

Type of Drug
Antiviral.

Prescribed for
Human immunodeficiency virus (HIV) infection, in combination with other antiviral drugs.

General Information

Delavirdine mesylate is a non-nucleoside reverse transcriptase inhibitor (NNRTI). Delavirdine inhibits the reverse transcriptase (RT) enzyme, necessary for reproduction of HIV in
body cells, by binding directly to RT. If delavirdine is not
taken with other antivirals, resistance to the drug may
develop as soon as 8 weeks after treatment begins. For this
reason, delavirdine is recommended only in combination
with other anti-HIV drugs.

Delavirdine is broken down in the liver. Delavirdine inhibits
the enzymes that break it down, so it actually stays in the
body longer as treatment continues. Women reach 30%
higher delavirdine blood levels than men.

Cautions and Warnings

Delavirdine **drug interactions may be serious or life threatening** (see "Drug Interactions"). Delavirdine is primarily broken
down in the liver; people with **liver disease** should use it with
caution. People taking delavirdine should have their liver
enzymes measured periodically. The chances of developing a
drug **rash** while taking delavirdine are almost 1 in 5. Anyone
who develops a severe rash, rash with fever, blisters, mouth
sores, eye irritation, swelling, or muscle or joint ache should
stop taking delavirdine and call the doctor.

Possible Side Effects

▼ Most common: nausea and rash.

▼ Common: headache and tiredness.

▼ Less common: diarrhea, vomiting, liver irritation,
itching. Other less common side effects can occur in
almost any part of the body. Contact your doctor if you
experience any side effect not listed above.

Drug Interactions

Some delavirdine drug interactions, which occur because
of delavirdine's effect on liver enzymes, are potentially life
threatening.

• Anticonvulsants, rifabutin, and rifampin may reduce the
amount of delavirdine in the blood.

• Antacids and didanosine may reduce the amount of
delavirdine in the blood by interfering with its absorption in

the blood; take these drugs and delavirdine at least 1 hour apart.

• When delavirdine and clarithromycin are combined, the amount of either drug in the blood may be doubled.

• Delavirdine interferes with the breakdown of protease inhibitors. A protease inhibitor dosage reduction may be needed.

• Fluoxetine and ketoconazole increase the amount of delavirdine in the blood by about 50%.

• Cimetidine, ranitidine, and similar drugs may reduce the amount of delavirdine absorbed. Do not combine these drugs with delavirdine for any length of time.

• Do not take delavirdine with certain antimicrobials, including clarithromycin, dapsone, and rifabutin; benzodiazepine tranquilizers and sleeping medication; cisapride; ergot drugs; quinidine; and warfarin.

Food Interactions

None known.

Usual Dose

Adult: 400 mg 3 times a day.

Overdosage

Little is known about the effects of delavirdine overdose. Overdose victims should be taken to a hospital emergency room for treatment. ALWAYS bring the prescription bottle or container.

Special Information

Delavirdine solution is somewhat better absorbed than the tablets. The amount of drug absorbed from delavirdine tablets can be increased by allowing them to disintegrate in water and then swallowing the mixture.

People with achlorhydria (absence of stomach acid) should take delavirdine with an acidic drink, such as orange or cranberry juice.

Delavirdine does not cure HIV. It will not prevent you from transmitting the HIV virus to another person; you must still practice safe sex. People taking delavirdine for HIV can still develop HIV-related conditions. The long-term effects of delavirdine are not known. People taking this drug should be under a doctor's care at all times.

If you develop a severe rash, or rash with fever, blisters, mouth sores, eye irritation, swelling, or muscle or joint ache, stop taking delavirdine and see your doctor.

Take the medication every day exactly as prescribed. It is important to follow your doctor's directions and not miss doses. If you forget to take a dose of delavirdine, take it as soon as you remember. If it is almost time for your next dose, skip the dose you forgot and continue with your regular schedule. Do not take a double dose.

Special Populations

Pregnancy/Breast-feeding
Delavirdine causes birth defects in laboratory animals. Of 7 unplanned pregnancies reported in delavirdine studies, 3 women had ectopic pregnancies, 3 had normal, healthy babies, and one baby was born prematurely with a heart valve defect. However, there are no specific studies of delavirdine in pregnant women. This drug should not be taken unless you have discussed the possible benefits and risks with your doctor.

Delavirdine passes into breast milk in concentrations that are 3 to 5 times the concentrations found in the mother's blood and should not be taken by nursing mothers. In any case, mothers who are HIV positive should bottle-feed their babies to avoid transmitting the virus through their milk.

Seniors
Seniors may take delavirdine without special precaution.

Depakote   *see Valproic Acid, page 1074*

Generic Name

Desmopressin (dez-moe-PRES-in) Ⓖ

Brand Names

DDAVP   Stimate

Type of Drug

Pituitary hormone replacement.

Prescribed for

Nighttime bed-wetting and diabetes insipidus (central or cranial diabetes). Desmopressin injection is used for hemophilia A and von Willebrand's disease.

General Information

Desmopressin is a synthetic version of antidiuretic hormone (ADH). When ADH is lacking, the body has difficulty retaining fluid. People lacking ADH experience excessive thirst, increased urination, and dehydration; desmopressin controls these symptoms. When used for nighttime bed-wetting, desmopressin should be used in conjunction with behavioral or other nondrug therapies.

Cautions and Warnings

People **allergic** to desmopressin should not take this drug.

People using desmopressin should only drink enough fluid to satisfy their thirst. Rarely, people taking it develop **water intoxication,** which can result in seizures.

Heart attacks and **strokes** after treatment with desmopressin have been reported in people at risk for them, but there is no definite link to desmopressin use.

People using desmopressin should have their urine checked regularly by their doctor. Other things your doctor will watch for are how the drug affects the heart, nasal swelling, congestion, and scarring.

Possible Side Effects

▼ Rare: slight increases in blood pressure, loss of sodium, water intoxication (symptoms include coma, confusion, drowsiness, continuing headache, decreased urination, rapid weight gain, and seizures), stomach or abdominal cramps, redness or flushing of the skin, and vulvar pain. A stuffy or runny nose may occur with use of the nasal solution.

Drug Interactions

• Desmopressin may increase the effects of other drugs that raise blood pressure. This only happens with large dosages.

• Chlorpropamide and carbamazepine may increase the effects of desmopressin.

Food Interactions

None known.

Usual Dose

Nasal Solution—Nighttime Bed-Wetting
   Adult and Child (age 6 and over): 20 mcg (0.2 ml) at bed-time.

Nasal Solution—Diabetes Insipidus
   Adult: 0.1–0.4 ml daily
   Child (age 3 months–12 years): 0.05–0.3 ml a day in 1–2 doses.

Tablets
   Adult: Begin with 0.05 mg 2 times a day. Daily dosage should be increased according to individual need, up to 1.2 mg a day divided into 2–3 doses.
   Child: Begin with 0.05 mg and adjust according to individual need.

Overdosage

Symptoms include headache, difficulty breathing, abdominal cramps, nausea, and facial flushing. Call your doctor or a hospital emergency room if you suspect an overdose. Because there is no known antidote to desmopressin, your dosage may be temporarily reduced until overdose symptoms subside.

Special Information

Call your doctor if you develop headache, breathing difficulties, heartburn, nausea, abdominal or stomach cramps, or vulvar pain.

The Stimate Nasal Solution spray pump must be primed before its first use. To prime the pump, press down 4 times. Stimate delivers 25 doses per bottle. Throw away the bottle after 25 doses have been used, because anything remaining after the 25th dose is likely to deliver less drug than is needed.

If you forget a dose of desmopressin, take it as soon as you remember. If you don't remember until your next dose, skip the forgotten dose and continue with your regular schedule.

Special Populations

Pregnancy/Breast-feeding

The safety of using desmopressin during pregnancy is not known, though it has been used to treat diabetes insipidus in pregnant women without apparent harm to the fetus. When this drug is considered crucial by your doctor, its potential benefits must be carefully weighed against its risks.

Desmopressin may pass into breast milk. Nursing mothers who must use this drug should consider bottle-feeding.

Seniors

Seniors may use desmopressin without special precaution. Avoid drinking too much fluid.

Desogen   *see Contraceptives, page 254*

Detrol   *see Tolterodine, page 1027*

Generic Name

Diazepam   (dye-AZ-uh-pam)   Ⓖ

Brand Names

Diastat   Valium
Diazepam Intensol

The information in this profile also applies to the following drugs:

Generic Ingredient: Halazepam
Paxipam

Generic Ingredient: Lorazepam Ⓖ
Ativan   Lorazepam Intensol

Generic Ingredient: Oxazepam Ⓖ
Serax

Generic Ingredient: Prazepam Ⓖ
Centrax

Type of Drug

Benzodiazepine tranquilizer.

Prescribed for

Anxiety, tension, fatigue, agitation, muscle spasm, and seizures; also prescribed for irritable bowel syndrome and panic attacks.

General Information

Diazepam and other benzodiazepines directly affect the brain. They can relax you and make you more tranquil or sleepy, or they can slow nervous system transmissions in such a way as to act as an anticonvulsant: Many doctors prefer benzodiazepines to other drugs that can be used to similar effect because they tend to be safer, have fewer side effects, and are usually as effective, if not more so.

Cautions and Warnings

Do not take diazepam if you know you are **sensitive** or **allergic** to it or to another benzodiazepine drug, including clonazepam.

Diazepam can aggravate narrow-angle **glaucoma,** but you may take it if you have open-angle glaucoma.

Other conditions in which diazepam should be avoided are severe **depression,** severe **lung disease, sleep apnea** (intermittent cessation of breathing during sleep), **liver disease, drunkenness,** and **kidney disease.** In all of these conditions, the depressive effects of diazepam may be enhanced or could be detrimental to your overall condition.

Diazepam should not be taken by **psychotic patients.** It is not effective for them and can trigger unusual excitement, stimulation, and rage.

Diazepam is not intended for more than 3 to 4 months of continuous use. Your condition should be reassessed before continuing your medication beyond that time.

Diazepam may be **addictive.** Drug withdrawal may develop if you stop taking it after only 4 weeks of regular use but is more likely after longer use. It may start with anxiety and progress to tingling in the hands or feet, sensitivity to bright light, sleep disturbances, cramps, tremors, muscle tension or twitching, poor concentration, flu symptoms, fatigue, appetite loss, sweating, and changes in mental state.

Possible Side Effects

▼ Most common: mild drowsiness during the first few days of therapy. Weakness and confusion may occur, especially in seniors and in those who are sickly. If these effects persist, contact your doctor.

▼ Less common: depression, lethargy, disorientation, headache, inactivity, slurred speech, stupor, dizziness, tremors, constipation, dry mouth, nausea, inability to control urination, sexual difficulties, irregular menstrual cycle, changes in heart rhythm, low blood pressure, fluid retention, blurred or double vision, itching, rash, hiccups, nervousness, inability to fall asleep, and occasional liver dysfunction. If you have any of these symptoms, stop taking the drug and contact your doctor at once.

▼ Rare: Rare side effects can affect your heart, stomach and intestines, urinary tract, blood, muscles, and joints. Contact your doctor if you experience any side effect not listed above.

Drug Interactions

• Diazepam is a central-nervous-system depressant. Avoid alcohol, other tranquilizers, narcotics, barbiturates, monoamine oxidase inhibitors (MAOIs), antihistamines, and antidepressants. Taking diazepam with these drugs may lead to excessive depression, drowsiness, or difficulty breathing.

• Smoking may reduce diazepam's effectiveness by increasing the rate at which it is broken down by the body.

• Effects of diazepam may be prolonged when taken with cimetidine, oral contraceptives, disulfiram, fluoxetine, isoniazid, ketoconazole, rifampin, metoprolol, probenecid, propoxyphene, propranolol, and valproic acid.

• Theophylline may reduce the sedative effects of diazepam.

• If you take antacids, separate them from your diazepam dose by at least 1 hour to prevent them from interfering with the passage of diazepam into the bloodstream.

• Diazepam may increase blood levels of digoxin and the chances for digoxin toxicity.

• Levodopa's effects may be decreased if it is taken with diazepam.

• Combining diazepam and phenytoin may increase phenytoin blood concentrations and the risk of phenytoin toxicity.

Food Interactions

Diazepam is best taken on an empty stomach, but it may be taken with food if it upsets your stomach.

Usual Dose

Solution or Tablets
Adult: 2–40 mg a day. Dosage must be adjusted to individual response for maximum effect. In seniors, less of the drug is usually required to control tension and anxiety.
Child (6 months and over): 1–2.5 mg 3 or 4 times a day; more may be needed to control anxiety and tension.
Child (under 6 months): not recommended.

Rectal Gel
Adult and Child (age 12 and over): 0.09 mg per lb. of body weight. Approximate dosage: 5 mg if 31–60 lbs., 10 mg if 61–110 lbs., 15 mg if 111–165 lbs., or 20 mg if 166–244 lbs.
Child (age 6–11): 0.14 mg per lb. of body weight. Approximate dosage: 5 mg if 22–40 lbs., 10 mg if 41–82 lbs., 15 mg if 83–121 lbs., or 20 mg if 122–163 lbs.
Child (age 2–5): 0.23 mg per lb. of body weight. Approximate dosage: 5 mg if 13–24 lbs., 10 mg if 25–49 lbs., 15 mg if 50–73 lbs., or 20 mg if 74–97 lbs.

An extra 2.5 mg of the rectal gel may be given if a more precise dosage is needed or as a partial replacement for people who do not retain the full dosage after it is first inserted rectally.

Overdosage

Symptoms of overdose include confusion, sleepiness, poor coordination, lack of response to pain, loss of reflexes, shallow breathing, low blood pressure, and coma. The victim should be taken to a hospital emergency room. ALWAYS bring the prescription bottle or container.

Special Information

Diazepam can cause tiredness, drowsiness, inability to concentrate, or similar symptoms. Be careful if you are driving, operating machinery, or performing other activities that require concentration.

People taking diazepam for more than 3 or 4 months at a time may develop drug withdrawal reactions if the medication is stopped suddenly (see "Cautions and Warnings").

If you forget a dose of diazepam, take it as soon as you remember. If it is almost time for your next dose, skip the one you forgot and continue with your regular schedule. Do not take a double dose.

Special Populations

Pregnancy/Breast-feeding

Diazepam may cause birth defects if taken during the first 3 months of pregnancy. Avoid taking any benzodiazepine if you are or might be pregnant.

Diazepam may pass into breast milk. Nursing mothers who must take this drug should bottle-feed.

Seniors

Seniors, especially those with liver or kidney disease, are more sensitive to the effects of diazepam and generally require smaller doses to achieve the same effect.

Generic Name

Diclofenac/Diclofenac Sodium

(dye-CLOE-fen-ak) G

Brand Names

Cataflam   Voltaren-XR
Voltaren

Combination Products

Generic Ingredients: Diclofenac + Misoprostol
Arthrotec

Type of Drug

Nonsteroidal anti-inflammatory drug (NSAID).

Prescribed for

Rheumatoid arthritis; osteoarthritis; ankylosing spondylitis; mild to moderate pain; juvenile rheumatoid arthritis; shoulder pain; menstrual pain and cramps; sunburn; and eye inflammation after cataract surgery—eyedrops only. The combination of diclofenac and misoprostol is intended for people with arthritis who are likely to develop an ulcer.

General Information

Diclofenac and other NSAIDs are used to relieve pain and inflammation. We do not know exactly how NSAIDs work, but they may achieve their effects by blocking the body's production of a hormone called prostaglandin and the action of other body chemicals. Pain relief comes within 1 hour after taking the first dose of diclofenac, but its anti-inflammatory effect takes several days to 2 weeks to become apparent and may take a month or more to reach maximum effect. Diclofenac is broken down in the liver and eliminated through the kidneys.

Cataflam, a newer version of diclofenac, has no sodium and is preferred for menstrual pain and cramps. Voltaren, the older version of diclofenac, has sodium; women taking Cataflam for menstrual problems should not switch to Voltaren. The combination of diclofenac and misoprostol is used to protect against stomach and intestinal irritation and ulcer. NSAID eyedrops are used during eye surgery to prevent movement of the eye muscles and for itching and redness due to seasonal allergies. After cataract surgery, they are used to prevent inflammation.

Cautions and Warnings

People **allergic** to diclofenac or any other NSAID and those with a history of **asthma** attacks brought on by an NSAID, iodides, or aspirin should not take diclofenac.

Diclofenac may cause **gastrointestinal (GI) bleeding**, **ulcers**, and **stomach perforation**. This can occur at any time, with or without warning, in people who take diclofenac regularly. People with a history of active GI bleeding should be cautious about taking any NSAID. People who develop bleeding or ulcers and continue NSAID treatment should be aware of the possibility of developing more serious side effects.

Diclofenac may affect platelets and **blood clotting** at high doses and should be avoided by people with clotting problems and those taking warfarin.

People with **heart problems** who use diclofenac may experience swelling in their arms, legs, or feet.

Diclofenac may cause severe toxic effects to the **kidney**. Report any unusual side effects to your doctor, who might need to periodically test your kidney function.

People taking diclofenac should have their **liver function** checked periodically.

Diclofenac may make you **unusually sensitive to the effects of the sun**.

Possible Side Effects

Tablets

▼ Most common: diarrhea, nausea, vomiting, constipation, stomach gas, stomach upset or irritation, and appetite loss, especially during the first few days of treatment.

▼ Less common: stomach ulcers, GI bleeding, hepatitis, gallbladder attacks, painful urination, poor kidney function, kidney inflammation, blood and protein in the urine, dizziness, fainting, nervousness, depression, hallucinations, confusion, disorientation, tingling in the hands or feet, light-headedness, itching, increased sweating, dry nose and mouth, heart palpitations, chest pain, breathing difficulties, and muscle cramps.

▼ Rare: severe allergic reactions including closing of the throat, fever and chills, changes in liver function, jaundice (yellowing of the skin or whites of the eyes), and kidney failure. People who experience such effects must be promptly treated in a hospital emergency room or doctor's office. NSAIDs have caused severe skin reactions; if this happens to you, see your doctor immediately.

Eyedrops

▼ Most common: temporary burning, stinging, or other minor eye irritation.

▼ Less common: nausea, vomiting, viral infections, and eye allergies including persistent redness, burning, itching, or tearing.

▼ Rare: The risk of developing bleeding problems or other systemic (whole-body) side effects is low because only a small amount of the drug is absorbed into the bloodstream.

Drug Interactions

Tablets

• Diclofenac may increase the effects of oral anticoagulant (blood-thinning) drugs such as warfarin. Your anticoagulant may need to be reduced.

• Taking diclofenac with cyclosporine may increase the kidney-related side effects of both drugs. Methotrexate side effects may be increased in people also taking diclofenac.

• Diclofenac may reduce the blood-pressure-lowering effect of beta blockers and loop diuretics.

• Diclofenac may increase phenytoin side effects. Lithium blood levels may be increased by diclofenac.

• Diclofenac blood levels may be affected by cimetidine.

• Probenecid may increase the risk of diclofenac side effects.

• Aspirin and other salicylates should never be combined with diclofenac.

Eyedrops
None known.

Food Interactions

Take diclofenac tablets with food or a magnesium/aluminum antacid if it upsets your stomach.

Usual Dose

Diclofenac Tablets
  Adult: 100–200 mg a day.
  Senior: starting dose—1/3–1/2 the usual dosage.

Diclofenac Eyedrops
1 drop 4 times a day for 2 weeks, beginning 24 hours after cataract surgery.

Diclofenac and Misoprostol
  Adult: one 50/200 tablet 3 or 4 times a day or one 75/200 tablet 3 times a day. For seniors, taking the combination product 4 times a day provides better ulcer protection, but arthritis relief does not improve.

Overdosage

People have died from oral NSAID overdoses. Common signs of overdose are drowsiness, nausea, vomiting, diarrhea, abdominal pain, rapid breathing, rapid heartbeat, increased sweating, ringing or buzzing in the ears, confusion, disorientation, stupor, and coma. Take the victim to a hospital emergency room at once. ALWAYS bring the prescription bottle or container.

Special Information

Tablets: Take each dose with a full glass of water and do not lie down for 15 to 30 minutes afterward.

Diclofenac can make you drowsy or tired: Be careful when driving or operating hazardous equipment. Do not take any over-the-counter products containing acetaminophen or aspirin while taking diclofenac. Avoid alcoholic beverages.

If you are taking Cataflam for menstrual problems, be sure not to substitute Voltaren.

Contact your doctor if you develop rash or itching, visual disturbances, weight gain, breathing difficulties, fluid retention, hallucinations, black or tarry stools, persistent headache, or any unusual or intolerable side effect.

If you forget a dose of oral diclofenac, take it as soon as you remember. If you take several doses a day and it is within 4 hours of your next dose, skip the one you forgot and continue with your regular schedule. Do not take a double dose.

Eyedrops: To prevent possible infection, do not allow the dropper to touch your fingers, eyelids, or any surface. Wait at least 5 minutes before using any other eyedrops.

If you forget to administer a dose of your eyedrops, do so as soon as you remember. If it is almost time for your next dose, skip the one you missed and continue with your regular schedule. Do not take a double dose.

Special Populations

Pregnancy/Breast-feeding

NSAIDs may affect fetal heart development during the second half of pregnancy. Pregnant women should not take diclofenac without their doctor's approval. Misoprostol can cause miscarriage and birth defects. The combination of diclofenac and misoprostol must not be taken by women who are or might be pregnant.

NSAIDs may pass into breast milk. There is a possibility that a nursing mother taking diclofenac could affect her baby's heart or cardiovascular system. Nursing mothers who must take this drug should bottle-feed.

Seniors

Seniors may be more susceptible to side effects, especially ulcer disease.

Generic Name

Dicyclomine (dih-SYE-kloe-meen) Ⓖ

Brand Names

Bemote   Byclomine
Bentyl   Di-Spaz

Type of Drug

Antispasmodic and anticholinergic.

Prescribed for

Irritable bowel, spastic colon, and similar digestive problems.

General Information

Dicyclomine hydrochloride has been used for many years to calm "nervous stomach." It and other anticholinergics work by blocking the effects of the neurohormone acetylcholine in the gastrointestinal (GI) tract. This reduces the mobility of the GI tract and slows the production of enzymes and other secretions.

Cautions and Warnings

Do not take dicyclomine if you are **allergic** to it or another belladonna-related drug. This drug should be used with caution if you have **heart disease, Down syndrome, reduced mobility of the stomach and lower esophagus, fever, stomach obstruction, glaucoma, acute bleeding, hiatal hernia, intestinal paralysis, myasthenia gravis, kidney or liver dysfunction, rapid heartbeat, high blood pressure,** or **ulcerative colitis**. Because this drug reduces your ability to sweat, its use in hot weather may cause **heat exhaustion**.

Possible Side Effects

▼ Common: constipation, decreased sweating, and dry mouth, throat, or skin.

▼ Less common: reduced breast-milk flow, difficulty swallowing, blurred vision, and sensitivity to bright light.

▼ Rare: drug allergy (symptoms include rash, itching, hives, and breathing difficulties), confusion, eye pain, dizziness when rising quickly from a sitting or lying position, a bloated feeling, difficult or painful urination, drowsiness, unusual tiredness or weakness, headache, memory loss, and nausea or vomiting.

Drug Interactions

• Antacids containing calcium or magnesium, citrates, sodium bicarbonate, and carbonic-anhydrase inhibitor drugs may increase dicyclomine's therapeutic effect and side effects.

• Combining dicyclomine with other anticholinergic drugs including atropine, belladonna, clidinium, glycopyrrolate, hyoscyamine, isopropamide, propantheline, and scopolamine may intensify side effects.

• Dicyclomine may reduce stomach acidity and blood levels of oral ketoconazole (an antifungal).

• Dicyclomine may counteract the effect of metoclopramide in reducing nausea and vomiting.

• Taking dicyclomine with a narcotic pain reliever may cause severe constipation.

• Taking this or any drug that slows the movement of stomach and intestinal muscles with a potassium chloride supplement—especially one in wax-matrix tablet form—may lead to excessive irritation of the stomach.

Food Interactions

Take dicyclomine on an empty stomach, a half hour before or 2 hours after a meal.

Usual Dose

Adult: 30–160 mg a day. Seniors should receive the lowest possible dosage and increase only as needed.

Child (age 2 and over): 10 mg 3–4 times a day.

Child (age 6 months–2 years): 5–10 mg 3–4 times a day.

Child (under 6 months): not recommended.

Overdosage

Symptoms include blurred vision; clumsiness; confusion; breathing difficulties; dizziness; drowsiness; dry mouth, nose, or throat; rapid heartbeat; fever; hallucinations; weakness; slurred speech; excitement, restlessness, or irritability; warmth; and dry or flushed skin. Take the victim to a hospital emergency room at once. ALWAYS bring the prescription bottle or container.

Special Information

Children taking dicyclomine may be more likely to develop high body temperature in hot weather and other side effects and should be carefully watched for side effects.

Call your doctor if you develop rash, flushing, eye pain, dry mouth, urinary difficulties, constipation, increased sensitivity to light, or any bothersome or persistent side effect.

Brush and floss your teeth regularly while taking this drug. Because dicyclomine may cause dry mouth, you may be more likely to develop cavities or other dental problems. Ice or hard candy may relieve dry mouth.

Constipation may be treated by using a laxative.

Dicyclomine may make you drowsy or tired and cause blurred vision. Be careful when driving or doing any task that requires concentration.

If you forget a dose, take it as soon as you remember. If it is almost time for your next dose, skip the dose you forgot and continue with your regular schedule. Do not take a double dose.

Special Populations

Pregnancy/Breast-feeding

A few cases of human malformation were linked to dicyclomine, but studies have shown that the drug has no effect on the fetus. As with all other drugs, dicyclomine should be used during pregnancy only when absolutely necessary.

Dicyclomine can reduce the amount of milk produced. Infants given dicyclomine may faint, go limp, and develop breathing problems and seizures. Nursing mothers who must take this drug should bottle-feed.

Seniors

Seniors may be more susceptible to side effects, especially memory loss, changes in mental state, and glaucoma. Seniors may obtain maximum benefit with smaller dosages.

Generic Name

Didanosine (dye-DAN-oe-zene)

Brand Name

Videx

Type of Drug

Antiviral.

Prescribed for

Acquired immunodeficiency syndrome (AIDS).

General Information

Didanosine, also known as ddI or dideoxyinosine, is typically used together with a protease inhibitor and another anti-HIV drug or as part of another "HIV drug cocktail." Didanosine can also be given to children 6 months and older with AIDS who cannot tolerate or do not respond to AZT.

Didanosine interferes with the life of the human immuno-deficiency virus (HIV) that causes AIDS by interrupting the internal DNA manufacturing process essential to the repro-duction of HIV. Didanosine was tested in patients with advanced AIDS. It was approved because of its ability to pro-long life and to delay the next AIDS-related opportunistic infection or other AIDS-defining event. Didanosine was also effective in increasing blood levels of CD4 cells, which repre-sent the level of immune function and are considered impor-tant indicators of the severity of an AIDS infection.

Cautions and Warnings

The most serious—and potentially fatal—side effects of didanosine are nervous system inflammation and inflamma-tion of the pancreas.

Up to 50% of patients who take didanosine experience symptoms of **nervous system inflammation** and about 33% need to reduce their dosage to control these symptoms. Symptoms generally manifest as numbness, tingling, and pain in the hands and feet. People who already have these signs of nerve damage should not take didanosine.

Potentially fatal **inflammation of the pancreas** has occurred in up to 3% of people taking didanosine. Of people with a history of pancreatic inflammation who take didanosine, 33% are likely to develop this problem again. Symptoms of inflammation of the pancreas include major changes in blood-sugar levels, increased triglyceride blood levels, a drop in blood calcium, nausea, vomiting, and abdominal pain. People who develop pancreatic inflammation must stop taking didanosine.

Liver failure may develop in people taking this drug; 15% to 20% will begin to test abnormally for liver function. A small number of these patients may develop fatal liver disease.

Four children taking didanosine developed **severe eye disease,** resulting in some loss of sight. The progress of the eye disease slowed or stopped when dosage was reduced. Children taking this drug should have an eye examination every 6 months or if vision starts to worsen.

Kidney and liver disease may interfere with the elimination of didanosine from the body. Reduced doses may be required to accommodate these conditions.

Do not take didanosine if you are **allergic** to it or any ingredient in the didanosine tablet.

Possible Side Effects

▼ Most common: diarrhea, nervous system inflammation, fever, chills, itching, rash, abdominal pain, weakness, pains, headache, nausea, vomiting, infection, pneumonia, and pancreatic inflammation.

▼ Less common: tumors, muscle pain, appetite loss, dry mouth, convulsions, abnormal thought patterns, breathing difficulties, drug allergy, anxiety, nervousness, twitching, confusion, depression, and blood component abnormalities.

▼ Rare: Rare side effects can occur in almost any part of the body. Contact your doctor if you experience any side effect not listed above.

Almost all children who take didanosine experience side effects. They are likely to experience many of the same reactions as adults, most commonly chills, fever, weakness, appetite loss, nausea and vomiting, diarrhea, liver dysfunction, pains, headache, nervousness, sleeplessness, cough, runny nose, asthma or breathing difficulties, rash, and skin problems.

Drug Interactions

• Other drugs that may cause inflammation of the nervous system such as chloramphenicol, cisplatin, dapsone, disulfiram, ethionamide, glutethimide, gold, hydralazine, isoniazid, metronidazole, nitrofurantoin, ribavirin, and vincristine should be avoided while you are taking didanosine.

• Didanosine should not be taken with zalcitabine.

• Drugs that may cause inflammation of the pancreas, including intravenous pentamidine, should not be taken with didanosine.

• Quinolone anti-infectives, tetracycline antibiotics, and other drugs whose absorption into the bloodstream may be affected by antacids should not be taken within 2 hours of taking didanosine because of its high magnesium and aluminum content.

Food Interactions

Food may prevent the absorption of a dose of didanosine by up to 50%. Take didanosine on an empty stomach.

Usual Dose

Adult: 167–250 mg every 12 hours.
Child: 50–250 mg a day.

Dosage should be adjusted to the patient's level of kidney and liver function.

Overdosage

Didanosine overdose will cause many of the drug's side effects, especially inflammation of the nervous system or pancreas, diarrhea, and liver failure. Overdose victims should be taken to a hospital emergency room for testing and monitoring. ALWAYS remember to bring the prescription bottle or container.

Special Information

Didanosine does not cure AIDS. It will not prevent you from transmitting the HIV virus to another person; you must still practice safe sex. People may still develop AIDS-related opportunistic infections while taking this drug.

Didanosine may affect components of the blood system. Your doctor should perform blood tests to check for any changes.

People taking didanosine should take good care of their teeth and gums to minimize the possibility of oral infections.

Call your doctor if you develop any of the following symptoms of didanosine toxicity: numbness and pain in the hands and feet, nausea, vomiting, or abdominal pain.

If you are taking didanosine in chewable tablets, be sure to thoroughly chew each tablet. You may also completely dissolve the tablets in about ¼ cup of water and drink the entire mixture immediately. Do not mix didanosine tablets with juice or any other acidic drink.

If you are using the powdered form of didanosine, make a solution by pouring the entire contents of a packet into ½ cup of water. Stir until dissolved and drink immediately. Do not mix didanosine powder with juice or any other acidic drink. For children, your pharmacist will prepare a mixture of 10 mg per ml of didanosine and an equal amount of Mylanta Double Strength Antacid or Maalox TC Antacid. This mixture must be stored in a refrigerator and can be kept for 30 days. Shake well before using. Spilled didanosine should be cleaned immediately to prevent accidental poisoning.

If you forget to take a dose of didanosine, take it as soon as you remember. If it is almost time for your next dose, allow 4 to 8 hours to pass between the dose you took late and your next dose, and then continue with your regular schedule. Call your doctor for more specific advice if you forget to take several doses.

Special Populations

Pregnancy/Breast-feeding
Didanosine was slightly toxic to pregnant animals receiving doses 12 times human levels. There are no studies of pregnant women taking this drug; however, women who are or might become pregnant should only take didanosine if absolutely necessary and should use effective contraception to avoid passing on the virus.

It is not known if didanosine passes into breast milk. In any case, mothers who are HIV positive should bottle-feed their babies to avoid transmitting the virus through their milk.

Seniors
People with reduced kidney or liver function—common in seniors—should receive smaller dosages of didanosine than those with normal function.

Diflucan   *see Fluconazole, page 437*

Generic Name

Diflunisal (dye-FLOO-nih-sal) Ⓖ

Brand Name

Dolobid

Type of Drug

Nonsteroidal anti-inflammatory drug (NSAID).

Prescribed for

Rheumatoid arthritis, osteoarthritis, and mild to moderate pain.

General Information

Diflunisal is chemically similar to aspirin and is used to relieve pain and inflammation. We do not know exactly how NSAIDs work, but they may achieve their effects by blocking the body's production of a hormone called prostaglandin and the action of other body chemicals. Pain relief occurs within 1 hour of the first dose of diflunisal, but the drug's anti-inflammatory effect takes several days to 2 weeks to become apparent and may take several months to reach its maximum.

Cautions and Warnings

People who are **allergic** to diflunisal or any other NSAID and those with a history of **asthma** attacks brought on by NSAIDs, by iodides, or by aspirin should not take diflunisal.

This drug can cause **gastrointestinal (GI) bleeding, ulcers, and perforation**. This can occur at any time with or without warning in people who regularly use diflunisal. People with a history of active GI bleeding should be cautious about taking any NSAID. Minor stomach upset, gas, or distress is common during the first few days of treatment. People who develop bleeding or ulcers and continue their NSAID treatment should be aware of the possibility of developing more serious drug toxicity.

High doses of diflunisal can affect blood platelets and **blood clotting**. This drug should be avoided by people with clotting problems and those taking warfarin.

People with **heart problems** who use diflunisal may find that their arms, legs, or feet swell.

Diflunisal can cause severe side effects to the **kidney**. Report any unusual side effects to your doctor, who may need to periodically test your kidney function.

Diflunisal can make you **unusually sensitive to the effects of the sun.**

Diflunisal should be used with **caution in children and adolescents;** because it is related to aspirin, it may cause Reye's syndrome.

Possible Side Effects

▼ Most common: diarrhea, nausea, vomiting, constipation, stomach gas, stomach upset or irritation, and appetite loss.

▼ Less common: stomach ulcers, GI bleeding, hepatitis, gallbladder attacks, painful urination, poor kidney function, kidney inflammation, blood and protein in the urine, dizziness, fainting, nervousness, depression, hallucinations, confusion, disorientation, tingling in the hands or feet, light-headedness, itching, increased sweating, dry nose and mouth, heart palpitations, chest pain, breathing difficulties, and muscle cramps.

▼ Rare: severe allergic reactions including closing of the throat, fever and chills, changes in liver function, jaundice (symptoms include yellowing of the skin or whites of the eyes), and kidney failure. People who experience such effects must promptly be treated in a hospital emergency room or doctor's office at once. NSAIDs have caused severe skin reactions; if this happens to you, see your doctor immediately.

Drug Interactions

• Diflunisal can increase the effects of oral anticoagulant (blood-thinning) drugs such as warfarin. Your anticoagulant dose may need to be reduced.

• Diflunisal may increase acetaminophen blood levels by as much as 50%. This can be a problem for people with liver disease.

• Diflunisal increases the effects of thiazide diuretics.

• Combining diflunisal with indomethacin can cause fatal GI bleeding.

Food Interactions

Take diflunisal with food or a magnesium/aluminum antacid if it upsets your stomach.

Usual Dose

Starting dosage—500–1000 mg. Maintenance dosage—250–500 mg every 8–12 hours. Do not take more than 1500 mg a day. Do not crush or chew diflunisal tablets.

Overdosage

People have died from diflunisal overdose. Common overdose signs are drowsiness, nausea, vomiting, diarrhea, abdominal pain, rapid breathing, rapid heartbeat, increased sweating, ringing or buzzing in the ears, confusion, disorientation, stupor, and coma. Take the victim to a hospital emergency room at once. ALWAYS bring the prescription bottle or container.

Special Information

Take each dose with a full glass of water and do not lie down for 15 to 30 minutes afterward. Diflunisal can make you drowsy or tired: Be careful when driving or operating hazardous equipment.

Do not take any over-the-counter products containing acetaminophen or aspirin while taking diflunisal; also, avoid alcoholic beverages.

Contact your doctor if you develop rash, itching, visual disturbances, weight gain, breathing difficulties, fluid retention, hallucinations, black stools, persistent headache, or any unusual or intolerable side effect.

If you forget a dose of diflunisal, take it as soon as you remember. If you take several diflunisal doses a day and it is within 4 hours of your next dose, skip the one you forgot and continue with your regular schedule. If you take diflunisal once a day and it is within 8 hours of your next dose, skip the dose you forgot and continue with your regular schedule. Never take a double dose.

Special Populations

Pregnancy/Breast-feeding

Diflunisal may affect the fetal heart if taken during the last 3 months of pregnancy. If you are or might be pregnant, do not take diflunisal without your doctor's approval. When the drug is considered crucial by your doctor, its potential benefits must be carefully weighed against its risks.

Diflunisal passes into breast milk. There is a possibility that a nursing mother taking diflunisal could affect her baby's heart or cardiovascular system. Nursing mothers who must take this drug should bottle-feed.

Seniors

Seniors may be more susceptible to side effects, especially ulcer disease.

Type of Drug

Digitalis Glycosides

(dih-jih-TAL-is GLYE-coe-sides) G

Brand Names

Generic Ingredient: Digitoxin
Crystodigin

Generic Ingredient: Digoxin G
Lanoxicaps   Lanoxin

Prescribed for

Congestive heart failure (CHF) and other heart conditions involving a very rapid heartbeat.

General Information

Digitalis glycosides work directly on heart muscle. They improve the heart's pumping ability or help to control its beating rhythm. People with heart failure often develop swelling of the lower legs, feet, and ankles; digitalis drugs improve these symptoms by improving blood circulation. Digitoxin is more useful than digoxin for people who have kidney problems because digitoxin is removed mostly by the liver, not the kidneys. Digitalis glycosides are generally used as part of the lifelong treatment of CHF.

Cautions and Warnings

Do not use digitalis glycosides if you are **allergic** or **sensitive** to them. Digitalis allergies are rare and often limited to 1 member of the group; another digitalis drug may work in its place.

Digitalis glycosides have been used to treat obesity. The risk of fatal heart rhythms associated with such treatment makes them extremely **dangerous as weight-loss medication**. Many **heart disease symptoms** may be associated with digitalis glycosides. Report any unusual side effects to your doctor at once. **Kidney disease** may increase blood levels of all digitalis glycosides except digitoxin. **Liver disease** may increase blood levels of digitoxin. Your dosage may need adjusting.

Long-term use of a digitalis glycoside may cause the body to lose **potassium,** especially since these drugs are generally used in combination with diuretics (agents that increase urination). For this reason, be sure to eat a balanced diet and high-potassium foods—bananas, citrus fruits, melons, and tomatoes.

Digitalis requirements vary with **thyroid status**. If you are taking a digitalis glycoside and your thyroid status changes, your doctor will have to change your digitalis dosage.

Possible Side Effects

Adults and Seniors

▼ Most common: appetite loss, nausea, vomiting, diarrhea, and blurred or disturbed vision. If you experience any of these problems, call your doctor immediately.

▼ Less common: headache, weakness, apathy, drowsiness, blurred or yellow-tinted vision, seeing halos around bright lights, depression, psychoses, confusion or disorientation, restlessness, hallucinations, delirium, seizure, nerve pain, abnormal heart rhythms, and slow pulse.

▼ Rare: Enlargement of the breasts has been reported after long-term use of a digitalis glycoside. Allergy or sensitivity to digitalis drugs is uncommon.

Children

Children are more likely to develop abnormal heart rhythms before they see yellow or green halos or spots and before they develop nausea, vomiting, diarrhea, or stomach pain. Any abnormal heart rhythms that develop while a child is taking a digitalis glycoside should be assumed to be a side effect.

Drug Interactions

• Drugs that may increase the effect of a digitalis glycoside are alprazolam, amiloride aminoglycoside antibiotics, amiodarone, anticholinergic drugs, benzodiazepines, bepridil, captopril, diltiazem, erythromycin, esmolol, felodipine, flecainide, hydroxychloroquine, ibuprofen, indomethacin, itraconazole, nifedipine, omeprazole, propafenone, propantheline, quinidine, quinine, tetracycline, tolbutamide, triamterene, and verapamil.

• Drugs that may decrease blood levels of a digitalis glycoside include aminoglutethimide, aminoglycosides, oral sulfonylurea antidiabetes medication, antihistamines, barbiturates, phenytoin and related anti-seizure drugs, phenylbutazone, rifampin, antacids, aminosalicylic acid, cholestyramine, colestipol, anti-cancer combinations, kaolin-pectin mixtures, sucralfate, sulfasalazine, oral kanamycin, metoclopramide, and oral neomycin.

• Disopyramide may alter the effects of digoxin, although the exact interaction is not well understood.

• Thiazide diuretics, furosemide, ethacrynic acid, and bumetanide increase a digitalis glycoside's effect and increase the risk of side effects.

• Spironolactone may increase or decrease the effect of a digitalis glycoside.

• Spironolactone may increase or decrease the side effects of digitalis glycosides; amiloride may reduce the effect of a digitalis glycoside on the force of heart contraction.

• The effects of a digitalis glycoside on the heart may be additive to those of ephedrine, epinephrine and other stimulants, beta blockers, calcium salts, procainamide, and rauwolfia drugs.

• The dosage of a digitalis glycoside must be adjusted when it is combined with a thyroid drug.

Food Interactions

These drugs may generally be taken without regard to meals. Taking your medication after a high-fiber meal reduces the amount of drug absorbed into your blood.

Usual Dose

Digitoxin
   Adult: Starting dosage—known as the digitalizing or loading dosage—is 2 mg over about 3 days or 0.4 mg a day for 4

days. Digitalization may also be accomplished with lower dosage over 10–14 days. Maintenance dosage—0.03–0.05 mg daily. For seniors, lower dosage is required.

Child: usually not recommended.

Digoxin

Adult and Child (age 11 and over): Starting dosage—known as the digitalizing or loading dosage—is about 4–7 mcg per lb. of body weight. Digitalization may also be accomplished with a lower dosage over 7 days. Maintenance dosage—0.125–0.5 mg; it must be corrected for kidney function. For seniors, lower dosage is required.

Child (under age 11): starting dosage—5–30 mcg per lb. of body weight. Maintenance dosage—20%–35% of the starting dosage. Careful measurement of your child's digoxin dosage is crucial to safe and effective treatment.

Overdosage

Adult: Symptoms include appetite loss, nausea, vomiting, diarrhea, headache, weakness, apathy, blurred vision, yellow or green spots or halos before the eyes, yellowing of the skin or whites of the eyes, and changes in heartbeat.

Senior: Vomiting, diarrhea, and eye trouble are frequently seen.

Child: An early sign is a change in heart rhythms.

Call your doctor immediately if any of these symptoms appear. Take the victim to a hospital emergency room. ALWAYS bring the prescription bottle or container.

Special Information

Take each day's dose at the same time of day.

Do not stop taking a digitalis glycoside without your doctor's knowledge.

Lanoxicaps are better absorbed than tablet forms of digoxin. For this reason, each dose of lanoxicaps is slightly lower than the corresponding digoxin tablet.

Avoid over-the-counter diet and cold medication containing stimulants.

Call your doctor at once if you develop side effects.

There may be some variation between digitalis glycoside tablets from different manufacturers. Do not change drug brands without telling your doctor.

Check your pulse every day—your doctor will teach you how—and call your doctor if it drops below 60 beats per minute.

If you forget a dose and remember at least 12 hours before your next dose, take it right away. If you do not remember until it is less than 12 hours before your next dose, skip the one you forgot and continue with your regular schedule. Do not take a double dose. Call your doctor if you miss a dose for 2 or more days.

Special Populations

Pregnancy/Breast-feeding

Digitalis glycosides cross into the fetal circulation. While digoxin is sometimes used during pregnancy to treat fetal heart disease, women who are or might be pregnant should not take any digitalis glycoside without their doctor's approval. When this drug is considered crucial by your doctor, its potential benefits must be carefully weighed against its risks.

Small amounts of digoxin pass into breast milk. It is not known if digitoxin passes into breast milk. Nursing mothers who must take either drug should consider bottle-feeding.

Seniors

Seniors are more sensitive to digitalis effects, especially appetite loss.

Dilantin   see Phenytoin, page 813

Generic Name

Diltiazem   (dil-TYE-uh-zem)   Ⓖ

Brand Names

Cardizem	Dilacor XR
Cardizem CD	Tiamate
Cardizem SR	Tiazac
Cartia-XT	

Type of Drug

Calcium channel blocker.

Prescribed for

Angina pectoris, Raynaud's disease, prevention of second heart attacks, tardive dyskinesia (severe side effects associated with antipsychotic and other drugs), and hypertension (high blood pressure).

General Information

Diltiazem hydrochloride is one of many calcium channel blockers available in the U.S. These drugs block the passage of calcium, an essential factor in muscle contraction, into the heart and smooth muscles. Such blockage of calcium interferes with the contraction of these muscles, which in turn dilates (widens) the veins and vessels that supply blood to them. This dilating effect reduces blood pressure, the amount of oxygen used by the heart muscles, and the risk of blood vessel spasm. Diltiazem is therefore useful in treating not only hypertension but also angina pectoris (a condition characterized by brief attacks of chest pain), a condition related to poor oxygen supply to the heart muscles.

Diltiazem affects the movement of calcium only into muscle cells; it has no effect on calcium in the blood.

Cautions and Warnings

Diltiazem can slow your heart and interfere with normal electrical conduction. For people with a condition called **sick sinus syndrome,** this can result in temporary heart stoppage.

Diltiazem should not be taken if you are having a **heart attack** or if you have **lung congestion**. Diltiazem should be taken with caution by people with **heart failure** because it can worsen that condition.

Low blood pressure may occur, especially in people also taking a beta blocker.

Diltiazem can cause severe **liver damage** and should be taken with caution if you have had hepatitis or any other liver condition.

Caution should also be exercised if you have a history of **kidney problems,** although no clear tendency toward causing kidney damage is seen with this drug.

Possible Side Effects.

▼ Common: dizziness, light-headedness, weakness, headache, and fluid accumulation in the hands, legs, or feet.

▼ Less common: low blood pressure, fainting, increase or decrease in heart rate, abnormal heart rhythm, heart failure, nervousness, fatigue, nausea, rash, tingling in the hands or feet, hallucinations, temporary memory loss, difficulty sleeping, diarrhea, vomiting, constipation, upset stomach, itching, unusual sensitivity to sunlight, painful or stiff joints, liver inflammation, and increased urination, especially at night.

Drug Interactions

• Diltiazem taken with a beta-blocking drug for hypertension is usually well tolerated, but may lead to heart failure in people with already weakened hearts.

• Calcium channel blockers, including diltiazem, may add to the effects of digoxin. This effect is not observed with any consistency, however, and only affects people with a large amount of digoxin already in their systems.

• Cimetidine and ranitidine increase the amount of diltiazem in the bloodstream and may account for a slight increase in the drug's effect.

• Diltiazem may increase blood levels of cyclosporine, carbamazepine, encainide, and theophylline, and thus increase the chance of side effects from these drugs.

• Diltiazem may cause a decrease in blood lithium levels, possibly undermining lithium's antimanic effect.

Food Interactions

Diltiazem is best taken on an empty stomach, at least 1 hour before or 2 hours after meals.

Usual Dose

Immediate-Release Products
30–60 mg 4 times a day.

Sustained-Release Products
Cardizem SR: 60–180 mg twice a day.

Cardizem CD: 120–480 mg once a day.
Dilacor XR: 240–480 mg once a day.
Tiamate: 120–240 mg once a day.
Tiazac: 180–360 mg once a day.

Overdosage

Symptoms of diltiazem overdose are very low blood pressure and reduced heart rate. Overdose victims must be made to vomit with ipecac syrup—available at any pharmacy—within 30 minutes of taking the overdose. DO NOT INDUCE VOMITING IF THE VICTIM HAS FAINTED OR IS CONVULSING. If overdose symptoms have developed or more than 30 minutes have passed, vomiting is of little value. Take the victim to a hospital emergency room immediately. ALWAYS bring the prescription bottle or container.

Special Information

Call your doctor if you develop any of the following symptoms: swelling of the hands, legs, or feet; severe dizziness; constipation or nausea; or very low blood pressure.

Do not open, chew, or crush sustained-release capsules of Dilacor XR.

If you take your diltiazem 3 or 4 times a day and forget a dose, take it as soon as you remember. Space the remaining doses throughout the rest of the day. If you take diltiazem 1 or 2 times a day and forget to take a dose, take it as soon as you remember. If it is almost time for your next dose, skip the one you forgot and continue with your regular schedule. Never take a double dose.

Special Populations

Pregnancy / Breast-feeding

In animal studies, high doses of diltiazem interfered with the development of the fetus. Diltiazem should not be taken by women who are or might be pregnant. When your doctor considers this drug crucial, its potential benefits must be carefully weighed against its risks.

Because diltiazem passes into breast milk, nursing mothers taking this drug should bottle-feed.

Seniors

Seniors may be more sensitive to the effects of this drug because it takes longer to pass out of their bodies.

Generic Name

Dimenhydrinate (dye-men-HYE-drih-nate) G

Brand Names

Dimetabs   Dramamine

The information in this profile also applies to the following drug:

Generic Ingredient: Meclizine G
Antivert   Meni-D
Antivert 25   Ru-Vert-M
Antrizine

Type of Drug

Antihistamine and antiemetic (an agent that prevents or relieves nausea and vomiting).

Prescribed for

Nausea, vomiting, and dizziness associated with motion sickness.

General Information

Dimenhydrinate, which depresses middle ear function, is a mixture of diphenhydramine—an antihistamine believed to be the active ingredient—and another ingredient. Meclizine is an antihistamine. It takes a little longer to start working than dimenhydrinate, but its effects last much longer. Meclizine does a better job of preventing motion sickness than treating its symptoms. It takes 30 minutes to 1 hour to work and lasts for 12 to 24 hours.

Cautions and Warnings

People with a **prostate condition, stomach ulcer, bladder problems, difficulty urinating, glaucoma, asthma,** or **abnormal heart rhythms** should use dimenhydrinate only while under a doctor's care. **Newborn babies** and people who are **allergic** or **sensitive** to dimenhydrinate should not be given this drug.

Because it controls nausea and vomiting, dimenhydrinate **may hide the symptoms of appendicitis and overdoses of other drugs.**

Possible Side Effects

▼ Most common: drowsiness.

▼ Less common: confusion; nervousness; excitation; restlessness; headache; sleeplessness, especially in children; tingling; heavy or weak hands; fainting; dizziness; tiredness; rapid heartbeat; low blood pressure; heart palpitations; blurred or double vision; difficult or painful urination; increased sensitivity to the sun; appetite loss; nausea; vomiting; diarrhea; upset stomach; constipation; nightmares; rash; drug reaction (symptoms include rash, itching, hives, and breathing difficulties); ringing or buzzing in the ears; dry mouth, nose, or throat; stuffy nose; wheezing; and increased chest phlegm or chest tightness.

Drug Interactions

• Taking dimenhydrinate with an alcoholic beverage, other antihistamine, tranquilizer, or other nervous-system depressant may cause excessive dizziness, drowsiness, or other signs of nervous-system depression.

• Taking dimenhydrinate with a drug that causes dizziness or other ear-related side effects may mask early signs of these side effects, especially in infants and children.

Food Interactions

Take dimenhydrinate with food or milk if it upsets your stomach.

Usual Dose

Dimenhydrinate

Adult and Child (age 13 and over): 50–100 mg—1 or 2 tablets or 4–8 tsp.—every 4–6 hours; do not take more than 400 mg a day.

Child (age 6–12): 25–50 mg—½ or 1 tablet or 2–4 tsp.— every 6–8 hours; do not take more than 150 mg a day.

Child (age 2–5): up to 25 mg—½ tablet or 2 tsp.—every 6–8 hours; do not take more than 3 doses a day.

Child (under age 2): Consult your doctor.

Meclizine
Adult and Child (age 13 and over): 25–50 mg 1 hour before travel; repeat every 24 hours for duration of journey. Up to 100 mg may be needed to control dizziness from other causes.
Child: not recommended.

Overdosage

Symptoms of overdose include drowsiness, clumsiness, unsteadiness, feeling faint, facial flushing, and dry mouth, nose, or throat. Convulsions, coma, and breathing difficulties may also develop. Overdose victims should be taken to a hospital emergency room for treatment. ALWAYS bring the prescription bottle or container.

Special Information

For maximum effectiveness against motion sickness, take dimenhydrinate 1 to 2 hours before traveling; it may still be effective if taken 30 minutes before traveling.

Dimenhydrinate may cause dry mouth, nose, or throat. Sugarless candy, gum, or ice chips can usually relieve these symptoms. Constant dry mouth may increase the likelihood of developing tooth decay or gum disease. Pay special attention to oral hygiene while you are taking dimenhydrinate, and contact your doctor if dry mouth lasts more than 2 weeks.

If you forget to take a dose of dimenhydrinate, take it as soon as you remember. If it is almost time for your next dose, skip the one you forgot and continue with your regular schedule. Do not take a double dose.

Special Populations

Pregnancy/Breast-feeding

Animal studies suggest that meclizine may cause birth defects. Do not take any antihistamine without your doctor's knowledge if you are or might be pregnant—especially during the last 3 months of pregnancy, because newborns may have severe reactions to antihistamines.

Small amounts of dimenhydrinate may pass into breast milk. Dimenhydrinate may also slow milk production. Nursing mothers who must take dimenhydrinate should bottle-feed.

Seniors

Seniors are more sensitive to antihistamine side effects and should take the lowest effective dose.

Diovan   *see Angiotensin II Blockers, page 72*

Generic Name

Diphenhydramine Hydrochloride

(dye-fen-HYE-druh-mene hye-droe-KLOR-ide) Ⓖ

Brand Names

Dytuss   Tusstat

Type of Drug

Antihistamine.

Prescribed for

Stuffy and runny nose, itchy eyes, and scratchy throat caused by seasonal allergy and for other symptoms of allergy such as itching, rash, and hives; also prescribed for motion sickness, insomnia, and Parkinson's disease.

General Information

Antihistamines generally work by blocking the release of histamine (a chemical released by body tissue during an allergic reaction) drying the nose, throat, and eye secretions. Diphenhydramine is the most common active ingredient found in nonprescription sleep-aids.

Cautions and Warnings

This drug should not be used if you are **allergic** to it. It should be avoided or used with extreme care if you have narrow-angle **glaucoma, stomach ulcer** or other **stomach problems, enlarged prostate,** or **problems passing urine**. It should not be used by people who have **deep-breathing problems such**

as asthma. Use with care if you have a history of **thyroid disease, heart disease, high blood pressure,** or **diabetes**.

Possible Side Effects

▼ Common: drowsiness, weakness.

▼ Less common: itching, rash, sensitivity to bright light, perspiration, chills, lowering of blood pressure, headache, rapid heartbeat, sleeplessness, dizziness, disturbed coordination, confusion, restlessness, nervousness, irritability, euphoria (feeling high), tingling and weakness of the hands or feet, blurred or double vision, ringing in the ears, upset stomach, appetite loss, nausea, vomiting, constipation, diarrhea, urinary difficulties, thickening of lung secretions, tightness of the chest, wheezing, nasal stuffiness, and dry mouth, nose, or throat.

Drug Interactions

• This drug should not be taken with a monoamine oxidase inhibitor (MAOI) antidepressant.

• The effects of tranquilizers, sedatives, and sleeping medication will be intensified when combined with diphenhydramine hydrochloride; it is extremely important that doses of these drugs are properly adjusted.

• This drug increases the intoxicating and sedating effects of alcohol.

Food Interactions

Take this drug with food if it upsets your stomach.

Usual Dose

Allergy
  Adult: 25–50 mg 3–4 times a day.
  Child (over 20 lbs.): 12.5–25 mg 3–4 times a day.

Nightime Sedation
  Adult: 25–50 mg at bedtime.

Overdosage

Symptoms of overdose include depression or stimulation—especially in children; dry mouth; fixed or dilated pupils; flushing; and upset stomach. Overdose victims should be made to vomit with ipecac syrup—available at any pharmacy.

Take the overdose victim to a hospital emergency room immediately if you cannot induce vomiting. ALWAYS bring the prescription bottle or container.

Special Information

This drug produces a depressant effect: Be extremely cautious when driving or operating heavy equipment.

If you forget to take a dose of diphenhydramine hydrochloride, take it as soon as you remember. If it is almost time for your next dose, skip the one you forgot and continue with your regular schedule. Do not take a double dose.

Special Populations

Pregnancy/Breast-feeding

Animal studies have shown that some antihistamines may cause birth defects. Do not take any antihistamine without your doctor's knowledge if you are or might be pregnant—especially during the last 3 months of pregnancy—because newborns may have severe reactions to antihistamines.

Small amounts of antihistamine pass into breast milk. Nursing mothers who must take this drug should bottle-feed.

Seniors

Seniors are more sensitive to antihistamine side effects.

Generic Name

Dipivefrin (dye-piv-EF-rin) [G]

Brand Names

AK-Pro   Propine

Type of Drug

Sympathomimetic.

Prescribed for

Glaucoma.

General Information

When applied to the eye, dipivefrin hydrochloride is converted to epinephrine, one of the cornerstone drugs of glaucoma treatment. Dipivefrin has the same effect on glaucoma as epinephrine but has fewer side effects. Epinephrine decreases the production of fluid inside the eye and opens the channels by which eye fluid naturally drains. Dipivefrin starts working about half an hour after it is applied and reaches maximum effect in about 1 hour.

Cautions and Warnings

Use this product with care if you have **reacted to dipivefrin** in the past. People who have reacted to epinephrine eyedrops in the past are not likely to react to dipivefrin and can probably use this product.

Dipivefrin eyedrops contain a sulfite preservative. If you are **sensitive to sulfites,** this product might cause irritation or allergic reactions.

Possible Side Effects

▼ Common: burning or stinging upon applying the eyedrops.

▼ Rare: conjunctivitis, drug allergies, rapid heartbeat, abnormal heart rhythms, and high blood pressure.

Drug Interactions

• Dipivefrin eyedrops may be taken with other antiglaucoma eyedrops.

Usual Dose

1 drop in the affected eye every 12 hours.

Overdosage

Possible symptoms of overdose are rapid heartbeat, excitement, or sleeplessness. Call your local poison control center or hospital emergency room for more information.

Special Information

To prevent infection, do not touch the dropper tip to your finger or eyelid. Wait 5 minutes before using any other eyedrop or ointment.

If you forget a dose of dipivefrin, take it as soon as you remember. If it is almost time for your next dose, skip the dose you forgot and then go back to your regular schedule. Do not take a double dose.

Special Populations

Pregnancy/Breast-feeding

Pregnant women should not use dipivefrin unless its possible benefits have been carefully weighed against its risks.

It is not known if this drug passes into breast milk. Nursing mothers who use dipivefrin should exercise caution.

Seniors

Seniors may use dipivefrin without any special precautions. Some older adults may have weaker eyelid muscles. This creates a small reservoir for the eyedrops and may actually increase the drug's effect by keeping it in contact with the eye for a longer period.

Generic Name

Dirithromycin (dye-rith-roe-MYE-sin)

Brand Name

Dynabac

Type of Drug

Macrolide antibiotic.

Prescribed for

Infections caused by streptococcus, staphylococcus, and other bacteria against which penicillin or tetracycline antibiotics cannot be used.

General information

Dirithromycin and other macrolide antibiotics are either bactericidal (bacteria-killing) or bacteriostatic (inhibiting bacterial growth), depending on the organism in question and amount of antibiotic present. Dirithromycin has been studied in bronchitis, sore throat, pneumonia, tonsillitis, and legionnaires' disease. The drug is not broken down by the liver and passes out of the body through the stool.

Cautions and Warnings

Do not take dirithromycin if you are **allergic** to it or any macrolide.

Dirithromycin should not be used for **serious blood infections** or ***Haemophilus influenzae,*** a very contagious infection that often affects children in daycare centers and their families.

Dosage changes are not needed for people with mild liver disease or with kidney disease. This drug has not been studied in people with **severe liver disease**.

Colitis (bowel inflammation) has been associated with all antibiotics (see "Possible Side Effects").

Possible Side Effects

▼ Most common: abdominal pain, headache, nausea, and diarrhea.

▼ Less common: increased blood-platelet count, vomiting, upset stomach, increased blood potassium, dizziness, fainting, pain, weakness, stomach disorders, increasing cough, gas, rash, breathing difficulties, itching, and sleeplessness. Blood tests can also be affected.

▼ Rare: Rare side effects can occur in almost any part of the body. Contact your doctor if you experience any side effect not listed above.

Drug Interactions

• The amount of dirithromycin absorbed into the blood increases slightly when it is taken immediately after an antacid or H_2-antagonist such as cimetidine, famotidine, nizatidine, or ranitidine. This effect is not considered important.

• Pimozide should not be taken with dirithromycin. Two people died after combining a macrolide and pimozide.

Food Interactions

For optimum effectiveness, take with food or within 1 hour of having eaten.

Usual Dose

Tablets
   Adult and Child (age 12 and over): 500 mg a day for 7–10 days.
   Child (under age 12): not recommended.

Overdosage

Overdose may result in nausea, vomiting, stomach cramps, and diarrhea. Call your local poison control center or a hospital emergency room for more information.

Special Information

Dirithromycin is not the antibiotic of choice for severe infections.

Do not crush, cut, or chew dirithromycin tablets.

Call your doctor if you develop nausea, vomiting, diarrhea, stomach cramps, severe abdominal pain, or any severe or persistent side effect.

If you forget a dose, take it as soon as you remember. If you do not remember until the next day, skip the dose you forgot and go back to your regular schedule. Call your doctor if you forget more than 1 dose.

Remember to take the full course of dirithromycin exactly as prescribed, even if you feel well sooner.

Special Populations

Pregnancy/Breast-feeding

Dirithromycin affected the fetus in animal studies. When this drug is considered crucial by your doctor, its potential benefits must be carefully weighed against its risks.

It is not known if dirithromycin passes into breast milk, but other macrolides do. Nursing mothers who take this drug should bottle-feed.

Seniors

Seniors may use dirithromycin without special restriction.

Generic Name

Disopyramide (die-soe-PIE-rah-mide) Ⓖ

Brand Names

Norpace   Norpace CR

Type of Drug

Antiarrhythmic.

Prescribed for

Abnormal heart rhythms.

General Information

Disopyramide phosphate slows the rate at which nerve impulses are carried through heart muscle, reducing the response of heart muscle to those impulses. It acts on the heart similarly to the more widely used antiarrhythmic medications procainamide hydrochloride and quinidine sulfate. Disopyramide is often prescribed for people who do not respond to other antiarrhythmic drugs.

Cautions and Warnings

This drug can worsen **heart failure** or trigger severely **low blood pressure**. It should be used in combination with another antiarrhythmic agent or beta blocker, only with caution.

In rare instances, disopyramide has caused a **reduction in blood-sugar levels**. Therefore, the drug should be used with caution by diabetics, older adults—who are more susceptible to this effect—and people with poor kidney or liver function. Ask your doctor if you should have your blood-sugar levels checked while taking this drug.

Because of its anticholinergic effects, men with a severe **prostate condition** and people who have **glaucoma, myasthenia gravis,** or severe **difficulty urinating** should use disopyramide with caution.

People with liver or kidney disease must take a reduced dose of disopyramide.

Possible Side Effects

▼ Most common: heart failure, low blood pressure, and urinary difficulty.

▼ Common: dry mouth, throat, or nose; constipation; and blurred vision.

▼ Less common: urination, dizziness, fatigue, headache, nervousness, breathing difficulties, chest pain, nausea, stomach pain or bloating, gas, appetite loss, diarrhea, vomiting, itching, rashes, muscle weakness, generalized aches and pains, not feeling well, low blood-potassium levels, increases in blood-cholesterol and triglyceride levels, and dry eyes.

> **Possible Side Effects** *(continued)*
>
> ▼ Rare: Rare side effects can occur in almost any part of the body. Contact your doctor if you experience any side effect not listed above.

Drug Interactions

• Phenytoin and rifampin may increase the rate at which the body removes disopyramide from the blood. Your disopyramide dose may need alteration if this combination is used. Other drugs known to increase drug breakdown by the liver, such as barbiturates and primidone, may also have this effect.

• Other antiarrhythmic drugs, such as procainamide and quinidine, may increase the effect of disopyramide, making dosage reduction necessary. At the same time, disopyramide may reduce the effectiveness of quinidine.

• When disopyramide is combined with a beta-blocking drug, increased disopyramide effects, additive effects, or depression of heart function may result.

• Erythromycin may increase the amount of disopyramide in your blood, causing abnormal heart rhythms or other cardiac effects.

• Disopyramide may reduce the effectiveness of oral anticoagulant (blood-thinning) drugs. Your doctor should check your anticoagulant dosage to be sure you are getting the right amount.

• Disopyramide may increase the amount of digoxin in your blood, though the amount of the increase is not likely to affect your heart.

Food Interactions

Disopyramide should be taken on an empty stomach at least 1 hour before or 2 hours after meals.

Usual Dose

Adult: 400–600 mg a day divided into 2 or 4 doses. In severe cases, 400 mg every 6 hours may be required. The sustained-release preparation is taken every 12 hours. People with reduced kidney function should receive a lower dosage, depending on the degree of kidney function present. People with liver failure should take 400 mg a day.

Child (age 13–18): 2.5–7 mg a day per lb. of body weight.
Child (age 5–12): 4.5–7 mg a day per lb. of body weight.
Child (age 1–4): 4.5–9 mg a day per lb. of body weight.
Child (under age 1): 4.5–13.5 mg a day per lb. of body weight.

Overdosage

Overdose symptoms are breathing difficulties, abnormal heart rhythms, and unconsciousness. In severe cases, overdosage can lead to death. Overdose victims should be made to vomit with ipecac syrup—available at any pharmacy—to remove any remaining drug from the stomach. Call your doctor or poison control center before doing this. If you must go to a hospital emergency room, ALWAYS bring the prescription bottle or container. Prompt and vigorous treatment can mean the difference between life and death in severe overdosage.

Special Information

Disopyramide may cause symptoms of low blood sugar: anxiety, chills, cold sweats, drowsiness, excessive hunger, nausea, nervousness, rapid pulse, shakiness, unusual weakness, tiredness, or cool, pale skin. If this happens to you, eat some chocolate, candy, or other high-sugar food, and call your doctor at once.

Disopyramide can cause dry mouth, urinary difficulty, constipation, or blurred vision. Call your doctor if these symptoms become severe or intolerable, but do not stop taking the medication without your doctor's approval.

If disopyramide is required for a child and capsules are not appropriate, your pharmacist can make a liquid product. Do not do this at home: This medication requires special preparation. The liquid should be refrigerated and protected from light and should be thrown away after 30 days.

If you forget to take a dose of disopyramide, take it as soon as possible. However, if it is within 4 hours of your next dose, skip the dose you forgot and go back to your regular schedule. Do not take a double dose.

Special Populations

Pregnancy/Breast-feeding
Do not take this drug if you are pregnant or planning to become pregnant while using it, because it will pass into the

fetus and may affect its development. When disopyramide is considered crucial by your doctor, its potential benefits must carefully be weighed against its risks.

Disopyramide passes into breast milk. Nursing mothers who must take this drug should bottle-feed.

Seniors
Seniors, especially those with liver or kidney disease, are more sensitive to the effects of this drug.

Generic Name

Donepezil (don-EP-eh-zil)

Brand Name
Aricept

Type of Drug
Cholinesterase inhibitor.

Prescribed for
Alzheimer's disease (degenerative condition of the central nervous system).

General Information
Donepezil hydrochloride works by increasing the function of certain receptors in the brain that are stimulated by the hormone acetylcholine. It does this by interfering with cholinesterase, the enzyme that breaks down acetylcholine. There is no evidence that donepezil reverses the degenerative effects of Alzheimer's, but it may slow the rate at which the disease worsens.

Cautions and Warnings
Do not take this drug if you are **allergic** to it or to piperidine-type drugs.

Donepezil must be discontinued prior to **surgery** because it increases the effects of anesthetic drugs.

People with **heart disease** should use donepezil with caution because it may slow heart rate.

Donepezil has not been linked to other effects caused by cholinesterase inhibitors, such as an increase in stomach acid that may lead to **ulcers** or **bleeding**—alcohol and non-steroidal anti-inflammatory drugs (NSAIDs) such as aspirin may worsen this effect. Use of cholinesterase inhibitors may also lead to **urinary blockage,** increase the risk of generalized **seizures,** and worsen **asthma or other pulmonary disease**.

Possible Side Effects

In studies, people taking donepezil experienced side effects at about the same rate as those taking a placebo (sugar pill).

▼ Most common: headache, pain, accidents, nausea, diarrhea, sleeplessness, and dizziness.

▼ Common: tiredness, vomiting, appetite loss, and muscle cramps.

▼ Less common: arthritis, depression, abnormal dreams, fainting, black-and-blue marks, and weight loss.

▼ Rare: Rare side effects can occur in almost any part of the body. Contact your doctor if you experience any side effect not listed above.

Drug Interactions

• Donepezil interferes with anticholinergic drugs (often prescribed for stomach disorders).

• Donepezil can be expected to increase the effects of surgical anesthetic drugs and drugs that irritate the stomach and intestines, such as aspirin or other NSAIDs.

• Ketoconazole and quinidine can slow the breakdown of donepezil in the liver. The importance of this interaction is unclear.

Food Interactions

None known.

Usual Dose

Adult: 5 or 10 mg once a day.

Overdosage

Overdose may be very serious. Symptoms include severe nausea, vomiting, salivation, sweating, slow heart rate, low blood pressure, slow breathing rate, convulsions, muscle weakness, and collapse. Take the victim to a hospital emer-

gency room at once. ALWAYS bring the prescription bottle or
container.

Special Information

Take donepezil just before bedtime.

If you forget a dose, take it as soon as you remember. If it is
almost time for your next dose, skip the dose you forgot and
continue with your regular schedule. Never take a double
dose.

Special Populations

Pregnancy/Breast-feeding

One animal study of donepezil indicated a small risk of birth
defects. When this drug is considered crucial by your doctor,
its potential benefits must be carefully weighed against its
risks.

It is not known if donepezil passes into breast milk. Nursing
mothers who must take this drug should consider bottle-
feeding.

Seniors

Seniors may take this drug without special precaution.

Brand Name

Donnatal

Generic Ingredients

Atropine Sulfate + Hyoscyamine Sulfate + Phenobarbital +
Scopolamine Hydrobromide G

Other Brand Names

Barbidonna   Spasmolin
Hyosophen   Susano

The information in this profile also applies to the following
drugs:

Generic Ingredient: Hyoscyamine Sulfate G
Donnamar

*Generic Ingredients: Belladonna Alkaloids +
Phenobarbital* G
Donnapine

Generic Ingredient: Propanthelene Ⓖ
Pro-Banthine

Type of Drug

Anticholinergic combination.

Prescribed for

Stomach spasm and gastrointestinal (GI) cramps; also used
to treat motion sickness.

General Information

Donnatal is a mild antispasmodic sedative. Its principal action
is to counteract the effect of acetylcholine, an important neurohormone. Donnatal is used only to relieve symptoms, not to
treat the underlying condition, and there is considerable
doubt among medical experts that this drug lives up to its
claims. In addition to the brand names listed above, there are
about 50 other anticholinergic combinations with similar
properties. All are used to relieve cramps and all are about
equally effective. Some have additional ingredients to reduce
or absorb excess gas in the stomach, to coat the stomach, or
to control diarrhea. Donnatal and products like it should not
be used for more than the temporary relief of symptoms.

Cautions and Warnings

Donnatal should not be used by people with **glaucoma**, **rapid
heartbeat**, severe **intestinal disease** such as **ulcerative colitis**,
serious **kidney or liver disease**, or a history of **allergy** to any
of the ingredients of this drug.

Donnatal can reduce your ability to sweat and may lead to
heat exhaustion. Avoid extended heavy exercise and limit
your exposure to high temperatures.

Possible Side Effects

▼ Most common: blurred vision, dry mouth, urinary
difficulties, flushing, and dry skin.

▼ Less common: rapid or unusual heartbeat,
increased sensitivity to bright light, loss of the sense of
taste, headache, nervousness, tiredness, weakness, dizziness, sleeplessness, nausea, vomiting, fever, stuffy nose,
heartburn, loss of sex drive, decreased sweating, constipation, feeling bloated, and allergic reactions such as
fever and rash.

Drug Interactions

• Although Donnatal contains only a small amount of phenobarbital, it is wise to avoid alcohol or other sedative drugs. Although unlikely, phenobarbital interactions are possible with anticoagulants, adrenal corticosteroids, tranquilizers, narcotics, sleeping pills, digitalis or other cardiac glycosides, and antihistamines.

• Some phenothiazine drugs, tranquilizers, tricyclic antidepressants, and narcotics may increase the side effects of the atropine sulfate ingredient in Donnatal, causing dry mouth, urinary difficulties, and constipation.

Food Interactions

Take Donnatal 30 to 60 minutes before meals.

Usual Dose

Donnatal
   Adult (age 13 and over): 1–2 tablets, capsules, or tsp. 3–4 times a day.
   Child (age 2–12): ½ the adult dosage.
   Child (under age 2): not recommended.

Propantheline
   Adult: 7.5–15 mg 3 times a day, and 30 mg at bedtime.
   Senior: 7.5 mg 3 times a day.
   Child (under age 12): not recommended.

Overdosage

Symptoms of overdose include dry mouth; difficulty swallowing; thirst; blurred vision; sensitivity to bright light; flushed, hot, or dry skin; rash; fever; abnormal heart rate; high blood pressure; urinary difficulties; restlessness; confusion; delirium; and breathing difficulties. The victim should be taken to a hospital emergency room immediately. ALWAYS bring the prescription bottle or container.

Special Information

Dry mouth usually can be relieved by chewing gum or sucking hard candy or ice chips. Constipation can be treated with a stool-softening laxative.

Donnatal may reduce the amount of saliva in your mouth, making it easier for bacteria to grow there. Pay special attention to dental hygiene while taking this medication to prevent cavities and gum disease.

Donnatal may cause drowsiness and blurred vision. Be careful when driving or operating hazardous equipment.

If you forget to take a dose of Donnatal, take it as soon as you remember. If it is almost time for your next dose, skip the one you forgot and continue with your regular schedule. Do not take a double dose.

Special Populations

Pregnancy/Breast-feeding

Donnatal may cause drug dependency or breathing problems in newborns and may interfere with labor and delivery. Check with your doctor before taking it if you are or might be pregnant.

Donnatal passes into breast milk and may reduce the amount of milk produced. It may cause tiredness, shortness of breath, and a slower-than-normal heartbeat in infants. Nursing mothers who must take this medication should consider bottle-feeding.

Seniors

Seniors are often more sensitive to the side effects of Donnatal, such as excitement, confusion, drowsiness, agitation, constipation, dry mouth, and urinary difficulties. Memory may be impaired and glaucoma worsened.

Generic Name

Doxazosin (dok-SAY-zoe-sin)

Brand Name

Cardura

Type of Drug

Antihypertensive.

Prescribed for

High blood pressure and benign prostatic hyperplasia (BPH); also used with digoxin and diuretic drugs to treat congestive heart failure.

General Information

Doxazosin mesylate and other alpha-adrenergic blocking agents, or alpha blockers, reduce blood pressure by dilating (widening) blood vessels. They achieve this effect by blocking nerve endings known as alpha$_1$ receptors. The maximum blood-pressure-lowering effect of doxazosin is seen between 2 and 6 hours after taking a dose. In BPH treatment, doxazosin works by relaxing smooth muscles in the prostate and neck of the bladder. Doxazosin reduces the symptoms of BPH, but the drug's long-term effect on the complications of BPH or the need for surgery is not known. Doxazosin's effect lasts for 24 hours. It is broken down in the liver; little passes out of the body via the kidneys.

Cautions and Warnings

Doxazosin may cause **dizziness** and **fainting,** especially the first few doses. This is known as a first-dose effect, which can be minimized by limiting the first dose to 1 mg at bedtime. First-dose effects occur in about 1% of people taking an alpha blocker and may recur if the drug is stopped for a few days and then started again.

Doxazosin should be taken with caution if you have **liver disease**.

People **allergic** or **sensitive** to any alpha blocker should avoid doxazosin.

Doxazosin may slightly reduce cholesterol levels and improve the ratio of high-density lipoprotein (HDL)/low-density lipoprotein (LDL), a positive step for people with a blood-cholesterol problem.

Red- and white-blood-cell counts may be slightly decreased in people taking doxazosin.

Possible Side Effects

▼ Most common: headache, dizziness, and weakness.

▼ Less common: heart palpitations, abnormal heart rhythms, chest pain, nausea, diarrhea, constipation, abdominal pain or discomfort, gas, breathing difficulties, nosebleed, sore throat, runny nose, muscle or joint pain, visual disturbances, conjunctivitis (pinkeye), ringing in the ears, fainting, depression, decreased sex drive or sexual function, tingling in the hands or feet, nervousness, tiredness, anxiety, sleeplessness, poor muscle coordination, muscle stiffness, poor bladder control, frequent urination, itching, rash, sweating, fluid retention, facial swelling and flushing, and back, neck, shoulder, arm, or leg pain.

Possible Side Effects (continued)

▼ Rare: vomiting, dry mouth, sinus irritation, bronchitis, cold or flu symptoms, worsening of asthma, coughing, hair loss, weight gain, and fever.

Drug Interactions

• Doxazosin may interact with beta blockers to increase the risk of dizziness or fainting after the first dose of doxazosin.
• The blood-pressure-lowering effect of doxazosin may be reduced by indomethacin.
• When taken with other blood-pressure-lowering drugs, doxazosin produces a severe reduction of blood pressure.
• The blood-pressure-lowering effect of clonidine may be reduced by doxazosin.

Food Interactions

None known.

Usual Dose

1 mg at bedtime to start; may be increased to a total daily dosage of 16 mg, taken once or twice a day.

Overdosage

Overdose may produce drowsiness, poor reflexes, and very low blood pressure. Overdose victims should be taken to a hospital emergency room at once. ALWAYS bring the prescription bottle or container.

Special Information

Take doxazosin exactly as prescribed. Do not stop taking it unless directed to do so by your doctor. Avoid over-the-counter drugs that contain stimulants because they may increase your blood pressure.

Doxazosin may cause dizziness, headache, and drowsiness, especially 2 to 6 hours after you take your first dose, although these effects can persist after the first few doses.

Call your doctor if you develop severe dizziness, heart palpitations, or any bothersome or persistent side effect.

Wait 12 to 24 hours after taking your first dose of doxazosin before driving or doing anything that requires concentration. Take your dose at bedtime to minimize this problem.

If you forget a dose, take it as soon as you remember. If it is almost time for your next dose, skip the dose you forgot and continue with your regular schedule. Do not take a double dose.

Special Populations

Pregnancy/Breast-feeding
The safety of using doxazosin during pregnancy is not known.

Small amounts of doxazosin pass into breast milk. Nursing mothers who must take this drug should bottle-feed.

Seniors
Seniors, especially those with liver disease, may be more sensitive to the effects and side effects of doxazosin.

Generic Name

Dronabinol (droe-NAB-ih-nol)

Brand Name
Marinol

Type of Drug
Antinauseant.

Prescribed for
Nausea and vomiting associated with cancer chemotherapy, and appetite stimulation and weight loss prevention in people with acquired immunodeficiency syndrome (AIDS).

General Information
Dronabinol is a legal form of marijuana. The psychoactive chemical in marijuana is delta-9-THC. Dronabinol has all of the psychological effects of marijuana and is therefore considered to be a highly abusable drug. It can cause personality changes, feelings of detachment, hallucinations, and euphoria (feeling "high"). Younger adults have reported a greater success rate with dronabinol, probably because they are better able to tolerate these effects.

Most people start taking dronabinol while in the hospital so their response to the drug and its possible adverse effects can be monitored. Dronabinol is also being studied as a glaucoma treatment.

Cautions and Warnings

Dronabinol should not be used to treat **nausea and vomiting** caused by anything other than cancer chemotherapy. It should not be used by people who are **allergic** to it, to marijuana, or to sesame oil. Dronabinol has a profound effect on **mental states;** it will impair your ability to operate complex equipment or engage in any activity that requires intense concentration, sound judgment, or coordination—such as driving a car.

Dronabinol produces **withdrawal symptoms** when the drug is stopped. These may develop within 12 hours of the drug's discontinuation and include restlessness, sleeplessness, and irritability. Within a day after the drug has been stopped, stuffy nose, hot flashes, sweating, loose stools, hiccups, or appetite loss may occur. The symptoms usually subside within a few days.

Dronabinol should be used with caution by people with a **manic-depressive or schizophrenic history** because it may aggravate the underlying disease.

Possible Side Effects

▼ Most common: drowsiness, euphoria, dizziness, anxiety, muddled thinking, perceptual difficulties, poor coordination, irritability, a separation in time and space, depression, weakness, sluggishness, headache, hallucinations, memory lapses, loss of muscle coordination, unsteadiness, paranoia, depersonalization, disorientation, confusion, rapid heartbeat, and dizziness when rising from a sitting or lying position.

▼ Less common: difficulty talking or slurred speech, facial flushing, excessive perspiration, nightmares, ringing or buzzing in the ears, fainting, diarrhea, loss of bowel control, and muscle pain.

Drug Interactions

• Dronabinol increases the effects of alcohol, tranquilizers, sleeping pills, sedatives, and other depressants. It also enhances the effects of psychoactive drugs including tricyclic antidepressants, amphetamines, cocaine, and other stimulants.

• Dronabinol may increase the effects of fluoxetine and disulfiram.

• The effects of theophylline drugs are reduced by dronabinol.

Food Interactions

This drug may be taken without regard to food or meals; as an appetite stimulant, it is often taken before meals.

Usual Dose

Antiemetic: 5–15 mg 1–3 hours before starting chemotherapy treatment and repeated every 2–4 hours after treatment, for a total of 4–6 doses a day. Dosage may be increased up to 30 mg a day if needed; psychiatric side effects increase greatly at higher dosages.

Appetite Stimulant: 2.5 mg before lunch or dinner or at bedtime. Dosage may be increased to 20 mg a day.

Overdosage

Overdose symptoms may occur at usual dosages or at higher dosages if the drug is being abused. The primary symptoms of overdose are the psychological symptoms listed above (see "Possible Side Effects"). In some cases, overdose may lead to panic reactions or seizure. Contact a hospital or local poison center for more information. Dronabinol therapy may be restarted at lower dosages if other drugs are ineffective.

Special Information

Be careful when driving or performing any task that requires concentration. Avoid alcohol and other nervous-system depressants.

Dronabinol may cause acute psychiatric or psychological effects. Call your doctor if any develop.

The capsules must be stored in the refrigerator.

If you forget a dose, take it as soon as you remember. If it is almost time for your next dose, skip the one you forgot and continue with your regular schedule. Do not take a double dose.

Special Populations

Pregnancy/Breast-feeding
Animal studies have shown no adverse effects on fetal development. However, dronabinol should not be taken by a pregnant woman unless it is absolutely necessary.

Dronabinol passes into breast milk. Nursing mothers who
must take this drug should bottle-feed.

Seniors
Seniors are more sensitive to this drug, especially its psychological effects.

Brand Name

Dyazide

Generic Ingredients

Hydrochlorothiazide + Triamterene Ⓖ

Other Brand Names
Maxzide   Maxzide-25MG

The information in this profile also applies to the following
drugs:

Generic Ingredients: Amiloride + Hydrochlorothiazide Ⓖ
Moduretic

Generic Ingredients: Spironolactone + Hydrochlorothiazide Ⓖ
Aldactazide

Type of Drug

Diuretic (an agent that increases urination).

Prescribed for

Hypertension (high blood pressure) or any condition where it
is desirable to eliminate excess water from the body.

General Information

Dyazide combines a thiazide diuretic and a potassium-sparing diuretic. The latter, triamterene, helps the body retain

potassium while producing a diuretic effect. This balances the other ingredient, hydrochlorothiazide, which normally causes a loss of potassium. Different products contain differing concentrations of these 2 drugs. Dyazide should be used only when you need its exact proportion of ingredients.

Cautions and Warnings

Do not use Dyazide if you have **nonfunctioning kidneys,** are **allergic** to this drug or any sulfa drug, or have a history of **allergy** or **bronchial asthma**.

Do not combine any **potassium supplement** and Dyazide without your doctor's knowledge.

Possible Side Effects

▼ Most common: appetite loss, drowsiness, lethargy, headache, gastrointestinal upset, cramping, and diarrhea.

▼ Less common: rash, mental confusion, fever, feeling unwell, impotence, bright red tongue, burning sensation in the tongue, tingling in the toes and fingers, restlessness, anemia or other effects on blood components, increased sensitivity to sunlight, and dizziness when rising quickly from a sitting position. Dyazide may also produce muscle spasms, gout, weakness, and blurred vision.

Drug Interactions

• Dyazide increases the effect of other blood-pressure-lowering drugs. This is positive and used regularly in blood-pressure treatment.

• Combining Dyazide and digitalis drugs, amphotericin B, or adrenal corticosteroids increases the risk of body-fluid imbalance. If you are taking insulin or an oral antidiabetic drug and begin taking Dyazide, the insulin or antidiabetic dosage may have to be modified.

• Dyazide may increase the risk of allopurinol side effects.

• Dyazide may decrease the effects of oral anticoagulant (blood-thinning) drugs.

• Antigout drug dosage may have to be modified since Dyazide raises uric-acid levels.

• Dyazide may prolong the effects of chemotherapy drugs on reducing white-blood-cell counts.

• Dyazide may increase the effects of diazoxide, which may lead to symptoms of diabetes.

• Dyazide should not be taken with loop diuretics because the combination can lead to an extreme diuretic effect and an extreme effect on blood-sodium levels.

• Dyazide may increase the effect of vitamin D, which may cause high blood-calcium levels.

• Propantheline and other anticholinergics may increase the diuretic effect of Dyazide.

• Lithium carbonate taken with Dyazide should be monitored carefully by a doctor due to an increased risk of lithium side effects.

• Cholestyramine and colestipol prevent Dyazide from being absorbed. Dyazide should be taken at least 2 hours before cholestyramine or colestipol.

• Methenamine and other urinary agents may reduce the effect of Dyazide.

• Some nonsteroidal anti-inflammatory drugs (NSAIDs), particularly indomethacin, may reduce the effect of Dyazide. Sulindac, another NSAID, may increase its effect.

Food Interactions

Take this drug with food if it upsets your stomach.

Usual Dose

1–2 capsules or tablets a day.

Overdosage

Symptoms may include tingling in the arms or legs, weakness, fatigue, changes in heartbeat, a sickly feeling, dry mouth, restlessness, muscle pain or cramps, urinary difficulties, nausea, and vomiting. Take the victim to a hospital emergency room immediately. ALWAYS bring the prescription bottle or container.

Special Information

Dyazide causes excess urination at first, but this subsides after several weeks of use. Diuretics are usually taken early in the day to prevent excessive nighttime urination that may interfere with sleep.

Dyazide may make you drowsy. Be careful when driving or performing any task that requires concentration.

Call your doctor if you develop muscle pain, sudden joint pain, weakness, cramps, nausea, vomiting, restlessness, excessive thirst, tiredness, drowsiness, increased heart or pulse rate, diarrhea, dizziness, headache, or rash.

People with diabetes may experience an increased blood-sugar level and require dosage adjustments of their antidiabetic medications.

Avoid other drugs while taking Dyazide unless otherwise directed by your doctor. Avoid alcohol.

If you are taking Dyazide for the treatment of hypertension or congestive heart failure (CHF), avoid over-the-counter cough, cold, or allergy medications, which may contain stimulants.

Take Dyazide exactly as prescribed. Be aware that all triamterene-hydrochlorothiazide products are not equal to each other and should not be freely substituted. Check with your doctor and pharmacist before switching brands.

If you forget a dose, take it as soon as you remember. If it is almost time for your next dose, skip the dose you forgot and continue with your regular schedule. Do not take a double dose.

Special Populations

Pregnancy/Breast-feeding

Dyazide may enter the fetal circulation, though it is sometimes used to treat specific conditions in pregnant women. When this drug is considered crucial by your doctor, its potential benefits must be carefully weighed against its risks.

The thiazide diuretic in Dyazide passes into breast milk. Nursing mothers who must take Dyazide should consider bottle-feeding.

Seniors

Seniors are more sensitive to the effects of Dyazide.

Generic Name

Econazole (ee-KON-uh-zole)

Brand Name

Spectazole

Type of Drug

Antifungal.

Prescribed for

Fungal infections of the skin, including athlete's foot and jock itch.

General Information

Econazole nitrate can kill fungal organisms that may have penetrated to deep layers of the skin. Very small amounts of econazole are absorbed into the bloodstream.

Cautions and Warnings

Do not use econazole if you have had an **allergic reaction** to it or any other ingredient in this product. Do not apply econazole cream in or near your **eyes**.

Long-term application of this product to large areas of skin may cause **liver damage**.

Possible Side Effects

▼ Most common: burning, itching, stinging, and redness in the areas to which the cream has been applied.

Drug Interactions

None known.

Usual Dose

Apply enough of the cream to cover affected areas with a thin layer 1–2 times a day.

Overdosage

Accidental ingestion may cause nausea, upset stomach, drowsiness, and liver inflammation or damage. Call your local poison control center for more information.

Special Information

Clean the affected areas before applying econazole cream unless otherwise directed by your doctor.

Call your doctor if the treated area burns, stings, or becomes red.

This product can be expected to relieve symptoms within 1 or 2 days after you begin using it. Follow your doctor's directions for the complete 2- to 4-week course of treatment to gain maximum benefit. Stopping the drug too soon can lead to a relapse.

If you forget a dose of econazole, apply it as soon as you remember. If it is almost time for your next dose, skip the one you forgot and continue with your regular schedule. Do not apply a double dose.

Special Populations

Pregnancy/Breast-feeding

When given by mouth to pregnant animals in high doses, econazole was toxic to the fetus. It should be strictly avoided during the first 3 months of pregnancy. During the last 6 months of pregnancy, it should be used only if absolutely necessary.

Econazole may pass into breast milk. Nursing mothers who must take this drug should consider bottle-feeding.

Seniors

Seniors may take this drug without special restriction.

Generic Name

Efavirenz (ef-ah-VIE-renz)

Brand Name

Sustiva

Type of Drug

Antiviral.

Prescribed for

Human immunodeficiency virus (HIV).

General Information

Efavirenz is a non-nucleoside reverse transcriptase inhibitor (NNRTI). It inhibits the reverse transcriptase (RT) enzyme, necessary for reproduction of HIV in body cells, by binding directly to it. The duration of any benefit from taking this drug may be limited because liver enzymes that break down efavirenz grow more potent as you continue to take it, removing it from your blood faster as time passes. The HIV virus can become resistant to efavirenz. For this reason, efavirenz is prescribed as part of a multi-drug anti-HIV "cocktail." Drug combinations containing efavirenz are just as effective in children as in adults.

Cautions and Warnings

Do not take this drug if you are **allergic** or **sensitive** to it.

HIV becomes **resistant** to efavirenz if it is used alone. Treatment must always include at least 1 other anti-HIV drug.

Efavirenz can be toxic to the **liver**. People with a history of hepatitis should have their liver function evaluated periodically and probably should use an alternate therapy. Efavirenz can raise blood **cholesterol** by 10% to 20%.

This drug has not been studied in **children** under age 3 or those who weigh less than 22 lbs.

Possible Side Effects

More than half of people who take efavirenz experience some side effects. About 2% have to stop treatment because of them. Children are more likely than adults to develop rash.

▼ Most common: nausea, dizziness, temporary rash, blisters, wet ulcers, and peeling skin.

▼ Common: headache, sleeplessness, abnormal dreaming, poor concentration, tiredness, and diarrhea.

▼ Less common: itching, sweating, stomach pain or gas, upset stomach, reduced sensitivity to stimulation, depression, appetite loss, and nervousness.

▼ Rare: blood in the urine, delusions, inappropriate behavior, and severe depression. Other rare side effects can occur in almost any part of the body. Contact your doctor if you experience any side effect not listed above.

Drug Interactions

• Combining efavirenz and astemizole; cisapride; midazolam, triazolam, or other benzodiazepine drugs; or ergot-containing products can lead to life-threatening abnormal heart rhythms, excessive sedation, or severe breathing difficulties. DO NOT COMBINE these drugs.

• Efavirenz increases the nervous-system effects of alcohol, tranquilizers, antidepressants, and other psychoactive drugs.

• Combining efavirenz with ritonavir increases blood levels of both drugs. This interaction increases the effectiveness of anti-HIV therapy as well as the risk of side effects.

• Efavirenz reduces indinavir blood levels. Your indinavir dosage may need to be increased.

• Efavirenz significantly reduces saquinavir blood levels.

• Combining efavirenz with clarithromycin, ethinyl estradiol, nelfinavir, rifampin, or rifabutin can alter blood levels of either drug. The importance of this interaction is unclear and dosage adjustments are unnecessary.

• Combining efavirenz and warfarin may increase the risk of excessive bleeding.

• The effect of efavirenz on oral contraceptives ("the pill") is not known. People combining these drugs should use an additional contraceptive method.

Food Interactions

High-fat meals increase the amount of efavirenz absorbed by 50%.

Usual Dose

Adult: 600 mg once a day at bedtime for the first 2–4 weeks. After that period, you may take it at any time of day.

Child (age 3 and over and more than 88 lbs.): 600 mg a day.
Child (age 3 and over and 71.5–87 lbs.): 400 mg a day.
Child (age 3 and over and 55–71.5 lbs.): 350 mg a day.
Child (age 3 and over and 44–54 lbs.): 300 mg a day.
Child (age 3 and over and 33–43 lbs.): 250 mg a day.
Child (age 3 and over and 22–32 lbs.): 200 mg a day.
Child (under age 3 or less than 22 lbs.): not recommended.

Overdosage

Symptoms may include dizziness, nausea, loss of concentration, and other nervous system effects. Take the victim to a hospital emergency room. ALWAYS bring the prescription bottle or container.

Special Information

It is imperative for you to take your HIV medication exactly as prescribed. Missing or skipping doses of efavirenz increases your risk of becoming resistant to the drug and losing the benefits of efavirenz therapy.

Efavirenz does not cure acquired immunodeficiency syndrome (AIDS). It does not prevent you from transmitting the HIV virus to another person; you must still practice safe sex.

About half of people taking efavirenz develop dizziness, loss of concentration, depression, delusions, or drowsiness. Call your doctor if this occurs or if strange behavior develops. Do not combine efavirenz with alcohol, tranquilizers, or other psychoactive drugs.

Be careful when driving or performing any task that requires concentration. Take your medication at bedtime to better tolerate the depressant effects of efavirenz.

If you forget a dose, take it as soon as you remember. Contact your doctor if you forget your medication for 1 day.

Special Populations

Pregnancy/Breast-feeding
Animal studies of efavirenz showed that it can cause birth defects. Before starting on efavirenz, women should be tested to ensure they are not pregnant. When this drug is considered crucial by your doctor, its potential benefits must be carefully weighed against its risks.

Efavirenz passes into breast milk. Nursing mothers with HIV should always bottle-feed, regardless of whether they take this drug, to avoid transmitting the virus.

Seniors
Seniors may take this drug without special precaution.

Effexor-XR *see Venlafaxine, page 1077*

see Venlafaxine, page 1077

Generic Name

Emedastine (em-ah-DAS-tine)

Brand Name

Emadine

Type of Drug

Antihistamine.

Prescribed for

Allergies.

General Information

Emedastine acts on histamine receptors in the eye to reduce allergic irritation and redness.

Cautions and Warnings

Do not use this drug if you are **sensitive** or **allergic** to it.

Possible Side Effects

▼ Common: headache.

▼ Less common: weakness, abnormal dreams, bad taste in the mouth, blurred vision, burning or stinging sensation in the eyes, staining of the cornea, rash, dry eyes, eye discomfort, sensation that something is in your eye, red eye, inflammation of the cornea, sinus irritation, runny nose, and tearing.

Drug Interactions

• If you use several different eyedrops, separate them by 5 minutes.

Usual Dose

Adult and Child (age 3 and over): 1 drop in each eye, up to 4 times a day.

Child (under age 3): not recommended.

Overdosage

Symptoms of accidental ingestion may include not feeling well and feeling weak. Call your local poison control center or a hospital emergency room for more information.

Special Information

Do not wear contact lenses if your eyes are red due to use of this drug.

If you forget a dose of emedastine, take it as soon as you remember. If it is almost time for your next dose, skip the forgotten dose and continue with your regular schedule.

To prevent possible infection, don't allow the dropper to touch your fingers, eyelids, or any surface. Wait at least 5 minutes before using any other eyedrops.

Special Populations

Pregnancy/Breast-feeding
At very high doses, emedastine taken orally caused birth defects in animal studies. Do not use any antihistamine drug without your doctor's knowledge if you are or might be pregnant—especially during the last 3 months of pregnancy, because newborns may have severe reactions to antihistamines.

It is unknown if emedastine passes into breast milk. Nursing mothers who must use this drug should consider bottle-feeding.

Seniors
Seniors may use this drug without any special precautions.

Brand Name
EMLA

Generic Ingredients
Lidocaine + Prilocaine

Type of Drug
Topical anesthetic.

Prescribed for
Skin pain.

General Information
EMLA—which stands for Eutectic Mixture of Local Anesthetics—is a mixture of anesthetics that turns to liquid on contact with the skin. EMLA penetrates all layers of skin, dulling nerve endings and providing a local anesthetic effect comparable with that produced by injectable drugs. EMLA can pre-

vent virtually any kind of skin pain and may be used by people of almost any age. The cream must be applied under an occlusive bandage (one that prevents contact with air or water), which intensifies the contact between skin and anesthetic. It works after being on the skin for at least 1 hour but may be more effective if left on for 2 or 3 hours. The anesthetic effect remains for 2 hours after the cream has been removed. EMLA is also available in patch form.

EMLA cream has been used to relieve the pain of intravenous catheter placement, minor plastic and skin surgery, shingles, and injections such as those used during vaccinations and blood donation.

Cautions and Warnings

Do not use EMLA cream if you are **allergic** to either of its anesthetics. People with **methemoglobinemia** (a rare blood condition) should not use EMLA.

Do not apply EMLA cream beyond the area prescribed by your doctor—otherwise, too much anesthetic may enter your blood and cause side effects. Do not put EMLA in your **eyes** or **ears**.

People with severe **liver disease** should use EMLA with caution because they may have difficulty removing the absorbed anesthetics from the blood.

Possible Side Effects

▼ Most common: irritation, redness, and swelling of the area to which it is applied.

▼ Common: skin pallor, patches of white skin, itching, rash, and changes in how you sense skin temperature.

▼ Rare: severe allergic reaction (symptoms include breathing difficulties, rash, intense itching, and elevated pulse). In rare cases when EMLA is applied in excess, is used too often, or too much anesthetic is absorbed, the following reactions may occur: nervous system excitation; nervousness; apprehension; light-headedness; euphoria (feeling "high"); confusion; dizziness; drowsiness; ringing or buzzing in the ears; blurred or double vision; vomiting; feelings of warmth, coldness, or numbness; twitching; tremors; convulsions; unconsciousness; or a very slow breathing rate or cessation of breathing.

Drug Interactions

• Drugs associated with causing methemoglobinemia should not be taken with EMLA. This interaction is generally limited to children under age 1. Some of these drugs are acetaminophen, sulfa drugs, oral antidiabetes drugs, thiazide diuretics, phenacetin, phenobarbital, phenytoin, primaquine, and quinine.

Usual Dose

Cream

Adult and Child (age 1 month and over): Apply a thick layer—2.5 g or ½ tsp.—and cover with the dressing provided in the package or some other occlusive bandage. Leave in place for at least 1–2 hours. The cream should be wiped away immediately before any surgical procedure or injection. Seniors should avoid multiple uses over a short period of time because of the risk of side effects.

Patch

Apply to designated area and leave in place for at least 1–2 hours before removing.

Overdosage

Accidental ingestion of EMLA may affect the heart by making it less efficient. Call your local poison control center or a hospital emergency room for more information. If you seek treatment, ALWAYS bring the prescription bottle or container.

Special Information

EMLA numbs the skin. Be careful not to accidentally scratch or burn yourself after the product has been applied.

When you apply the cream, place the entire dose in the center of the designated area. Then cover it with the occlusive dressing and allow the pressure of the dressing to spread the cream.

Call your doctor if you develop severe, persistent, or bothersome side effects.

If you forget to apply EMLA, do so as soon as you can.

Special Populations

Pregnancy/Breast-feeding

The safety of using EMLA cream during pregnancy is not known, though there is no evidence that it interferes with fetal development. When this drug is considered crucial by your doctor, its potential benefits must be carefully weighed against its risks.

The anesthetics in EMLA cream pass into breast milk. Nursing mothers who must use this drug should consider bottle-feeding.

Seniors

Seniors may be more sensitive to side effects, especially after repeated applications.

Generic Name

Enalapril (uh-NAL-uh-pril)

Brand Name

Vasotec

Combination Products

Generic Ingredients: Enalapril + Hydrochlorothiazide
Vaseretic

Generic Ingredients: Enalapril + Felodipine
Lexxel (see page 581)

Type of Drug

Angiotensin-converting enzyme (ACE) inhibitor.

Prescribed for

Hypertension (high blood pressure) and heart failure; also prescribed for diabetic kidney disease and heart attack treatment when the function of the left ventricle has been affected.

General Information

Enalapril maleate and other ACE inhibitors work by preventing the conversion of a hormone called angiotensin I to another hormone called angiotensin II, a potent blood-vessel constrictor. Preventing this conversion relaxes blood vessels, thus reducing blood pressure and relieving symptoms of heart failure. Enalapril also affects the production of other hormones and enzymes that participate in the regulation of blood-vessel dilation. Enalapril begins working about 1 hour after you take it and continues to work for 24 hours.

Some people who start taking enalapril after they are already on a diuretic (an agent that increases urination) experience a rapid drop in blood pressure after their first doses or when their dosage is increased. To prevent this from happening, your doctor may tell you to stop taking your diuretic 2 or 3 days before starting enalapril or to increase your salt intake during that time. The diuretic may then be restarted gradually.

Cautions and Warnings

Do not take enalapril if you are **allergic** to it.

Enalapril occasionally causes **very low blood pressure**.

Enalapril may affect your **kidney function,** especially if you have congestive **heart failure**. Your doctor should check your urine for protein content during the first few months of treatment. Dosage adjustment of enalapril is necessary if you have reduced kidney function.

Enalapril can affect white-blood-cell counts, possibly increasing your susceptibility to **infection**. Your doctor should monitor your blood counts periodically.

Possible Side Effects

▼ Most common: dizziness, fatigue, headache, nausea, and chronic cough. The cough usually goes away a few days after you stop taking the medication.

▼ Less common: chest tightness or pain, dizziness when rising from a sitting or lying position, fainting, abdominal pain, nausea, vomiting, diarrhea, bronchitis, urinary tract infection, breathing difficulties, weakness, and rash.

▼ Rare: Rare side effects can occur in almost any part of the body. Contact your doctor if you experience any side effect not listed above.

Drug Interactions

• The blood-pressure-lowering effect of enalapril is additive with diuretic drugs and beta blockers. Any other drug that causes a rapid drop in blood pressure should be used with caution if you are taking enalapril.

• Enalapril may increase blood-potassium levels, especially when taken with Dyazide or other potassium-sparing diuretics.

• Enalapril may increase the effects of lithium; this combination should be used with caution.

• Antacids and enalapril should be taken at least 2 hours apart.

• Capsaicin may trigger or aggravate the cough associated with enalapril therapy.

• Indomethacin may reduce the blood-pressure-lowering effects of enalapril.

• Phenothiazine tranquilizers and antiemetics may increase the effects of enalapril.

• Rifampin may reduce the effects of enalapril.

• The combination of allopurinol and enalapril increases the chance of side effects. Avoid this combination.

• Enalapril increases blood levels of digoxin, which may increase the chance of digoxin-related side effects.

Food Interactions

You may take enalapril with food if it upsets your stomach.

Usual Dose

2.5–40 mg once a day. Some people may take their daily dosage in 2 doses. People with poor kidney function need less medication.

Overdosage

The principal effect of enalapril overdose is a rapid drop in blood pressure, as evidenced by dizziness or fainting. Take the overdose victim to a hospital emergency room immediately. ALWAYS bring the prescription bottle or container.

Special Information

Enalapril can cause swelling of the face, lips, hands, or feet. This swelling can also affect the larynx (throat) or tongue and interfere with breathing. If this happens, go to a hospital emergency room at once. Call your doctor if you develop a sore throat, mouth sores, abnormal heartbeat, chest pain, persistent rash, or loss of taste perception.

You may get dizzy if you rise to your feet too quickly from a sitting or lying position.

Avoid strenuous exercise or very hot weather because heavy sweating or dehydration can cause a rapid drop in blood pressure.

While taking enalapril, avoid over-the-counter diet pills, decongestants, and other stimulants that can raise blood pressure.

If you take enalapril once a day and forget to take a dose, take it as soon as you remember. If it is within 8 hours of your next dose, skip the one you forgot and continue with your regular schedule. If you take enalapril twice a day and miss a dose, take it right away. If it is within 4 hours of your next dose, take 1 dose immediately and another in 5 or 6 hours, then go back to your regular schedule. Never take a double dose.

Special Populations

Pregnancy/Breast-feeding
ACE inhibitors can cause fetal injury or death. Women who are or might become pregnant should not take ACE inhibitors. Sexually active women of childbearing age who must take enalapril must use an effective contraceptive method to prevent pregnancy. If you become pregnant, stop taking the medication and call your doctor immediately.

Small amounts of enalapril pass into breast milk. Nursing mothers who must take this drug should consider bottle-feeding.

Seniors
Seniors may be more sensitive to the effects of this drug due to age-related losses in kidney or liver function.

Brand Name
Entex

Generic Ingredients
Guaifenesin + Phenylpropanolamine + Phenylephrine

Other Brand Names
Coldloc   Entac
Contuss   Guiafenex
Dura-Gest   Guiatex
Enomine

The information in this profile also applies to the following drugs:

Generic Ingredients: Guaifenesin + Phenylpropanolamine Ⓖ

Ami-Tex LA	Guaitex LA
Coldloc-LA	Partuss LA
Dura-Vent	Phenylfenesin LA
Entex LA	Rymed-TR
Exgest LA	Stamoist LA
Guaipax	ULR-LA

Generic Ingredients: Guaifenesin + Pseudoephedrine Ⓖ

Duratuss	H 9600 SR
Entex PSE	Histalet X
Guai-Vent PSE	PanMist LA
Guaifenex PSE	Ru-Tuss DE
Guaifed	Sudal
Guaifed-PD	Zephrex LA
Guaimax-D	

Generic Ingredients: Caramiphen Edisylate + Phenylpropanolamine Hydrochloride Ⓖ

Ordrine AT	Tussogest
Rescaps-D S.R.	Tuss-Ornade
Tuss-Allergine Modified T.D.	

Type of Drug

Decongestant and expectorant combination.

Prescribed for

Cold or allergy and for nasal congestion, stuffy nose, and runny nose associated with other upper respiratory conditions.

General Information

The decongestant ingredient in Entex, phenylpropanolamine, dramatically reduces congestion and stuffiness. The expectorant, guaifenesin, is used to help loosen thick mucus that may contribute to chest congestion; the effectiveness of guaifenesin and other expectorants has not been established. There are other drugs on the market using this same general formula—an expectorant plus a decongestant—but they use different decongestant ingredients or a combination of decongestants plus guaifenesin. Nothing cures a cold or allergy, but Entex may provide relief from symptoms.

Cautions and Warnings

Entex may cause **anxiety** or **nervousness** or interfere with **sleep**.

Do not use Entex if you have **diabetes, heart disease, hypertension** (high blood pressure), **thyroid disease, glaucoma,** stomach ulcer, urinary blockage, or **prostate condition.**

Entex should not be used over extended periods of time to treat **persistent or chronic cough,** especially one that may be caused by cigarette smoking, asthma, or emphysema.

Possible Side Effects

▼ Most common: fear, anxiety, restlessness, sleeplessness, tension, excitation, nervousness, dizziness, drowsiness, hallucinations, headache, psychological disturbances, tremor, and convulsions.

▼ Less common: nausea, vomiting, upset stomach, low blood pressure, heart palpitations, chest pain, rapid heartbeat, abnormal heart rhythms, irritability, euphoria (feeling "high"), eye irritation and tearing, hysterical reaction, appetite loss, urinary difficulties in men with a prostate condition, weakness, loss of facial color, and breathing difficulties.

Drug Interactions

• Entex should be avoided if you are taking a monoamine oxidase inhibitor (MAOI) antidepressant for depression or hypertension because the MAOI may cause a very rapid rise in blood pressure or increase side effects such as dry mouth or nose, blurred vision, and abnormal heart rhythms.

• The decongestant in Entex may interfere with blood-pressure-lowering medication.

Food Interactions

Take Entex with food if it upsets your stomach.

Usual Dose

Capsules: 1 twice a day.

Liquid: 2 tsp. 4 times a day.

Overdosage

Most cases of overdose are not severe. Symptoms include sedation, sleepiness, increased sweating, and increased blood pressure. Hallucinations, convulsions, nervous-system depression, and breathing difficulties are more prominent in older adults. Most cases of overdose are not severe. Induce vomiting with ipecac syrup—available at any pharmacy. Call you local poison control center or a hospital emergency room before doing this. If you seek treatment, ALWAYS bring the prescription bottle or container.

Special Information

Call your doctor if your side effects are severe or gradually become intolerable.

If you forget a dose, take it as soon as you remember. If it is almost time for your next dose, skip the one you forgot and continue with your regular schedule. Do not take a double dose.

Special Populations

Pregnancy/Breast-feeding

Women who are or might be pregnant should avoid Entex. When your doctor considers this drug crucial, its potential benefits must be carefully weighed against its risks.

The decongestant in Entex may pass into breast milk. Nursing mothers who must take Entex should consider bottle-feeding.

Seniors

Seniors are more sensitive to the effects of Entex.

Brand Name

Equagesic

Generic Ingredients

Aspirin + Meprobamate

Type of Drug

Analgesic combination.

Prescribed for

Pain from muscle spasms, sprains, strains, or bad backs.

General Information

Equagesic is one of several combination products containing a tranquilizer and an analgesic; it is used to relieve pain associated with muscle spasms.

Cautions and Warnings

Do not take this combination if you are **allergic** to any of its ingredients or to other salicylates or carisoprodol.

Aspirin can worsen **kidney function** in people who already have a kidney condition, and meprobamate should be used with caution by people with **liver or kidney disease**. Aspirin can irritate your stomach and should be avoided by people with **gastritis** or **ulcers**. Also, aspirin should be used with caution by people with mild **diabetes** or **bleeding tendencies**.

The meprobamate in this product can become habit-forming and possibly addictive, especially when taken with other tranquilizers or depressant drugs. Avoid using this product for more than a few weeks at a time. Abruptly stopping this medicine can lead to drug withdrawal (symptoms include anxiety, appetite loss, insomnia, vomiting, tremors, muscle weakness or twitching, confusion, and hallucinations) or recurrence of symptoms. The dose should be gradually reduced over a period of 1 to 2 weeks.

Possible Side Effects

▼ Most common: nausea, vomiting, stomach upset, dizziness, and drowsiness.

▼ Less common: allergy, itching, rash, fever, swelling in the arms or legs, occasional fainting spells, and bronchial spasms leading to breathing difficulties.

▼ Rare: changes in blood components and blurred vision.

Drug Interactions

• In high doses, meprobamate can cause sleepiness, drowsiness, or difficulty breathing. Avoid taking this medication with other nervous system depressants, including alcohol, barbiturates, narcotics, sleeping pills, tranquilizers, and some antihistamines.

• If you are taking an anticoagulant (blood-thinner) and begin taking an aspirin-meprobamate combination, your doctor may need to adjust your anticoagulant dosage because aspirin affects the ability of blood to clot.

Food Interactions

An aspirin-meprobamate combination may be taken with food if it upsets your stomach.

Usual Dose

Adult and Child (age 17 and over): 1–2 tablets 3–4 times a day.

Child (under age 17): not recommended.

Overdosage

Overdoses are serious. Symptoms are drowsiness, light-headedness, sleepiness, nausea, and vomiting. Victims should be taken to a hospital emergency room immediately. ALWAYS bring the prescription bottle or container.

Special Information

Be careful when driving or performing complex tasks while taking this medication.

Call your doctor if drug side effects become bothersome or persistent.

If you forget a dose, take it as soon as you remember. If it is almost time for your next dose, skip the one you forgot and continue with your regular schedule. Do not take a double dose.

Special Populations

Pregnancy/Breast-feeding

These drugs cross into the fetal blood circulation. They have not caused birth defects, although meprobamate has been known to increase the risk of birth defects if taken during the first 3 months of pregnancy. When this medication is considered essential by your doctor, its potential benefits must be carefully weighed against its risks.

These drugs pass into breast milk. Nursing mothers taking this medication should consider bottle-feeding.

Seniors
Seniors are more sensitive to the effects of this combination, especially drowsiness or sleepiness.

Generic Name

Ergoloid Mesylates

(ER-goe-loid MES-il-ates) Ⓖ

Brand Names

Gerimal   Hydergine LC
Hydergine

Type of Drug

Psychotherapeutic agent.

Prescribed for

Age-related decline in mental capacity.

General Information

Ergoloid mesylates is used to treat decreased mental capacity of unknown cause in people over age 60. This drug should not be used for any condition that is treatable with another drug or that may be reversible. People who respond to ergoloid mesylates are likely to have Alzheimer's disease or some other cause of dementia. Nobody knows exactly how ergoloid mesylates produces its effect, but it improves the supply of blood to the brain in test animals, reduces heart rate, and improves muscle tone in blood vessels. Some studies show the drug to be very effective in relieving mild symptoms of mental impairment, while others find it to be only moderately effective. It is most beneficial in people whose symptoms are due to the effects of high blood pressure in the brain.

Cautions and Warnings

Ergoloid mesylates should not be taken if you are **allergic** or **sensitive** to it or have **psychotic symptoms** or **psychosis**.

Possible Side Effects

▼ Common: Ergoloid mesylates does not produce serious side effects. When taken under the tongue, this drug may cause irritation, nausea, or upset stomach. Other side effects are drowsiness, slow heartbeat, and rash.

Drug Interactions

None known.

Food Interactions

Do not eat, drink, or smoke while you have an ergoloid mesylates pill under your tongue.

Usual Dose

1 mg 3 times a day. Do not exceed 12 mg a day.

Overdosage

Symptoms include blurred vision, dizziness, fainting, flushing, headache, appetite loss, nausea, vomiting, stomach cramps, and stuffy nose. Take the victim to a hospital emergency room. ALWAYS bring the prescription bottle or container.

Special Information

The effects of ergoloid mesylates are gradual and frequently not seen for up to 6 months. A 6-month period of treatment with ergoloid mesylates is recommended before your doctor can fully evaluate your response to the drug. Your doctor should periodically reevaluate your condition to determine if ergoloid mesylates is still needed and that it is working for you.

Dissolve sublingual tablets under the tongue. Do not chew or crush them; they are not effective if swallowed whole.

If you forget a dose, skip it and go back to your regular schedule. Do not take a double dose. Call your doctor if you miss 2 or more consecutive doses.

Special Populations

Pregnancy/Breast-feeding
Ergoloid mesylates may interfere with fetal development. When this drug is considered crucial by your doctor, its potential benefits must be carefully weighed against its risks.

Ergoloid mesylates passes into breast milk. Nursing mothers who must take this drug should bottle-feed.

Seniors
Seniors are more likely to develop side effects, especially hypothermia (low body temperature).

Generic Name

Erythromycin (eh-rith-roe-MYE-sin) [G]

Brand Names

A/T/S	Erymax
Akne-mycin	Ery-Tab
Benzamycin	Erythra-Derm
Del-Mycin	Erythromycin Filmtabs
E-Base	Ilotycin
E-Mycin	PCE Dispertab
Eryc	Staticin
Erycette	Theramycin Z
Eryderm	T-Stat
Erygel	

The information in this profile also applies to all forms of erythromycin:

Generic Ingredient: Erythromycin Estolate [G]

Ilosone	Ilosone Pulvules

Generic Ingredient: Erythromycin Ethylsuccinate [G]

E.E.S. 200	EryPed 400
E.E.S. 400	EryPed Drops
EryPed	Erythromycin ES
EryPed 200	

Generic Ingredient: Erythromycin Stearate [G]
Erythrocin Stearate

Type of Drug

Macrolide antibiotic.

Prescribed for

Infections of virtually any part of the body: upper and lower respiratory tract infections; sexually transmitted diseases; urinary tract infections; infections of the mouth, gums, or teeth; and infections of the nose, ears, or sinuses. It is prescribed for acne and may be used for mild to moderate skin infections. Erythromycin is effective against diphtheria and dysentery. It is also prescribed for legionnaires' disease, rheumatic fever, and bacterial endocarditis. The eye ointment is used to prevent newborn gonococcal or chlamydial eye infections.

General Information

Erythromycin and other macrolide antibiotics are either bactericidal (bacteria-killing) or bacteriostatic (inhibiting bacterial growth) depending on the organism in question and amount of antibiotic present. Erythromycin is deactivated by stomach acid, so the tablet form is made to bypass the stomach and dissolve in the intestine.

Since the action of this antibiotic depends on its concentration in the invading bacteria, it is crucial that you follow your doctor's directions regarding the spacing of doses as well as the number of days you must take the medication—otherwise this antibiotic may be much less effective.

Cautions and Warnings

Do not take erythromycin if you are **allergic** to it or any macrolide.

Erythromycin is excreted primarily through the liver. People with **liver disease or damage** should consult their doctors. Those on long-term therapy with erythromycin should have periodic blood tests. If you restart erythromycin after having experienced liver damage, it is likely that symptoms will recur within 48 hours.

Erythromycin estolate has occasionally produced **liver problems** (symptoms include fatigue, nausea, vomiting, abdominal cramps, and fever). If you are susceptible to stomach problems, erythromycin may cause mild to moderate **stomach upset;** discontinuing the drug will reverse this condition.

Colitis (bowel inflammation) has been associated with all antibiotics (see "Possible Side Effects").

Possible Side Effects

▼ Most common: nausea, vomiting, stomach cramps, and diarrhea. Colitis (symptoms include severe abdominal cramps and severe, persistent, and possibly bloody diarrhea) may develop.

▼ Less common: hairy tongue, itching, and irritation of the anal or vaginal region. If any of these symptoms appear, call your physician immediately.

▼ Rare: hearing loss—which reverses itself after the drug is stopped and occurs most often in people with liver and kidney problems—and abnormal heart rhythms.

Drug Interactions

• Antacids may slightly affect the release of erythromycin from your body. This effect is not considered important.

• Erythromycin may slow the breakdown of carbamazepine (an anticonvulsant prescribed for seizures). Avoid this combination.

• Mixing erythromycin with rifabutin or rifampin can interfere with the antibiotic's effect and increase the risk of intestinal side effects.

• Do not mix erythromycin with sparfloxacin (a fluoroquinolone antibiotic). This mixture can lead to severe, possibly fatal, abnormal heart rhythms. Grepafloxacin (another fluoroquinolone) should only be mixed with erythromycin in hospitalized patients whose hearts can be monitored during treatment.

• Do not combine erythromycin and pimozide. Two people died after combining pimozide and a macrolide.

• Do not mix erythromycin with cisapride—serious heart rhythm abnormalities, some fatal, can result.

• Erythromycin may neutralize penicillin. It may also neutralize the antibiotics lincomycin and clindamycin.

• Erythromycin interferes with the elimination of theophylline from the body, possibly leading to theophylline overdose. It may also increase the effects of caffeine.

• Mixing erythromycin with a statin cholesterol-lowering drug increases the risk of developing a potentially fatal condition involving severe muscle pain and destruction.

• Combining erythromycin and alfentanil (an injectable pain reliever), bromocriptine, buspirone, digoxin, disopyramide, ergotamine, cyclosporine, methylprednisolone (a corticosteroid), tacrolimus, vinblastine, or benzodiazepines (such as alprazolam, diazepam, midazolam, and triazolam), increases the risk of drug side effects.

• Erythromycin estolate may increase the liver side effects of other drugs that affect the liver.

• Erythromycin may increase the anticoagulant (blood-thinning) effects of warfarin in people who take it regularly, especially older adults. People taking this combination should be tested regularly.

Food Interactions

For optimum effectiveness, take erythromycin base and erythromycin stearate on an empty stomach, 1 hour before or 2 hours after meals. Other forms of erythromycin can be taken without regard to food or meals.

Usual Dose

Tablet and Suspension
  Adult: 250–500 mg every 6 hours.
  Child: 50–200 mg per lb. of body weight a day in divided doses depending on age, weight, and severity of infection.

Eye Ointment
½ in. 2–3 times a day.

Topical Solution
Apply morning and night.

Doses of erythromycin ethylsuccinate are 60% higher due to differences in chemical composition.

Overdosage

Overdose may cause severe side effects, especially nausea, vomiting, stomach cramps, and diarrhea. Mild hearing loss, ringing or buzzing in the ears, or fainting may also occur. Call your local poison control center or a hospital emergency room for more information.

Special Information

Erythromycin is used instead of penicillin for mild to moderate infections in people who are allergic to penicillin. Erythromycin is not the antibiotic of choice for severe infections.

Erythromycin products should be stored at room temperature, except for oral and topical liquids, which should be kept in the refrigerator.

Take each oral dose of erythromycin with 6 to 8 oz. of water.

Call your doctor if you develop nausea; vomiting; diarrhea; stomach cramps; severe abdominal pain; rash, itching, or redness; dark or amber-colored urine; yellowing of the skin or whites of the eyes; or any severe or persistent side effect.

If you forget a dose of oral erythromycin, take it as soon as you remember. If it is almost time for your next dose, space the next 2 doses over 4 to 6 hours, then continue with your regular schedule. Do not take a double dose.

Remember to complete the full course of therapy prescribed even if you feel well before you finish the medication.

Special Populations

Pregnancy/Breast-feeding

Erythromycin passes into the fetal circulation. Erythromycin estolate has caused mild liver inflammation in about 10% of pregnant women who took it and should not be used if you are or might be pregnant. Other forms of erythromycin have been used safely without difficulty.

Erythromycin passes into breast milk. Nursing mothers who must take erythromycin should bottle-feed.

Seniors

Seniors with liver disease should use caution.

Generic Name

Estazolam (es-TAZ-oe-lam) G

Brand Name

ProSom

Type of Drug

Benzodiazepine sedative.

Prescribed for

Insomnia and sleep disturbances.

General Information

Estazolam is a member of the group of drugs known as benzodiazepines. They work by a direct effect on the brain. Benzodiazepines make it easier to go to sleep and decrease the number of times you wake up during the night. Estazolam is considered an intermediate-acting sedative and generally remains in your body long enough to give you a good night's sleep with minimal "hangover."

Cautions and Warnings

People with **respiratory disease** taking estazolam may experience **sleep apnea** (intermittent cessation of breathing during sleep).

People with **kidney or liver disease** should be carefully monitored while taking estazolam. Take the lowest possible dose to help you sleep.

Clinical **depression** may be increased by estazolam, which can depress the nervous system. Intentional overdose is more common among depressed people who take sleeping pills than among those who do not.

All benzodiazepines can be **addictive** if taken for long periods of time and can cause drug withdrawal symptoms if discontinued suddenly. Withdrawal symptoms include tremors, muscle cramps, insomnia, agitation, diarrhea, vomiting, sweating, and convulsions.

Possible Side Effects

▼ Common: drowsiness, headache, dizziness, talkativeness, nervousness, apprehension, poor muscle coordination, light-headedness, daytime tiredness, muscle weakness, slowness of movement, hangover, and euphoria (feeling high).

▼ Less common: nausea, vomiting, rapid heartbeat, confusion, temporary memory loss, upset stomach, stomach cramps and pain, depression, blurred or double vision and other visual disturbances, constipation, changes in sense of taste, appetite changes, stuffy nose, nosebleeds, common cold symptoms, asthma, sore throat, cough, breathing difficulties, diarrhea, dry mouth, allergic reaction, fainting, abnormal heart rhythm, itching, acne, dry skin, sensitivity to bright light or to the sun, rash, nightmares or strange dreams, sleeplessness, tingling in the hands or feet, ringing or buzzing in the ears, ear or eye pain, menstrual cramps, frequent urination and other urinary difficulties, blood in the urine, discharge from the penis or vagina, lower back and joint pain, muscle spasms and pain, fever, swollen breasts, and weight changes.

Possible Side Effects *(continued)*

▼ Rare: Rare side effects can affect your heart, stomach and intestines, urinary tract, blood, muscles, and joints. Contact your doctor if you experience any side effect not listed.

Drug Interactions

• As with all benzodiazepines, the effects of estazolam are enhanced if it is taken with an alcoholic beverage, antihistamine, tranquilizer, barbiturate, anticonvulsant medication, antidepressant, or monoamine oxidase inhibitor drug (MAOI).

• Oral contraceptives, cimetidine, disulfiram, and isoniazid may increase the effect of estazolam by interfering with the drug's breakdown in the liver. Probenecid also increases estazolam's effects.

• Cigarette smoking, rifampin, and theophylline may reduce the effect of estazolam.

• Levodopa's effectiveness may be decreased by estazolam.

• Estazolam may increase the amount of zidovudine (an AIDS drug—also known as AZT), phenytoin, or digoxin in your bloodstream, increasing the chances of side effects.

• The combination of clozapine and benzodiazepines has led to respiratory collapse in a few people. Estazolam should be stopped at least 1 week before starting clozapine treatment.

Food Interactions

Estazolam may be taken with food if it upsets your stomach.

Usual Dose

Adult (age 18 and over): 1–2 mg about 60 minutes before you want to go to sleep.

Senior: starting dose—0.5–1 mg. Dosage should be increased cautiously.

Child (under age 18): not recommended.

Overdosage

The most common overdose symptoms are confusion, sleepiness, depression, loss of muscle coordination, and slurred speech. Coma may also occur. People who take an estazolam overdose must be made to vomit with ipecac syrup—available at any pharmacy—to remove any remaining drug from the stomach: Call your doctor or a poison control center before doing this. The victim must be taken to a hospital emergency room for treatment if 30 minutes have passed since the overdose was taken or if symptoms have begun to develop. ALWAYS bring the prescription bottle or container.

Special Information

Never take more estazolam than your doctor has prescribed.

Avoid alcoholic beverages and other nervous system depressants while taking estazolam.

Exercise caution while performing tasks that require concentration and coordination; estazolam may make you tired, dizzy, or light-headed.

If you take estazolam daily for 3 or more weeks, you may experience some withdrawal symptoms when you stop taking the drug.

If you forget to take a dose of estazolam and remember within about 1 hour of your regular time, take it right away. If you do not remember until later, skip the dose you forgot and go back to your regular schedule. Do not take a double dose.

Special Populations

Pregnancy/Breast-feeding

Estazolam absolutely should not be used by pregnant women or by women who may become pregnant.

Estazolam passes into breast milk. The drug should not be taken by nursing mothers.

Seniors

Seniors are more susceptible to the effects of estazolam.

Type of Drug

Estrogens (ES-troe-jens)

Brand Names

Generic Ingredient: Chlorotrianisene
TACE

Generic Ingredient: Conjugated Estrogens
Premarin

Generic Ingredient: Conjugated Estrogens (Synthetic)
Cenestin

Generic Ingredients: Conjugated Estrogens +
Medroxyprogesterone
Prempro   Premphase

Generic Ingredient: Dienestrol
Ortho Dienestrol

Generic Ingredient: Esterified Estrogens
Estratab   Menest

Generic Ingredient: Estradiol G
Alora   FemPatch
Climara   Gynodiol
Esclim   Innofem
Estrace   Vagifem
Estraderm   Vivelle
Estring   Vivelle-Dot

Generic Ingredients: Estradiol + Norgestimate
Ortho-Prefest

Generic Ingredient: Estropipate G
Ogen   Ortho-Est

Generic Ingredient: Ethinyl Estradiol
Estinyl

Generic Ingredients: Ethinyl Estradiol + Norethindrone
Acetate
femhrt 1/5

Prescribed for

Menopausal symptoms and heart disease and osteoporosis
in postmenopausal women; also prescribed for ovarian failure, breast cancer in women and men, advanced prostate
cancer, abnormal bleeding of the uterus, vaginal irritation,
female castration, Turner's syndrome, and birth control.

General information

Six estrogens have been identified in women but only 3 are
present in large amounts: estradiol, estrone, and estriol.

Estradiol is the most potent and important. Other estrogens are produced by chemical conversions in the body. Estradiol, for example, is transformed into estrone, which in turn becomes estriol. Estrogens all have the same actions and side effects; only potency varies. More potent types require smaller dosages to produce the same effect.

Estrogens are largely responsible for the growth and maintenance of the female reproductive system and sex characteristics. They affect the release of hormones from the pituitary gland (controller of hormone production and regulator of basic bodily functions). These hormones control the functioning of capillaries (smallest blood vessels), may cause fluid retention, affect protein breakdown in the body, prevent ovulation and breast engorgement after childbirth, and influence the shaping and maintenance of the skeleton through an effect on calcium.

Estrogen products differ in their hormone content and dosage. Some may affect one part of the body more than another. Generally, though, estrogens are interchangeable as long as dosage differences are taken into account.

Cautions and Warnings

Women with **blood clotting problems** and those who are **allergic** to estrogens should not take them.

Estrogens may increase the risk of **endometrial cancer** by 4.5 to 14 times in postmenopausal women taking them without progestin for prolonged periods of time; the risk depends on duration of treatment and dosage. Adding a progestin such as medroxyprogesterone to long-term estrogen therapy reduces the risk of endometrial cancer and other problems. Combination products such as Prempro, are also available. Women who have had a hysterectomy do not need a progestin.

Women with **breast cancer** should not take estrogens, except some being treated for breast cancer that has spread, nor should those with an estrogen-dependent cancer or **abnormal vaginal bleeding** whose cause is unknown. Women who have a strong family **history of breast cancer** or who have **breast nodules or cysts** or an **abnormal mammogram** should be cautious about using estrogens. Women taking an estrogen for breast cancer that has spread to their bones can develop large increases in blood **calcium**.

Oral contraceptives ("the pill") containing norgestrel and ethinyl estradiol have been used as emergency **"morning-after" contraception**. The drug must be taken no more than 72 hours after intercourse to be effective and can harm the fetus if pregnancy is not prevented.

Postmenopausal women taking estrogen are 2 to 3 times more likely to develop **gallbladder disease**.

Estrogens can raise **blood pressure**. Pressure usually returns to normal when the drug is stopped.

People with **thrombophlebitis** should avoid these drugs. The risk is greatest with very high dosages. Low dosages may not be a problem.

Estrogens should not be used to treat painful **breast enlargement** that sometimes develops after giving birth.

Estrogens can cause significant increases in blood **triglycerides** and **pancreas inflammation** in women with inherited **blood-fat disorders**.

Vaginal estrogen cream may stimulate **bleeding of the uterus**. It may also cause **breast tenderness, vaginal discharge,** and **withdrawal bleeding** if the product is suddenly stopped. Women with **endometriosis** may experience heavy vaginal bleeding.

Possible Side Effects

▼ Most common: breast enlargement or tenderness, ankle and leg swelling, appetite loss, weight changes, water retention, nausea, vomiting, abdominal cramps, and a feeling of abdominal bloating. The estrogen patch may cause rash, irritation, and redness where it is applied.

▼ Less common: bleeding gums, breakthrough vaginal bleeding, vaginal spotting, changes in menstrual flow, painful menstruation, premenstrual syndrome (PMS), absence of menstrual periods during and after estrogen use, uterine fibroid enlargement, vaginal *Candida* infection, a cystitis-like condition, mild diarrhea, yellowing of the skin or whites of the eyes, eye lesions, contact-lens intolerance, rash, hair loss, development of new hairy patches, migraine, mild dizziness, depression, increased sex drive (women), and decreased sex drive (men).

Possible Side Effects *(continued)*

▼ Rare: stroke, blood-clot formation, dribbling or sudden passage of urine, loss of coordination, chest pain, leg pain, breathing difficulties, slurred speech, and changes in vision. Men who take large estrogen dosages for prostate cancer have a greater risk of heart attack, phlebitis, and blood clots in the lungs.

Drug Interactions

• Phenytoin, ethotoin, and mephenytoin may interfere with estrogen's effects.

• Estrogens may reduce the effect of oral anticoagulant (blood-thinning) drugs. Your anticoagulant dosage may need an adjustment.

• Estrogens increase the amount of calcium absorbed from the stomach. This interaction is used to help women with osteoporosis increase their calcium level.

• Estrogens may increase the side effects of antidepressants and phenothiazine tranquilizers.

• Low estrogen dosages may increase phenothiazine's effectiveness.

• Estrogens may increase cyclosporine and corticosteroid blood levels. Dosage adjustments of the non-estrogen drugs may be needed.

• Rifampin, barbiturates, and other drugs that stimulate the liver to break down drugs may reduce estrogen blood levels.

• Estrogens may interfere with tamoxifen and bromocriptine.

• Women, especially those over age 35, who smoke cigarettes and take estrogen have a much greater risk of developing stroke, hardening of the arteries, and blood clots in the lungs. The risk increases with age and tobacco use.

• Estrogens interfere with many diagnostic tests. Make sure your doctor knows you are taking estrogen before conducting any blood tests or other diagnostic procedures.

Food Interactions

Estrogens may be taken with food to reduce nausea and upset stomach. Avoid drinking grapefruit juice if you are taking this drug.

Usual Dose

Dosage varies. All of these products, including the transdermal skin patch, may be taken continuously or on a cyclic schedule of 3 weeks on, 1 week off.

Tablets
Chlorotrianisene: 12–200 mg.
   Conjugated estrogens: 0.3–30 mg.
   Conjugated estrogens, synthetic: 0.625–1.25 mg.
   Esterified estrogens: 0.3–30 mg.
   Estradiol: 0.5–30 mg.
   Estropipate: 0.625–7.5 mg.
   Ethinyl estradiol: 0.02–3.0 mg.

Estradiol Transdermal Patch (0.025, 0.0375, 0.05, 0.075, or 0.1 mg)
Alora, Estraderm, and Esclim: 1 patch twice a week; or use 1 patch twice a week for 3 weeks, stop for 1 week, then start again.
   Climara and Fempatch: 1 patch every week; or use 1 patch once a week for 3 weeks, stop for 1 week, then start again.

Vaginal Cream
Conjugated estrogens: 0.5–2.0 g a day for 3 weeks; stop for 1 week, then start again.
   Dienestrol: 1 applicatorful 1–2 times a day for 1–2 weeks, half the original dosage for another 1–2 weeks, then 1 applicatorful 1–3 times a week.
   Estradiol: 2–4 g a day for 2 weeks, half the starting dosage for another 2 weeks, then 1 g 1–3 times a week.
   Estropipate: 2–4 g a day for 3 weeks; stop for 1 week, then start again.

Estradiol Ring
Insert once every 3 months.

Overdosage

Symptoms may include nausea and vaginal bleeding in adult women. Call your local poison control center or a hospital emergency room for information. If you seek treatment, ALWAYS bring the prescription bottle or container.

Special Information

Call your doctor if you develop breast pain or tenderness, swelling of the feet and lower legs, rapid weight gain, chest pain, breathing difficulties, pain in the groin or calves, unusual or persistent vaginal bleeding, missed menstrual period, lumps in the breast, sudden severe headache, dizziness or fainting, disturbances in speech or vision, weakness or numbness in the arms or legs, abdominal pain, depression, yellowing of the skin or whites of the eyes, or jerky or involuntary muscle movement.

Your doctor should reevaluate your need for estrogen vaginal cream every 3–6 months. Do not stop using the drug suddenly because this may increase your risk of developing unpredicted or breakthrough vaginal bleeding.

Women using the cream who develop breast tenderness, start to bleed, or have other vaginal discharge should contact their doctors at once.

Women who smoke cigarettes and take estrogen have a greater risk of cardiovascular side effects including stroke and blood clotting.

Estrogen skin patches should be applied to a clean, dry, non-oily, hairless area of intact skin, preferably on the abdomen. Do not apply them to your breasts or waist, or to any area where tight-fitting clothes may loosen the patch from your skin. The application site should be rotated to prevent irritation and each site should have a patch-free period for 7 days.

Good dental hygiene is important while taking estrogen because estrogen may increase your risk of oral infection. Dental work should be completed prior to starting estrogen, if possible.

Vaginal estrogen cream should be inserted high into the vagina, about 2/3 of the length of the applicator.

Press the vaginal ring into an oval and insert as deeply as possible in the upper 1/3 of the vagina.

Some of these products contain tartrazine (a commonly used orange dye and food-coloring). If you are allergic to tartrazine or have asthma, check with your pharmacist to find out if your estrogen product contains this coloring agent.

If you forget a dose, take it as soon as you remember. If it is almost time for your next dose, skip the one you forgot and continue with your regular schedule. Do not take a double dose.

Special Populations

Pregnancy/Breast-feeding
Estrogens harm the fetus and should never be used during pregnancy for any reason.

Estrogens pass into breast milk and reduce its flow. Nursing mothers who must take them should bottle-feed.

Seniors
The risk of side effects increases with age, especially if you smoke.

Generic Name
Etanercept (ee-TAN-er-sept)

Brand Name
Enbrel

Type of Drug
Anti-TNF therapy.

Prescribed for
Rheumatoid arthritis.

General Information
Etanercept works by blocking the effects of tumor necrosis factor (TNF), a protein that plays an important role in the body's inflammatory process. Etanercept, which is used in adults and children age 4 and older who have not responded to other treatments, reduces inflammation by binding to TNF and preventing it from combining with cells.

Cautions and Warnings
Do not use this drug if you are **allergic** to it.

Etanercept compromises the body's ability to fight **infection** and should not be used if you have an infection of any kind. Stop taking etanercept if you develop an infection. Treatment may be restarted once the infection is gone.

People taking etanercept may become allergic to it over time, but the seriousness of this reaction is not known.

In theory, anti-TNF therapies like etanercept could interfere with the body's ability to prevent **malignancies**. It is not known if long-term etanercept treatment increases the risk of malignancy.

People taking etanercept should not receive any **vaccination** or **immunization** because etanercept may increase their susceptibility to the immunization. Make sure your vaccinations are up to date before starting etanercept.

Possible Side Effects

In studies, serious side effects were about the same for people taking etanercept and those taking a placebo (sugar pill). Abdominal pain and vomiting are much more common in children than in adults.

▼ Most common: infection, injection site reactions, headache, and runny nose.

▼ Common: dizziness, sore throat, cough, weakness, abdominal pain, rash, and respiratory problems.

▼ Less common: upset stomach, sinus irritation, and vomiting.

▼ Rare: heart failure, heart attack, chest pain, blood pressure changes, reduced blood supply to the brain, gallbladder inflammation, inflammation of the pancreas, stomach bleeding, bursitis, depression, and breathing difficulties.

Drug Interactions

• Do not combine etanercept with any other injectable drug.

Food Interactions

None known.

Usual Dose

Adult: 25 mg twice a week by injection under the skin.

Child (age 4–17): 0.18 mg per lb. of body weight, up to 25 mg, twice a week.

Child (under age 4): not recommended.

Overdosage

Overdose is unlikely to be serious. Call your local poison control center or a hospital emergency room for more information. If you seek treatment, ALWAYS bring the prescription bottle or container.

Special Information

Etanercept is taken by injection under the skin.

To mix and inject etanercept: Withdraw all the water supplied with the medicine into a syringe and slowly inject it into the vial containing etanercept. Swirl the mixture gently to avoid excess foaming in the vial. *Do not shake the vial*.

Do not combine etanercept with any other injectable drug.

Etanercept should be mixed just before you inject it, but may be stored in a refrigerator for up to 6 hours after it is mixed. The mixed vial must be discarded if not used in 6 hours.

You may inject yourself in the thigh, abdomen, or upper arm. Rotate injection sites and do not inject into skin that is bruised, tender, red, or hard.

Before using etanercept, clean the injection site with an alcohol swab or soap and water. Let the area dry before you inject the drug.

Hold an alcohol swab near the needle when you pull it out of the skin. Press the swab against the injection area for several seconds. Do not rub.

If you forget to administer a dose, do so as soon as you remember. If it is time for your next dose, take 1 dose right away and another in 48 hours, then resume your regular schedule. Do not take a double dose. Call your doctor if you miss 2 or more consecutive doses.

Special Populations

Pregnancy/Breast-feeding

The safety of using etanercept during pregnancy is not known. When this drug is considered crucial by your doctor, its potential benefits must be carefully weighed against its risks.

It is not known if this drug passes into breast milk. Nursing mothers who must take it should bottle-feed to avoid possible effects on the nursing infant.

Seniors

Seniors may use this drug without special restriction.

Generic Name

Etodolac (ee-TOE-doe-lak) [G]

Brand Names

Lodine   Lodine XL

Type of Drug

Nonsteroidal anti-inflammatory drug (NSAID).

Prescribed for

Osteoarthritis; may also be used to treat rheumatoid arthritis, ankylosing spondylitis, mild to moderate pain, tendinitis, bursitis, painful shoulder, and gout.

General Information

Etodolac and other NSAIDs are used to relieve pain and inflammation. We do not know exactly how NSAIDs work, but they may achieve their effects by blocking the body's production of a hormone called prostaglandin and the action of other body chemicals. Etodolac starts relieving pain in about 30 minutes and its effects last for 4 to 12 hours. Etodolac is broken down in the liver and eliminated through the kidneys.

Cautions and Warnings

People who are **allergic** to etodolac or any other NSAID and those with a history of **asthma** attacks brought on by an NSAID, iodides, or aspirin should not take etodolac.

Etodolac may cause **gastrointestinal (GI) bleeding, ulcers, and stomach perforation**. This can occur at any time, with or without warning, in people who take etodolac regularly. People with a history of active GI bleeding should be cautious about taking any NSAID. People who develop bleeding or ulcers and continue NSAID treatment should be aware of the possibility of developing more serious side effects.

Etodolac may affect platelets and **blood clotting** at high doses, and should be avoided by people with clotting problems and those taking warfarin.

People with **heart problems** who use etodolac may experience swelling in their arms, legs, or feet.

Etodolac may cause severe toxic effects to the **kidney**. Report any unusual side effects to your doctor, who may need to periodically test your kidney function.

Etodolac may make you **unusually sensitive to the effects of the sun**.

Possible Side Effects

▼ Most common: diarrhea, nausea, vomiting, constipation, gas, stomach upset or irritation, and appetite loss, especially during the first few days of treatment.

▼ Less common: stomach ulcers, GI bleeding, hepatitis, gallbladder attacks, painful urination, poor kidney function, kidney inflammation, blood and protein in the urine, dizziness, fainting, nervousness, depression, hallucinations, confusion, disorientation, tingling in the hands or feet, light-headedness, itching, increased sweating, dry nose and mouth, heart palpitations, chest pain, breathing difficulties, and muscle cramps.

▼ Rare: severe allergic reactions including closing of the throat, fever and chills, changes in liver function, jaundice (yellowing of the skin or whites of the eyes), and kidney failure. People who experience such effects must be promptly treated in a hospital emergency room or doctor's office. NSAIDs have caused severe skin reactions; if this happens to you, see your doctor immediately.

Drug Interactions

• Etodolac may increase the effects of oral anticoagulant (blood-thinning) drugs such as warfarin. Your anticoagulant dose may need to be reduced.

• Taking etodolac with cyclosporine may increase the kidney-related side effects of both drugs. Methotrexate side effects may be increased in people also taking etodolac.

• Etodolac may increase phenytoin side effects. Lithium blood levels may be increased by etodolac.

• Etodolac blood levels may be affected by cimetidine.

• Probenecid may increase the risk of etodolac side effects.

• Aspirin and other salicylates should never be combined with etodolac.

Food Interactions

Take etodolac with food or a magnesium-aluminum antacid if it upsets your stomach.

Usual Dose

200–400 mg every 6–8 hours, not to exceed 1200 mg a day. People weighing 132 lbs. or less should not take more than 20 mg for every 2.2 lbs. of body weight.

Overdosage

People have died from NSAID overdoses. Common signs of overdose are drowsiness, nausea, vomiting, diarrhea, abdominal pain, rapid breathing, rapid heartbeat, increased sweating, ringing or buzzing in the ears, confusion, disorientation, stupor, and coma. Take the victim to a hospital emergency room at once. ALWAYS bring the prescription bottle or container.

Special Information

Take each dose with a full glass of water and do not lie down for 15 to 30 minutes afterward.

Etodolac can make you drowsy or tired: Be careful when driving or operating hazardous equipment. Do not take any over-the-counter products containing acetaminophen or aspirin while taking etodolac. Avoid alcoholic beverages.

Contact your doctor if you develop rash or itching, visual disturbances, weight gain, breathing difficulties, fluid retention, hallucinations, black or tarry stools, persistent headache, or any unusual or intolerable side effect.

If you forget a dose of etodolac, take it as soon as you remember. If you take etodolac once a day and it is within 8 hours of your next dose, or if you take several doses a day and it is within 4 hours of your next dose, skip the dose you forgot and continue with your regular schedule. Never take a double dose.

Special Populations

Pregnancy/Breast-feeding

NSAIDs may affect the fetal heart during the second half of pregnancy. Pregnant women should not take etodolac without their doctor's approval. When the drug is considered crucial by your doctor, its potential benefits must be carefully weighed against its risks.

NSAIDs may pass into breast milk. There is a possibility that a nursing mother taking etodolac might affect her baby's heart or cardiovascular system. Nursing mothers who must take this drug should bottle-feed.

Seniors
Seniors may be more susceptible to side effects, especially ulcer disease.

Evista   see **Raloxifene**, page 871

Generic Name
Exemestane (ex-eh-MES-tane)

Brand Name
Aromasin

Type of Drug
Aromatase inactivator.

Prescribed for
Breast cancer.

General Information

In women, aromatase is the principal enzyme that converts androgen (male hormone) to estrogen, the female hormone often responsible for fueling breast cancer growth. Exemestane, which is prescribed for postmenopausal women whose condition worsens despite treatment with tamoxifen, reduces estrogen levels by interfering with this conversion process. In postmenopausal women, whose ovaries no longer produce estrogen, most of this hormone is produced via conversion from androgen. Exemestane is broken down in the liver.

Cautions and Warnings

Do not take this drug if you are **sensitive** or **allergic** to it.
Exemestane may be prescribed only for postmenopausal women.

Possible Side Effects

▼ Most common: fatigue, hot flashes, pain, depression, sleeplessness, anxiety, nausea, and breathing difficulties.

▼ Common: flu-like symptoms, leg swelling, high blood pressure, dizziness, headache, vomiting, abdominal pain, appetite loss, constipation, and coughing.

▼ Less common: increased appetite due to the effects of diarrhea, fever, weakness, tingling in the hands or feet, broken bones, bronchitis, sinus irritation, rash, itching, urinary infection, and swollen lymph glands.

Drug Interactions

Knowledge of exemestane interactions is limited.

• Estrogen-containing drugs reduce exemestane's effectiveness. Do not combine these drugs.

Food Interactions

Take this drug after a meal.

Usual Dose

Adult: 25 mg once a day.
Child: not recommended.

Overdosage

Volunteers have taken up to 800 mg of exemestane in a single dose. Accidental overdose symptoms may include drug side effects but they are not likely to be serious. Take the victim to a hospital emergency room for evaluation and treatment. ALWAYS bring the prescription bottle or container.

Special Information

If you forget a dose, take it as soon as you remember. If it is almost time for your next dose, skip the forgotten dose and continue with your regular schedule.

Special Populations

Pregnancy/Breast-feeding

Exemestane is intended only for postmenopausal women. Pregnant women taking this drug risk damaging the fetus and losing their pregnancy.

Exemestane passes into breast milk. Nursing mothers who must take it should bottle-feed.

Seniors
Seniors may take this drug without special precaution.

Generic Name

Famciclovir (fam-SYE-kloe-vere)

Brand Name

Famvir

Type of Drug

Antiviral.

Prescribed for

Herpes zoster (shingles) and recurrent genital herpes.

General Information

Famciclovir is absorbed into the body and converted to the antiviral penciclovir, the drug that actually works against shingles by interfering with the reproduction of DNA in the herpes virus. Penciclovir does not affect DNA in uninfected body cells. Penciclovir is broken down by the liver and eliminated from the body through the kidneys.

Cautions and Warnings

People **sensitive** or **allergic** to famciclovir should not take this drug. Those with **reduced kidney function** should have their dosage adjusted accordingly. **Severe liver disease** reduces the maximum possible concentration of penciclovir in the blood and increases the time it takes to reach this maximum level; however, dosage adjustment is not normally required.

Possible Side Effects

▼ Most common: headache, nausea, and diarrhea.
▼ Less common: fever, fatigue, pain, vomiting, constipation, appetite loss, dizziness, tingling in the hands or feet, sleepiness, sore throat, sinus irritation, itching, and signs of shingles.

Possible Side Effects *(continued)*

▼ Rare: chills, abdominal pain, back or joint pain, and upset stomach.

Drug Interactions

• Probenecid, cimetidine, and theophylline interfere with the elimination of penciclovir from the body, possibly leading to higher levels of penciclovir in the blood.

• People who took famciclovir and digoxin together experienced increased digoxin in their blood.

Food Interactions

None known.

Usual Dose

Shingles

Adult (age 18 and over): 500 mg every 8 hours for 1 week. People with reduced kidney function may require a reduced dose taken as infrequently as once a day.

Child (under age 18): not recommended.

Genital Herpes

Adult (age 18 and over): 125 mg twice a day for 5 days. People with reduced kidney function take the same dose but less often, as infrequently as once every 2 days.

Child (under age 18): not recommended.

Overdosage

Little is known about the effects of famciclovir overdose. Overdose victims should be taken to a hospital emergency room for treatment. ALWAYS bring the prescription bottle or container.

Special Information

Famciclovir treatment should be started as soon as shingles is diagnosed. For maximum benefit, be sure to complete the full week of treatment.

Famciclovir is not a cure for genital herpes and it is not known if it will prevent the transmission of the herpes virus to another person. Avoid sexual intercourse when herpes lesions are present even while taking famciclovir for genital herpes.

Begin taking famciclovir at the first sign of a herpes attack (symptoms include pain, tenderness, burning, itching, tingling, ulcers, or scabs). The effectiveness of starting famciclovir 6 hours or more after symptoms or lesions appear has not been established.

Call your doctor if you experience any unusual or intolerable side effects.

If you forget a dose of famciclovir, take it as soon as you remember. If it is almost time for your next dose, skip the dose you forgot. Do not take a double dose. Call your doctor if you forget more than 2 doses in a row.

Special Populations

Pregnancy/Breast-feeding

Famciclovir should only be taken by a pregnant woman if it is absolutely necessary and the possible benefits outweigh the risks to the fetus.

In animal studies, penciclovir (the active form of famciclovir) passed into breast milk in high concentrations but it is not known if this holds true for humans. Nursing mothers who must take this drug should bottle-feed.

Seniors

Seniors clear penciclovir from the bloodstream more slowly than younger people and should have their dosage adjusted according to their level of kidney function.

Generic Name

Famotidine (fam-OE-tih-dine)

Brand Names

Pepcid   Pepcid AC

Type of Drug

Histamine H_2 antagonist.

Prescribed for

Ulcers of the stomach and duodenum (upper intestine). This drug is also used to treat gastroesophageal reflux disease (GERD), stress ulcer, and other conditions characterized by the production of large amounts of gastric fluids; to prevent

stress ulcer and stomach and upper intestinal bleeding; and
to stop the production of stomach acid during surgery. Pepcid AC is approved for heartburn.

General Information

Histamine H_2 antagonists work by turning off the system that
produces stomach acid and other secretions. Famotidine is
effective in treating the symptoms of ulcer and preventing
complications of the disease, although an ulcer that does not
respond to another histamine H_2 antagonist will probably not
respond to famotidine. Histamine H_2 antagonists differ only
in their potency. Cimetidine is the least potent; 1000 mg are
roughly equal to 300 mg of either nizatidine or ranitidine, or
40 mg of famotidine. All these drugs have roughly equivalent
success rates in treating ulcer disease and comparable risk of
side effects.

Cautions and Warnings

Do not take famotidine if you have had an **allergic reaction** to
it or any histamine H_2 antagonist.

People with **kidney or liver disease** should take famotidine
with caution because ⅓ of each dose is broken down in the
liver and the rest passes out of the body through the kidneys.

Possible Side Effects

▼ Most common: headache.

▼ Less common: dizziness, mild diarrhea, and constipation.

▼ Rare: Rare side effects can occur in almost any part
of the body. Contact your doctor if you experience any
side effect not listed above.

Drug Interactions

• Enteric-coated tablets should not be taken with famotidine. The change in stomach acidity that famotidine produces causes the tablets to disintegrate prematurely in the
stomach.

• Antacids, anticholinergics, and metoclopramide may
slightly reduce the amount of famotidine absorbed into the
blood. No special precaution is needed.

Food Interactions

Famotidine may be taken without regard to food or meals.

Usual Dose

Adult: 20–40 mg at bedtime, or 20 mg twice a day. Dosage should be reduced in people with severe kidney disease.

Overdosage

Little is known about the effects of famotidine overdose, but victims may experience exaggerated side effects. Your local poison control center may advise giving ipecac syrup—available at any pharmacy—to induce vomiting and remove any remaining drug from the stomach. Victims who have definite symptoms should be taken to a hospital emergency room. ALWAYS bring the prescription bottle or container.

Special Information

Take famotidine exactly as directed and follow your doctor's instructions regarding diet and other treatment in order to get the maximum benefit from the drug. Antacids may be taken together with famotidine if needed.

Cigarettes worsen stomach ulcers and may reduce famotidine's effectiveness.

Call your doctor at once if you develop any unusual side effects such as bleeding or bruising, tiredness, diarrhea, dizziness, or rash. Black, tarry stools or vomiting material that resembles coffee grounds may indicate your ulcer is bleeding.

If you forget a dose of famotidine, take it as soon as you remember. If it is almost time for your next dose, skip the one you forgot and continue with your regular schedule. Do not take a double dose.

Special Populations

Pregnancy/Breast-feeding

Although animal studies revealed no damage to the fetus, famotidine should be avoided by women who are or might be pregnant. When this drug is considered crucial by your doctor, its possible benefits must be carefully weighed against its risks.

Famotidine may pass into breast milk. Nursing mothers who must take this drug should consider bottle-feeding.

Seniors

Seniors may need lower doses due to loss of kidney function and may be more susceptible to side effects.

Generic Name

Felbamate (FEL-bam-ate)

Brand Name

Felbatol

Type of Drug

Anticonvulsant.

Prescribed for

Partial seizure and Lennox-Gastaut syndrome in children.

General Information

Felbamate is related to the older tranquilizer-sedative meprobamate (Miltown). Exactly how felbamate works is not known, but it raises the seizure threshold and prevents the seizure impulse from spreading in the brain, as do other anticonvulsants. Felbamate should only be used when other seizure drugs have failed because of the risks associated with it. About half of each dose passes out of the body through the kidneys; the other half is broken down and eliminated by the liver.

Cautions and Warnings

Rarely, **aplastic anemia** (potentially fatal condition characterized by a reduction in white-blood-cell count) has occurred in people taking felbamate for 5 weeks or more, resulting in several deaths. About 2 to 5 in 1 million people are affected. Possibly fatal **liver failure** occurs in people taking felbamate much more often than normal. Regular liver function tests are recommended.

Felbamate should never be **suddenly stopped** or seizures may become more frequent. Dosage should be gradually reduced or replaced by another anticonvulsant.

People who are **allergic** to felbamate or related drugs should not take it.

Felbamate may cause **increased sensitivity to the sun**. Wear protective clothing and use sunscreen while taking this drug. People with **kidney disease** may require lower doses.

Possible Side Effects

Adults

▼ Most common: sleeplessness, sleepiness, fatigue, headache, dizziness, nervousness, upset stomach, vomiting, constipation, nausea, appetite loss.

▼ Common: anxiety, tremors, walking unusually, depression, tingling in the hands or feet, diarrhea, liver inflammation, abdominal pains, respiratory infections, abnormal vision, taste changes.

▼ Less common: weakness, dry mouth, stupor, abnormal thinking, rash, sinus irritation, sore throat, muscle aches, fever, chest pain.

▼ Rare: Rare side effects can occur in almost any part of the body. Contact your doctor if you experience any side effect not listed above.

Children

▼ Most common: abdominal pain, fever, respiratory infections, sleeplessness, sleepiness, nervousness, vomiting, constipation, black and blue marks.

▼ Common: headache, appetite loss, hiccups, sore throat, coughing, middle ear infections, fatigue, weight loss, temporary loss of urine control, pain, walking unusually, weakness, abnormal thinking, emotional instability, pinpoint pupils, rash, upset stomach, low white blood cell count.

▼ Rare: Rare side effects can occur in almost any part of the body. Contact your doctor if your child experiences any side effect not listed above.

Drug Interactions

• Combining felbamate and other antiseizure drugs usually requires dosage adjustments due to the risk of drug interaction.

• Combining felbamate and carbamazepine reduces blood levels of both drugs by roughly half. Dosage adjustments are necessary.

• Combining phenobarbital and felbamate increases the amount of phenobarbital in the blood and decreases felbamate levels. Dosage adjustments are necessary.

• If you combine felbamate and phenytoin, your phenytoin dosage may have to be reduced by as much as 30%. This combination also decreases felbamate blood levels by almost 50%.

• Felbamate increases blood levels of valproic acid and methsuximide.

Food Interactions

Felbamate is best taken on an empty stomach but may be taken with food if it causes upset stomach.

Usual Dose

Adult and Child (age 14 and over): 1200–3600 mg a day, divided into 3–4 doses.

Child (age 2–13): 6.8–20.5 mg per lb. a day, divided into 3–4 doses.

Overdosage

Overdose symptoms may include upset stomach, increased heart rate, and felbamate side effects. Call your local poison control center or a hospital emergency room for more information. If you seek treatment, ALWAYS bring the prescription bottle or container.

Special Information

Do not take more felbamate than your doctor has prescribed.

Felbamate can cause drowsiness; be careful when driving or performing tasks that require concentration.

Avoid prolonged exposure to the sun while taking felbamate.

Call your doctor if you develop any bothersome or persistent side effect.

Maintain good dental hygiene while taking felbamate and use extra care when brushing or flossing because this drug can cause swollen gums. See your dentist regularly.

If you forget a dose, take it as soon as you remember. If it is almost time for your next dose, take 1 dose right away and another in 3 or 4 hours, then go back to your regular schedule. Do not take a double dose.

Special Populations

Pregnancy/Breast-feeding

This drug may cross into fetal circulation. When the drug is considered crucial by your doctor, its potential benefits must be carefully weighed against its risks.

Felbamate passes into breast milk. Nursing mothers who must take this drug should consider bottle-feeding.

Seniors

Seniors, especially those with liver, kidney, or heart disease, may be more sensitive to the effects of this drug and should receive lower doses.

Generic Name

Felodipine (feh-LOE-dih-pene)

Brand Name

Plendil

Type of Drug

Calcium channel blocker.

Prescribed for

High blood pressure.

General Information

Felodipine is one of many calcium channel blockers available in the U.S. Its once-daily dosage schedule makes it particularly suited to treating high blood pressure. Felodipine blocks the passage of calcium, an essential factor in muscle contraction, into the heart and smooth muscles. Such blockage interferes with the contraction of these muscles, which in turn dilates (widens) the veins and vessels that supply blood to them. This dilating effect reduces blood pressure, the amount of oxygen used by the heart muscle, and the risk of blood vessel spasm. Felodipine is therefore useful in treating not only high blood pressure but also angina pectoris (brief attacks of chest pain), a condition related to poor oxygen supply to the heart muscles.

Felodipine only affects the movement of calcium into muscle cells; it has no effect on calcium in the blood.

Cautions and Warnings

Felodipine should not be taken if you have had an **allergic reaction** to it in the past.

On rare occasions, felodipine may cause very **low blood pressure** that may lead to stimulation of the heart and rapid heartbeat and can worsen angina. This reaction may happen when treatment is first started, when dosage is increased, or if the drug is rapidly withdrawn; it may be avoided by reducing dosage gradually.

Studies have shown that people taking calcium channel blockers—usually those taken several times a day, not those taken only once daily—have a greater chance of having a **heart attack** than do people taking beta blockers or other medications for the same purpose. Discuss this with your doctor to be sure you are receiving the best possible treatment.

Patients taking a beta-blocking drug who begin taking felodipine may develop **heart failure** or increased **angina**.

People with severe **liver disease** may require dosage adjustments.

People taking felodipine who have had a **heart attack** and have **lung congestion** may experience worsened heart failure, since this drug can actually slow the force of each heartbeat.

Possible Side Effects

Side effects produced by calcium channel blockers are generally mild and rarely cause people to stop taking them. Side effects are more common with higher doses and in older patients.

▼ Most common: swelling in the ankles, feet, or legs; dizziness; light-headedness; muscle weakness or cramps; facial flushing; and headache.

▼ Less common: respiratory infections, cough, tingling in the hands or feet, upset stomach, abdominal pains, chest pains, nausea, constipation, diarrhea, heart palpitations, sore throat, runny nose, back pain, and rash.

▼ Rare: Rare side effects can affect the heart, stomach, blood and joints. It can affect your mood, sex drive, and urinary tract. Contact your doctor if you experience any side effect not listed above.

Drug Interactions

• Felodipine may increase the amount of beta-blocking drugs in the bloodstream. This can lead to heart failure, very low blood pressure, or an increased incidence of angina. However, in many cases these drugs have been taken together with no problem.

• Felodipine increases the effects of other blood-pressure-lowering drugs. Such drug combinations are often used to treat hypertension.

• Cimetidine and ranitidine increase the amount of felodipine in the blood and may account for a slight increase in the drug's effect.

• Phenytoin and other hydantoin antiseizure medicines, carbamazepine, and barbiturate sleeping pills and sedatives may decrease the amount of felodipine in the blood, reducing its effect on the body.

• Erythromycin may increase the side effects of felodipine.

• Felodipine may increase the effects of digoxin, theophylline (prescribed for asthma and other respiratory problems), and oral anticoagulant (blood-thinning) drugs.

• Felodipine may also interact with quinidine (prescribed for abnormal heart rhythm) to produce low blood pressure, very slow heart rate, abnormal heart rhythms, and swelling in the arms or legs.

Food Interactions

You may take felodipine with food if it upsets your stomach. Avoid taking felodipine with concentrated grapefruit juice—it doubles the amount of drug absorbed.

Usual Dose

5–10 mg a day. No patient should take more than 20 mg a day. Do not stop taking felodipine abruptly. The dosage should be reduced gradually over a period of time.

Overdosage

Felodipine overdose can cause low blood pressure. If you think you have taken an overdose of felodipine, call your doctor or go to a hospital emergency room. ALWAYS bring the prescription bottle or container.

Special Information

Call your doctor if you develop constipation, nausea, very low blood pressure, breathing difficulties, increased heart pain, dizziness, or light-headedness, or if other side effects are bothersome or persistent.

Swelling of the hands or feet may develop within 2 or 3 weeks of starting felodipine. The chances of this happening depend on age and dosage. It occurs in less than 10% of people under age 50 taking 5 mg a day and in more than 30% of those over age 60 taking 20 mg a day.

Be sure to continue taking your medication even if you feel well, and follow any instructions for diet restriction or other treatments to help maintain lower blood pressure.

Do not break or crush felodipine tablets.

It is important to maintain good dental hygiene while taking felodipine and to use extra care when using your toothbrush or dental floss because of the chance that the drug will make you more susceptible to certain infections.

If you forget to take a dose of felodipine, take it as soon as you remember. If it is almost time for your next dose, skip the dose you forgot and continue with your regular schedule. Do not take a double dose.

Special Populations

Pregnancy/Breast-feeding
Animal studies of felodipine have shown that it crosses into the fetal circulation and causes birth defects. Women who are or who might become pregnant while taking this drug should not take it without their doctor's approval. The potential benefit of taking felodipine must be carefully weighed against its risks.

It is not known if felodipine passes into breast milk. Before breast-feeding, you must consider the drug's potential effect on the nursing infant.

Seniors
Seniors, especially those with liver disease, are more sensitive to the effects of this drug.

Generic Name

Fenofibrate (fen-oe-FIH-brate)

Brand Name

Tricor

Type of Drug

Anti-hyperlipidemic (blood-fat reducer).

Prescribed for

High blood triglycerides.

General Information

Fenofibrate works by interfering with the body's ability to make triglyceride. It also reduces uric acid levels. This drug should only be used in people with very high triglyceride levels who are at risk for pancreatitis (inflammation of the pancreas) and have not responded to other treatments.

Cautions and Warnings

People taking fenofibrate and other triglyceride-lowering drugs are more likely to die from causes unrelated to triglyceride levels. It has not been established whether fenofibrate helps people live longer. For both these reasons, fenofibrate should **only be used if absolutely necessary.**

People with **liver or severe kidney disease** should avoid fenofibrate. People with less severe kidney disease require reduced dosage.

People taking fenofibrate are more likely to develop **gallstones.**

Fenofibrate can destroy muscle cells, leading to **kidney failure,** especially when combined with a statin cholesterol-lowering drug (see "Drug Interactions").

Possible Side Effects

▼ Most common: infections and pain.

▼ Common: rash, headache, upset stomach, weakness, tiredness, and flu-like symptoms.

▼ Less common: joint pain, abnormal heart rhythms, reduced sex drive, dizziness, increased appetite, sleeplessness, tingling in the hands or feet, nausea, vomiting, diarrhea, abdominal pain, constipation, stomach noise or gas, frequent urination, vaginal irritation, runny nose, cough, sinus irritation, eye irritation, blurred vision, conjunctivitis (pinkeye), earache, and tiny particles inside the eye ("floaters").

Possible Side Effects *(continued)*

▼ Rare: allergic reactions including severe rash, itching, liver inflammation or enlargement, gallstones, gallbladder disease, muscle aches, and increased sensitivity to the sun.

Drug Interactions

• Combining fenofibrate and a statin cholesterol-lowering drug (atorvastatin, cerivastatin, fluvastatin, lovastatin, pravastatin, or simvastatin) can lead to severe muscle pain, muscle cell destruction, and kidney failure. If you have extremely high blood-fat levels, the potential benefits of this combination may outweigh the risks. In people taking this combination, the health of muscles and kidneys must be monitored regularly via blood tests.

• Fenofibrate increases the effects of anticoagulant (blood-thinning) drugs. Your anticoagulant dosage may need an adjustment.

• Combining fenofibrate and cyclosporine can increase the risk of kidney disease. This combination should only be used if it is absolutely necessary and the lowest possible dosage is taken.

• If you are taking cholestyramine or colestipol (both are used to reduce blood-fat levels) as well as fenofibrate, take the fenofibrate at least 1 hour before or 4 to 6 hours after these drugs.

Food Interactions

Take fenofibrate with food to get the best effect from it.

Usual Dose

Adult: 1–3 capsules (67 mg each) a day.
Senior: Begin with 1 capsule a day. This dosage also applies to people with kidney disease.
Child: not recommended.

Overdosage

Little is known about the effects of fenofibrate overdose. Victims should be taken to a hospital emergency room. ALWAYS bring the prescription bottle or container.

Special Information

People should take fenofibrate only after a triglyceride-lowering diet and other medications have failed. While taking fenofibrate, follow the diet recommended by your doctor.

If you forget a dose, take it as soon as you remember. If it is almost time for your next dose, skip the forgotten dose and continue with your regular schedule.

Special Populations

Pregnancy/Breast-feeding

Fenofibrate causes fetal injury and death in animal studies. When this drug is considered crucial by your doctor, its potential benefits must be carefully weighed against its risks.

This drug should not be taken by nursing mothers because of its potential to affect the nursing infant.

Seniors

Seniors are more likely to experience side effects and should never start with more than 1 capsule (67 mg) a day.

Generic Name

Fenoprofen (fen-oe-PROE-fen) Ⓖ

Brand Names

Nalfon   Nalfon 200

Type of Drug

Nonsteroidal anti-inflammatory drug (NSAID).

Prescribed for

Rheumatoid arthritis, juvenile rheumatoid arthritis, osteoarthritis, mild to moderate pain, sunburn, and migraine.

General Information

Fenoprofen calcium and other NSAIDs are used to relieve pain and inflammation. We do not know exactly how NSAIDs work, but they may achieve their effects by blocking the body's production of a hormone called prostaglandin and the action of other body chemicals. Fenoprofen starts relieving pain within 24 hours, but its anti-inflammatory effect takes about 2 days to begin and 2 to 3 weeks to reach maximum effect. Fenoprofen is broken down in the liver and eliminated through the kidneys.

Cautions and Warnings

People **allergic** to fenoprofen or any other NSAID and those with a history of **asthma** attacks brought on by an NSAID, iodides, or aspirin should not take fenoprofen.

Fenoprofen may cause **gastrointestinal (GI) bleeding, ulcers,** and **stomach perforation**. This can occur at any time, with or without warning, in people who take fenoprofen regularly. People with a history of active GI bleeding should be cautious about taking any NSAID. People who develop bleeding or ulcers and continue NSAID treatment should be aware of the possibility of developing more serious side effects.

Fenoprofen can affect platelets and **blood clotting** at high doses, and should be avoided by people with clotting problems and those taking warfarin.

People with **heart problems** who use fenoprofen may experience swelling in their arms, legs, or feet.

People with **impaired hearing** may be affected by fenoprofen and should have periodic hearing tests.

Fenoprofen may actually cause **headaches**. If this happens, you might have to stop taking the drug or switch to another NSAID.

Fenoprofen may cause severe toxic effects to the **kidney**. Report any unusual side effects to your doctor, who might need to periodically test your kidney function. People with kidney disease should not take fenoprofen.

Fenoprofen can make you **unusually sensitive to the effects of the sun**.

Possible Side Effects

▼ Most common: diarrhea, vomiting, nausea, constipation, stomach gas, stomach upset or irritation, and appetite loss, especially during the first few days of treatment.

Possible Side Effects *(continued)*

▼ Less common: stomach ulcers, GI bleeding, hepatitis, gallbladder attacks, painful urination, poor kidney function, kidney inflammation, blood and protein in the urine, dizziness, fainting, nervousness, depression, hallucinations, confusion, disorientation, tingling in the hands or feet, light-headedness, heart palpitations, chest pain, itching, increased sweating, dry nose and mouth, breathing difficulties, and muscle cramps.

▼ Rare: severe allergic reactions including closing of the throat, fever and chills, changes in liver function, jaundice (yellowing of the skin or whites of the eyes), and kidney failure. People who experience such effects must be promptly treated in a hospital emergency room or doctor's office. NSAIDs have caused severe skin reactions; if this happens to you, see your doctor immediately.

Drug Interactions

• Fenoprofen may increase the effects of oral anticoagulant (blood-thinning) drugs such as warfarin. Your anticoagulant dose may need to be reduced.

• Combining fenoprofen with cyclosporine may increase the kidney-related side effects of both drugs. Methotrexate toxicity may be increased in people also taking fenoprofen.

• Fenoprofen may reduce the blood-pressure-lowering effect of beta blockers and loop diuretics.

• Fenoprofen may increase phenytoin side effects. Lithium blood levels may be increased by fenoprofen.

• Fenoprofen blood levels may be affected by cimetidine.

• Probenecid may increase the risk of fenoprofen side effects.

• Aspirin and other salicylates should never be combined with fenoprofen.

Food Interactions

Take fenoprofen with food or a magnesium-aluminum antacid if it upsets your stomach.

Usual Dose

Adult: mild to moderate pain—200 mg every 4–6 hours. Arthritis—300–600 mg 3–4 times a day to start, individual-

ized to your needs. Total daily dosage should not exceed
3200 mg.

Child: not recommended.

Overdosage

People have died from NSAID overdoses. Common signs of
overdose are drowsiness, nausea, vomiting, diarrhea,
abdominal pain, rapid breathing, rapid heartbeat, increased
sweating, ringing or buzzing in the ears, confusion, disorientation, stupor, and coma. Take the victim to a hospital emergency room at once. ALWAYS bring the prescription bottle or
container.

Special Information

Take each dose with a full glass of water and do not lie down
for 15 to 30 minutes afterward.

Fenoprofen can make you drowsy or tired: Be careful when
driving or operating hazardous equipment. Do not take any
over-the-counter products containing acetaminophen or
aspirin while taking fenoprofen.

Contact your doctor if you develop rash or itching, visual
disturbances, weight gain, breathing difficulties, fluid retention, hallucinations, black or tarry stools, persistent
headache, or any unusual or intolerable side effect.

If you forget a dose of fenoprofen, take it as soon as you
remember. If you take fenoprofen once a day and it is within
8 hours of your next dose, or if you take several doses a day
and it is within 4 hours of your next dose, skip the dose you
forgot and continue with your regular schedule. Never take a
double dose.

Special Populations

Pregnancy/Breast-feeding

Fenoprofen may affect the fetal heart during the second half
of pregnancy. Pregnant women should not take fenoprofen
without their doctor's approval. When the drug is considered
crucial by your doctor, its potential benefits must be carefully
weighed against its risks.

Fenoprofen may pass into breast milk. There is a possibility
that a nursing mother taking fenoprofen could affect her
baby's heart or cardiovascular system. If you must take fenoprofen, talk to your doctor about bottle-feeding your baby.
Nursing mothers who must take this drug should bottle-feed.

Seniors

Seniors may be more susceptible to side effects, especially ulcer disease.

Generic Name

Finasteride (fin-ASS-ter-ide)

Brand Names

Proscar   Propecia

Type of Drug

Alpha-reductase inhibitor.

Prescribed for

Benign prostatic hyperplasia (BPH) and male pattern baldness.

General Information

A gradual reduction in urine flow in men over age 50 usually leads to gradual enlargement of the prostate gland. This condition is known as BPH. Finasteride works by interfering with the action of the enzyme alpha-reductase, which is essential to the process of converting testosterone into a much more potent substance called 5-dihydrotestosterone (DHT). By suppressing DHT levels, finasteride dramatically reduces the size of the prostate in most men who take the drug for PBH. You may need to take finasteride for 6 to 12 months before its effects can be assessed.

Urine flow improves in about 60% of men taking finasteride for BPH and symptoms improve in about 30%. In one study, men experienced a significant regression in prostate size after 3 months and the reduction was maintained through the 12-month study period; these men experienced a significant improvement in urine flow that could be maintained up to 36 months.

Studies of finasteride for hair loss on the top and back-middle of the scalp show new hair growth in 60% to 80% of men taking the drug continuously for 2 years. The drug must be taken for 3 months or more before it begins to have an effect and must be taken continuously to maintain hair growth. Once you stop taking this drug, any new hair you have grown is likely to fall out in the next 12 months. Seventeen percent of men taking the drug continued to lose hair throughout the study period.

Finasteride has been studied as therapy following radical prostatectomy surgery and in the prevention of first-stage prostate cancer, acne in women, and unusual hairiness.

Cautions and Warnings

Do not take finasteride if you are **allergic** to any of its ingredients. This drug must not be used in **women** or **children**.

People who do not respond to finasteride may have a condition that causes BPH-like symptoms, such as prostate cancer, bladder or nerve disorders, or physical obstruction of the urinary tubes. Finasteride cannot be used to treat these conditions.

Because it is broken down in the liver, finasteride must be used with caution by people with **liver disease**.

Finasteride may mask symptoms of **prostate cancer** by causing a reduction in the level of prostate-specific antigen (PSA), an increasingly acknowledged indicator of prostate cancer.

Possible Side Effects

Side effects are generally mild and often subside with continued use of the drug.

▼ Most common: impotence, loss of sex drive, decreased amount of semen, breast tenderness and enlargement, and drug sensitivity reaction including lip swelling and rash.

Drug Interactions

• Finasteride may reduce the effectiveness of theophylline and aminophylline, though dosage adjustments usually are not required.

• Finasteride affects the PSA blood test used for prostate cancer screening. Be sure your doctor knows you are taking this drug if you have a PSA test done or are being tested for prostate cancer.

Food Interactions

You may take finasteride with food if it upsets your stomach.

Usual Dose

BPH
  Adult: 5 mg once a day.
  Child: Do not use.

Male Pattern Baldness
  Adult: 1 mg once a day.
  Child: Do not use.

  Women should not take finasteride.

Overdosage

Side effects are unlikely. Call your local poison control center or a hospital emergency room for more information. If you seek treatment, ALWAYS bring the prescription bottle or container.

Special Information

Women who are or might be pregnant should not handle crushed finasteride tablets because small amounts of the drug may be absorbed into the blood, possibly affecting the fetus.

  If your sexual partner is or might be pregnant and you start taking finasteride, you must wear a condom during sex to avoid directly exposing her to finasteride in the semen.

  Semen volume may decrease while on finasteride. Impotence or reduced sex drive is also a risk.

  If you forget a dose, take it as soon as you remember. If it is almost time for your next dose, skip the one you forgot and continue with your regular schedule. Do not take a double dose. Call your doctor if you miss a dose for 2 or more days.

Special Populations

Pregnancy/Breast-feeding
This drug is not intended for women. Finasteride will harm the fetus if taken during pregnancy. It is not known if finasteride passes into breast milk.

Seniors
Seniors with liver disease should use this drug with caution.

Brand Name

Fioricet

Generic Ingredients

Acetaminophen + Butalbital + Caffeine Ⓖ

Other Brand Names
Esgic   Fiorpap
Esgic-Plus   Isocet
Femcet   Repan

Type of Drug

Barbiturate and analgesic (pain reliever) combination.

Prescribed for

Migraine and other pain.

General Information

Fioricet is one of many combination products containing a barbiturate—butalbital—and an analgesic—acetaminophen. Products of this kind also often contain a tranquilizer or a narcotic. Other analgesic combinations, such as Fiorinal, substitute aspirin for acetaminophen.

Cautions and Warnings

Do not take Fioricet if you are **allergic** or **sensitive** to it. Use this drug with extreme caution if you suffer from **asthma or other breathing problems,** have **kidney or liver disease,** or a **viral infection of the liver**. Chronic (long-term) use of Fioricet may lead to drug dependence or **addiction**.

Butalbital is a respiratory depressant and affects the central nervous system (CNS), producing **drowsiness, tiredness,** and an **inability to concentrate**.

Possible Side Effects

▼ Most common: light-headedness, dizziness, sedation, nausea, vomiting, sweating, appetite loss, and mild stimulation.

Possible Side Effects *(continued)*

▼ Less common: weakness, headache, upset stomach, sleeplessness, agitation, tremor, uncoordinated muscle movement, mild hallucinations, disorientation, visual disturbances, euphoria (feeling "high"), dry mouth, constipation, facial flushing, changes in heart rate, palpitations, feeling faint, urinary difficulties, rash, itching, confusion, rapid breathing, and diarrhea.

Drug Interactions

• Combining Fioricet with alcohol, tranquilizers, barbiturates, sleeping pills, or other nervous-system depressants may cause tiredness, drowsiness, and trouble concentrating.

Food Interactions

Fioricet is best taken on an empty stomach but may be taken with food if it upsets your stomach.

Usual Dose

1–2 tablets or capsules every 4 hours or as needed; do not exceed 6 doses a day.

Overdosage

Symptoms include breathing difficulties, nervousness progressing to stupor or coma, pinpointed pupils, cold and clammy skin and lowered heart rate or blood pressure, nausea, vomiting, dizziness, ringing in the ears, facial flushing, sweating, and thirst. Take the victim to a hospital emergency room immediately. ALWAYS bring the prescription bottle or container.

Special Information

Be careful when driving or performing any task that requires concentration. Alcohol may increase the risk of acetaminophen-related liver toxicity and butalbital-related drowsiness.

Call your doctor if you develop side effects that are bothersome or persistent.

If you forget a dose, take it as soon as you remember. If it is almost time for your next dose, skip the one you forgot and continue with your regular schedule. Do not take a double dose.

Special Populations

Pregnancy/Breast-feeding
Fioricet should be avoided during pregnancy. It is associated with birth defects, prolonged labor and delayed delivery, and breathing problems in newborns. Regular use of Fioricet during the last 3 months of pregnancy may also cause drug dependency in the newborn.

Fioricet passes into breast milk. Breast-feeding while using Fioricet may cause babies to become tired, short of breath, or have a slow heartbeat. Nursing mothers who must take this drug should consider bottle-feeding.

Seniors
Fioricet may have a greater depressant effect on seniors. Other effects that may be more prominent are light-headedness and dizziness or fainting when rising suddenly from a sitting or lying position.

Brand Name
Fiorinal

Generic Ingredients
Aspirin + Butalbital + Caffeine Ⓖ

Other Brand Names

Amaphen	Fiorital
Anoquan	Lanorinal
Endolor	Margesic
Esgic	Medigesic
Femcet	Triad

Type of Drug
Barbiturate and analgesic (pain reliever) combination.

Prescribed for
Migraine and other pain.

General Information

Pain relief products often combine an analgesic with a sedative. The analgesic ingredient in Fiorinal is aspirin; other brand-name products, such as Esgic and Fioricet, contain acetaminophen. The sedative ingredient in pain-relief combinations may be a barbiturate, narcotic, or other tranquilizer. Fiorinal contains the barbiturate butalbital. Fiorinal also contains caffeine, which is often used in analgesic combinations that treat headache because it enhances the pain-relieving effect of aspirin.

Cautions and Warnings

Do not take Fiorinal if you are **allergic** or **sensitive** to any of its ingredients, including aspirin, or to any salicylate or nonsteroidal anti-inflammatory drug (NSAID). Fiorinal and other aspirin-containing products should not be taken by **children under age 16**. People with **liver damage** should avoid Fiorinal.

Use Fiorinal with extreme caution if you suffer from **asthma or other breathing problems**. Long-term use of this drug may cause drug dependence and **addiction**. Butalbital is a respiratory depressant and affects the central nervous system (CNS), producing **drowsiness, tiredness,** and **inability to concentrate**.

Alcohol may aggravate stomach irritation caused by aspirin and increases the risk of aspirin-related ulcers. Alcohol also increases the nervous system depression caused by butalbital.

Do not take any aspirin-containing product if you develop **dizziness, hearing loss,** or **ringing or buzzing in the ears**. Aspirin may interfere with **blood coagulation** (clotting) and should be avoided for 1 week before surgery. Talk to your surgeon or dentist before taking an aspirin-containing product for pain after surgery.

Possible Side Effects

▼ Most common: light-headedness, dizziness, sedation, nausea, vomiting, sweating, upset stomach, appetite loss, and mild stimulation.

Possible Side Effects *(continued)*

▼ Less common: weakness, headache, sleeplessness, agitation, tremor, uncoordinated muscle movements, mild hallucinations, disorientation, visual disturbances, euphoria (feeling "high"), dry mouth, constipation, facial flushing, changes in heart rate, palpitations, faintness, urinary difficulties, rash, itching, confusion, rapid breathing, and diarrhea.

Drug Interactions

• Combining Fiorinal with alcohol, tranquilizers, barbiturates, sleeping pills, or other nervous system depressants may cause tiredness, drowsiness, and trouble concentrating.

• Combining Fiorinal with prednisone or other corticosteroids, phenylbutazone, or alcohol may irritate your stomach and increase the risk of developing an ulcer.

• Your anticoagulant (blood thinner) dosage must be changed if you begin taking Fiorinal.

• Fiorinal counteracts the effect of probenecid and sulfinpyrazone on the elimination of uric acid. Fiorinal may counteract the blood-pressure-lowering effects of angiotensin-converting enzyme (ACE) inhibitors and beta blockers.

• Fiorinal may counteract the effects of diuretics in people with severe liver disease.

• Fiorinal may increase methotrexate or valproic acid blood levels and the risk of side effects.

• Combining Fiorinal and nitroglycerin tablets may lead to an unexpected drop in blood pressure.

• Do not take Fiorinal together with an NSAID. There is no benefit to the combination, and the risk of side effects, especially stomach irritation, is vastly increased.

Food Interactions

Fiorinal is best taken on an empty stomach but may be taken with food if it upsets your stomach.

Usual Dose

1–2 tablets or capsules every 4 hours or as needed. Do not exceed 6 doses a day.

Overdosage

Symptoms include breathing difficulties, nervousness progressing to stupor or coma, pinpointed pupils, cold and clammy skin, lowered heart rate or blood pressure, nausea, vomiting, dizziness, ringing in the ears, flushing, sweating, and thirst. Symptoms of mild overdose are rapid and deep breathing, nausea, vomiting, dizziness, ringing or buzzing in the ears, flushing, sweating, thirst, headache, drowsiness, diarrhea, and rapid heartbeat. Severe overdose may cause fever, excitement, confusion, convulsions, liver or kidney failure, coma, and bleeding. Take the victim to a hospital emergency room immediately. ALWAYS bring the prescription bottle or container.

Special Information

Fiorinal may cause drowsiness. Be careful when driving or performing any task that requires concentration.

Call your doctor if you develop any bothersome or persistent side effect.

If you forget a dose, take it as soon as you remember. If it is almost time for your next dose, skip the dose you forgot and continue with your regular schedule. Do not take a double dose.

Special Populations

Pregnancy/Breast-feeding

Fiorinal should be avoided during pregnancy. Pregnant women taking it may experience prolonged labor, delayed delivery, and bleeding problems. Fiorinal increases the risk of birth defects and may cause breathing or bleeding problems in newborns. Regular use of Fiorinal during the last 3 months of pregnancy may also cause drug dependency in the newborn.

Fiorinal passes into breast milk. Breast-feeding while using Fiorinal may cause tiredness, shortness of breath, or slowed heartbeat in the baby. Nursing mothers who must take Fiorinal should consider bottle-feeding.

Seniors

Fiorinal may have a greater depressant effect on seniors. Other side effects that may be more prominent are lightheadedness and dizziness or fainting when rising suddenly from a sitting or lying position.

Brand Name

Fiorinal with Codeine

Generic Ingredients

Aspirin + Butalbital + Caffeine + Codeine Phosphate Ⓖ

Type of Drug

Barbiturate, narcotic, and analgesic (pain reliever) combination.

Prescribed for

Migraine or other pain.

General Information

Fiorinal with Codeine is one of many combination products containing a barbiturate, an analgesic, and a narcotic. In Fiorinal with Codeine, butalbital is the barbiturate, aspirin is the analgesic, and codeine is the narcotic. These products often also contain a tranquilizer, and acetaminophen may be substituted for aspirin.

Cautions and Warnings

Do not take Fiorinal with Codeine if you are **allergic** or **sensitive** to any of its ingredients. Use this drug with extreme caution if you suffer from **asthma or other breathing problems**. Long-term use of this drug may cause drug dependence or **addiction**. Fiorinal with Codeine is a respiratory depressant and affects the central nervous system (CNS), producing **sleepiness, tiredness,** or **inability to concentrate**.

Do not take this drug if you are allergic to aspirin, any salicylate, or any nonsteroidal anti-inflammatory drug (NSAID). This and other aspirin-containing drugs should not be taken by **children under age 16**. People with **liver damage** should avoid this drug.

Alcohol may aggravate the stomach irritation caused by aspirin and increases the risk of aspirin-related ulcer. Alcohol also increases the nervous-system depression caused by codeine and butalbital.

Do not use any aspirin-containing drug if you develop **dizziness, hearing loss,** or **ringing or buzzing in the ears**. Aspirin may interfere with **blood coagulation** (clotting) and should be avoided for 1 week before surgery. Ask your surgeon or dentist for advice before taking an aspirin-containing drug for pain after surgery.

Possible Side Effects

▼ Most common: light-headedness, dizziness, sleepiness, nausea, vomiting, appetite loss, and sweating. If these occur, ask your doctor to consider lowering the dosage. Usually the side effects disappear if you lie down.

▼ Less common: euphoria (feeling "high"), breathing difficulties, weakness, sleepiness, headache, agitation, uncoordinated muscle movement, minor hallucinations, disorientation and visual disturbances, dry mouth, constipation, facial flushing, rapid heartbeat, palpitations, feeling faint, urinary difficulties or hesitancy, reduced sex drive or potency, itching, rash, anemia, lowered blood sugar, and yellowing of the skin or whites of the eyes. Narcotic analgesics may aggravate convulsions in those who have had them.

Drug Interactions

• Interaction with alcohol, tranquilizers, barbiturates, sleeping pills, or other drugs that produce depression may cause tiredness, drowsiness, and trouble concentrating.

• Combining this drug with prednisone or other corticosteroids, alcohol, or phenylbutazone may irritate your stomach.

• Your anticoagulant (blood thinner) dosage must be changed if you begin taking Fiorinal with Codeine.

• This drug counteracts the uric acid-eliminating effects of probenecid and sulfinpyrazone.

• Fiorinal with Codeine may counteract the blood-pressure-lowering effects of angiotensin-converting enzyme (ACE) inhibitor and beta-blocker drugs.

• Fiorinal with Codeine may counteract the effects of diuretics (agents that increase urination) in people with severe liver disease.

• This drug may increase methotrexate or valproic acid blood levels and the risk of side effects.

• Combining Fiorinal with Codeine and nitroglycerin tablets may lead to an unexpected drop in blood pressure.

• Do not take this drug together with any NSAID drug. There is no benefit to the combination and the risk of side effects, especially stomach irritation, is significantly increased.

Food Interactions

Fiorinal with Codeine is best taken on an empty stomach but may be taken with food if it upsets your stomach.

Usual Dose

1–2 tablets or capsules every 4 hours or as needed; do not exceed 6 doses a day.

Overdosage

Usual overdose symptoms include breathing difficulties, nervousness progressing to stupor or coma, pinpointed pupils, cold clammy skin and lowered heart rate or blood pressure, nausea, vomiting, dizziness, ringing in the ears, flushing, sweating, and thirst. Symptoms of mild overdose include rapid and deep breathing, nausea, vomiting, dizziness, ringing or buzzing in the ears, flushing, sweating, thirst, headache, drowsiness, diarrhea, and rapid heartbeat. Severe overdose may cause fever, excitement, confusion, convulsions, liver or kidney failure, coma, or bleeding. Take the victim to a hospital emergency room immediately. ALWAYS bring the prescription bottle or container.

Special Information

This drug may cause drowsiness. Be careful when driving or performing any task that requires concentration.

Call your doctor if you develop any side effects that are bothersome or persistent.

If you forget a dose, take it as soon as you remember. If it is almost time for your next dose, skip the one you forgot and continue with your regular schedule. Do not take a double dose.

Special Populations

Pregnancy/Breast-feeding

Fiorinal with Codeine should not be used during pregnancy. Pregnant women taking it may experience prolonged labor, delayed delivery, and bleeding problems.

This drug increases the risk of birth defects and may cause breathing or bleeding problems in newborns. Regular use of Fiorinal with Codeine during the last 3 months of pregnancy may also cause drug dependency in the newborn.

Fiorinal with Codeine passes into breast milk. Breast-feeding while using this drug may cause tiredness, shortness of breath, or a slow heartbeat in the baby. Nursing mothers who must take this drug should consider bottle-feeding.

Seniors
This drug may have a greater depressant effect on seniors. Other effects that may be more prominent are light-headedness and dizziness or fainting when rising suddenly from a sitting or lying position.

Generic Name

Flecainide (FLEH-kan-ide)

Brand Name
Tambocor

Type of Drug
Antiarrhythmic.

Prescribed for
Abnormal heart rhythm.

General Information
Flecainide is prescribed in situations where the abnormal rhythm is so severe as to be life-threatening and does not respond to other drug treatments. Like other antiarrhythmic drugs, flecainide works by affecting the movement of nervous impulses within the heart. Flecainide's effects may not become apparent for 3 to 4 days after you start taking it.

Cautions and Warnings
As with other antiarrhythmic drugs, there is no proof that flecainide helps people live longer or avoid sudden death. Do not take flecainide if you are **allergic** or **sensitive** to it or if you have **heart block,** unless you have a cardiac pacemaker.

Flecainide causes **new arrhythmias** or worsens already existing ones in 7% of people who take it; this risk increases with certain kinds of underlying heart disease and higher doses of the drug. Flecainide causes or worsens **heart failure** in about 5% of people taking it because it tends to reduce the force and rate of each heartbeat.

Flecainide is extensively broken down in the liver. People with **poor liver function** should not take flecainide unless the benefits clearly outweigh the risks.

Possible Side Effects

▼ Most common: dizziness, fainting, light-headedness, unsteadiness, visual disturbances including blurred vision and seeing spots before the eyes, breathing difficulties, headache, nausea, fatigue, heart palpitations, chest pain, tremors, weakness, constipation, bloating, and abdominal pain.

▼ Less common: new or worsened heart arrhythmias or heart failure, heart block, slowed heart rate, vomiting, diarrhea, upset stomach, loss of appetite, stomach gas, a bad taste in your mouth, dry mouth, tingling in the hands or feet, partial or temporary paralysis, loss of muscle control, flushing, sweating, ringing or buzzing in the ears, anxiety, sleeplessness, depression, not feeling well, twitching, weakness, convulsions, speech disorders, stupor, memory loss, personality loss, nightmares, apathy, eye pain, unusual sensitivity to bright light, sagging eyelids, reduced white-blood-cell or blood-platelet counts, impotence, reduced sex drive, frequent urination, urinary difficulty, itching, rash, fever, muscle ache, closing of the throat, and swollen lips, tongue, or mouth.

Drug Interactions

• The combination of propranolol and flecainide may cause an exaggerated lowering in heart rate. Other drugs that slow the heart may also interact with flecainide to produce an excessive slowing of heart rate.

• Avoid megadoses of vitamin C while taking this drug.

• The amount of flecainide in your blood and its effect on your heart may be increased if it is taken together with amiodarone, cimetidine, disopyramide, or verapamil.

• Smokers may need a larger dose of flecainide than nonsmokers.

• Flecainide may increase the amount of digoxin in the bloodstream, increasing the chance of side effects.

Food Interactions

None known.

Usual Dose

Starting dose—50–100 mg every 12 hours. Maximum dosage is 600 mg a day.

Overdosage

Flecainide overdose affects heart function, causing slower heart rate, low blood pressure, and possible death from respiratory failure. Victims of flecainide overdose should be taken to a hospital emergency room for treatment. ALWAYS bring the prescription bottle or container.

Special Information

Flecainide can make you dizzy, light-headed, or disoriented. Take care while driving or performing complex tasks.

Call your doctor if you develop chest pains, an abnormal heartbeat, breathing difficulties, bloating in your feet or legs, tremors, fever, chills, sore throat, unusual bleeding or bruising, yellowing of the whites of your eyes, or any other intolerable side effect.

If you forget to take a dose of flecainide and remember within 6 hours, take it as soon as possible. If you do not remember until later, skip the dose you forgot and continue with your regular schedule. Do not take a double dose.

Special Populations

Pregnancy/Breast-feeding

At high doses, flecainide damages an animal fetus. When this drug is considered crucial by your doctor, its potential benefits must be weighed against its risks.

Flecainide passes into breast milk. Nursing mothers who must take this drug should bottle-feed.

Seniors

Seniors with reduced kidney or liver function are more likely to develop side effects and require a lower dosage.

Flonase *see Corticosteroids, Nasal, page 274*

Flovent *see Corticosteroids, Inhalers, page 270*

Generic Name

Fluconazole (flue-KON-uh-zole)

Brand Name

Diflucan

Type of Drug

Antifungal.

Prescribed for

Infections of the blood, mouth, throat, vagina, or central nervous system due to *Candida, aspergillus,* or *cryptococcus.*

General Information

Fluconazole is effective against a variety of fungal organisms. It works by inhibiting important enzyme systems in the organisms it attacks. Fluconazole can be used to treat opportunistic fungal infections that afflict many people with AIDS.

Cautions and Warnings

Do not take fluconazole if you are **allergic** to it. People who are allergic to similar antifungals—ketoconazole, miconazole, and itraconazole—may also be allergic to fluconazole, but cross-reactions are not common and serious allergic reaction is rare.

Rarely, fluconazole causes **liver damage**. The drug should be used with caution in people with preexisting liver disease.

Rash may be an important sign of drug toxicity, especially in people with acquired immunodeficiency syndrome (AIDS) or others with compromised immune function. Report any rashes, especially ones that do not heal readily, to your doctor.

Possible Side Effects

Side effects are generally more common among AIDS patients.

▼ Most common: nausea, headache, rash, vomiting, abdominal pain, and diarrhea.

▼ Less common: liver toxicity, as measured by increases in specific lab tests. These changes in lab values are more common in people with AIDS or cancer, who are more likely to be taking several drugs, some of which may also be toxic to the liver; these include rifampin, phenytoin, isoniazid, valproic acid, and oral antidiabetes agents.

▼ Rare: People with AIDS or cancer who take fluconazole for fungal infections rarely develop severe liver or skin problems.

Drug Interactions

• Cimetidine and rifampin may reduce blood levels of fluconazole, but the importance of these interactions is not known.

• Fluconazole may increase the amount of the oral antidiabetes drugs tolbutamide, glyburide, and glipizide in the blood, causing low blood-sugar. Cyclosporine, phenytoin, theophylline, warfarin, and zidovudine (an AIDS drug—also known as AZT) are similarly affected. Dosage adjustments of these drugs may be required.

• Fluconazole may interfere with oral contraceptive drugs. Use special precautions.

• Hydrochlorothiazide may increase blood levels of fluconazole up to 40%.

Food Interactions

None known.

Usual Dose

Adult and Child (age 14 and over): 100–400 mg once a day.

Child: 1.3–5.5 mg per lb. of body weight once a day; no more than 400 mg a day.

Overdosage

Symptoms of a very large overdose may include breathing difficulties, lethargy, excess tearing, droopy eyelids, excess salivation, loss of bladder control, convulsions, and blue discoloration of the skin under the nails. Overdose victims should be taken to a hospital emergency room for treatment. ALWAYS bring the prescription bottle or container.

Special Information

Regular doctor visits are necessary to monitor liver function and general progress.

Call your doctor if you develop reddening, loosening, blistering, or peeling of the skin; darkening of the urine; yellowing of the skin or whites of the eyes; loss of appetite; or abdominal pain, especially on the right side. Report other symptoms that are bothersome or persistent.

If you forget a dose of fluconazole, take it as soon as you remember. If it is almost time for your next dose, skip the one you forgot and continue with your regular schedule. Do not take a double dose. .

Special Populations

Pregnancy/Breast-feeding

Animal studies of fluconazole show effects on the fetus that have not been seen in humans. Pregnant women should not use fluconazole unless the possible benefits outweigh the risks.

Fluconazole passes into breast milk. Nursing mothers who must take this drug should bottle-feed.

Seniors

Seniors may require a reduced dosage due to loss of kidney function.

Generic Name

Flucytosine (floo-SYE-toe-sene)

Brand Name

Ancobon

Type of Drug

Antifungal.

Prescribed for

Serious blood-borne fungal infections.

General Information

Flucytosine is meant for fungal infections—*Candida, chromomycoses,* and *cryptococcus*—carried in the blood that affect the urinary tract, respiratory tract, central nervous system, heart, and other organs. It is not meant for fungal infections of the skin, such as common athlete's foot.

Cautions and Warnings

Do not take this drug if you are **allergic** to it. Flucytosine can worsen **bone-marrow depression** in people whose immune systems are already compromised. Liver and kidney function and blood composition should be monitored while you are taking this drug.

People with **kidney disease** must be closely monitored by their doctors and should take this medication with extreme caution; daily dosage must be reduced.

Possible Side Effects

▼ Most common: unusual tiredness or weakness, liver inflammation, yellowing of the eyes or skin, abdominal pain, diarrhea, loss of appetite, nausea, vomiting, rash, redness, itching, sore throat, fever, and unusual bleeding or bruising.

▼ Less common: chest pains, breathing difficulties, sensitivity to the sun or bright light, dry mouth, duodenal ulcers, severe bowel irritation, stomach bleeding, interference with kidney function, kidney failure, reduced red- and white-blood-cell counts or other changes in blood composition, headache, hearing loss, confusion, dizziness, weakness, shaking, sedation or tiredness, psychosis, hallucinations, heart attack, and low blood-sugar and potassium levels.

Drug Interactions

• Amphotericin B increases flucytosine's effectiveness; this combination is generally used to produce better results.

• Flucytosine may interfere with some routine blood tests.

Food Interactions

Take flucytosine with food if it upsets your stomach.

Usual Dose

22–66 mg per lb. a day, in divided doses.

Overdosage

Little is known about the effects of flucytosine overdose, but it may cause exaggerated drug side effects.

Special Information

Take the capsules a few at a time over 15 minutes to avoid nausea and vomiting.

Call your doctor if you develop unusual tiredness or weakness; yellowing of the skin or whites of the eyes; rash, redness, or itching; sore throat or fever; unusual bleeding or bruising; or any persistent or intolerable side effect.

Maintain good dental hygiene while taking flucytosine. Use extra care when using your toothbrush or dental floss because of the risk that flucytosine will make you more susceptible to infection. Dental work should be completed prior to starting on this drug.

If you forget a dose, take it as soon as you remember. If it is almost time for your next dose, take 1 dose right away and another in 3 or 4 hours, then go back to your regular schedule. Do not take a double dose.

Special Populations

Pregnancy/Breast-feeding

Flucytosine causes birth defects in animals and crosses the placenta. Flucytosine should be used by pregnant women only when its potential benefits clearly outweigh its risks.

It is not known if flucytosine passes into breast milk. Nursing mothers who must take this drug should bottle-feed.

Seniors

Dosage adjustment may be required due to loss of kidney function.

Type of Drug

Fluoroquinolone Anti-Infectives

(flor-oe-QUIN-oe-lone)

Brand Names

Generic Ingredient: Ciprofloxacin G
Ciloxan   Cipro

Generic Ingredient: Enoxacin
Penetrex

Generic Ingredient: Gatifloxacin
Tequin

Generic Ingredient: Levofloxacin
Levaquin

Generic Ingredient: Lomefloxacin
Maxaquin

Generic Ingredient: Moxifloxacin
Avelox

Generic Ingredient: Norfloxacin
Chibroxin   Noroxin

Generic Ingredient: Ofloxacin
Floxin

Generic Ingredient: Sparfloxacin
Zagam

Generic Ingredient: Trovafloxacin
Trovan

Prescribed for

Infections of the lower respiratory system, sinuses, urinary tract, skin, bone and joints, lungs, and prostate; also prescribed for sexually transmitted diseases, prostatitis, infectious diarrhea, bronchitis, pneumonia, and traveler's diarrhea. The eyedrops are used to treat ocular infections.

General Information

Fluoroquinolone anti-infectives work against many organisms that traditional antibiotics have trouble killing. They do not work against the common cold, flu, or other viral infections. These medications are chemically related to an older antibacterial called nalidixic acid but work better than 'that drug against urinary infections. Some fluoroquinolone drugs such as ciprofloxacin are used to treat a variety of infections all over the body. Others are used for more specific purposes.

Cautions and Warnings

Do not take a fluoroquinolone if you are **allergic** to any drug in this group or have had a reaction to related medications like nalidixic acid. Severe, possibly fatal, allergic reactions can occur even after the very first dose. These reactions include cardiovascular collapse, loss of consciousness, tingling, swelling of the face or throat, breathing difficulties, itching, and rash. Stop taking the drug if this happens and seek medical help at once.

Fluoroquinolones may cause increased pressure on parts of the brain, leading to **convulsions** and **psychotic reactions**. Other possible effects include **tremors, restlessness, lightheadedness, confusion,** and **hallucinations**. Fluoroquinolones should be used with caution in people with **head trauma, seizure disorders,** or other nervous system conditions.

Moxifloxacin should not be used by people with **liver disease**. It and gatifloxacin should be avoided by people with **heart rhythm problems** or those taking drugs that can affect heart rhythm. Dosage of trovafloxacin must be reduced in people with **chronic liver disease**. People taking trovafloxacin have developed **severe liver damage or liver failure leading to death**. Trovafloxacin should be reserved for treating severe infections when other drugs have failed.

People with **kidney disease** require reduced dosage of these drugs, except in the case of trovafloxacin and moxifloxacin.

People taking fluoroquinolones may be unusually **sensitive to the sun**. Avoid the sun while taking this drug and for several days following therapy, EVEN IF YOU ARE USING SUNSCREEN.

People taking a fluoroquinolone may develop **colitis** that could range from mild to very serious. Contact your doctor if you develop diarrhea or cramps.

Prolonged fluoroquinolone use can lead to **fungal overgrowth**. Follow your doctor's directions exactly.

Possible Side Effects

Side effects are rarely serious.

▼ Most common: nausea (most likely with ciprofloxacin), vomiting (most likely with enoxacin), and diarrhea (may be most likely with ofloxacin).

▼ Less common: dizziness, vomiting, abdominal pain, headache, and liver inflammation. Taking trovafloxacin-alatrofloxacin for more than 2 weeks increases the risk of serious liver injury.

▼ Rare: Rare side effects can occur in almost any part of the body. Contact your doctor if you experience any side effect not listed above.

Drug Interactions

• Separate your fluoroquinolone dose from that of antacids, didanosine, iron supplements, sucralfate, or zinc by at least 2 hours. These drugs decrease the amount of fluoroquinolone absorbed. Moxifloxacin must be taken 4 hours before or 8 hours after antacids, iron, or zinc.

• Probenecid may increase the risk of fluoroquinolone side effects (excepting moxifloxacin). Cimetidine may also increase fluoroquinolone blood levels (excepting gatifloxacin).

• Fluoroquinolones (excepting moxifloxacin and gatifloxacin) may increase the effect of oral anticoagulant drugs such as warfarin. Your anticoagulant dosage may have to be reduced.

• Fluoroquinolones may increase the toxic effects of cyclosporine (used for organ transplants) on your kidneys.

• Fluoroquinolones (excepting moxifloxacin and gatifloxacin) may increase theophylline blood levels and the risk of side effects.

• Azlocillin may increase the risk of ciprofloxacin side effects.

• Ciprofloxacin, enoxacin, and norfloxacin may increase caffeine's effects.

• Anticancer drugs may decrease fluoroquinolone blood levels.

• Nitrofurantoin may antagonize norfloxacin's antibacterial effects. Do not take these drugs together.

• Ciprofloxacin may reduce blood levels of phenytoin (an antiseizure drug), requiring alteration of your daily dosage.

• Fluoroquinolones may reduce blood levels of sulfony-lurea antidiabetes drugs, though dosage adjustments are unnecessary.

• Moxifloxacin and gatifloxacin can increase the effects of other drugs that also affect heart rhythm. Do not combine moxifloxacin or gatifloxacin with any of these drugs, which include cisapride, erythromycin, tricylic antidepressants, and antipsychotic drugs.

Food Interactions

Gatifloxacin, levofloxacin, lomefloxacin, moxifloxacin, and sparfloxacin may be taken with or without food. Take enoxacin, ofloxacin, norfloxacin, and trovafloxacin at least 2 hours before or 2 hours after meals or antacids. Ciprofloxacin is best taken 1 hour before or 2 hours after meals, but may be taken with food. Dairy products inter-fere with the absorption of ciprofloxacin and should be avoided.

Usual Dose

Tablets (Adults, age 18 and over; not recommended for use in children)
Ciprofloxacin: 250–750 mg twice a day.
   Enoxacin: 200–400 mg every 12 hours; a single dose of 400 mg may be taken for gonorrhea.
   Gatifloxacin: 400 mg a day.
   Levofloxacin: 250–500 mg once a day.
   Lomefloxacin: 400 mg a day.
   Moxifloxacin: 400 mg a day.
   Norfloxacin: 400 mg every 12 hours; a single dose of 800 mg may be taken for gonorrhea.
   Ofloxacin: 200–400 mg every 12 hours.
   Sparfloxacin: two 200-mg tablets on the first day, then one 200-mg tablet a day.
   Trovafloxacin: 100–200 mg once a day for up to 28 days.

Dosage of most fluoroquinolones must be reduced in the presence of kidney failure. In the case of trovafloxacin-ala-trofloxacin, dosage adjustment is unnecessary.

Eyedrops
Ciprofloxacin or norfloxacin: 1–2 drops in the affected eye several times a day.

Overdosage

Symptoms generally include drug side effects. Overdose may cause kidney failure and, in the case of moxifloxacin, abnormal heart rhythms. Call your local poison control center or a hospital emergency room for more information. You may be told to induce vomiting with ipecac syrup—available at any pharmacy—before taking the victim to an emergency room. If you seek treatment, ALWAYS bring the prescription bottle or container.

Special Information

Take each dose with a full glass of water. Be sure to drink at least 8 glasses of water a day while taking this drug to help avoid side effects.

If you are taking an antacid, didanosine, sucralfate, or an iron or zinc supplement while taking a fluoroquinolone, separate the doses by at least 4 hours to avoid a drug interaction. Moxifloxacin must be taken 4 hours before or 8 hours after antacids, iron, or zinc.

Drug sensitivity reactions can develop even after only 1 dose. Stop taking the drug and get immediate medical attention if you feel faint or develop itching, rash, facial swelling, breathing difficulties, convulsions, depression, visual disturbances, dizziness, headache, light-headedness, or any sign of a drug reaction.

Colitis can be caused by any anti-infective medication. If diarrhea develops, call your doctor at once.

Avoid excessive sunlight. Call your doctor if you become sensitive to the sun.

Follow your doctor's directions exactly. Complete the full course of drug therapy, even if you feel well.

To avoid infection, do not let the eyedropper tip touch your finger, eyelid, or any surface. Wait 5 minutes before using another eyedrop or eye ointment.

Call your doctor at once if your vision declines or if eye stinging, itching or burning, redness, irritation, swelling, or pain worsens.

Fluoroquinolones can cause changes in vision, dizziness, drowsiness, and light-headedness. Be careful when driving or performing any task that requires concentration.

If you forget to administer a dose, do so as soon as you remember. If it is almost time for your next dose, skip the missed dose and continue with your regular schedule. Do not take a double dose.

Special Populations

Pregnancy/Breast-feeding

Animal studies have shown that fluoroquinolones may damage the fetus or reduce the likelihood of a successful pregnancy. When a fluoroquinolone is considered crucial by your doctor, its potential benefits must be carefully weighed against its risks.

Fluoroquinolones pass into breast milk. Nursing mothers who must take them should bottle-feed.

Seniors

With the exception of moxifloxacin and gatifloxacin, seniors may require reduced dosage due to decreases in kidney function. In the case of eyedrops, seniors may also need less medication.

Generic Name

Fluoxetine (flue-OX-eh-tene)

Brand Name

Prozac

Type of Drug

Selective serotonin reuptake inhibitor (SSRI).

Prescribed for

Depression, bulimic binge-eating and vomiting, and obsessive-compulsive disorder (OCD); also prescribed for obesity, alcoholism, anorexia, attention-deficit hyperactivity disorder (ADHD), bipolar affective disorder, borderline personality disorder, cataplexy and narcolepsy, kleptomania, migraine, chronic daily headache, tension headaches, post-traumatic stress disorder, schizophrenia, Tourette's syndrome, dyskinetic side effects of levodopa, and social phobias.

General Information

Fluoxetine and other SSRIs, which are chemically unrelated to the older tricyclic and tetracyclic antidepressant drugs, work by preventing the movement of the neurohormone serotonin into nerve endings. This forces serotonin to remain in the spaces surrounding nerve endings, where it works. Fluoxetine is effective in treating common symptoms of depression. It can help improve mood and mental alertness, increase physical activity, and improve sleep patterns. Fluoxetine takes about 4 weeks to work and stays in the body for several weeks after you stop taking it. This may be important as your doctor considers when to start or stop treatment.

Cautions and Warnings

Do not take fluoxetine if you are **allergic** to it or other SSRIs. Some people have experienced serious **drug reactions** to fluoxetine.

Serious, **potentially fatal reactions** may occur if fluoxetine and a **monoamine oxidase inhibitor (MAOI)** antidepressant are taken together (see "Drug Interactions").

About 1 in 25 people taking fluoxetine develop an **itchy rash,** ⅓ of whom have to stop taking the medication. Other symptoms associated with the rash are fever, joint pain, swelling, wrist and hand pain, breathing difficulties, swollen lymph glands, and laboratory abnormalities. In most people, these symptoms go away when they stop taking fluoxetine and receive antihistamine or corticosteroid treatments.

People with severe **liver or kidney disease** should be cautious about taking fluoxetine and should be treated at below-normal doses.

As many as ⅓ of people taking an SSRI experience **anxiety, sleeplessness,** and **nervousness.**

Underweight depressed people who take fluoxetine may lose more weight. About 9% of people taking fluoxetine experience appetite loss, while 13% lose more than 5% of their body weight.

SSRIs may affect **blood platelets,** though their exact effect is not known. Some people have had abnormal bleeding while taking these drugs.

Less than 2 in 1000 people taking fluoxetine experience **seizures** or **convulsions.** This effect is similar to that seen with other antidepressants.

The possibility of **suicide** exists in severely depressed patients and may be present until the condition is significantly improved. Severely depressed people should be

allowed to carry only small quantities of fluoxetine to limit
the risk of overdose.

Possible Side Effects

▼ Most common: headache, anxiety, nervousness,
sleeplessness, drowsiness, tiredness, weakness,
tremors, sweating, dizziness, light-headedness, dry
mouth, upset or irritated stomach, appetite loss, nausea,
vomiting, diarrhea, gas, rash, and itching.

▼ Less common: changes in sex drive, abnormal ejaculation, impotence, abnormal dreams, difficulty concentrating, increased appetite, acne, hair loss, dry skin, chest
pain, allergy, runny nose, bronchitis, abnormal heart
rhythms, bleeding, blood pressure changes, dizziness or
fainting when rising suddenly from a sitting position,
bone pain, bursitis, twitching, breast pain, fibrocystic disease of the breast, cystitis, urinary pain, double vision,
eye or ear pain, conjunctivitis, anemia, swelling, low
blood sugar, and low thyroid activity.

▼ Rare: Rare side effects can occur in almost any part
of the body. Contact your doctor if you experience any
side effect not listed above.

Drug Interactions

• At least 5 weeks should elapse between stopping fluoxetine and starting an MAOI antidepressant. Two weeks should
elapse between stopping an MAOI and starting fluoxetine.
Taking these drugs too close together or at the same time
may cause serious, life-threatening reactions.

• Fluoxetine blood levels may be increased if the drug is
taken with a tricyclic antidepressant.

• Fluoxetine may increase lithium's side effects. Your
lithium dosage may need to be adjusted.

• Cyproheptadine (an antihistamine) may reverse the
effects of fluoxetine.

• Hallucinations have occurred after combining fluoxetine
with dextromethorphan (the most common cough suppressant in over-the-counter products).

• Combining fluoxetine with phenytoin can lead to possible side effects.

• Fluoxetine can raise blood levels of the antipsychotic drugs clozapine (for schizophrenia), haloperidol, and pimozide; and of cyclosporine (an immune suppressant used in organ transplants).

• People who combine l-tryptophan and fluoxetine may become agitated, restless, and have an upset stomach.

• Alcohol may increase tiredness and other depressant effects of fluoxetine.

• Fluoxetine may reduce the effectiveness of buspirone, which has led to a worsening of OCD in people taking this combination to treat OCD.

• Fluoxetine may increase the risk of carbamazepine side effects.

• Fluoxetine may increase the effect of benzodiazepine antianxiety drugs.

• People taking warfarin and fluoxetine may experience increased bleeding, although without testing differently for prothrombin time (a rate used to measure bleeding tendency).

Food Interactions

This drug may be taken without regard to food or meals.

Usual Dose

20–80 mg a day. Seniors, people with kidney or liver disease, and people taking several different drugs may need a lower dosage.

Overdosage

Overdose symptoms may include seizures, nausea, vomiting, agitation, restlessness, and nervous system excitation. Any person suspected of having taken a fluoxetine overdose should be taken to a hospital emergency room at once. ALWAYS bring the prescription bottle or container.

Special Information

Fluoxetine can make you dizzy or drowsy. Take care when driving or performing other tasks that require alertness and concentration. Avoid alcohol.

Be sure your doctor knows if you are pregnant, breast-feeding, or taking other drugs, including OTC drugs, while taking fluoxetine.

Call your doctor if you develop rash or hives, become excessively nervous or anxious, lose your appetite—especially if you are already underweight—or experience any unusual side effects.

If you forget a dose, take it as soon as you remember. If it is almost time for your next dose, skip the dose you forgot and continue with your regular schedule. Do not take a double dose.

Special Populations

Pregnancy/Breast-feeding

In one study, approximately 5% of women who took fluoxetine during pregnancy had babies with major abnormalities. In addition, women taking this drug were more likely to deliver prematurely. Do not take fluoxetine if you are or might be pregnant without first seeing your doctor and weighing its potential benefits against its risks.

Fluoxetine passes into breast milk. Nursing mothers who must take this drug should consider bottle-feeding.

Seniors

Seniors with liver or kidney disease must receive a lower dose.

Generic Name

Fluoxymesterone (flue-OX-ee-MES-ter-one) [G]

Brand Name

Halotestin

Type of Drug

Androgen (male hormone).

Prescribed for

Men: hormone replacement or augmentation and male menopause; also prescribed as male contraception for up to 12 months.

Women: breast pain and fullness in women who have given birth, and inoperable breast cancer.

General Information

Fluoxymesterone is an androgen. Androgens are responsible for the normal growth and development of male sex organs and for maintaining secondary sex characteristics including hair distribution, vocal cord thickening, muscle development, and fat distribution.

Cautions and Warnings

Androgens do not improve athletic performance.

Women taking any androgen may develop **deepening of the voice, oily skin, acne, hairiness, increased sex drive,** and **menstrual irregularities**. Androgens should be avoided if possible by young boys who have not gone through puberty.

Fluoxymesterone worsens **gynecomastia** (a condition characterized by swollen male breast tissue).

Men with unusually **high blood levels of calcium,** known or suspected **prostate cancer** or **prostate destruction,** or **breast cancer** should not use fluoxymesterone, nor should anyone with severe **liver, heart, or kidney disease**.

Long-term, high-dose androgen therapy may cause severe **liver disease,** including hepatitis and cancer, **reduced sperm count,** and water retention. **Blood cholesterol** may be raised by androgens. This can be a problem for people who have heart disease.

Possible Side Effects

Men

▼ Most common: inhibition of testicle function, impotence, chronic erection, and painful enlargement of breast tissue.

Women

▼ Most common: unusual hairiness, male pattern baldness, deepening of the voice, and enlargement of the clitoris. These changes are usually IRREVERSIBLE once they occur. Increased blood calcium and menstrual irregularities may also develop.

Men and Women

▼ Most common: changes in sex drive, headache, anxiety, depression, a tingling feeling, sleep apnea (condition characterized by intermittent cessation of breathing during sleep), flushing, rash, acne, habituation (the drug may be habit forming), excitation, chills, sleeplessness,

> **Possible Side Effects** *(continued)*
>
> water retention, nausea, vomiting, diarrhea, hepatitis (symptoms include yellowing of the skin or whites of the eyes), liver inflammation, and liver cancer. Symptoms resembling those of a stomach ulcer may also develop.

Drug Interactions

• Fluoxymesterone may increase the effect of an oral anticoagulant (blood thinner); dosage of the anticoagulant may have to be reduced. It may also have an effect on the glucose-tolerance test, a blood test used to screen for diabetes. Androgens may interfere with tests of thyroid function.

• Combining an androgen and imipramine or another tricyclic antidepressant may result in a severe paranoid reaction.

Food Interactions

Take fluoxymesterone with meals if it upsets your stomach.

Usual Dose

2.5–40 mg a day.

Overdosage

Symptoms include nausea, vomiting, and diarrhea. Call your local poison control center or a hospital emergency room for more information. If you seek treatment, ALWAYS bring the prescription bottle or container.

Special Information

Androgens must be taken only under the close supervision of your doctor. The dosage and clinical effects of fluoxymesterone vary widely and require constant monitoring.

Call your doctor if you develop nausea or vomiting, swelling of the legs or feet, yellowing of the skin or whites of the eyes, or a painful or persistent erection. Women should call their doctors immediately if they develop a deep or hoarse voice, acne, hairiness, male pattern baldness, or menstrual irregularities.

If you forget a dose, take it as soon as you remember. If it is almost time for your next dose, skip the one you forgot and continue with your regular schedule. Do not take a double dose.

Special Populations

Pregnancy/Breast-feeding
Fluoxymesterone should never be taken by pregnant or nursing women because it can affect the developing fetus and nursing infant:

Seniors
Seniors are more likely to develop prostate enlargement or prostate cancer. A marked increase in sex drive may also occur.

Generic Name

Flurazepam (fluh-RAZ-uh-pam) G

Brand Name
Dalmane

Type of Drug
Benzodiazepine sedative.

Prescribed for
Insomnia and sleep disturbances.

General Information
Flurazepam is a member of the group of drugs known as benzodiazepines. Benzodiazepines work by a direct effect on the brain. They make it easier to go to sleep and decrease the number of times you wake up during the night. Flurazepam and quazepam remain in your bloodstream longer than other drugs in this class, thus resulting in the greatest incidence of morning "hangover."

Cautions and Warnings
People with **kidney or liver disease** should be carefully monitored while taking flurazepam. Take the lowest possible dose to help you sleep.

People with **respiratory disease** may experience **sleep apnea** (intermittent cessation of breathing during sleep) while taking flurazepam.

Clinical **depression** may be increased by flurazepam, which can depress the nervous system. Intentional overdose is more common among depressed people who take sleeping pills than among those who do not.

All benzodiazepines can be **addictive** if taken for long periods of time and can cause drug withdrawal symptoms if discontinued suddenly. Withdrawal symptoms include tremors, muscle cramps, insomnia, agitation, diarrhea, vomiting, sweating, and convulsions.

Possible Side Effects

▼ Common: drowsiness, headache, dizziness, talkativeness, nervousness, apprehension, poor muscle coordination, light-headedness, daytime tiredness, muscle weakness, slowness of movement, hangover, and euphoria (feeling high).

▼ Less common: nausea, vomiting, rapid heartbeat, confusion, temporary memory loss, upset stomach, stomach cramps and pain, depression, blurred or double vision and other visual disturbances, constipation, changes in sense of taste, appetite changes, stuffy nose, nosebleeds, common cold symptoms, asthma, sore throat, cough, breathing difficulties, diarrhea, dry mouth, allergic reaction, fainting, abnormal heart rhythm, itching, rash, acne, dry skin, sensitivity to the sun, nightmares or strange dreams, sleeplessness, tingling in the hands or feet, ringing or buzzing in the ears, ear or eye pain, menstrual cramps, frequent urination and other urinary difficulties, blood in the urine, discharge from the penis or vagina, lower back and other pain, muscle spasms and pain, fever, swollen breasts, and weight changes.

▼ Rare: Rare side effects can affect your heart, stomach and intestines, urinary tract, blood, muscles and joints. Contact your doctor if you experience any side effect not listed above.

Drug Interactions

• As with all benzodiazepines, the effects of flurazepam are enhanced if it is taken with an alcoholic beverage, antihistamine, tranquilizer, barbiturate, anticonvulsant medication, antidepressant, or monoamine oxidase inhibitor (MAOI).

• Oral contraceptives, cimetidine, disulfiram, and isoniazid may increase the effect of flurazepam by reducing the drug's breakdown in the liver. Probenecid also increases flurazepam's effects.

• Cigarette smoking, rifampin, and theophylline may reduce the effect of flurazepam on your body by increasing the rate at which it is broken down by the liver.

• Levodopa's effectiveness may be decreased by flurazepam.

• Flurazepam may increase the amount of zidovudine (an AIDS drug—also known as AZT), phenytoin, or digoxin in your bloodstream, increasing the chances of side effects.

• Mixing clozapine with a benzodiazepine has led to respiratory collapse in a few people. Flurazepam should be stopped at least 1 week before starting clozapine treatment.

Food Interactions

Flurazepam may be taken with food if it upsets your stomach.

Usual Dose

Adult and Child (age 15 and over): 15–30 mg at bedtime. Dosage must be individualized for maximum benefit.

Senior: starting dose—15 mg at bedtime.

Child (under age 15): not recommended.

Overdosage

The most common overdose symptoms are confusion, sleepiness, depression, loss of muscle coordination, and slurred speech. Coma may also occur. Patients who overdose on this drug must be made to vomit with ipecac syrup—available at any pharmacy—to remove any remaining drug from the stomach: Call your doctor or a poison control center before doing this. If 30 minutes have passed since the overdose was taken or if symptoms have begun to develop, take the victim immediately to a hospital emergency room for treatment. ALWAYS bring the prescription bottle or container.

Special Information

Never take more flurazepam than your doctor has prescribed.

Avoid alcoholic beverages and other nervous system depressants while taking flurazepam.

Exercise caution while performing tasks that require concentration and coordination. Flurazepam may make you tired, dizzy, or light-headed.

If you take flurazepam daily for 3 or more weeks, you may experience some withdrawal symptoms when you stop taking the drug.

If you forget a dose and remember within 1 hour, take it as soon as you remember. If you do not remember until later, skip the dose you forgot and go back to your regular schedule. Do not take a double dose.

Special Populations

Pregnancy/Breast-feeding
Flurazepam absolutely should not be used by pregnant women or by women who may become pregnant.

Flurazepam passes into breast milk. The drug should not be taken by nursing mothers.

Seniors
Seniors are more susceptible to the effects of flurazepam.

Generic Name

Flurbiprofen (flur-bih-PROE-fen) G

Brand Names

Ansaid   Ocufen

Type of Drug

Nonsteroidal anti-inflammatory drug (NSAID).

Prescribed for

Rheumatoid arthritis, osteoarthritis, ankylosing spondylitis, mild to moderate pain, menstrual pain, tendinitis, bursitis, painful shoulder, gout, sunburn, and migraine headache. Flurbiprofen eyedrops are used to prevent movement of the eye muscles during eye surgery.

General Information

Flurbiprofen sodium and other NSAIDs are used to relieve pain and inflammation. We do not know exactly how NSAIDs work, but they may achieve their effects by blocking the body's production of a hormone called prostaglandin and the action of other body chemicals. Pain relief comes within 1 hour after taking the first dose of flurbiprofen, but its anti-inflammatory effect generally takes several days to 2 weeks to become apparent and may take a month or more to reach maximum effect. Flurbiprofen is broken down in the liver and eliminated through the kidneys.

Cautions and Warnings

People **allergic** to flurbiprofen or any other NSAID and those with a history of **asthma** attacks brought on by an NSAID, iodides, or aspirin should not take flurbiprofen.

Flurbiprofen may cause **gastrointestinal (GI) bleeding, ulcers,** and **stomach perforation**. This can occur at any time, with or without warning, in people who take flurbiprofen regularly. People with a history of active GI bleeding should be cautious about taking any NSAID. People who develop bleeding or ulcers and continue NSAID treatment should be aware of the possibility of developing more serious side effects.

Flurbiprofen may affect platelets and **blood clotting** at high doses, and should be avoided by people with clotting problems and those taking warfarin.

People with **heart problems** who use flurbiprofen may experience swelling in their arms, legs, or feet.

Flurbiprofen may cause toxic effects to the **kidneys**. Report any unusual side effects to your doctor, who might need to periodically test your kidney function.

Flurbiprofen may make you **unusually sensitive to the effects of the sun**.

Possible Side Effects

Tablets

▼ Most common: diarrhea, nausea, vomiting, constipation, stomach gas, stomach upset or irritation, and appetite loss, especially during the first few days of treatment.

▼ Less common: stomach ulcers, GI bleeding, hepatitis, gallbladder attacks, painful urination, poor kidney function, kidney inflammation, blood and protein in the urine, dizziness, fainting, nervousness, depression, hallucinations, confusion, disorientation, tingling in the hands or feet, light-headedness, itching, increased sweating, dry nose and mouth, heart palpitations, chest pain, breathing difficulties, and muscle cramps.

▼ Rare: severe allergic reactions including closing of the throat, fever and chills, changes in liver function, jaundice (yellowing of the skin or whites of the eyes), and kidney failure. People who experience such effects must be promptly treated in a hospital emergency room or doctor's office. NSAIDs have caused severe skin reactions; if this happens, see your doctor immediately.

Eyedrops
▼ Most common: temporary burning, stinging, or other minor eye irritation.
▼ Less common: nausea, vomiting, viral infections, and eye allergies including redness, burning, itching, or tearing. The risk of developing bleeding problems or other systemic (whole-body) side effects with flurbiprofen eyedrops is low because only a small amount of the drug is absorbed into the bloodstream.

Drug Interactions

Tablets
• Flurbiprofen may increase the effects of oral anticoagulant (blood-thinning) drugs such as warfarin. Your anticoagulant dose may need to be reduced.
• Combining flurbiprofen with cyclosporine may increase the kidney-related side effects of both drugs. Methotrexate side effects may be increased in people also taking flurbiprofen.
• Flurbiprofen may reduce the blood-pressure-lowering effect of beta blockers and loop diuretics.
• Flurbiprofen may increase phenytoin side effects. Lithium blood levels may be increased by flurbiprofen.
• Flurbiprofen blood levels may be affected by cimetidine.
• Probenecid may increase the risk of flurbiprofen side effects.
• Aspirin and other salicylates should never be combined with flurbiprofen.

Eyedrops
• Flurbiprofen eyedrops may inactivate acetylcholine or carbachol eyedrops.

Food Interactions

Take flurbiprofen with food or a magnesium-aluminum antacid if it upsets your stomach.

Usual Dose

Tablets: 200–300 mg a day. Seniors and people with kidney problems should start with a lower dose.

Eyedrops: 1 drop every ½ hour for 2 hours before eye surgery.

Overdosage

Common signs of overdose are drowsiness, nausea, vomiting, diarrhea, abdominal pain, rapid breathing, rapid heartbeat, increased sweating, ringing or buzzing in the ears, confusion, disorientation, stupor, and coma. Take the victim to a hospital emergency room at once. ALWAYS bring the prescription bottle or container.

Special Information

Tablets: Take each dose with a full glass of water and do not lie down for 15 to 30 minutes afterward.

Flurbiprofen can make you drowsy or tired: Be careful when driving or operating hazardous equipment. Do not take any over-the-counter products containing acetaminophen or aspirin while taking flurbiprofen. Avoid alcoholic beverages.

Contact your doctor if you develop rash or itching, visual disturbances, weight gain, breathing difficulties, fluid retention, hallucinations, black or tarry stools, persistent headache, or any unusual or intolerable side effect.

If you forget a dose of oral flurbiprofen, take it as soon as you remember. If you take flurbiprofen once a day and it is within 8 hours of your next dose, of if you take several doses a day and it is within 4 hours of your next dose, skip the dose you forgot and continue with your regular schedule. Never take a double dose.

Eyedrops: To prevent possible infection, do not allow the dropper to touch your fingers, eyelids, or any surface. Wait at least 5 minutes before using any other eyedrops.

If you forget to administer a dose of the eyedrops, do so as soon as you remember. If it is almost time for your next dose, skip the dose you forgot and continue with your regular schedule. Do not take a double dose.

Special Populations

Pregnancy/Breast-feeding

NSAIDs may affect the fetal heart during the second half of pregnancy. Pregnant women should not take flurbiprofen without their doctor's approval. When the drug is considered crucial by your doctor, its potential benefits must be carefully weighed against its risks.

NSAIDs may pass into breast milk. There is a possibility that a nursing mother taking flurbiprofen could affect her baby's heart or cardiovascular system. Nursing mothers who must take this drug should bottle-feed.

Seniors

Seniors may be more susceptible to side effects, especially ulcer disease.

Generic Name

Flutamide (FLUE-tuh-mide)

Brand Name

Eulexin

Type of Drug

Antiandrogen.

Prescribed for

Prostate cancer.

General Information

Flutamide works by slowing the uptake of androgen (male) hormone or by interfering with the binding of androgen to body tissues. Prostatic cancer is sensitive to anything that removes the source of androgen. It is always prescribed together with a luteinizing hormone-releasing hormone (LHRH) drug.

Cautions and Warnings

Do not take flutamide if you are **allergic** to it.

This drug may cause **jaundice** and a severe blood condition called **hemolytic anemia**. Severe **liver toxicity** may also occur; your doctor should check your liver function.

Two men taking this drug have developed **breast cancer**.
Flutamide may **reduce sperm counts**.

Possible Side Effects

▼ Most common: diarrhea, cystitis, and bleeding from
the rectum.

▼ Common: rectal irritation, blood in the urine, hot
flashes, nausea, rash, and swollen breasts.

▼ Less common: drowsiness, confusion, depression,
anxiety, nervousness, appetite loss, stomach problems,
anemia, low white-blood-cell and blood-platelet counts,
arm or leg swelling, urinary and muscle problems, and
high blood pressure.

▼ Rare: hepatitis, jaundice, and lung problems.

Food and Drug Interactions

None known.

Usual Dose

Adult: 250 mg (2 capsules) every 8 hours, 3 times a day.

Overdosage

Overdose symptoms may include tiredness or low activity
levels, slow breathing, weakness, tearing, appetite loss,
vomiting, swollen and tender breasts, and liver inflammation. Overdose victims should be taken to a hospital
emergency room. ALWAYS bring the prescription bottle or
container.

Special Information

Report anything unusual to your doctor, especially severe
itching, dark urine, persistent appetite loss, yellowing of the
skin or whites of the eyes, unexplained flu symptoms, and
unexplained abdominal pain. These may be signs of severe
liver toxicity.

Flutamide can turn your urine amber or yellow-green and
cause unusual sun sensitivity. Use sunscreen and wear long-
sleeved protective clothing while you are taking flutamide.

Flutamide must be taken exactly as prescribed. Call your
doctor if you miss a dose of this drug.

Special Populations

Pregnancy/Breast-feeding
This drug is not intended for use by women.

Seniors
Seniors may take this drug without special precaution.

Generic Name

Fluvoxamine (flue-VOX-uh-mene)

Brand Name

Luvox

Type of Drug

Selective serotonin reuptake inhibitor (SSRI).

Prescribed for

Obsessive-compulsive disorder (OCD) and depression.

General Information

Fluvoxamine and other SSRIs, which are chemically unrelated to the older tricyclic and tetracyclic antidepressant drugs, work by preventing the movement of the neurohormone serotonin into nerve endings. This forces serotonin to remain in the spaces surrounding nerve endings, where it works. Fluvoxamine is effective in treating common symptoms of OCD. The drug takes several weeks to work and stays in the body for several weeks after you stop taking it. This fact may be important as your doctor considers when to start or stop treatment.

Cautions and Warnings

Do not take fluvoxamine if you are **allergic** to it or other SSRIs. Some people have experienced serious **drug reactions** to fluvoxamine.

Serious, **potentially fatal reactions** may occur if fluvoxamine and a **monoamine oxidase inhibitor (MAOI)** antidepressant are taken together (see "Drug Interactions").

SSRIs may affect **blood platelets,** though their exact effect is not known. Some people have had abnormal bleeding while taking these drugs.

People with severe **liver disease** should use caution with this drug and be treated at lower doses.

Possible Side Effects

▼ Most common: headache, weakness, sleeplessness, tiredness, nervousness, dizziness, nausea, upset stomach, diarrhea, dry mouth, and constipation.

▼ Common: anxiety, tremors, respiratory infection, gas, appetite loss, vomiting, and excessive sweating.

▼ Less common: allergy or allergic reactions, flu-like symptoms, chills, palpitations, flushing, dizziness when rising from a sitting or lying position, high blood pressure, fainting, rapid heartbeat, depression, reduced sex drive or function, muscle twitching, agitation, muscle stiffness, nervous system stimulation, fatigue, not feeling well, memory loss, emotional upset, apathy, mood changes, manic or psychotic reaction, swelling, weight changes, stomach irritation, cavities or other teeth disorders, swallowing difficulties, liver inflammation, cough, sinus irritation, breathing difficulties, bronchitis, and yawning.

▼ Rare: Rare side effects can occur in almost any part of the body. Contact your doctor if you experience any side effect not listed above.

Drug Interactions

• Allow at least 5 weeks between stopping fluvoxamine and starting an MAOI antidepressant. Two weeks should pass between stopping an MAOI and starting fluvoxamine. Taking these drugs too close together or at the same time may cause serious, life-threatening reactions.

• Fluvoxamine blood levels may be increased if taken together with a tricyclic antidepressant.

• Lithium may increase fluvoxamine side effects. Your dosage may need to be adjusted.

• People who combine L-tryptophan and fluvoxamine may develop agitation, restlessness, and upset stomach.

• Alcohol may increase the tiredness and other depressant effects of fluvoxamine.

• Fluvoxamine may increase the side effects of clozapine, diltiazem, methadone, sumatriptan, carbamazepine, and theophylline. Dosage adjustment may be needed.

• Fluvoxamine may increase the effects of the beta-blocking drugs propranolol and metoprolol.

• Cigarette smoking may increase the speed at which the body breaks down fluvoxamine by 25%.

• Blood levels of the non-sedating antihistamines astemizole and terfenadine may be increased if taken with fluvoxamine, increasing the risk of potentially fatal cardiac reactions to those drugs. Haloperidol blood levels may also be increased, which can affect memory.

• Fluvoxamine may increase the effect of diazepam and other benzodiazepines.

• People taking warfarin may experience an increase in its effect if they start taking fluvoxamine; your doctor should reevaluate your warfarin dosage.

Food Interactions

None known.

Usual Dose

50–300 mg at bedtime. Seniors, people with liver disease, and people taking several different drugs should start with a lower dosage.

Overdosage

Symptoms of overdose include drowsiness, diarrhea, vomiting, and dizziness. Other signs are coma, change in heart rate, low blood pressure, convulsions, and liver or cardiac abnormalities. Fluvoxamine overdose victims should be taken to a hospital emergency room at once. ALWAYS bring the prescription bottle or container.

Special Information

Fluvoxamine can make you dizzy or drowsy. Take care when driving or doing tasks that require alertness and concentration. Avoid alcohol.

Be sure your doctor knows if you are pregnant, breast-feeding, or taking other drugs, including over-the-counter drugs, while taking fluvoxamine.

Call your doctor if you develop rash or hives, become excessively nervous or anxious, or lose your appetite—especially if you are already underweight—or experience any unusual side effect.

If you forget a dose, take it as soon as you remember. If it is almost time for your next dose, skip the dose you forgot and continue with your regular schedule. Do not take a double dose.

Special Populations

Pregnancy/Breast-feeding
Animal studies indicate that fluvoxamine may affect the fetus. If you are or might be pregnant, do not take this drug without first weighing its potential benefits against its risks with your doctor.

Fluvoxamine passes into breast milk. Nursing mothers who must take this drug should consider bottle-feeding.

Seniors
Seniors should begin with a 25-mg dose, to be increased as needed every 4 to 7 days.

Fosamax *see Bisphosphonates, page 131*

Generic Name

Fosfomycin (fos-foe-MYE-sin)

Brand Name
Monurol

Type of Drug
Urinary anti-infective.

Prescribed for
Uncomplicated urinary infections.

General Information
Fosfomycin kills a variety of bacteria. It works by preventing bacteria from sticking to the wall of the urinary tract and by interfering with bacterial cell division. In the body, it is converted to its active form—free fosfomycin. Generally, bacteria that are resistant to other antibiotics are not resistant to fosfomycin, so this drug may work where others have failed.

Cautions and Warnings

Do not take fosfomycin if you are **allergic** to it. Fosfomycin is meant to be taken once, in a single dose. Taking more than 1 packet of fosfomycin only **increases side effects;** it does not improve the drug's effectiveness.

Possible Side Effects

▼ Less common: diarrhea, vaginal irritation, runny nose, nausea, and headache.

▼ Rare: Rare side effects can occur in almost any part of the body. Contact your doctor if you experience any side effect not listed above.

Drug Interactions

• Metoclopramide reduces fosfomycin blood levels.

Food Interactions

You may take fosfomycin with or without food.

Usual Dose

Adult: 1 packet.
Child (under age 18): not recommended.

Overdosage

Little is known about the effects of fosfomycin overdose. Call your local poison control center or a hospital emergency room for more information. If you seek treatment, ALWAYS bring the prescription bottle or container.

Special Information

Do not take fosfomycin powder in its dry form. Mix the contents of the packet with 3 to 4 oz. of cool or cold water until it dissolves. Then drink the solution immediately.

Call your doctor if your infection does not improve within 2 or 3 days.

Special Populations

Pregnancy/Breast-feeding

The safety of using fosfomycin during pregnancy is not known. When this drug is considered crucial by your doctor, its potential benefits must be carefully weighed against its risks.

It is not known if fosfomycin passes into breast milk. Nursing mothers who must take this drug should bottle-feed.

Seniors
Seniors may take fosfomycin without special restriction.

Generic Name

Fosinopril (fos-IN-oe-pril)

Brand Name
Monopril

Type of Drug
Angiotensin-converting enzyme (ACE) inhibitor.

Prescribed for
High blood pressure.

General Information
Fosinopril sodium and other ACE inhibitors work by preventing the conversion of a hormone called angiotensin I to another hormone called angiotensin II, a potent blood-vessel constrictor. Preventing this conversion relaxes blood vessels, thus reducing blood pressure and relieving the symptoms of heart failure. Fosinopril also affects the production of other hormones and enzymes that participate in the regulation of blood vessel dilation. Fosinopril begins working 2 to 6 hours after you take it.

Some people who start taking an ACE inhibitor after they are already on a diuretic (agent that increases urination) experience a rapid drop in blood pressure after their first doses or when the dosage is increased. To prevent this from happening, you may be told to stop taking the diuretic 2 or 3 days before starting the ACE inhibitor or to increase your salt intake during that time. The diuretic may then be restarted gradually.

Cautions and Warnings
Do not take fosinopril if you have had an **allergic reaction** to it.

Fosinopril occasionally causes **very low blood pressure** or affects your **kidneys**. Your doctor should check your urine for changes during the first few months of treatment.

ACE inhibitors can affect your white-blood-cell count, possibly increasing your susceptibility to **infection**. Blood counts should be checked periodically.

Possible Side Effects

▼ Most common: headache and chronic cough. The cough usually goes away a few days after you stop taking the medicine.

▼ Less common: chest pain; low blood pressure; dizziness, especially when rising from a sitting or lying position; fatigue; diarrhea; vomiting; and nausea.

▼ Rare: Rare side effects can affect your heart, sleeping, stomach and intestines, skin, sex drive, and joints. Contact your doctor if you experience any side effect not listed above.

Drug Interactions

• The blood-pressure-lowering effect of fosinopril is additive with diuretic drugs and beta blockers. Any other drug that causes a rapid drop in blood pressure should be used with caution if you are taking an ACE inhibitor.

• Fosinopril may increase potassium levels in your blood, especially when taken with Dyazide or other potassium-sparing diuretics.

• Fosinopril may increase the effects of lithium; this combination should be used with caution.

• Antacids and fosinopril should be taken at least 2 hours apart.

• Capsaicin may trigger or aggravate the cough associated with fosinopril therapy.

• Indomethacin may reduce the blood-pressure-lowering effects of fosinopril.

• Phenothiazine tranquilizers and antivomiting drugs may increase the effects of fosinopril.

• The combination of allopurinol and fosinopril increases the chance of side effects.

• ACE inhibitors increase blood levels of digoxin, possibly increasing the chance of digoxin-related side effects.

Food Interactions

You may take fosinopril with food if it upsets your stomach.

Usual Dose

10–80 mg once a day. People with liver disease may require lower dosages.

Overdosage

The principal effect of ACE inhibitor overdose is a rapid drop in blood pressure, as evidenced by dizziness or fainting. Take the overdose victim to a hospital emergency room immediately. ALWAYS bring the prescription bottle or container.

Special Information

Call your doctor if you develop swelling of the face or throat, if you have sudden difficulty in breathing, or if you develop a sore throat, mouth sores, abnormal heartbeat, chest pain, persistent rash, or loss of taste perception. Unexplained swelling of the face, lips, hands, and feet can also affect the larynx (throat) and tongue and interfere with breathing. If this happens, the victim should be taken to a hospital emergency room at once.

You may get dizzy if you rise to your feet quickly from a sitting or lying position.

Avoid strenuous exercise or very hot weather, because heavy sweating or dehydration can cause a rapid decrease in blood pressure.

Avoid over-the-counter diet pills, decongestants, and other stimulants that can raise blood pressure.

If you forget to take a dose of fosinopril, take it as soon as you remember. If it is within 8 hours of your next dose, skip the one you forgot and continue with your regular schedule. Do not take a double dose.

Special Populations

Pregnancy/Breast-feeding

ACE inhibitors can cause fetal injury or death. Women who are or might be pregnant should not take ACE inhibitors. Stop taking the drug and contact your doctor if you become pregnant.

Large amounts of fosinopril pass into breast milk. Nursing mothers who must take this drug should bottle-feed.

Seniors
Seniors may be more sensitive to the effects of fosinopril.

Generic Name

Ganciclovir (gan-SYE-kloe-vere)

Brand Names

Cytovene   Vitrasert

Type of Drug

Antiviral.

Prescribed for

Cytomegalovirus (CMV) infections of the eye and CMV infections in other parts of the body, in people with compromised immune systems.

General Information

Ganciclovir works by preventing reproduction of the virus CMV. Unlike other antiviral drugs, it works only against this virus and no others. Because viral resistance develops more quickly to the capsules, the capsule form of ganciclovir is restricted to follow-up treatment in people who have received intravenous treatment for CMV infections. The drug is eliminated through the kidneys.

Though most often used for CMV retinitis (eye infection), ganciclovir has also been used for CMV infections of the urine, blood, throat, and semen. It is also used to prevent CMV infection. Ganciclovir is helpful in controlling CMV infection in heart or bone marrow transplant patients.

Cautions and Warnings

Ganciclovir causes **anemia, reduced white-blood-cell count,** and **blood platelet loss**. Regular monitoring of blood and platelet counts is recommended while taking this drug.

Oral ganciclovir is linked to a faster progression of CMV eye infection than the intravenous form of the drug. The **risk of rapid progression of eye infection** should be balanced against the benefits of taking oral CMV.

People **allergic** to acyclovir or ganciclovir should not take ganciclovir.

Ganciclovir is intended only for people who are immuno-compromised. It is not intended to treat or prevent CMV infections in **newborns**.

Detachment of the retina has been noted in people taking ganciclovir, as well as in people with CMV who have not taken the drug. The relationship between ganciclovir and this effect is not well known.

Ganciclovir causes increased **sensitivity to the sun;** use a sunscreen or wear protective clothes when you go outside.

Studies of ganciclovir in African Americans, Hispanics, and Caucasians showed a trend toward higher blood levels among Caucasians than other groups.

Intravenous ganciclovir has been given to a small number of children under age 12 with mixed results. Side effects were similar to those experienced by adults taking the drug.

Possible Side Effects

▼ Most common: fever, diarrhea, abdominal pain, reduced white-blood-cell counts, anemia, rash, sweating, nausea, vomiting, and appetite loss.

▼ Common: infection; chills; stomach gas; low platelet counts (symptoms include bleeding or oozing blood); tingling; burning; numbness or pain in the hands, arms, legs, or feet; itching; pneumonia; weakness; and headache.

▼ Less common: Less common side effects can occur in almost any part of the body. Contact your doctor if you experience any side effect not listed above.

Drug Interactions

• Dapsone, pentamidine, flucytosine, vincristine, vinblastine, adriamycin, amphotericin B, trimethoprim-sulfamethoxazole, and other antiviral drugs may increase the side effects of ganciclovir and should be used together only if absolutely necessary, and only if the potential benefits outweigh the risks.

• People taking imipenem-cilastatin together with ganciclovir have experienced seizures. Avoid this combination.

• Mixing ganciclovir with other drugs that can be damaging to the kidneys may increase the rate and extent of kidney damage.

• Probenecid interferes with ganciclovir release through the kidneys and substantially increases blood levels of ganciclovir.

• Mixing ganciclovir with the anti-HIV drugs didanosine or zidovudine (AZT) may increase didanosine or AZT levels and reduce ganciclovir levels. Because AZT and ganciclovir both cause anemia and low white-blood-cell counts, many people cannot tolerate this combination.

Food Interactions

High-fat, high-calorie meals can increase the amount of ganciclovir absorbed into the blood. Take this drug with food.

Usual Dose

Adult and Child (age 13 and over): 3000 mg a day, divided into 3 or 6 equal doses. People with reduced kidney function will need to have their dosage reduced accordingly, possibly to as little as 500 mg 3 times a week.

Child (under age 13): not recommended.

Overdosage

Little is known about the effects of ganciclovir overdose. As much as 6000 mg a day has been taken with only temporary lowering of white-blood-cell count. Call your hospital emergency room for instructions in case of ganciclovir overdose.

Special Information

Ganciclovir does not cure CMV eye infection, and immunocompromised people taking this drug may find their disease worsening. Dosage reductions or discontinuation of the drug may be necessary if white-blood-cell or platelet counts get too low.

Ganciclovir may cause infertility in men and women. Pregnant women taking this drug should use effective contraception. Men should use a condom while taking the drug and for at least 90 days afterward to avoid passing the drug to their partners.

Good dental hygiene is important while taking ganciclovir to minimize the risk of infection. If you have dental work done while taking this drug, expect the healing process to take longer.

Regular blood tests are necessary to watch for white-blood-cell or platelet-level alterations.

It is very important to take ganciclovir exactly as directed. If you forget a dose, take it as soon as you remember and continue with your regular schedule. If you take ganciclovir 3 times a day and it is almost time for your next dose, take one dose immediately, another in 6 hours, and then continue with your regular schedule. If you take it 6 times a day and it is almost time for your next dose, skip the dose you forgot and continue with your regular schedule.

Special Populations

Pregnancy/Breast-feeding

Animal studies showed ganciclovir to be toxic to the fetus. There is no reliable information about its effect in pregnant women, but it should be taken only when the possible benefits outweigh the risks. Women who are likely to become pregnant while taking this drug should use reliable contraception.

It is not known if ganciclovir passes into breast milk, but the possible side effects of this drug on a nursing infant should be kept in mind. Nursing mothers who must take this drug should bottle-feed.

Seniors

Seniors often have reduced kidney function; dosage adjustments may be needed.

Generic Name

Gemfibrozil (jem-FYE-broe-zil) [G]

Brand Name

Lopid

Type of Drug

Anti-hyperlipidemic (blood-fat reducer).

Prescribed for

High blood triglycerides.

General Information

Gemfibrozil consistently reduces blood triglycerides and may reduce the risk of heart disease in people with high levels of triglycerides, low levels of high-density lipoprotein (HDL) cholesterol, and high levels of low-density lipoprotein (LDL) cholesterol. It works by affecting the breakdown of body fats and by reducing the amount of triglyceride manufactured by the liver. It is usually prescribed only for people with very high blood-fat levels who have not responded to dietary changes or other therapies. Gemfibrozil usually has little effect on blood-cholesterol levels, although it may reduce blood cholesterol in some people.

Cautions and Warnings

Do not take gemfibrozil if you are **allergic** to it or have severe **liver or kidney disease**. Some people taking gemfibrozil have experienced worsening of kidney function. Gemfibrozil users may have an increased risk of developing **gallbladder disease**. People taking gemfibrozil may develop **muscle aches and inflammation**. Tell your doctor if you experience muscle tenderness or weakness.

Estrogen drugs may cause massive increases in triglyceride levels and may have to be discontinued when using gemfibrozil.

Gemfibrozil may cause a moderate rise in **blood sugar** and mild decreases in **white-blood-cell counts**.

Possible Side Effects

▼ Most common: abdominal and stomach pain, gas, diarrhea, nausea, and vomiting.

▼ Less common: rash, itching, dizziness, blurred vision, anemia, reduced levels of white blood cells, increased blood sugar, and muscle pain—especially in the arms or legs.

▼ Rare: dry mouth, constipation, appetite loss, upset stomach, sleeplessness, tingling in the hands or feet, ringing or buzzing in the ears, back pain, painful muscles or joints, swollen joints, fatigue, feeling unwell, reduction in blood potassium, and abnormal liver function.

Drug Interactions

• Gemfibrozil increases the effects of oral anticoagulant (blood-thinning) drugs. Your anticoagulant dosage must be reduced when starting gemfibrozil.

• Combining gemfibrozil with a statin cholesterol-lowering drug (atorvastatin, cerivastatin, fluvastatin, lovastatin, pravastatin, or simvastatin) has led to the destruction of skeletal muscles. This effect may begin as early as 3 weeks after you start taking the combination or may not appear for months.

Food Interactions

Gemfibrozil is best taken on an empty stomach 30 minutes before meals but may be taken with food if it upsets your stomach. It is important that you follow your doctor's dietary instructions.

Usual Dose

1200 mg a day, divided into 2 doses taken 30 minutes before breakfast and dinner.

Overdosage

Little is known about the effects of gemfibrozil overdose. Symptoms may include severe side effects. Induce vomiting with ipecac syrup—available at any pharmacy—but call your doctor or local poison control center before doing this. If you go to a hospital emergency room, ALWAYS bring the prescription bottle or container.

Special Information

Your doctor should perform periodic blood counts during the first year of gemfibrozil treatment to check for anemia or other changes in blood components. Liver-function tests are also necessary. Blood-sugar levels should be checked periodically while you are taking gemfibrozil, especially if you are diabetic or have a family history of diabetes.

Gemfibrozil may cause dizziness or blurred vision. Be careful when driving or doing any task that requires concentration.

Call your doctor if side effects become severe or intolerable, especially diarrhea, nausea, vomiting, or stomach pain or gas. These may disappear if your doctor reduces the dosage.

If you forget a dose, take it as soon as you remember. If it is almost time for your next dose, skip the one you forgot and continue with your regular schedule. Do not take a double dose.

Special Populations

Pregnancy/Breast-feeding

The safety of using gemfibrozil during pregnancy is not known. When this drug is considered crucial by your doctor, its potential benefits must be carefully weighed against its risks.

This drug passes into breast milk and should not be taken by a nursing mother.

Seniors

Seniors are more likely to develop side effects.

Generic Name

Glatiramer (glah-TYE-ram-er)

Brand Name

Copaxone

Type of Drug

Relapsing-remitting multiple sclerosis (MS) therapy.

Prescribed for

MS.

General Information

Glatiramer is a random mixture of several amino acids. It is thought to work by modifying the immune processes responsible for MS. In studies, people who took the drug for over a year were twice as likely to be relapse-free as those who took a placebo (sugar pill).

Cautions and Warnings

Do not use this drug if you are **allergic** to it or mannitol.

About 10% of people who self-administer glatiramer experience a **post-injection reaction** with symptoms that include flushing, chest pain, heart palpitations, anxiety, breathing difficulties, closing of the throat, and an itchy rash. These symptoms usually go away without treatment. This reaction generally occurs after several months of drug therapy, though it may occur earlier.

About half of the people who took glatiramer in drug studies had **chest pain,** but the exact relationship of this pain to use of glatiramer could not be determined. Report any chest pain to your doctor at once.

Because it interferes with immune response, glatiramer may increase your risk of developing **infections** and **tumors.**

Glatiramer may interfere with **kidney function.**

Possible Side Effects

▼ Most common: infections, weakness, pain, chest pain, flu-like symptoms, back pain, flushing, heart palpitations, anxiety, muscle stiffness or spasticity, an urgent need to urinate, swollen lymph glands, injection-site reactions (including pain, inflammation, itching, an unknown mass at the injection site, welts, skin marks, and bleeding), breathing difficulties, runny nose, and joint pain.

▼ Common: fever, neck pain, facial swelling, bacterial infection, migraine, fever, rapid heartbeat, tremors, fainting, appetite loss, vomiting, general stomach disorders, vaginal infection, painful menstruation, black-and-blue marks, swelling in the arms or legs, bronchial irritation, spasm of the larynx, and ear pain.

▼ Less common: chills, cysts, agitation, foot drop, nervousness, rolling eyeballs, confusion, speech problems, cold sores, redness, itchy rash, skin nodules, stomach pain and irritation, weight gain, and eye disorders.

▼ Rare: Rare side effects can occur in almost any part of the body. Contact your doctor if you experience any side effect not listed above.

Food and Drug Interactions

None known.

Usual Dose

Adult (age 18 and over): 20 mg a day by injection under the skin.

Child: not recommended.

Overdosage

Little is known about the effects of glatiramer overdose. Call you local poison control center or a hospital emergency room for information. If you seek treatment, ALWAYS bring the prescription bottle or container.

Special Information

Store unused glatiramer in the refrigerator before it is mixed with the diluent supplied by the manufacturer. Do not use any other diluent. The mixed injection must be used right away.

Suggested injection sites are the arms, abdomen, hips, and thighs. Be sure to rotate injection sites.

If you forget to administer a dose, do so as soon as you remember. If it is almost time for your next dose, skip the dose you forgot and continue with your regular schedule. Do not take a double dose. Call your doctor if you miss more than 2 doses in a row.

Special Populations

Pregnancy/Breast-feeding
The safety of using glatiramer during pregnancy is not known. When this drug is considered crucial by your doctor, its potential benefits must be carefully weighed against its risks.

It is not known if glatiramer passes into breast milk. Nursing mothers who must take it should consider bottle-feeding.

Seniors
Seniors may use glatiramer without special restriction.

Glucophage   *see Metformin, page 637*

Glucotrol XL   *see Sulfonylurea Antidiabetes Drugs,*
page 957

Generic Name

Guanabenz   (GWAN-uh-benz) Ⓖ

Brand Name

Wytensin

Type of Drug

Antihypertensive.

Prescribed for

High blood pressure.

General Information

Guanabenz acetate works by depressing the central nervous system by stimulating certain receptors. Initially, guanabenz reduces blood pressure without a major effect on blood vessels; however, long-term use of guanabenz may result in the dilation (widening) of blood vessels and a slight slowing of pulse rate. Guanabenz may be taken alone or with a thiazide diuretic.

Cautions and Warnings

Do not take guanabenz if you are **sensitive** or **allergic** to it. People with **severe kidney or liver disease** should take this drug with caution.

Possible Side Effects

Risk and severity of side effects increase with dosage.

▼ Most common: drowsiness, sedation, dry mouth, dizziness, weakness, and headache.

▼ Less common: chest pain; swelling in the hands, legs, or feet; heart palpitations or abnormal heart rhythms; stomach or abdominal pain or discomfort; nausea; diarrhea; vomiting; constipation; anxiety; poor muscle control; depression; difficulty sleeping; stuffy nose; blurred vision; muscle aches and pains; breathing difficulties; frequent urination; impotence; unusual taste in the mouth; and swollen and painful breasts in men.

Drug Interactions

• Other blood-pressure-lowering agents increase the effect of guanabenz.

• The sedating effects of guanabenz are increased by combining it with tranquilizers, sleeping pills, or other nervous system depressants, including alcohol.

• People taking this drug for high blood pressure should avoid over-the-counter drugs that might aggravate their condition, including decongestants, cold and allergy remedies, and diet pills—all of which may contain stimulants.

Food Interactions

This drug is best taken on an empty stomach, but it may be taken with food if it upsets your stomach.

Usual Dose

4 mg twice a day to start; increased gradually to a maximum dose of 32 mg twice a day—though doses this large are rarely needed.

Overdosage

Overdose causes sleepiness, lethargy, low blood pressure, irritability, pinpoint pupils, and reduced heart rate. Overdose victims should be made to vomit with ipecac syrup—available at any pharmacy—but call your doctor or poison control center first. If you must go to a hospital emergency room, ALWAYS bring the prescription bottle or container.

Special Information

Take guanabenz exactly as prescribed for maximum benefit. If any side effect becomes severe or intolerable, contact your doctor.

Guanabenz often causes tiredness or dizziness; avoid alcohol because it increases these effects. Take care when driving or doing anything that requires concentration.

Do not stop taking guanabenz without your doctor's approval. Suddenly stopping this drug may cause a rapid increase in blood pressure. Dosage must be gradually reduced by your doctor.

If you forget a dose, take it as soon as you remember. If it is almost time for your next dose, skip the one you forgot and continue with your regular schedule. Do not take a double dose. Call your doctor if you miss 2 or more consecutive doses.

Special Populations

Pregnancy/Breast-feeding
Guanabenz may affect the fetus. It should be avoided by women who are or might be pregnant. When guanabenz is considered crucial by your doctor, its potential benefits must be carefully weighed against its risks.

It is not known if guanabenz passes into breast milk. Nursing mothers who must take this drug should bottle-feed.

Seniors
Seniors are more sensitive to the sedating and blood-pressure-lowering effects of guanabenz.

Generic Name
Halofantrine (hay-loe-FAN-treen)

Brand Name
Halfan

Type of Drug
Antimalarial.

Prescribed for
Malaria.

General Information
Halofantrine hydrochloride kills malaria organisms circulating in the blood. It does not affect forms of malaria that reside in the liver or its immature forms. Halofantrine, which does not prevent malaria, is only intended for the treatment of mild to moderate infections. Severe or life-threatening malaria should be treated with other, more potent drugs.

Cautions and Warnings
Do not take this drug if you are **sensitive** or **allergic** to it.

Halofantrine affects the **heart**. This drug is associated with potentially fatal changes in heart ventricle rhythm. People with ventricular disorders should not take this drug and it should not be combined with other drugs that affect the ventricles (see "Drug Interactions"). People who have taken **mefloquine** (another antimalarial) should not take halofantrine because of the increased risk of heart problems.

People treated with halofantrine experience **relapse** more often than those treated with other malaria drugs.

Possible Side Effects

▼ Common: abdominal pain and diarrhea.

▼ Less common: nausea, vomiting, dizziness, cough, headache, itching, chills, and muscle aches.

▼ Rare: Rare side effects can occur in almost any part of the body. Contact your doctor if you experience any side effect not listed above.

Drug Interactions

• Combining halofantrine and mefloquine can lead to a fatal effect on heart ventricles. Do not combine these drugs. People who have already taken mefloquine should not take halofantrine to treat malaria.

Food Interactions

To avoid severe side effects, take this drug on an empty stomach at least 1 hour before or 2 hours after meals.

Usual Dose

Adult and Child (over 81.5 lbs.): 500 mg every 6 hours for 3 doses.

Child (68.25–81.5 lbs.): 375 mg every 6 hours for 3 doses.

Child (50.5–68.25 lbs.): 250 mg every 6 hours for 3 doses.

Child (under 50.5 lbs.): Dosage not established.

If necessary, treatment with halofantrine is repeated after 1 week.

Overdosage

Symptoms include abdominal pain, stomach and intestinal problems, vomiting, cramping, and diarrhea. Palpitations may also develop. Induce vomiting with ipecac syrup—available at any pharmacy—then take the victim to a hospital emergency room. If you seek treatment, ALWAYS bring the prescription bottle or container.

Special Information

Contact your doctor immediately if you develop anxiety; black-colored urine or decreased urine volume; chest or lower back pain; rapid and irregular heartbeat; restlessness; flushing; or rapid breathing.

Call your doctor if symptoms do not improve after taking this drug.

Tell your doctor if you have any medical problems, especially abnormal heartbeat or other heart conditions, thiamine deficiency, or unexplained fainting. These conditions increase the risk of cardiac side effects, including fast or irregular heartbeat.

Complete the full course of drug therapy. Your symptoms may return if you stop treatment too early. Your doctor may also recommend a second course of treatment.

It is important that your doctor check your progress after treatment to ensure that the infection is completely gone.

If you forget a dose, take it as soon as possible. If it is almost time for your next dose, skip the dose you forgot and go back to your regular schedule. Do not take a double dose.

Special Populations

Pregnancy/Breast-feeding

Animal studies with halofantrine reveal that it may harm the fetus. When this drug is considered crucial by your doctor, its potential benefits must be carefully weighed against its risks.

It is not known if halofantrine passes into breast milk, though it did in animal studies. Nursing mothers who must take it should bottle-feed.

Seniors

Seniors may take halofantrine without special precaution.

Generic Name

Haloperidol (hal-oe-PER-ih-dol) G

Brand Name

Haldol

Type of Drug

Butyrophenone antipsychotic.

Prescribed for

Psychotic disorders, including Tourette's syndrome; severe behavioral problems in children; short-term treatment of hyperactive children; chronic schizophrenia; vomiting; treatment of acute psychiatric situations; and phencyclidine (PCP) psychosis.

General Information

Haloperidol is one of many nonphenothiazine agents used to treat psychosis. These drugs are equally effective when given in therapeutically equivalent doses. The major differences are in the type and severity of side effects. Some people may respond well to one and not at all to another. Haloperidol acts on a portion of the brain called the hypothalamus. It affects parts of the hypothalamus that control metabolism, body temperature, alertness, muscle tone, hormone balance, and vomiting. Haloperidol is available in liquid form for those who have trouble swallowing tablets.

Cautions and Warnings

Haloperidol should not be used by people who are **allergic** to it.

People with very **low blood pressure, Parkinson's disease,** or **blood, liver, or kidney disease** should avoid this drug.

If you have **glaucoma, epilepsy, ulcers,** or **difficulty urinating,** haloperidol should be used with caution and under strict supervision of your doctor.

Avoid **exposure to extreme heat** because this drug can upset your body's temperature-regulating mechanism.

Possible Side Effects

▼ Most common: drowsiness, especially during the first or second week of therapy. If the drowsiness becomes troublesome, contact your doctor.

▼ Less common: jaundice (yellowing of the whites of the eyes or skin), which may occur in the first 2 to 4 weeks. The jaundice usually goes away when the drug is discontinued, but there have been cases in which it did not. If you notice this effect, develop fever, or generally feel unwell, contact your doctor immediately. Other less common side effects are changes in components of the blood, including anemias; raised or lowered blood pressure; abnormal heartbeat; heart attack; and feeling faint or dizzy.

Possible Side Effects *(continued)*

▼ Rare: neurological effects such as spasms of the neck muscles, severe stiffness of the back muscles, rolling back of the eyes, convulsions, difficulty in swallowing, and symptoms associated with Parkinson's disease. These effects usually disappear after the drug has been withdrawn; however, symptoms of the face, tongue, or jaw may persist for years, especially in seniors with a long history of brain disease. If you experience any of these effects, contact your doctor immediately. Other rare side effects can occur in almost any part of the body. Contact your doctor if you experience any side effect not listed above.

Drug Interactions

• Be cautious about taking haloperidol with barbiturates, sleeping pills, narcotics or other tranquilizers, alcohol, or any other medication that may produce a depressive effect.

• Anticholinergic drugs may reduce the effectiveness of haloperidol and increase the risk of side effects.

• The blood-pressure-lowering effect of guanethidine may be counteracted by haloperidol.

• Taking lithium together with haloperidol may lead to disorientation, loss of consciousness, or uncontrolled muscle movements.

• Combining propranolol and haloperidol may lead to unusually low blood pressure.

• Combining tricyclic antidepressant drugs and haloperidol can lead to antidepressant side effects.

Food Interactions

Haloperidol is best taken on an empty stomach, but you may take it with food if it upsets your stomach.

Usual Dose

Adult: starting dose—0.5–2 mg 2 or 3 times a day. Your doctor may later increase your dose up to 100 mg a day, according to your needs. Seniors generally need smaller doses.

Child (age 3–12 or 33–88 lbs.): starting dose—0.5 mg a day. Dosage may be increased in 0.5-mg steps every 5–7 days until a satisfactory effect is realized.

Child (under age 3): not recommended.

Overdosage

Symptoms of overdose are depression, extreme weakness, tiredness, desire to sleep, coma, lowered blood pressure, uncontrolled muscle spasms, agitation, restlessness, convulsions, fever, dry mouth, and abnormal heart rhythm. The victim should be taken to a hospital emergency room immediately. ALWAYS bring the prescription bottle or container.

Special Information

This medication may cause drowsiness. Use caution when driving or operating hazardous equipment; also, avoid alcoholic beverages while taking it.

Haloperidol may cause unusual sensitivity to the sun. It may also turn your urine reddish-brown or pink.

If dizziness occurs, avoid sudden changes in posture and avoid climbing stairs. Use caution in hot weather. This medication may make you more prone to heat stroke.

If you forget to take a dose of haloperidol, take it as soon as you remember. Take the rest of the day's doses evenly spaced throughout the day. Do not take a double dose.

Special Populations

Pregnancy/Breast-feeding
Serious problems have been seen in pregnant animals given large amounts of haloperidol. Although haloperidol has not been studied in pregnant women, you should avoid this drug if you are or might be pregnant.

Haloperidol passes into breast milk. Nursing mothers who must use this medication should bottle-feed.

Seniors
Seniors are more sensitive to the effects of this medication and usually require $\frac{1}{2}$ to $\frac{1}{4}$ the usual adult dose. Seniors are also more likely to develop side effects.

Brand Name

Helidac

Generic Ingredients

Bismuth Subsalicylate + Metronidazole + Tetracycline

Type of Drug

Antibacterial combination.

Prescribed for

Duodenal ulcers.

General Information

Research has shown that the bacterium *Helicobacter pylori* is usually present in ulcer disease and some forms of gastritis. This discovery changed the treatment of these diseases. Drugs used to treat the *H. pylori* infection are now prescribed along with a drug that alleviates ulcer symptoms by blocking stomach acid. Doctors have developed a variety of approaches to treating ulcers by using combinations of various antibiotic and acid-blocking drugs. Helidac combines 3 drugs with antibacterial or antibiotic action. This combination generally works by disrupting the cell walls of the bacterium and interfering with its ability to make proteins or duplicate itself. It is often prescribed together with ranitidine, cimetidine, or another acid blocker. Other treatments use other drug combinations.

Cautions and Warnings

Do not take Helidac if you are **sensitive** or **allergic** to any of its ingredients.

Rarely, bismuth causes severe **nervous-system toxicity.** Symptoms go away after the drug is stopped. Bismuth subsalicylate can cause dark stools or darkening of the tongue. This darkening of stools is not dangerous; however, be aware that blood in the stool often manifests as blackening of the stool.

Children or teenagers who have or are recovering from chickenpox should not use Helidac because it contains a small amount of salicylate, which is related to aspirin. Children or teenagers who take aspirin or a salicylate may develop Reye's syndrome, symptoms of which include nausea and vomiting.

Metronidazole can cause convulsive **seizures** and **nervous system effects** including numbness or tingling in the arms, legs, hands, or feet. The risk of developing these effects increases with dosage and duration of use. Call your doctor at once if you experience any of these effects.

Metronidazole should be taken with caution by people who have had **blood diseases**.

Candida infections may worsen while you are taking metronidazole. People with **liver disease** may require reduced dosage.

Tetracycline should be avoided by people with severe **kidney disease**. Other infections, called superinfections, can develop while you are taking tetracycline. If this happens, your doctor will discontinue Helidac and prescribe a different drug to treat your *H. pylori* infection, as well as another drug to treat the superinfection. People taking tetracycline can develop **pseudotumor cerebri** (pressure inside the brain), the symptoms of which are usually headache and blurred vision. Symptoms usually go away when the drug is stopped, but permanent damage can result. Tetracycline may increase your **sensitivity to the sun;** use sunscreen and wear protective clothing.

Possible Side Effects

For more information on possible side effects, see "Metronidazole" and "Tetracycline."

▼ Most common: nausea and diarrhea.

▼ Less common: abdominal pain, blood in the stool, anal discomfort, appetite loss, dizziness, tingling in the hands or feet, vomiting, muscle weakness, constipation, sleeplessness, pain, and respiratory infections.

Drug Interactions

• Tetracycline antibiotics, which are bacteriostatic, may interfere with the action of bactericidal (bacteria-killing) agents such as penicillin. You should not take both kinds of antibiotics for the same infection.

• Antacids, mineral supplements, and multivitamins containing bismuth, calcium, zinc, magnesium, and iron can reduce the effectiveness of tetracycline. Separate doses of your antacid, mineral supplement, vitamin with minerals, or sodium bicarbonate and Helidac by at least 2 hours.

• Tetracycline and metronidazole may each increase the effect of anticoagulant (blood-thinning) drugs such as warfarin. An adjustment in the anticoagulant dosage may be required.

- Cimetidine, ranitidine, and other H_2 antagonists may reduce tetracycline's effectiveness.
- Cimetidine can increase metronidazole blood levels. Your metronidazole dosage may be reduced if you are also taking cimetidine.
- Tetracycline may increase blood levels of digoxin in a small number of people, leading to possible digoxin side effects. In some people this interaction with digoxin can occur for months after tetracycline has been stopped. If you are taking this combination, watch carefully for digoxin side effects and call your doctor if any develop.
- Tetracycline may reduce diabetic insulin requirements. If you are using this combination, be sure to carefully monitor your blood-sugar level.
- Tetracycline may increase or decrease lithium blood levels. Metronidazole raises lithium blood levels, effects, and toxicity.
- Combining alcohol and metronidazole may cause abdominal cramps, nausea, vomiting, headaches, and flushing. Modification of the taste of alcohol has also been reported. Metronidazole should not be used if you are taking disulfiram (a drug used to maintain alcohol abstinence) because the combination can cause confusion and psychotic reactions.
- Phenobarbital and other barbiturates can decrease metronidazole's effectiveness.
- Drugs that cause nervous system toxicity, such as mexiletine, ethambutol, isoniazid, lincomycin, lithium, pemoline, quinacrine, and long-term high-dose pyridoxine (vitamin B_6) should not be taken with metronidazole because of the increased risk of nervous system side effects.
- Metronidazole may increase phenytoin blood levels and the risk of phenytoin side effects; your doctor may need to adjust your phenytoin dosage.

Food Interactions

Do not take this drug with milk or dairy products. Helidac should be taken with meals and at bedtime.

Usual Dose

Adult: Each dose consists of 4 pills. Take all 4 pills, 4 times a day for 14 days. Take your acid blocker according to your doctor's directions.

Child: not recommended.

Overdosage

All 3 ingredients in Helidac can be dangerous if taken in overdose, but salicylate poisoning is the most threatening. Symptoms of salicylate toxicity are rapid or heavy breathing, nausea, vomiting, ringing or buzzing in the ears, high fever, lethargy, rapid heartbeat, and confusion. Other more serious symptoms may develop. Take the victim to a hospital emergency room at once. ALWAYS bring the prescription bottle or container.

Special Information

Each Helidac dose consists of 2 pink, round, chewable tablets (bismuth subsalicylate); 1 white tablet (metronidazole); and 1 pale orange and white capsule (tetracycline). Chew the 2 bismuth tablets and then swallow the other 2 pills with a full glass (8 oz.) of water. Take the acid blocker according to your doctor's directions.

Tetracycline can reduce the effectiveness of oral contraceptives ("the pill"); you should use backup contraception while taking Helidac. Breakthrough bleeding is also possible.

Bismuth can cause a temporary darkening of your tongue or stool. This is a harmless effect. Stool darkening should not be confused with blood in the stool, which turns it black.

Avoid alcohol while taking Helidac and for 1 day after you stop taking it.

Call your doctor if you develop ringing in the ears. This can be a sign of salicylate toxicity from the bismuth subsalicylate.

If you forget a dose, take it as soon as you remember. If it is almost time for your next dose, skip the dose you forgot and continue with your regular schedule. Never take a double dose. If you have any doses left after 14 days, continue to take them at your regular times until you have used up all the medication. Call your doctor if you forget more than 4 doses in 14 days.

Special Populations

Pregnancy/Breast-feeding

Helidac should not be taken by pregnant women. Tetracycline affects bone and tooth development in the fetus.

Tetracycline and metronidazole pass into breast milk. Tetracycline interferes with the development of the child's skull, bones, and teeth, and metronidazole also may cause side effects in the baby. Nursing mothers who must take Helidac should bottle-feed.

Seniors
Seniors may take this drug without special restriction.

Generic Name

Hydralazine (hye-DRAL-uh-zene) Ⓖ

Brand Names

Apresoline

Type of Drug

Antihypertensive.

Prescribed for

High blood pressure, aortic insufficiency after heart valve replacement, and congestive heart failure.

General Information

Although its mechanism of action is not completely understood, hydralazine hydrochloride is believed to lower blood pressure by enlarging blood vessels throughout the body. This also helps to improve heart function and blood flow to the kidneys and brain.

Cautions and Warnings

Long-term administration of more than 200 mg a day of hydralazine may produce **lupus erythematosus** (a chronic condition affecting the body's connective tissue). Symptoms include muscle and joint pain, skin reactions, fever, and anemia, although they usually disappear when the drug is discontinued. Report any fever, chest pain, feelings of ill health, or other unexplained symptoms to your doctor. The risk of developing lupus increases with higher dosages; 10% to 20% of people taking 400 mg a day of hydralazine develop lupus.

Hydralazine may actually improve kidney blood flow and kidney function in people who have below-normal function. It should be used with caution in people with advanced **kidney damage**.

Hydralazine may worsen heart problems and should be used with care in people with a history of **heart disease**. It can cause angina pain and may cause heart attacks.

Tingling in the hands or feet caused by hydralazine may be relieved by taking pyridoxine (vitamin B$_6$).

People taking hydralazine may develop **reduced hemoglobin and red-blood-cell counts. Reduced white-blood-cell and platelet counts** may also occur. Periodic blood counts are recommended while taking hydralazine.

Possible Side Effects

▼ Most common: headache, appetite loss, nausea, vomiting, diarrhea, rapid heartbeat, and chest pain.

▼ Less common: stuffy nose, flushing, tearing of the eyes, itching or redness of the eyes, numbness or tingling in the hands or feet, dizziness, tremors, muscle cramps, depression, disorientation, anxiety, itching, rash, fever, chills, occasional hepatitis (symptoms include yellowing of the skin or whites of the eyes), constipation, urinary difficulties, and adverse effects on normal blood composition.

Drug Interactions

• Taking hydralazine with the beta blockers metoprolol or propranolol may result in increased blood levels of both hydralazine and the beta blocker.

• Indomethacin may reduce the effects of hydralazine.

• Do not use over-the-counter cough, cold, or allergy medications. These products often contain stimulant ingredients that can increase blood pressure.

Food Interactions

Take hydralazine with food.

Hydralazine may counteract the benefits of vitamin B$_6$, which can result in tremors and tingling and numbness of the fingers, toes, or extremities. If these symptoms occur, your doctor may consider pyridoxine supplements.

Usual Dose

Adult: 40 mg a day for the first few days; increased to 100 mg a day for the rest of the first week. Dosage is then increased until the maximum effect is seen.

Child: 0.34 mg per lb. of body weight a day; increased up to 200 mg a day.

Overdosage

Symptoms include extreme lowering of blood pressure, rapid heartbeat, headache, flushing, chest pain, and abnormal heart rhythms. If you experience any of these symptoms, contact your doctor immediately. If you go to a hospital emergency room, ALWAYS bring the prescription bottle or container.

Special Information

Take hydralazine exactly as prescribed.

Call your doctor if you experience prolonged and unexplained tiredness, fever, muscle or joint aching, or chest pain while taking this drug.

If you forget a dose, take it as soon as you remember. If it is almost time for your next dose, skip the one you forgot and continue with your regular schedule. Do not take a double dose.

Special Populations

Pregnancy/Breast-feeding

High doses of hydralazine caused birth defects in animal studies, and temporary blood-related problems have been seen in newborns whose mothers took hydralazine during pregnancy. Women who are or might be pregnant should not take hydralazine unless its possible benefits have been carefully weighed against its risks.

Hydralazine passes into breast milk. Nursing mothers who must take this drug should consider bottle-feeding.

Seniors

Seniors are more sensitive to the blood-pressure-lowering effects of hydralazine and its side effects, especially low body temperature.

Generic Name

Hydroxyzine (hye-DROK-suh-zene) Ⓖ

Brand Names

Atarax   Vistaril

Type of Drug

Antihistamine and antianxiety agent.

Prescribed for

Nausea, vomiting, anxiety, tension, agitation, itching caused by allergy, and sedation; also prescribed in injectable form for acute adult psychiatric emergency including acute alcoholism, surgical sedation, and sedation before or after delivery.

General Information

Hydroxyzine is an antihistamine with antianxiety, muscle-relaxing, antiemetic (antivomiting), bronchial-dilation, pain-relieving, and antispasmodic properties. Hydroxyzine has been used to treat a variety of problems including stress related to dental or other minor surgical procedures, acute emotional problems, anxiety associated with stomach and digestive disorders, skin problems, and behavior difficulties in children.

Cautions and Warnings

Hydroxyzine should not be used if you are **sensitive** or **allergic** to it.

Changes in **heart rhythm** have occurred in people taking this drug to relieve anxiety.

Hydroxyzine may worsen **porphyria,** a rare condition. People with this condition should not take hydroxyzine.

Possible Side Effects

Wheezing, chest tightness, and breathing difficulties are signs of a drug-sensitivity reaction.

▼ Most common: dry mouth and drowsiness. These usually disappear after a few days of continuous use or when the dose is reduced.

▼ Rare: occasional tremors or convulsions at higher doses.

Drug Interactions

• Hydroxyzine depresses the nervous system, producing drowsiness and sleepiness. Do not take this drug with alcohol, tranquilizers, sedatives, or other antihistamines or depressants. When hydroxyzine is taken with one of these drugs, the dose of the latter should be cut in half.

Food Interactions

Take hydroxyzine with food if it upsets your stomach.

Usual Dose

Adult: 25–100 mg 3–4 times a day.
Child (age 6 and over): 5–25 mg 3–4 times a day.
Child (under age 6): 5–10 mg 3–4 times a day.

Overdosage

The most common sign of overdose is sleepiness. Overdose victims should be taken to a hospital emergency room for treatment. ALWAYS bring the prescription bottle or container.

Special Information

Be aware of the depressive effect of hydroxyzine: Be careful when driving, operating hazardous machinery, or doing anything that requires concentration.

The dry mouth associated with taking hydroxyzine may increase your risk of dental cavities and decay. Pay attention to dental hygiene while taking this drug.

If you develop a drug-sensitivity reaction to hydroxyzine (see "Possible Side Effects"), call your doctor.

If you forget a dose of hydroxyzine, take it as soon as you remember. If it is almost time for your next dose, skip the one you forgot and continue with your regular schedule. Do not take a double dose.

Special Populations

Pregnancy/Breast-feeding

Animal studies have shown that regular treatment with hydroxyzine during the first few months of pregnancy may cause birth defects. Do not take any antihistamine without your doctor's knowledge if you are or might be pregnant—especially during the last 3 months of pregnancy—because newborns may have severe reactions to antihistamines.

Hydroxyzine may reduce the amount of breast milk you produce and may pass into breast milk. Nursing mothers who must take hydroxyzine should bottle-feed.

Seniors
Seniors are more sensitive to side effects.

Hytrin   see *Terazosin, page 976*

Hyzaar   see *Angiotensin II Blockers, page 72*

Generic Name
Ibuprofen (EYE-bue-PROE-fen) Ⓖ

Brand Names

Advil*	Ibuprohm
Arthritis Foundation	Menadol
Bayer Select Pain Relief Formula	IBU
	Midol-IB
Children's Advil*	Motrin*
Children's Motrin*	Motrin IB
Dynafed 1B	Nuprin
Genpril	Pediacare Fever Ⓐ
Haltran	Saleto
Ibuprin	

Some products in this brand-name group are alcohol- or sugar-free. Consult your pharmacist.

Type of Drug

Nonsteroidal anti-inflammatory drug (NSAID).

Prescribed for

Rheumatoid arthritis, osteoarthritis, mild to moderate pain, juvenile rheumatoid arthritis, sunburn, menstrual pain, and fever.

General Information

NSAIDs relieve pain and inflammation. NSAIDs may work by blocking the body's production of a hormone called prostaglandin and the action of other body chemicals. They also block both types of cyclooxygenase, COX 1 and COX 2. Most NSAIDs are broken down in the liver and eliminated through the kidneys. Over-the-counter (OTC) doses of ibuprofen provide pain relief within 1 hour; however, anti-inflammatory effects are not usually seen at OTC dosage levels. Ibuprofen's anti-inflammatory effects occur with doses in the prescription range—400 or more mg per dose—and take a week or more to appear.

Cautions and Warnings

People **allergic** to ibuprofen or any other NSAID and those with a history of **asthma** attacks brought on by an NSAID, iodides, or aspirin should not take ibuprofen.

Ibuprofen may cause **gastrointestinal (GI) tract bleeding, ulcers, and perforation**. This can occur at any time, with or without warning, in people who take ibuprofen regularly. People with a history of active GI bleeding should be cautious about taking any NSAID. People who develop these symptoms and continue NSAID treatment should be aware of the possibility of developing more serious side effects.

Ibuprofen can affect platelets and **blood clotting** at high doses and should be avoided by people with clotting problems and those taking warfarin.

People with **heart problems** who use ibuprofen may experience swelling in their arms, legs, or feet.

People taking ibuprofen, especially those with a **collagen disease such as systemic lupus erythematosus,** may experience an unusually severe drug-sensitivity reaction. Report any unusual symptoms to your doctor at once.

Ibuprofen may cause severe toxic effects to the **kidney**. Report any unusual side effects to your doctor, who might need to periodically test your kidney function.

Ibuprofen may make you **unusually sensitive to the effects of the sun**.

Possible Side Effects

▼ Common: diarrhea, nausea, vomiting, constipation, and minor stomach upset, distress, or gas, especially during the first few days of treatment.

▼ Less common: stomach ulcers, GI bleeding, appetite loss, hepatitis, gallbladder attacks, painful urination, poor kidney function, kidney inflammation, blood and protein in the urine, dizziness, fainting, nervousness, depression, hallucinations, confusion, disorientation, tingling in the hands or feet, light-headedness, itching, sweating, dry nose and mouth, heart palpitations, chest pain, breathing difficulties, and muscle cramps.

▼ Rare: severe allergic reactions including closing of the throat, fever and chills, changes in liver function, jaundice (yellowing of the skin and whites of the eyes), and kidney failure. These people must be treated in a hospital emergency room or doctor's office. NSAIDs have caused severe skin reactions; see your doctor immediately if this happens to you.

Drug Interactions

• Ibuprofen may increase the effects of oral anticoagulant (blood-thinning) drugs such as warfarin. Your anticoagulant dose may need to be reduced.

• Ibuprofen may reduce the blood-pressure-lowering effect of beta blocker drugs.

• Combining ibuprofen with cyclosporine may increase the kidney-related side effects of both drugs.

• Ibuprofen may increase digoxin blood levels and toxicity.

• Ibuprofen may increase phenytoin side effects.

• Lithium blood levels and side effects may be increased by ibuprofen.

• Methotrexate side effects may be increased in people also taking ibuprofen.

• Ibuprofen blood levels may be affected by cimetidine.

• Probenecid may increase the risk of NSAID side effects.

• Aspirin and other salicylates should never be combined with ibuprofen in the treatment of arthritis.

Food Interactions

Take ibuprofen with food or a magnesium/aluminum antacid if it upsets your stomach.

Usual Dose

Adult: 200–800 mg 4 times a day depending on the condition being treated; follow your doctor's directions. 200 mg every 4–6 hours is appropriate for mild to moderate pain.

Child: juvenile arthritis—9–18 mg per lb. of body weight a day, divided into several doses.

Overdosage

People have died from NSAID overdoses. Common signs of overdose are drowsiness, nausea, vomiting, diarrhea, abdominal pain, rapid breathing, rapid heartbeat, sweating, ringing or buzzing in the ears, confusion, disorientation, stupor, and coma. Take the victim to a hospital emergency room at once for treatment. ALWAYS bring the prescription bottle or container.

Special Information

Take each dose with a full glass of water and do not lie down for 15 to 30 minutes afterward.

Ibuprofen may make you drowsy or tired: Be careful when driving or operating hazardous equipment. Do not take OTC products containing acetaminophen or aspirin while taking ibuprofen. Avoid alcohol.

Contact your doctor if you develop rash, itching, visual disturbances, weight gain, breathing difficulties, fluid retention, hallucinations, black stools, persistent headache, or any unusual or intolerable side effect.

If you forget a dose of ibuprofen, take it as soon as you remember. If you take several doses a day and it is within 4 hours of your next dose, skip the dose you forgot and continue with your regular schedule. Do not take a double dose.

Special Populations

Pregnancy/Breast-feeding

NSAIDs may affect the developing fetal heart during the last half of pregnancy. Women who are or might become pregnant should not take ibuprofen without their doctor's approval. When the drug is considered crucial by your doctor, its potential benefits must be carefully weighed against its risks.

NSAIDs may pass into breast milk. There is a possibility that a nursing mother taking ibuprofen could affect her baby's heart or cardiovascular system. Nursing mothers who must take this drug should bottle-feed.

Seniors

Seniors, especially those with poor kidney or liver function, may be more susceptible to side effects.

Imdur   see Isorbide Dinitrate, page 530

Generic Name

Imiquimod (ih-MIH-kwih-mod)

Brand Name

Aldara

Type of Drug

Immune modifier.

Prescribed for

Genital warts, perianal warts, and condyloma acuminata.

General Information

Imiquimod has no direct antiviral activity. Animal studies suggest that imiquimod stimulates the skin to produce cytokines, potent natural chemicals that fight the warts, but its actual effect on genital warts and condyloma is not known. In studies of the drug, 50% of people who used it had complete clearance of their warts. But imiquimod is not a cure for genital warts—new ones may develop while others are being treated. Only minimal amounts of imiquimod enter the bloodstream.

Cautions and Warnings

Do not use this product if you are **sensitive** or **allergic** to it.

Imiquimod has not been studied in other viral diseases of the skin, such as papilloma virus, and should not be used to treat them, since its effect is unknown.

Do not apply imiquimod to any area until it has healed from any previous drug or surgery. Imiquimod can worsen skin that is already inflamed.

Possible Side Effects

▼ Most common: redness, itching, erosion of the skin, burning, flaking, abrasions, swelling, and fungal infections in women.

▼ Common: pain, marks on the skin, ulcers, skin scabbing, and headache.

▼ Less common: skin soreness, flu-like symptoms, skin discoloration, muscle aches, fungal infections in men, and diarrhea.

Drug Interactions

• Do not apply imiquimod with other drugs that may cause skin irritation.

Usual Dose

Adult: Apply a thin layer of the cream to external warts and rub it in until the cream disappears. Leave it on the skin for 6–10 hours, then remove the cream with mild soap and water. Do this 3 times a week—for example, Monday, Wednesday, and Friday. Continue treatment for up to 16 weeks or until the warts go away.

Child (under age 18): not recommended.

Overdosage

Overdose is not likely because such a small amount of imiquimod is absorbed through the skin. Accidental ingestion of imiquimod may cause low blood pressure. Anyone who has swallowed imiquimod should be taken to a hospital emergency room. ALWAYS bring the prescription bottle or container.

Special Information

Wash your hands before each application of imiquimod.

Most skin reactions are mild. If you develop a severe skin reaction to imiquimod, call your doctor and remove the cream with a mild soap and water. You can resume treatment with imiquimod after the reaction has completely subsided.

Imiquimod may weaken condoms and vaginal diaphragms. These birth control methods may prove undependable while you are using imiquimod cream. Avoid sexual contact while the cream is on your skin.

Uncircumcised men who use imiquimod to treat warts under the foreskin should retract the foreskin and cleanse the area every day.

Imiquimod is meant to be applied to the skin only. Do not let it get into your eyes, mouth, nose, or other mucous membranes. If you forget to apply a dose of imiquimod, do it as soon as you remember. If you don't remember until your next scheduled application, space the remaining doses equally throughout the rest of the week and continue with your regular schedule.

Special Populations

Pregnancy/Breast-feeding
The safety of using imiquimod during pregnancy is not known. When this drug is considered crucial by your doctor, its potential benefits must be carefully weighed against its risks.

It is not known if imiquimod passes into breast milk. Nursing mothers who must use this drug should consider bottle-feeding.

Seniors
Seniors may use this drug without special precaution.

Imitrex see Triptan-Type Antimigraine Drugs, page 1058

Generic Name
Indinavir (in-DIN-uh-vere)

Brand Name
Crixivan

Type of Drug
Protease inhibitor.

Prescribed for
Human immunodeficiency virus (HIV) infection.

General Information

Part of the multidrug cocktail responsible for the most important gains in the fight against acquired immunodeficiency syndrome (AIDS), indinavir sulfate belongs to a group of anti-HIV drugs called protease inhibitors. Triple-drug cocktails were considered responsible for the first overall reduction in the AIDS death rate, recorded in 1996. Protease inhibitors work in a unique way but are not a cure for HIV infection or AIDS. When the HIV virus attacks a cell, it must be converted into viral DNA. Older drugs, known as reverse transcriptase inhibitors, interfere with this step, but they need help in fighting HIV. Protease inhibitors work at the end of the HIV reproduction process, when proteins are "cut" into strands of exactly the right size to duplicate HIV. The protein is cut by a protease enzyme. Protease inhibitors prevent the mature HIV virus from being formed by interfering with this cutting process. Proteins that are cut to the wrong length or that remain uncut are inactive.

Protease inhibitors are always taken with 1 or 2 other nucleoside antiviral drugs such as AZT, ddI, ddC, or 3TC. Protease inhibitors revolutionized HIV treatment because, when taken in combination, they reduce the amount of HIV virus in the bloodstream to levels that are undetectable by current methods—CD_4 cell (immune system cell) counts and viral load (amount of virus in the blood) measurements. Multiple drug therapy has changed the current view of HIV from a fatal disease to a manageable chronic illness. Newer approaches are exploring multiple protease-inhibitor treatment.

People taking a protease inhibitor may still develop infections or other conditions associated with HIV disease. Because of this, it is very important for you to remain under the care of a doctor or other health care provider. The long-term effects of indinavir are not known. You may be able to pass the HIV virus to others even if you are on triple-drug therapy.

Cautions and Warnings

Do not take indinavir if you are **allergic** to it. People with mild or moderate **liver disease** or **cirrhosis** break down indinavir more slowly than those with normal liver function and may be more likely to develop side effects. People with cirrhosis should receive a reduced dose of indinavir.

About 4 of every 100 people taking indinavir can develop a **kidney stone,** indicated by pain in the middle to lower abdomen or back, or painful urination. Drinking at least 6 full glasses of liquid—48 oz.—a day will reduce your risk of developing a stone.

Indinavir may raise blood sugar, worsen diabetes, or bring out latent diabetes. Diabetics who take indinavir may have to have the dose of their antidiabetes medication adjusted against this effect.

Indinavir interferes with the liver's ability to break down terfenadine, astemizole, cisapride, triazolam, and midazolam. Do not combine indinavir with any of these drugs, as severe side effects may result.

Possible Side Effects

▼ Most common: nausea, abdominal pain, and headache.

▼ Common: weakness or fatigue, pain in the side, diarrhea, vomiting, changes in sense of taste, acid regurgitation, and sleeplessness.

▼ Less common: dizziness, drowsiness, and back pain.

▼ Rare: Rare side effects can occur in almost any part of the body. Contact your doctor if you experience any side effect not listed above.

Drug Interactions

• Rifampin reduces the amount of indinavir in the blood. Do not combine these drugs.

• Indinavir interferes with the liver's ability to break down terfenadine, astemizole, cisapride, triazolam, and midazolam. Do not combine indinavir with any of these drugs, as severe side effects may result.

• Combining indinavir with clarithromycin or with zidovudine increases the amount of each drug in the blood. Combining indinavir with isoniazid increases the amount of isoniazid in the blood.

• Combining indinavir with rifabutin can reduce the amount of indinavir absorbed into the blood by ⅓ and double the amount of rifabutin absorbed.

• Didanosine (ddI) interferes with the absorption of indinavir into the body. If you need both of these medications, take them at least 1 hour apart.

• Combining fluconazole with indinavir reduces the amount of indinavir in the blood by about 20%.

• Combining indinavir with ketoconazole increases the amount of indinavir in the blood by about 65%.

• Combining indinavir with quinidine raises indinavir levels by about 10%.

• Taking indinavir with zidovudine and lamivudine results in ⅓ more zidovudine in the blood and small decreases in lamivudine blood levels.

• Indinavir raises the amount of stavudine absorbed into the blood by 25% and the amount of trimethoprim by about 20%.

• Combining indinavir with oral contraceptives can result in higher blood hormone levels. This may lead to an excess of hormone-related side effects. If this happens to you, your doctor may be able to lower the dose of your contraceptive pills.

Food Interactions

Indinavir is best taken with water—or liquids such as skim milk, juice, coffee—at least 1 hour before or 2 hours after a meal. You should not eat meals that are high in calories, fat, and protein from 1 hour before to 2 hours after taking indinavir. You may take indinavir with a light meal.

Usual Dose

Adult: 800 mg every 8 hours, around the clock. People with cirrhosis should take 600 mg every 8 hours.

Child: not recommended.

Overdosage

Little is known about the effects of indinavir overdose except that it may cause severe drug side effects. Take overdose victims to a hospital emergency room at once. ALWAYS bring the prescription bottle or container.

Special Information

Indinavir does not cure HIV. It will not prevent you from transmitting HIV to another person; you must still practice safe sex.

It is imperative to take your HIV medication exactly as prescribed. Missing doses of indinavir makes you more likely to become resistant to the drug and to lose the benefits of therapy.

- Call your doctor if you develop pains in the middle to lower abdomen, back pain, or painful urination. Drink at least 48 oz. of liquid each day—for example, six 8-oz. glasses.

Stay in close touch with your doctor while taking indinavir and report anything unusual.

If you forget a dose of indinavir, take it as soon as you remember. If it is almost time for your next dose, skip the dose you forgot and continue with your regular schedule. Do not take a double dose.

Special Populations

Pregnancy/Breast-feeding

There is little information on how indinavir affects pregnant women and their fetuses. Pregnant women should take this drug with caution.

Indinavir passes into breast milk. Women with HIV and nursing mothers who must take indinavir should bottle-feed.

Seniors

Seniors may take indinavir without special restriction.

Generic Name

Indomethacin (IN-doe-METH-uh-sin) G

Brand Names

Indochron E-R   Indocin SR
Indocin

Type of Drug

Nonsteroidal anti-inflammatory drug (NSAID).

Prescribed for

Rheumatoid arthritis; osteoarthritis; ankylosing spondylitis; menstrual pain; tendinitis; bursitis; painful shoulder; gout—except Indocin SR; sunburn; migraine and cluster headache—except Indocin SR. Indomethacin has been used to prevent premature labor, to treat a rare condition in premature infants called patent ductus arteriosus, and (in eyedrop form) to treat a severe and unusual inflammation in the retina.

General Information

Indomethacin and other NSAIDs are used to relieve pain and inflammation. We do not know exactly how NSAIDs work, but they may achieve their effects by blocking the body's production of a hormone called prostaglandin and the action of other body chemicals. Pain relief comes about 30 minutes after taking the first dose of indomethacin and lasts for 4 to 6 hours, but its anti-inflammatory effect takes a week to become apparent and may take 2 weeks to reach maximum effect. Indomethacin is broken down in the liver and eliminated through the kidneys.

Cautions and Warnings

People **allergic** to indomethacin or any other NSAID and those with a history of **asthma** attacks brought on by an NSAID, iodides, or aspirin should not take indomethacin.

Indomethacin may cause **gastrointestinal (GI) bleeding, ulcers,** and **stomach perforation,** which can occur at any time, with or without warning, in people who take indomethacin regularly. People with a history of active GI bleeding should be cautious about taking any NSAID. People who develop bleeding or ulcers and continue NSAID treatment may develop more serious side effects.

Indomethacin may affect platelets and **blood clotting** at high doses and should be avoided by people with clotting problems and those taking warfarin.

People with **heart problems** who use indomethacin may experience swelling in their arms, legs, or feet.

Indomethacin should not be used by people who have had **ulcers or other stomach lesions**.

Indomethacin may worsen **depression or other psychiatric disorders, epilepsy, and parkinsonism.**

Indomethacin should never be used as "first therapy" for any disorder, with the possible exception of ankylosing spondylitis, because of the severe side effects associated with this drug.

Indomethacin may cause severe toxic effects to the **kidney.** Report any unusual side effects to your doctor, who might need to periodically test your kidney function.

Indomethacin may make you **unusually sensitive to the effects of the sun**.

Possible Side Effects

▼ Most common: diarrhea, nausea, vomiting, constipation, stomach gas, stomach upset or irritation, and appetite loss, especially during the first few days of treatment.

▼ Less common: stomach ulcers, GI bleeding, hepatitis, gallbladder attacks, painful urination, poor kidney function, kidney inflammation, blood and protein in the urine, dizziness, fainting, nervousness, depression, hallucinations, confusion, disorientation, tingling in the hands or feet, light-headedness, itching, increased sweating, dry nose and mouth, heart palpitations, chest pain, breathing difficulties, and muscle cramps.

▼ Rare: severe allergic reactions including closing of the throat, fever and chills, changes in liver function, jaundice (yellowing of the skin or whites of the eyes), and kidney failure. People who experience such effects must be promptly treated in a hospital emergency room or doctor's office. NSAIDs have caused severe skin reactions; if this happens to you, see your doctor immediately.

Drug Interactions

• Indomethacin may increase the effects of oral anticoagulant (blood-thinning) drugs such as warfarin. Your anticoagulant dose may need to be reduced.

• Indomethacin may reduce the effects of thiazide diuretics.

• Combining diflunisal and indomethacin has resulted in fatal GI hemorrhage.

• Indomethacin may reduce the blood-pressure-lowering effect of beta blockers, angiotensin-converting enzyme (ACE) inhibitor drugs, and loop diuretics.

• Taking indomethacin with cyclosporine may increase the kidney-related side effects of both drugs. Methotrexate side effects may be increased in people also taking indomethacin.

• Indomethacin may increase digoxin levels in the blood.

• Combining indomethacin with phenylpropanolamine—found in many over-the-counter (OTC) drug products—may cause an increase in blood pressure.

• Combining indomethacin and dipyridamole may increase water retention.

• Indomethacin may increase phenytoin's side effects.

• Lithium blood levels may be increased by indomethacin.

• Indomethacin blood levels may be affected by cimetidine.

• Probenecid may increase the risk of indomethacin side effects.

• Aspirin and other salicylates should never be combined with indomethacin to treat arthritis.

Food Interactions

Take indomethacin with a glass of water, food, or a magnesium/aluminum antacid to avoid an upset stomach.

Usual Dose

Adult and Child (age 15 and over): 50–200 mg a day, individualized to your needs.

Child (under age 15): not recommended.

Overdosage

People have died from NSAID overdoses. Common signs of overdose are drowsiness, nausea, vomiting, diarrhea, abdominal pain, rapid breathing, rapid heartbeat, increased sweating, ringing or buzzing in the ears, confusion, disorientation, stupor, and coma. Take the victim to a hospital emergency room at once. ALWAYS bring the prescription bottle or container.

Special Information

Take each dose with a full glass of water and do not lie down for 15 to 30 minutes afterward.

Indomethacin can make you drowsy or tired: Be careful when driving or operating hazardous equipment. Do not take any OTC products containing acetaminophen or aspirin while taking indomethacin. Avoid alcohol.

Contact your doctor if you develop rash or itching, visual disturbances, weight gain, breathing difficulties, fluid retention, hallucinations, black or tarry stools, persistent headache, or any unusual or intolerable side effect.

If you forget a dose of indomethacin, take it as soon as you remember. If you take indomethacin once a day and it is within 8 hours of your next dose, or if you take several doses a day and it is within 4 hours of your next dose, skip the dose you forgot and continue with your regular schedule. Never take a double dose.

Special Populations

Pregnancy/Breast-feeding
Indomethacin may affect the developing fetal heart if used during the second half of pregnancy. Pregnant women should not take indomethacin without their doctor's approval. When the drug is considered crucial by your doctor, its potential benefits must be carefully weighed against its risks.

Indomethacin may pass into breast milk. There is a possibility that the heart of a nursing baby could be affected by indomethacin. Nursing mothers who must take indomethacin should bottle-feed.

Seniors
Seniors may be more susceptible to side effects, especially ulcer disease.

Generic Name

Infliximab (in-FLIX-ih-mab)

Brand Name

Remicade

Type of Drug

Monoclonal antibody.

Prescribed for

Crohn's disease.

General Information

High levels of tumor necrosis factor (TNFα), which plays an important role in the inflammatory process, are linked to the worsening of Crohn's disease. Infliximab neutralizes TNFα so that it cannot exert its effects. TNFα levels have been found to correlate with the severity of Crohn's disease.

Cautions and Warnings

Do not take infliximab if you are **allergic** to it.

The safety and effectiveness of more than 3 infliximab infusions are not known.

Infliximab may cause **allergic reactions** including itching, breathing difficulties, and low blood pressure (symptoms include dizziness and fainting). These reactions may require emergency treatment. **Lupus erythematosus** may develop but goes away once drug treatment is stopped.

People with **compromised immune systems** should be cautious about using this drug because it can suppress immune function.

Possible Side Effects

Most people (8 of 10) experience more than 1 side effect. Sixteen percent develop a reaction to the drug within 2 hours. Those reactions include fever, chills, itching, rash, chest pain, low blood pressure, and breathing difficulties.

▼ Most common: headache, nausea, upper respiratory infection, abdominal pain, fatigue, and fever.

▼ Common: sore throat, vomiting, pain, dizziness, bronchitis, rash, runny nose, chest pain, coughing, itching, sinus inflammation, muscle aches, back pain, and fungus infection.

▼ Less common: Less common side effects can occur in almost any part of the body. Contact your doctor if you experience any side effect not listed above.

Drug Interactions

• Infliximab should not be combined with any drug infused into the bloodstream.

Food Interactions

None known.

Usual Dose

Adult: 2.25 mg per lb. of body weight. Another dose may be given 2 and 6 weeks after the first injection.

Child: not recommended.

Overdosage

Symptoms may include drug side effects. Take the victim to a hospital emergency room.

Special Populations

Pregnancy/Breast-feeding

The safety of taking infliximab during pregnancy is not known. When this drug is considered crucial by your doctor, its potential benefits must be carefully weighed against its risks.

It is not known if infliximab passes into breast milk. Nursing mothers who must take it should bottle-feed.

Seniors

Seniors may be more likely to develop infections while taking this drug.

Generic Name

Insulin (IN-suh-lin)

Most Common Brand Names

Humalog	Humulin 70/30
Humulin N	Novolin 70/30
Humulin R (regular insulin)	

Type of Drug

Antidiabetic.

Prescribed for

Type I and type II diabetes mellitus; may also be prescribed for hyperkalemia (high blood-potassium levels) and for severe complications of diabetes such as ketoacidosis (diabetic coma).

General Information

Insulin, a hormone made in the pancreas, helps the body turn food into energy. Also, insulin helps us store energy that we can use later. Insulin works by helping sugar enter body cells to make fat, sugar, and protein. Between meals, insulin helps us use the fat, sugar, and protein we have stored. In diabetes mellitus, the body does not make enough insulin to meet its needs or does not properly use the insulin it makes. Without insulin, glucose cannot get into body cells and the cells will not work properly. Insulin dosage must be balanced against the amount and type of food eaten and the amount of exercise you do. Blood glucose can drop too low or rise too high if diet and/or exercise change without modifying insulin dosage. The most widely used variety is human insulin. It is identical to natural human insulin but it is manufactured by semisynthetic or recombinant DNA methods. Semisynthetic insulins start with an animal product and may contain some impurities. Other types of insulin can be obtained from beef or pork pancreas glands. At present, all types of insulin must be injected because insulin is destroyed by stomach acid. An inhalable insulin is being developed.

People whose diabetes is well controlled by insulin derived from an animal source should not automatically be switched to a human insulin product, but people newly diagnosed with the disease are usually treated with highly purified synthetic human insulin. Human insulin is also the product of choice for people allergic to other insulin products, pregnant women with diabetes, and people who require insulin only during surgery or for short periods of time.

Regular insulin starts to work quickly and lasts only 6 to 8 hours. Prompt Insulin Zinc Suspension—also called Semilente Insulin—is also considered rapid-acting. It starts to work in 30 to 60 minutes and lasts 12 to 16 hours. The intermediate-acting insulins—NPH or Isophane Insulin and Lente or Insulin Zinc Suspension—start working 1 to 2½ hours after injection and continue to work for 24 hours. Long-acting insulins—PZI or Protamine Zinc Insulin Suspension and Ultralente or Extended Insulin Zinc Suspension—begin working in 4 to 8 hours and last for 36 hours or more. Other factors that influence insulin response include diet, exercise, and the use of other drugs.

Cautions and Warnings

Take the **exact dose** of insulin prescribed. Too much insulin will excessively lower blood sugar, and too little will not control diabetes. **Do not change insulin brands or types** unless you are under direct medical supervision. Follow the diet prescribed by your doctor and avoid alcohol.

Low blood sugar (see "Overdosage" for symptoms) can result from taking too much insulin, doing excess physical work or exercise without eating, not absorbing food normally because meals are postponed or skipped, or because of illness with vomiting, fever, or diarrhea. You may be able to correct the imbalance by eating sugar, food with sugar, or a commercial 40% glucose product. The symptoms of low blood sugar are less pronounced if you are taking human insulin.

Possible Side Effects

▼ Most common: allergic reactions, a depression in the skin at the site of injection, and accumulation of fat under the skin from repeatedly using the same injection site.

Drug Interactions

• Your insulin dosage may need to be raised if you are taking drugs that increase blood-sugar levels. These include corticosteroids, oral contraceptives ("the pill"), dextrothyroxine, diltiazem, dobutamine, epinephrine, cigarettes, thiazide-type diuretics, thyroid hormones, estrogens, furosemide, molindone, phenytoin, and ethacrynic acid.

• Other drugs can lower blood sugar and may require a reduced insulin dosage. These include alcohol, anabolic steroids, beta-blocking drugs, clofibrate, fenfluramine, phenylbutazone, sulfinpyrazone, tetracycline, guanethidine, monoamine oxidase inhibitor (MAOI) antidepressants, and large doses of aspirin.

• Oral antidiabetes drugs also lower blood sugar and should be taken with insulin only under the direct supervision of a doctor. Nonsteroidal anti-inflammatory drugs (NSAIDs) may also increase the blood-sugar-lowering effect of insulin.

• Beta-blocking drugs can mask the symptoms of low blood sugar and thus increase the risk of taking insulin.

• Quitting smoking—regardless of whether you are using a nicotine patch or gum, or another smoking deterrent—can also lower blood sugar. Lowering insulin dosage may be necessary if you stop smoking.

• Insulin may affect blood-potassium levels and digitalis drugs.

Food Interactions

Follow your doctor's directions for diet restrictions.

Usual Dose

Dosage must be individualized. Insulin is generally injected 30 minutes before meals; the longer-acting forms are taken a half hour before breakfast. People with diabetes must self-administer insulin subcutaneously (under the skin) or have a family member or friend give them injections. Hospitalized patients may receive insulin injection directly into a vein.

Overdosage

Accidental ingestion has little or no effect. Injecting too much insulin causes an insulin reaction or low blood sugar. Symptoms occur suddenly and include weakness, fatigue, nervousness, confusion, headache, double vision, convulsions, dizziness, psychoses, unconsciousness, rapid and shallow breathing, numbness or tingling around the mouth, hunger, nausea, loss of skin color, dry skin, and pulse changes. Overdose victims should eat chocolate, candy, or another sugar source at once to raise blood-sugar levels.

The symptoms of an insulin reaction are different from those of ketoacidosis coma. Insulin coma develops in hours or days; the symptoms are drowsiness, dim vision, a feeling that you cannot get enough air, thirst, nausea, vomiting, breath that smells like acetone (nail polish remover), abdominal pain, loss of appetite, dry and red skin, and rapid pulse. Go to an emergency room or call your doctor immediately if either of these groups of symptoms occur.

Special Information

Use the same brand and strength of insulin and insulin syringes or administration devices to avoid dosage errors. Rotate injection sites to prevent fat loss at the site.

Mix insulins according to your doctor's directions; do not change the method or order of mixing.

You may develop low blood sugar (see "Overdosage" for symptoms) if you take too much insulin, work or exercise more strenuously than usual, skip a meal, take insulin too long before a meal, or vomit before a meal. To help raise low blood sugar, eat a candy bar or lump of sugar, which you should carry with you at all times. If the signs of low blood sugar do not clear up within 30 minutes, call your doctor. You may need further treatment.

Your insulin requirements may change if you get sick, especially if you vomit or have a fever.

If your insulin is in suspension form, you must evenly distribute the particles throughout the liquid before taking the dose out. Do this by gently rotating the vial and turning it over several times. Do not shake the vial.

People with diabetes must maintain good dental hygiene because of their increased risk of developing oral infections. Be sure your dentist knows you have diabetes.

Have your eyes checked regularly.

Read and follow all patient information provided with insulin products. Monitor your blood and urine regularly for sugar and ketones.

Insulin products are generally stable at room temperature for about 2 years. They must be kept away from direct sunlight and extreme temperatures. Most manufacturers recommend that insulin be stored in a refrigerator or another cool place though it should not be put in a freezer. Partly used vials of insulin should be thrown away after several weeks if not used. Do not use any insulin that looks lumpy or grainy or that sticks to the bottle. Regular insulin should be clear and colorless; do not use it if it is thick or cloudy.

Some insulin products can be mixed. Mix 2 or more different insulins only if you have been so directed by your doctor. Your pharmacist may also mix your insulins to ensure accuracy. Insulin for injection may be mixed with Isophane Insulin Suspension and Protamine Zinc Insulin in any proportion. Insulin Zinc Suspension, Insulin Zinc Suspension (Prompt), and Insulin Zinc Suspension (Extended) may also be mixed in any proportion. Insulin for injection and Insulin Zinc Suspension must be mixed immediately before using.

If you forget a dose, take it as soon as you remember. If it is almost time for your next dose, or if you completely forget 1 or more doses, call your doctor for exact instructions.

Special Populations

Pregnancy/Breast-feeding

Insulin (human) is the preferred method for controlling diabetes in pregnant women. These women must follow their doctor's directions for insulin use exactly, because insulin requirements normally decrease during the first half of pregnancy and then increase during the second half.

Insulin does not pass into breast milk. Breast-feeding can reduce your insulin needs, so your doctor should closely monitor your insulin dosage during this period.

Seniors
Seniors may use insulin without special restriction.

Generic Name

Interferon Alfa-n1 (in-ter-FEER-on AL-fuh)

Brand Name
Wellferon

Type of Drug
Antiviral.

Prescribed for
Hepatitis C.

General Information

Interferon alfa-n1 lymphoblastoid attaches to the surface of an infected cell and stimulates a complicated set of reactions. These reactions lead to the production of enzymes inside the cell that prevent the hepatitis C virus from reproducing. Other causes of hepatitis do not respond to interferon treatment.

Cautions and Warnings

People taking this drug must be closely monitored by their doctors and receive periodic blood tests and liver and thyroid function tests.

Serious and life-threatening **allergic or drug-sensitivity reactions** can develop including an itchy rash, swelling, and breathing difficulties.

People with **kidney or heart disease** should use this drug with caution. If heart disease worsens during treatment, the drug should be discontinued.

Interferon alfa-n1 may worsen **liver disease**.

By affecting the nervous system, interferon alfa-n1 may cause **seizures, coma, dizziness, memory loss, agitation, psy-**

chosis, and complete loss of sensation. These effects generally go away when the drug is stopped.

Interferon alfa-n1 may cause **menstrual problems** or interfere with **ovulation**.

People who develop **severe side effects** or become **depressed** while taking this drug should have their dosage temporarily lowered. The drug should be stopped if depression is severe.

It is not known if this drug is safe for **children**.

Possible Side Effects

▼ Most common: anxiety, sleep disturbances, depression, hair loss, nausea, diarrhea, abdominal pain, muscle or joint pain, weakness, headache, fever, chills, injection-site reactions, back pain, and generalized pain.

▼ Common: dizziness, confusion, abnormal thought patterns, memory loss, tingling in the hands or feet, rash, dry skin, sweating, vomiting, appetite loss, weight loss, cough, bronchitis, breathing difficulties, pneumonia, pleurisy, lung problems, runny nose, and sore throat.

▼ Less common: poor vision, abnormal heart rhythms, high blood pressure, chest pain, high blood sugar, thyroid problems, urinary infection, low sex drive, accidental injury, liver problems, migraine, increased sensitivity to the sun, psoriasis, attempted suicide, seizures, and a ruptured spleen.

▼ Rare: blood in the urine, eye problems, rheumatoid arthritis, lupus and other autoimmune conditions, painful spasms of blood vessels in the legs, and worsening of diabetes and thyroid problems.

Drug Interactions

• Interferon alfa-n1 may interfere with the breakdown of vinblastine, zidovudine (also known as AZT), and theophylline.

Food Interactions

None known.

Usual Dose

Adult: One 3-megaunit (MU) subcutaneous or intramuscular injection 3 times a week for 1 year. People who cannot tolerate this dosage should have it reduced by half.

Overdosage

Symptoms may include increased side effects and changes in lab test results. Seizures have occurred at high dosages. Repeated overdose may cause lethargy or coma. Call your local poison control center or a hospital emergency room for more information. If you seek treatment, ALWAYS bring the prescription bottle or container.

Special Information

This drug does not prevent you from giving hepatitis C to others through unprotected sex or contact with blood or other body fluids.

People who do not respond to interferon alfa-n1 treatment in 1 year are not likely to benefit from this medication.

People who have a seizure disorder or other nervous system problem, low white-blood-cell or blood-platelet count, or asthma or other breathing problems, or who take drugs that depress bone marrow function may be especially sensitive to the effects of interferon alfa-n1.

Properly dispose of medication needles and syringes. Do not reuse them.

Ibuprofen, aspirin, and other anti-inflammatory drugs may alleviate some of the discomfort associated with starting interferon alfa-n1.

This drug must be stored in the refrigerator and protected from light. Do not shake or freeze it.

Special Populations

Pregnancy/Breast-feeding

Animal studies suggest that interferon alfa-n1 may harm the fetus and cause spontaneous abortion. When this drug is considered crucial by your doctor, its potential benefits must be carefully weighed against its risks.

It is not known if this drug passes into breast milk. Nursing mothers who must take it should bottle-feed.

Seniors

Seniors with liver, kidney, or heart conditions should use this drug with caution.

Generic Name

Interferon Beta (in-ter-FEER-on BAY-tuh)

Brand Names

Avonex (interferon beta-1a)
Betaseron (interferon beta-1b)

Type of Drug

Multiple sclerosis (MS) therapy.

Prescribed for

MS.

General Information

MS is an inflammatory disease in which protective myelin sheaths of the central nervous system are broken down by immune-system abnormalities. This leads to gradual and progressive loss of muscle tone and function, progressive weakness, and paralysis. Exacerbations—episodes of MS in which the disease worsens—develop slowly and may not recede for weeks or months. Interferon beta drugs are used to treat the relapsing-remitting form of the disease—about 66% of MS sufferers have it—in which stable periods are followed by periods of worsening. Until now, MS treatment has been aimed at controlling symptoms. Interferon beta can help reduce the number and severity of MS flare-ups.

Interferon beta is also being studied for acquired immunodeficiency syndrome (AIDS), AIDS-related Kaposi's sarcoma, cancer, herpes, and hepatitis.

Cautions and Warnings

Do not take interferon beta if you are **allergic** to it or human albumin.

The safety and benefit of interferon beta in **chronic progressive MS** is unproven.

People taking interferon beta in studies had potentially severe **depression** and suicidal tendencies, but the drug was judged not to be the cause.

People with **seizure** disorders may be more likely to develop a seizure while taking interferon beta.

Up to 75% of people who take interferon beta are likely to develop **flu-like symptoms** including fever, chills, muscle aches, sweating, and feeling unwell. These symptoms may prove stressful to people with **heart disease**.

Interferon beta may cause **increased sensitivity to the sun**. Wear protective clothing and use sunscreen.

Possible Side Effects

In general, interferon beta-1a has fewer side effects than interferon beta-1b.

Interferon Beta-1a

▼ Most common: respiratory infection, sinusitis, headache, fever, weakness, chills, dizziness, muscle aches, abdominal pain, flu-like symptoms, painful menstruation, diarrhea, nausea, upset stomach, and sleeping difficulties.

▼ Less common: swelling, pelvic pain, cyst, thyroid goiter, heart palpitations, bleeding, laryngitis, breathing difficulties, joint pain, stiffness, tiredness, speech problems, convulsions, uncontrolled movements, hair loss, urinary urgency, and cystitis. Pain, burning, or stinging at the injection site may also occur.

▼ Rare: Rare side effects can occur in almost any part of the body. Contact your doctor if you experience any side effect not listed above.

Interferon Beta-1b

▼ Most common: pain, burning, or stinging at the injection site, sinusitis, headache, migraine, fever, weakness, chills, muscle ache, abdominal pain, flu-like symptoms, menstrual disorders, painful menstruation, constipation, vomiting, liver inflammation, sweating, and reduced white-blood-cell count.

▼ Less common: itching, swelling, pelvic pain, cyst, thyroid goiter, heart palpitations, high blood pressure, rapid heartbeat, bleeding, laryngitis, breathing difficulties, muscle weakness, stiffness, tiredness, speech problems, convulsions, uncontrolled movements, visual disturbances or conjunctivitis (pinkeye), urinary urgency, cystitis, breast pain, cystic breast disease, breast cancer, and weight changes.

▼ Rare: Rare side effects can occur in almost any part of the body. Contact your doctor if you experience any side effect not listed above.

Food and Drug Interactions

None known.

Usual Dose

Interferon Beta-1a: 30 mcg once a week by intramuscular injection.

Interferon Beta-1b: 8 million units (250 mcg) every other day by subcutaneous injection.

This drug may be self-administered.

Overdosage

Little is known about the effects of interferon beta overdose. Symptoms may include exaggerated side effects. Call your local poison control center or a hospital emergency room for more information. If you seek treatment, ALWAYS bring the prescription bottle or container.

Special Information

Interferon Beta-1a: Interferon beta-1a may be associated with severe depression. Mood swings or changes, lack of interest in daily activities, excessive sleep, and other possible signs of depression should be reported to your doctor at once.

If you forget to administer a dose, do so as soon as you remember. If it is almost time for your next dose, skip the one you forgot and continue with your regular schedule. Do not take a double dose.

Interferon Beta-1b: Interferon beta-1b may be associated with severe depression. Mood swings or changes, lack of interest in daily activities, excessive sleep, and other possible signs of depression should be reported to your doctor at once.

If you forget to administer a dose, do so as soon as you remember. If it is almost time for your next dose, skip the one you forgot and continue with your regular schedule. Do not take a double dose.

Special Populations

Pregnancy/Breast-feeding

Animal studies show that interferon beta may cause abortion. Women who are or might be pregnant should not use this drug.

It is not known if interferon beta passes into breast milk. Nursing mothers who must take it should consider bottle-feeding.

Seniors
Seniors may use this drug without special restriction.

Generic Name

Ipratropium (ipe-ruh-TROE-pee-um) [G]

Brand Name

Atrovent

Combination Product

Generic Ingredients: Ipratropium Bromide + Albuterol Sulfate
Combivent

Type of Drug

Anticholinergic.

Prescribed for

Bronchospasm associated with bronchitis, emphysema, and other chronic lung diseases; also prescribed for runny nose.

General Information

Ipratropium bromide is related to atropine sulfate, another anticholinergic drug. Ipratropium works against natural acetylcholine in the bronchial muscles, causing them to dilate. It has little effect on other parts of the body. Much of each inhaled dose is swallowed and passes out of the body in the stool. Like all anticholinergic drugs, ipratropium has a drying effect; the nasal spray provides relief from runny nose.

Cautions and Warnings

Do not use ipratropium if you are **allergic** to atropine or to any related product. It should be used with caution if you have **glaucoma, prostate disease,** or **bladder obstruction**.

Ipratropium is not meant for the treatment of acute bronchospasm. This drug should be used only to prevent bronchospasm associated with chronic lung diseases.

Possible Side Effects

Generally, ipratropium side effects are infrequent and mild.

Inhalation
 ▼ Most common: nervousness, dizziness, headache, nausea, upset stomach, blurred vision, sensitivity to bright light, dry mouth, throat irritation, cough, worsening of symptoms, heart palpitations, rash, and mouth irritation.
 ▼ Less common: rapid heartbeat, urinary difficulties, tingling in the hands or feet, poor coordination, itching, hives, flushing, loss of hair, constipation, tremors, fatigue or sleeplessness, and hoarseness.
 ▼ Rare: worsening of glaucoma, eye pain, low blood pressure, and severe skin reactions.

Nasal Spray
 ▼ Most common: nosebleeds and nasal dryness.
 ▼ Less common: dry mouth or throat and stuffed nose.
 ▼ Rare: changes in sense of taste, nasal burning, red and itchy eyes, coughing, dizziness, hoarseness, heart palpitations, rapid heartbeat, thirst, ringing or buzzing in the ears, blurred vision, and difficulty urinating.

Drug Interactions

None known.

Food Interactions

Do not inhale a dose of ipratropium if you have any food in your mouth.

Usual Dose

Inhalation
 Adult and Child (age 12 and over): 2 inhalations—36 mcg—4 times a day; no more than 12 inhalations every 24 hours.
 Child (under age 12): not recommended.

Nasal Spray
 Adult and Child (age 5 and over): 2 sprays of 0.03% solution per nostril up to 4 times a day.

Overdosage

The risk of overdose is small because very little ipratropium is absorbed into the bloodstream. Ipratropium accidentally sprayed into the eye will cause blurred vision. ALWAYS bring the prescription bottle or container with you if you go to an emergency room for treatment.

Special Information

Use this product according to your doctor's instructions. Do not stop taking ipratropium without your doctor's approval even if you feel well.

Call your doctor if you develop rash or hives, sores on the mouth or lips, blurred vision, or other side effects that are bothersome or persistent.

Call your doctor if you stop responding to your usual dose of ipratropium: This may be a sign that your condition has worsened.

Prolonged use of ipratropium may decrease or stop the flow of saliva produced in your mouth. This can expose you to an increased chance of cavities, gum disease, oral infections, and other problems. Dry mouth can be relieved with hard candies or regular fluids. Increased attention to dental hygiene is important.

If, in addition to ipratropium, you use a corticosteroid inhaler or cromolyn sodium for lung disease, use the ipratropium about 5 minutes before the other inhaler.

If you take ipratropium and albuterol, metaproterenol, or another beta-stimulating aerosol product for bronchial disease, use the beta stimulator about 5 minutes before ipratropium unless otherwise instructed by your doctor. Ipratropium solution for inhalation can be mixed with albuterol or metaproterenol for inhalation so long as the mixture is used within 1 hour. The combination product Combivent (a mixture of ipratropium and albuterol) is also available.

The first use of each ipratropium nasal pump requires 7 pumps to prime the spray. Regular use of the spray should prevent the need to prime the pump again. If you do not use the spray for a day, you will have to pump twice to prime the spray. If you do not use the spray for a week, you will have to prime the spray again with 7 pumps.

If you forget to administer a dose of ipratropium, do so as soon as you remember. If it is almost time for your next dose, skip the one you forgot and continue with your regular schedule. Do not take a double dose.

Store this product at room temperature—59° to 86°F—and avoid freezing. Unused vials of the solution for inhalation should be stored in their foil wrapper.

Special Populations

Pregnancy/Breast-feeding
Massive oral doses of ipratropium have caused birth defects in animals. Ipratropium should be used during pregnancy only if clearly needed.

It is not known if ipratropium passes into breast milk. Nursing mothers who must take this drug should consider bottle-feeding.

Seniors
Seniors, especially those with prostate disease, may be more sensitive to the side effects of this drug and may require a dosage adjustment.

Type of Drug
Iron Supplements

Brand Names

Generic Ingredient: Carbonyl Iron, 100% Iron
Feosol

Generic Ingredient: Ferrous Fumarate ⬜G*, 33% Iron*

Femiron	Ircon
Feostat	Nepmo-Fer ⬜$
Ferro-Sequels	Vitron-C ⬜$
Hemocyte	

Generic Ingredient: Ferrous Gluconate ⬜G*, 12% Iron*
Fergon

Ferrous Sulfate ⬜G*, 20% to 30% Iron*

ED-IN-SOL	Fer-In-Sol
Feosol	Slow-FE
Feratab	FE^{50}
Fer-Gen-Sol	

Generic Ingredient: Polysaccharide Iron Complex

Hytinic   Nu-Iron ⑤
Niferex ⑤   Nu-Iron 150
Niferex-150

Prescribed for

Iron-deficiency anemia.

General Information

Iron supplements are used to treat anemias that result from iron deficiency. Iron is incorporated into red blood cells, which carry oxygen throughout the body. Iron is absorbed only in a small section of the gastrointestinal (GI) tract called the duodenum, the upper part of the small intestine. Sustained-release iron products should be used only to help minimize the stomach discomfort that iron supplements can cause, as some of the drug in these forms may bypass the duodenum and not be absorbed. Other products combining iron with vitamins or special extracts may also be used to treat iron-deficiency anemia. Iron supplements are available in many different forms and they all have different amounts of iron. When choosing an iron supplement, you must be sure to take one that gives you the amount of elemental iron you need.

Cautions and Warnings

Do not take an iron supplement if you have **hemochromatosis, hemosiderosis,** or a **hemolytic anemia**.

Do not take iron supplements if you have a history of **stomach problems, peptic ulcer,** or **ulcerative colitis**. People with normal iron levels should not take any iron product on a regular basis.

Possible Side Effects

▼ Common: stomach upset or irritation, nausea, diarrhea, constipation, appetite loss, and darkened stools.

Drug Interactions

• Iron and tetracycline interfere with each other. Separate doses of these by at least 2 hours.

• Iron interferes with the absorption of levodopa, methyldopa, penicillamine, and quinolone antibacterials.

- Antacids and cimetidine interfere with iron absorption.
- Ascorbic acid (vitamin C) and chloramphenicol increase the amount of iron absorbed.

Food Interactions

Iron supplements are best taken on an empty stomach, but they may be taken with food if they upset your stomach. Eggs and milk interfere with iron absorption. Coffee or tea consumed with a meal or within an hour of eating reduces the amount of iron absorbed into the blood. Do not take iron products together with calcium supplements and food. If you need both iron and calcium, take calcium carbonate (Tums) and use it between meals.

Usual Dose

Iron dosage is the same regardless of type. Read the product label to determine iron content.

Adult and Child (age 13 and over): 0.9–1⅓ mg per lb. of body weight a day.

Pregnant Women: 30 mg of iron daily. Do not take with food or meals.

Child (age 3–12): 1⅓ mg per lb. of body weight a day.

Child (age 6 months–2 years): up to 2¾ mg per lb. of body weight a day.

Child (under age 2): 10–25 mg a day.

Overdosage

Overdose symptoms usually appear after 30 minutes to several hours; they include tiredness, vomiting, diarrhea, upset stomach, weak and rapid pulse, and lowered blood pressure—or, after massive doses, shock, black and tarry stools due to massive bleeding in the stomach or intestine, and pneumonia. In case of overdose, call your local poison control center of a hospital emergency room. You may be told to induce vomiting with ipecac syrup—available at any pharmacy—and to give the victim eggs and milk before seeking treatment. Time is a critical factor in emergency care: Stomach pumping should not be performed after the first hour of iron ingestion due to the risk of stomach perforation. If you seek treatment ALWAYS bring the prescription bottle or container.

Special Information

Iron often causes black discoloration of stools and is slightly constipating. However, stools that are black or tarry may also indicate bleeding in the stomach or intestine. If you experience this symptom, discuss it with your doctor at once.

Do not chew or crush sustained-release iron products. Liquid iron products may stain your teeth. Drink lots of water or juice with them and sip the iron through a straw to prevent tooth contact.

If you forget a dose, take it as soon as you remember. If it is almost time for your next dose, skip the one you forgot and continue with your regular schedule. Do not take a double dose.

Special Populations

Pregnancy/Breast-feeding
This drug is safe for use during pregnancy and breast-feeding and is frequently prescribed for pregnant and nursing women. If you are pregnant, however, you should check with your doctor before taking any medication.

Seniors
Seniors may require larger dosages.

Generic Name

Isosorbide Dinitrate

(eye-soe-SORE-bide dih-NYE-trate) G

Brand Names

Dilatrate-SR	Isordil Titradose
Isordil Tembids	Sorbitrate

The information in this profile also applies to the following drug:

Generic Ingredient: Isosorbide Mononitrate G

Imdur	Monoket
ISMO	

Type of Drug

Antianginal agent.

Prescribed for

Heart or chest pain associated with angina pectoris; also prescribed in congestive heart failure and similar conditions to prevent the recurrence of chest or heart pain and to reduce stress on the heart.

General Information

Isosorbide dinitrate and other nitrates are used to treat pain associated with heart problems. While the exact nature of their action is not fully understood, they are believed to relax muscles in blood vessels. Isosorbide dinitrate sublingual tablets begin working in 2 to 5 minutes and last for 1 to 3 hours. The regular tablets begin working in 20 to 40 minutes and continue for 4 to 6 hours. The sustained-release form may take up to 4 hours to begin working and lasts for 6 to 8 hours. Isosorbide mononitrate begins working in 30 to 60 minutes and lasts for an undetermined period of time.

Cautions and Warnings

If you are **allergic** or **sensitive** to this drug or to other drugs used for heart pain such as nitroglycerin, do not use it.

If you have or recently have had a **head injury,** use this drug with caution.

This drug may be inappropriate for you if you have had a recent **heart attack** or have severe **anemia, glaucoma,** severe **liver disease, overactive thyroid, cardiomyopathy** (loss of blood-pumping ability due to damaged heart muscle), **low blood pressure,** severe **kidney problems,** or an **overactive gastrointestinal tract**.

Possible Side Effects

▼ Common: headache and flushing, which should disappear after your body adjusts to the drug. You may experience dizziness and weakness during this process. There is a risk of blurred vision and dry mouth; if either occurs, stop taking the drug and call your doctor.

▼ Less common: nausea, vomiting, weakness, sweating, and rash with itching, redness, and peeling. If these symptoms appear, discontinue the medication and consult your doctor.

Drug Interactions

• If you take isosorbide dinitrate, do not self-medicate with over-the-counter cough and cold remedies, since many contain ingredients that may aggravate heart disease.

• Taking this drug with large amounts of alcohol may rapidly lower blood pressure, resulting in weakness, dizziness, and fainting.

• Nitrates raise dihydroergotamine blood levels, which may elevate blood pressure or block isosorbide's effects.

• Aspirin and calcium channel blockers can increase isosorbide blood levels and the risk of side effects.

Food Interactions

Take isosorbide on an empty stomach with a glass of water unless you get a persistent headache. If this occurs, the drug can be taken with meals.

Usual Dose

Isosorbide Dinitrate: 10–20 mg 4 times a day. If needed, the drug may be given in doses of 5–40 mg. Sustained-release dosage is 40–80 mg every 8–12 hours.

Isosorbide Mononitrate: 20 mg twice a day, with the 2 doses taken 7 hours apart. Usually, the first dose is taken upon waking and the second dose is taken 7 hours later.

Overdosage

Overdose can result in low blood pressure; very rapid heartbeat; flushing; perspiration followed by cold, bluish, and clammy skin; headache; heart palpitations; blurred vision and other visual disturbances; dizziness; nausea; vomiting; difficult, slow breathing; slow pulse; confusion; moderate fever; and paralysis. Take the victim to a hospital emergency room at once. ALWAYS bring the prescription bottle or container.

Special Information

If you take this drug sublingually (under the tongue), be sure the tablet is fully dissolved before you swallow the drug. Do not crush or chew sustained-release capsules or tablets. Avoid alcohol.

Do not switch brands of isosorbide without consulting your doctor or pharmacist—they may not be equivalent.

Call your doctor if you develop a persistent headache, dizziness, facial flushing, blurred vision, or dry mouth.

If you take isosorbide on a regular schedule and forget a dose, take it as soon as you remember. If you take isosorbide more than once a day and it is within 2 hours of your next dose, skip the dose you forgot and continue with your regular schedule. If you take the sustained-release form once a day and it is within 6 hours of your next dose, skip the dose you forgot and continue with your regular schedule. Never take a double dose.

Special Populations

Pregnancy/Breast-feeding

Isosorbide crosses into the fetal circulation. When this drug is considered crucial by your doctor, its potential benefits must be carefully weighed against its risks.

This drug passes into breast milk. Nursing mothers who must take it should consider bottle-feeding.

Seniors

Seniors may take isosorbide without special restriction.

Generic Name

Isotretinoin (EYE-soe-TRET-ih-noin)

Brand Name

Accutane

Type of Drug

Antiacne.

Prescribed for

Severe cystic acne that has not responded to other treatment.

General Information

It is not known exactly how isotretinoin, which is related to vitamin A, works in cases of severe cystic acne. It reduces the amount of sebum (the skin's natural oily lubricant), shrinks the skin glands that produce sebum, and inhibits keratinization (hardening of the skin cells)—key to the problem of severe acne because it leads to the buildup of sebum within skin follicles and causes the formation of closed comedones (whiteheads). Sebum production may be permanently reduced after isotretinoin treatment.

Isotretinoin is also being studied as a treatment for keratinization and mycosis fungoides.

Cautions and Warnings

People **allergic or sensitive to vitamin A** (or any vitamin A product) or to paraben preservatives—used in isotretinoin—should not use isotretinoin.

Isotretinoin has been associated with **pseudotumor cerebri** (increased pressure in the brain). The symptoms of this condition include severe headaches, nausea, vomiting, and visual disturbances.

Diabetics taking this drug may have their diabetes drugs re-evaluated by their doctors. Some new cases of diabetes were found in people taking isotretinoin, but no direct relationship to drug therapy has been found.

Isotretinoin may cause temporary opaque spots on the cornea of your eye, causing **visual disturbances**. These are usually gone by 2 months after the drug is stopped.

Difficulty seeing at night or in the dark can develop suddenly while taking isotretinoin.

Several cases of **severe bowel inflammation** (symptoms include abdominal discomfort and pain, severe diarrhea, or bleeding from the rectum) have developed in people taking isotretinoin.

About 25% of people who take isotretinoin develop **high blood-triglyceride levels**. Fifteen percent have lower high-density lipoprotein (HDL)—"good" cholesterol—and 7% have higher total cholesterol.

Several cases of **hepatitis** have been linked to this drug. Fifteen percent of people who take it develop signs of **liver inflammation**.

Possible Side Effects

Side effects increase with dosage.

▼ Most common: dry, chapped, or inflamed lips; dry mouth; dry nose; nosebleeds; eye irritation; conjunctivitis (pinkeye); dry or flaky skin; rash; itching; peeling skin on the face, palms, or soles; unusual sensitivity to the sun; temporary skin discoloration; brittle nails; inflammation of the nailbed or bone under toes or fingernails;

Possible Side Effects *(continued)*

temporary hair thinning; nausea; vomiting; abdominal pain; tiredness; lethargy; sleeplessness; headache; tingling in the hands or feet; dizziness; protein, blood, or white blood cells in the urine; urinary difficulties; blurred vision; bone and joint aches or pains; and muscle pain or stiffness. Isotretinoin causes extreme elevations of blood-triglyceride levels and milder elevations of other blood-fat levels including cholesterol. It also can raise blood-sugar or uric-acid levels and can increase liver-function-test values.

▼ Less common: wound crusting caused by an exaggerated healing response stimulated by the drug, hair problems other than thinning, appetite loss, upset stomach or intestinal discomfort, severe bowel inflammation, stomach or intestinal bleeding, weight loss, visual disturbances, contact lens intolerance, pseudotumor cerebri, mild bleeding or easy bruising, fluid retention, and lung or respiratory system infection. Several people taking isotretinoin have developed widespread herpes simplex infections.

Drug Interactions

• Vitamin A supplements increase isotretinoin's side effects and must be avoided while taking this drug. Avoid alcohol because this combination can severely raise blood-triglyceride levels.

• Combining tetracycline antibiotics and isotretinoin may increase the risk of pseudotumor cerebri.

• Isotretinoin may reduce the amount of carbamazepine (an anticonvulsant) in the blood.

Food Interactions

Isotretinoin should be taken with food or meals. Avoid eating beef or chicken liver while taking isotretinoin, because liver contains very large amounts of vitamin A. Limit your intake of foods containing moderate to large amounts of vitamin A.

Usual Dose

0.22–0.9 mg per lb. of body weight a day in 2 divided doses for 15–20 weeks. Lower doses may be effective, but relapses are more common. Isotretinoin, like vitamin A, dissolves in body fat. People weighing more than 155 lbs. may need doses at the high end of the usual range.

If the total acne lesion count drops by 70% in 15–20 weeks, the drug may be discontinued. Stop taking isotretinoin for 2 months after 15–20 weeks of treatment. A second course of treatment may be needed if the acne does not clear.

Overdosage

Isotretinoin overdose is likely to cause nausea, vomiting, lethargy, and other common drug side effects. Overdose victims must be made to vomit with ipecac syrup—available at any pharmacy—to remove any remaining drug from the stomach. Call your doctor or poison control center before doing this. If you must go to a hospital emergency room, ALWAYS bring the prescription bottle or container.

Special Information

Women of childbearing age should not take isotretinoin unless their severe, disfiguring acne has not responded to any other treatment, they are using effective contraception, and they have had a negative pregnancy test during the 2 weeks before taking isotretinoin. You should start taking isotretinoin on day 2 or 3 of your next period. Be sure your doctor knows if you plan to become pregnant while taking isotretinoin, are breast-feeding, diabetic, taking a vitamin A supplement—as a multivitamin or vitamin A alone—or if you or any family member has a history of high blood-triglyceride levels.

Your skin may become unusually sensitive to the sun while you are taking this drug. Use sunscreen and wear protective clothing until your doctor can determine if you are likely to develop this effect.

Call your doctor if you develop any severe or unusual side effects, such as abdominal pain; bleeding from the rectum; severe diarrhea; headache; nausea or vomiting; visual difficulties; severe muscle, bone, or joint aches or pains; or unusual sensitivity to sunlight or to ultraviolet light.

Your acne may worsen when isotretinoin treatment begins, but then it should improve. Do not be alarmed if this happens, but tell your doctor.

Do not donate blood during isotretinoin treatment—or for at least 30 days after you have stopped—because of the risk to the fetus of a pregnant woman who may receive the blood.

If you forget a dose of isotretinoin, take it as soon as you remember. If it is almost time for your next dose, skip the one you forgot and continue with your regular schedule. Do not take a double dose.

Special Populations

Pregnancy/Breast-feeding
Pregnant women should NEVER take isotretinoin because it will injure the fetus. You must confirm that you are not pregnant before starting isotretinoin. You must also be absolutely certain that you are using effective birth control starting 1 month before treatment and continued at least 1 month after isotretinoin is stopped. Accidental pregnancy during isotretinoin therapy may be grounds for an abortion due to the severe effects of this drug on the fetus. Call your doctor immediately.

It is not known if isotretinoin passes into breast milk. Nursing mothers should not take isotretinoin because of the possibility that it will affect the nursing infant.

Seniors
Seniors may take this medication without special restriction.

Generic Name

Isradipine (is-RAD-ih-pene)

Brand Names

DynaCirc   DynaCirc CR

Type of Drug

Calcium channel blocker.

Prescribed for

High blood pressure; also prescribed for chronic stable angina pectoris.

General Information

Isradipine is one of many calcium channel blockers available in the U.S. These drugs block the passage of calcium, an essential factor in muscle contraction, into heart and smooth muscle cells. Blocking calcium interferes with contraction of these muscles, which in turn dilates (widens) the veins and vessels that supply blood to them. This dilating effect reduces blood pressure, the amount of oxygen used by the heart muscle, and the risk of blood vessel spasm. Isradipine is therefore useful in treating not only high blood pressure but also angina pectoris (brief attacks of chest pain), a condition related to poor oxygen supply to the heart muscle.

Isradipine affects the movement of calcium into muscle cells only; it has no effect on calcium in the blood.

Cautions and Warnings

Do not take this drug if you have had an **allergic reaction** to it.

Abruptly stopping this medication can cause increased **chest pain**. If you must stop, the drug dose should be gradually reduced.

Use isradipine with caution if you have **heart failure,** since the drug may worsen this condition.

On rare occasions, isradipine may cause very **low blood pressure**. This may lead to stimulation of the heart and rapid heartbeat and can worsen angina in some people.

Isradipine may cause **angina** when treatment is first started, when dosage is increased, or if the drug is rapidly withdrawn. This can be avoided by reducing dosage gradually.

Studies have shown that people taking calcium channel blockers—usually those taken several times a day, not those taken only once daily—have a greater chance of having a **heart attack** than do people taking beta blockers or other medication for the same purposes. Discuss this with your doctor to be sure you are receiving the best possible treatment.

People with severe **liver disease** may require dosage adjustments.

Possible Side Effects

Isradipine side effects are generally mild and self-limiting.

▼ Most common: headache.

▼ Less common: low blood pressure, chest pain, rapid heartbeat, dizziness, diarrhea, a feeling of warmth, nausea, light-headedness, fatigue and lethargy, itching, rash, flushing, changes in certain blood-cell components, and swelling of the legs, ankles, or feet.

Possible Side Effects *(continued)*

▼ Rare: Rare side effects can occur in almost any part of the body. Contact your doctor if you experience any side effect not listed above.

Drug Interactions

• Isradipine may interact with beta-blocking drugs to cause heart failure, very low blood pressure, or an increased incidence of angina pain. However, in many cases these drugs have been taken together with no problem.

• Combining isradipine with fentanyl (a narcotic pain reliever) can result in very low blood pressure.

Food Interactions

Taking isradipine with food has a minor effect on the absorption of the drug. You may take it with food if it upsets your stomach. Avoid drinking grapefruit juice if you are taking this medication.

Usual Dose

5–20 mg a day in 2 doses. Do not stop taking the drug abruptly. The dosage should be reduced gradually over a period of time.

Overdosage

Overdose of isradipine can cause nausea, dizziness, weakness, drowsiness, confusion, slurred speech, very low blood pressure, reduced heart efficiency, and unusual heart rhythms. Victims of an isradipine overdose should be taken to a hospital emergency room. ALWAYS bring the prescription bottle or container.

Special Information

Call your doctor if you develop swelling in the arms or legs, breathing difficulties, abnormal heartbeat, increased heart pains, dizziness, constipation, nausea, light-headedness, or very low blood pressure.

If you forget to take a dose of isradipine, take it as soon as you remember. If it is almost time for your next dose, skip the dose you forgot and continue with your regular schedule. Do not take a double dose.

Special Populations

Pregnancy/Breast-feeding

Isradipine affects the development of animal fetuses. Women who are or might be pregnant should not take isradipine without their doctor's approval. When the drug is considered crucial by your doctor, its potential benefits must be carefully weighed against its risks.

It is not known if isradipine passes into breast milk. Nursing mothers who must take isradipine should consider bottle-feeding.

Seniors

Seniors may absorb more isradipine than younger adults and may release the drug more slowly from their bodies.

Generic Name

Itraconazole (ih-trah-KON-uh-zole)

Brand Name

Sporanox

Type of Drug

Antifungal.

Prescribed for

Fungal infections—blastomycosis and histoplasmosis—of the blood, skin, or nails.

General Information

Itraconazole is effective against a variety of fungal organisms, some of which do not respond to other drugs. It is an important therapy for people with acquired immunodeficiency syndrome (AIDS) or cancer whose immune systems are compromised. It works by inhibiting important enzyme systems in the organisms it attacks. Drug treatment must be continued for at least 3 months until the fungal infection subsides. Itraconazole is broken down in the liver.

Cautions and Warnings

The combination of itraconazole and either astemizole or terfenadine (nonsedating antihistamines) can cause severe **cardiac side effects**.

Do not take itraconazole if you have had an **allergic reaction** to it. People who are allergic to similar antifungals—ketoconazole, miconazole, and fluconazole—may also be allergic to itraconazole, although cross-reactions are uncommon.

Rarely, itraconazole causes reversible **liver damage**. It should be used with caution by people who already have liver disease.

Possible Side Effects

▼ Most common: nausea, vomiting, and rash.

▼ Less common: diarrhea, abdominal pain, appetite loss, swelling in the legs or feet, fatigue, fever, feeling unwell, itching, headache, dizziness, reduced sex drive, tiredness, high blood pressure, liver or kidney function abnormalities, low blood potassium, and impotence.

▼ Rare: gas, sleeplessness, depression, ringing or buzzing in the ears, and swollen or painful breasts in men or women.

Drug Interactions

• People who have taken terfenadine or astemizole with itraconazole have experienced severe cardiac side effects. DO NOT TAKE THESE COMBINATIONS.

• Combining itraconazole and cisapride, digoxin, sulfonylurea-type antidiabetes drugs, phenytoin, quinidine, tacrolimus, or warfarin can lead to possible side effects. Important dosage adjustments may be required before you start on itraconazole.

• People taking itraconazole with the calcium channel blockers amlodipine and nifedipine can retain fluid. These combinations should be avoided.

• Rarely, people who combine itraconazole with a blood-fat-lowering drug of the statin type experience muscle pain and destruction. Some people who have experienced this interaction were also taking cyclosporine, the dose of which should be lowered if it is being taken with itraconazole and an HMG-CoA inhibitor.

• Cimetidine, ranitidine, famotidine, nizatidine, isoniazid, phenytoin, and rifampin may interfere with the effectiveness of itraconazole.

Food Interactions

Itraconazole should be taken with or after a full meal.

Usual Dose

Adult: 200–600 mg once a day.

Child (age 3–16): 100 mg a day has been prescribed, but the long-term effects of itraconazole in children are not known.

Overdosage

Symptoms of overdose may include any of the drug's side effects; liver toxicity is especially important. Call your local poison control center or hospital emergency room for more information. ALWAYS take the prescription bottle or container with you if you seek treatment.

Special Information

Itraconazole must be taken for at least 3 months to determine its effectiveness; otherwise, the infection may return.

Call your doctor if you develop unusual fatigue, yellowing of the skin or whites of the eyes, nausea or vomiting, appetite loss, dark urine or pale stools, or if you develop bothersome or persistent side effects.

If you forget a dose of itraconazole, take it as soon as you remember. If it is almost time for your next dose, skip the one you forgot and continue with your regular schedule. Do not take a double dose.

Special Populations

Pregnancy/Breast-feeding

Animal studies have shown that high doses of itraconazole damage the fetus. Pregnant women should not use itraconazole unless the possible benefits outweigh the risks.

Itraconazole passes into breast milk. Nursing mothers who must take this drug should bottle-feed.

Seniors

Seniors may use this drug without special restriction.

K-Dur   *see Potassium Replacements, page 831*

Generic Name

Ketoconazole (kee-toe-KON-uh-zole) Ⓖ

Brand Name

Nizoral

Type of Drug

Antifungal.

Prescribed for

Thrush and other systemic fungal infections, including candidiasis, histoplasmosis, and blastomycosis. Ketoconazole may also be prescribed for fungal infections of the skin, fingernails, and vagina. High-dose ketoconazole may be effective in treating fungal infections of the brain. The drug has been studied for the treatment of advanced prostate cancer and Cushing's syndrome. Ketoconazole shampoo is used to treat dandruff.

General Information

This drug is effective against a variety of fungal organisms. It kills fungus cells by disrupting the cell membrane.

Cautions and Warnings

At least 1 of every 10,000 people who take ketoconazole develop **liver inflammation and damage**. In most cases, the inflammation subsides when the drug is discontinued.

Do not take ketoconazole if you have had an **allergic reaction** to it.

Ketoconazole should not be used to treat **fungal infections of the nervous system**.

Ketoconazole reduces levels of testosterone and **corticosteroid hormone**.

In studies of ketoconazole in **prostate cancer,** 11 people died within 2 weeks of starting high-dose ketoconazole treatment. The reasons for these deaths are not known but may be related to the fact that the medication can suppress the body's natural production of adrenal corticosteroid hormones.

On rare occasions, people taking ketoconazole for the first time experience serious, **life-threatening reactions** including itching, rash, and breathing difficulties. Victims must receive emergency treatment at once.

Possible Side Effects

▼ Common: nausea, vomiting, upset stomach, abdominal pain or discomfort, itching, and swollen breasts in men. Most of these side effects are mild, and only a small number of people—1.5%—have to stop taking the drug because of severe side effects.

▼ Less common: headache, dizziness, drowsiness or tiredness, fever, chills, unusual sensitivity to bright light, diarrhea, impotence, and reduced levels of blood platelets. Reduced sperm counts have been associated with ketoconazole, but only at dosages above 400 mg a day.

Drug Interactions

• Antacids, histamine H_2 antagonists including cimetidine and ranitidine, and other drugs that reduce stomach acid counteract the effects of ketoconazole.

• Combining ketoconazole and rifampin may reduce the effects of both.

• Combining isoniazid and ketoconazole neutralizes ketoconazole's effects. This interaction occurs even when doses of the 2 drugs are separated by 12 hours.

• Ketoconazole increases the amount of cyclosporine in the bloodstream and the chances for kidney damage caused by cyclosporine. It also increases the effect of oral anticoagulant (blood-thinning) drugs. Ketoconazole increases blood levels of cisapride and the antihistamines terfenadine and astemizole, which leads to an increased chance of developing serious cardiac side effects from those drugs.

• Combining ketoconazole and phenytoin may increase or decrease either drug's effect.

• Combining ketoconazole and theophylline may trigger an asthma attack. Your doctor may adjust your theophylline dose.

• Ketoconazole may increase the side effects of oral corticosteroid drugs.

Food Interactions

Take ketoconazole with food or meals to improve absorption and avoid stomach upset.

Usual Dose

Tablets
Adult: 200–400 mg once a day. Treatment may continue for several months, depending on the type of infection being treated.
Child (age 2 and over): 1.5–3 mg per lb. of body weight once a day.
Child (under age 2): not recommended.

Cream
Apply to affected and immediate surrounding areas 1–2 times a day for 14 days.

Overdosage

Symptoms of overdose are liver damage and exaggerated side effects. Victims should immediately be given bicarbonate of soda or any other antacid to reduce the amount of ketoconazole absorbed into the blood. Call your local poison control center for more information. If you take the victim to a hospital emergency room for treatment, ALWAYS bring the prescription bottle or container.

Special Information

If you must take antacids or other ulcer treatments, separate doses of these medications from ketoconazole by at least 2 hours. Anything that reduces stomach-acid levels will reduce this drug's effectiveness.

Ketoconazole may cause headaches, dizziness, and drowsiness. Use caution while doing anything that requires intense concentration, like driving or operating machinery.

Call your doctor if you develop pains in the stomach or abdomen, severe diarrhea, high fever, unusual tiredness, appetite loss, nausea, vomiting, yellowing of the skin or whites of the eyes, pale stools, or dark urine.

If you forget to take a ketoconazole tablet, take it as soon as you remember. If it is almost time for your next dose, take 1 dose immediately and the next dose in 10 to 12 hours. Then go back to your regular schedule. Do not take a double dose.

Special Populations

Pregnancy/Breast-feeding

At high doses, ketoconazole causes damage in animal fetuses. Ketoconazole should not be taken by women who are or might be pregnant unless its potential benefits have been carefully weighed against its risks.

This drug passes into the breast milk. Nursing mothers who must take ketoconazole should bottle-feed.

Seniors

Seniors may take this drug without special restriction.

Generic Name

Ketoprofen (KEE-toe-PROE-fen) G

Brand Names

Orudis   Oruvail

Type of Drug

Nonsteroidal anti-inflammatory drug (NSAID).

Prescribed for

Rheumatoid arthritis, juvenile rheumatoid arthritis, osteoarthritis, mild to moderate pain, menstrual pain, menstrual headache, sunburn, and migraine. Controlled-release ketoprofen is prescribed only for arthritis.

General Information

Ketoprofen and other NSAIDs are used to relieve pain and inflammation. We do not know exactly how NSAIDs work, but they may achieve their effects by blocking the body's production of a hormone called prostaglandin and the action of other body chemicals. Pain relief comes within 1 hour after taking the first dose of ketoprofen, but its anti-inflammatory effect generally takes several days to 2 weeks to become apparent and may take a month or more to reach maximum effect. Controlled-release ketoprofen is not recommended for acute pain relief because it can take up to 7 hours to reach its maximum concentration in the blood. Ketoprofen is broken down in the liver and eliminated from the body through the kidneys.

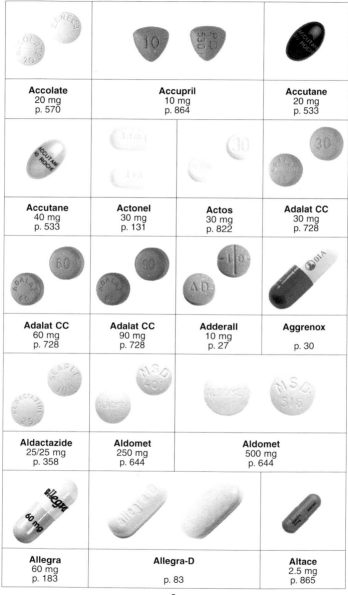

Accolate 20 mg p. 570	**Accupril** 10 mg p. 864	**Accutane** 20 mg p. 533

Accutane 40 mg p. 533	**Actonel** 30 mg p. 131	**Actos** 30 mg p. 822	**Adalat CC** 30 mg p. 728

Adalat CC 60 mg p. 728	**Adalat CC** 90 mg p. 728	**Adderall** 10 mg p. 27	**Aggrenox** p. 30

Aldactazide 25/25 mg p. 358	**Aldomet** 250 mg p. 644	**Aldomet** 500 mg p. 644

Allegra 60 mg p. 183	**Allegra-D** p. 83	**Altace** 2.5 mg p. 865

A

Altace 5 mg p. 865	**Amaryl** 2 mg p. 957	**Ambien** 5 mg p. 1108	**Ambien** 10 mg p. 1108
Amoxil 250 mg p. 785	**Amoxil** 500 mg p. 785	**Amoxil Chewable** 125 mg p. 785	**Ancobon** 500 mg p. 439
Ansaid 50 mg p. 457	**Antivert** 12.5 mg p. 334	**Aricept** 5 mg p. 347	**Aricept** 10 mg p. 347
Arthrotec 50 mg p. 311		**Asendin** 25 mg p. 1051	**Asendin** 50 mg p. 1051
Atarax 25 mg p. 495	**Atarax** 50 mg p. 495	**Ativan** 0.5 mg p. 307	**Ativan** 1 mg p. 307

B

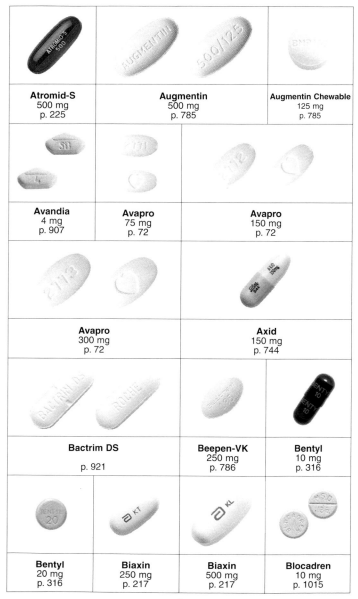

Atromid-S 500 mg p. 225	**Augmentin** 500 mg p. 785	**Augmentin Chewable** 125 mg p. 785
Avandia 4 mg p. 907	**Avapro** 75 mg p. 72	**Avapro** 150 mg p. 72
Avapro 300 mg p. 72		**Axid** 150 mg p. 744
Bactrim DS p. 921	**Beepen-VK** 250 mg p. 786	**Bentyl** 10 mg p. 316
Bentyl 20 mg p. 316	**Biaxin** 250 mg p. 217	**Biaxin** 500 mg p. 217	**Blocadren** 10 mg p. 1015

C

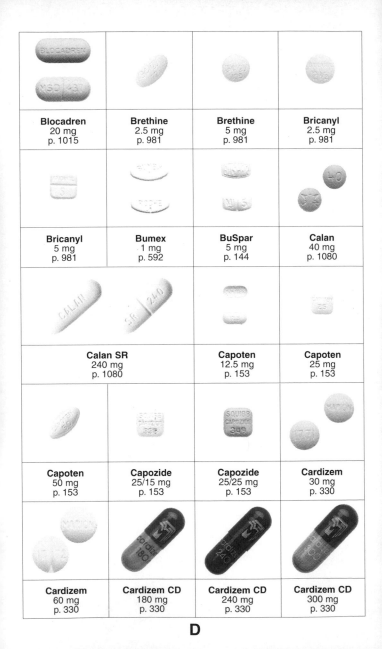

Blocadren 20 mg p. 1015	**Brethine** 2.5 mg p. 981	**Brethine** 5 mg p. 981	**Bricanyl** 2.5 mg p. 981
Bricanyl 5 mg p. 981	**Bumex** 1 mg p. 592	**BuSpar** 5 mg p. 144	**Calan** 40 mg p. 1080
Calan SR 240 mg p. 1080		**Capoten** 12.5 mg p. 153	**Capoten** 25 mg p. 153
Capoten 50 mg p. 153	**Capozide** 25/15 mg p. 153	**Capozide** 25/25 mg p. 153	**Cardizem** 30 mg p. 330
Cardizem 60 mg p. 330	**Cardizem CD** 180 mg p. 330	**Cardizem CD** 240 mg p. 330	**Cardizem CD** 300 mg p. 330

D

Cardizem SR 60 mg p. 330	**Cardizem SR** 90 mg p. 330	**Cardizem SR** 120 mg p. 330	**Cardura** 2 mg p. 352
Cartia XT 180 mg p. 330	**Cartia XT** 240 mg p. 330	**Cartrol** 2.5 mg p. 166	**Cartrol** 5 mg p. 166
Catapres 0.1 mg p. 231	**Catapres** 0.2 mg p. 231	**Ceclor** 500 mg p. 178	**Ceftin** 125 mg p. 178
Ceftin 500 mg p. 178		**Cefzil** 500 mg p.178	
CellCept 250 mg p. 696	**Celebrex** 100 mg p. 174	**Celexa** 20 mg p. 213	**Cipro** 250 mg p. 442

E

Cipro 500 mg p. 442	**Cipro** 750 mg p. 442	**Claritin** 10 mg p. 600	**Claritin Reditabs** 10 mg p. 600
Claritin-D 12-hour 5/120 mg p. 83	**Claritin-D 24-hour** 10/240 mg p. 83	**Clinoril** 150 mg p. 766	**Clozaril** 100 mg p. 243
Cogentin 1 mg p. 112	**Cogentin** 2 mg p. 112	**Compazine** 10 mg p. 845	**Compazine Spansule** 15 mg p. 845
Cordarone 200 mg p. 55		**Corgard** 40 mg p. 1015	
Corgard 80 mg p. 1015		**Coumadin** 5 mg p. 1084	**Covera HS** 180 mg p. 1080

F

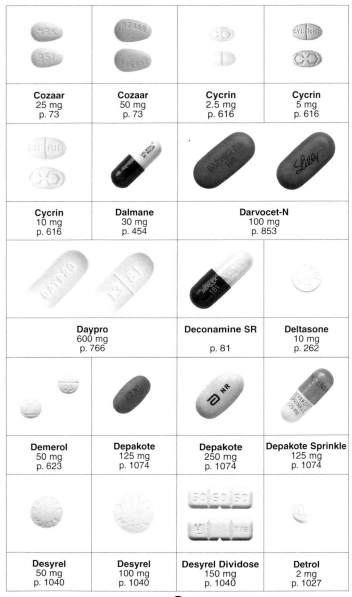

Cozaar 25 mg p. 73	Cozaar 50 mg p. 73	Cycrin 2.5 mg p. 616	Cycrin 5 mg p. 616
Cycrin 10 mg p. 616	Dalmane 30 mg p. 454	Darvocet-N 100 mg p. 853	
Daypro 600 mg p. 766		Deconamine SR p. 81	Deltasone 10 mg p. 262
Demerol 50 mg p. 623	Depakote 125 mg p. 1074	Depakote 250 mg p. 1074	Depakote Sprinkle 125 mg p. 1074
Desyrel 50 mg p. 1040	Desyrel 100 mg p. 1040	Desyrel Dividose 150 mg p. 1040	Detrol 2 mg p. 1027

G

DiaBeta 5 mg p. 957	**Diabinese** 100 mg p. 957	**Diabinese** 250 mg p. 957	**Diflucan** 100 mg p. 437
Diflucan 150 mg p. 437	**Dilacor XR** 120 mg p. 330	**Dilacor XR** 180 mg p. 330	**Dilacor XR** 240 mg p. 330
Dilantin 100 mg p. 813	**Diovan** 80 mg p. 73	**Diovan** 160 mg p. 73	**Ditropan** 5 mg p. 771
Diuril 500 mg p. 999		**Doral** 15 mg p. 1048	**Duricef** 500 mg p. 178
Dyazide p. 358	**Dynabac** 250 mg p. 341	**DynaCirc** 2.5 mg p. 537	**E.E.S.** 400 mg p. 382

H

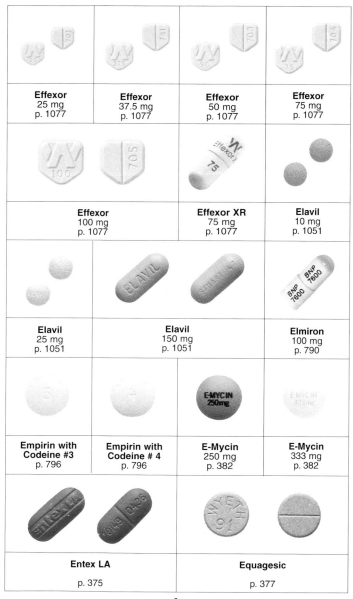

| **Effexor** 25 mg p. 1077 | **Effexor** 37.5 mg p. 1077 | **Effexor** 50 mg p. 1077 | **Effexor** 75 mg p. 1077 |

| **Effexor** 100 mg p. 1077 | **Effexor XR** 75 mg p. 1077 | **Elavil** 10 mg p. 1051 |

| **Elavil** 25 mg p. 1051 | **Elavil** 150 mg p. 1051 | **Elmiron** 100 mg p. 790 |

| **Empirin with Codeine #3** p. 796 | **Empirin with Codeine # 4** p. 796 | **E-Mycin** 250 mg p. 382 | **E-Mycin** 333 mg p. 382 |

| **Entex LA** p. 375 | **Equagesic** p. 377 |

I

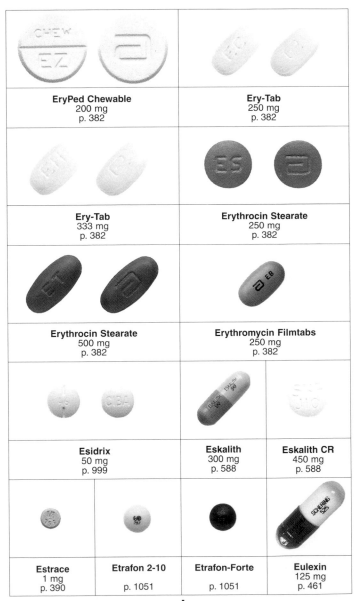

EryPed Chewable
200 mg
p. 382

Ery-Tab
250 mg
p. 382

Ery-Tab
333 mg
p. 382

Erythrocin Stearate
250 mg
p. 382

Erythrocin Stearate
500 mg
p. 382

Erythromycin Filmtabs
250 mg
p. 382

Esidrix
50 mg
p. 999

Eskalith
300 mg
p. 588

Eskalith CR
450 mg
p. 588

Estrace
1 mg
p. 390

Etrafon 2-10
p. 1051

Etrafon-Forte
p. 1051

Eulexin
125 mg
p. 461

J

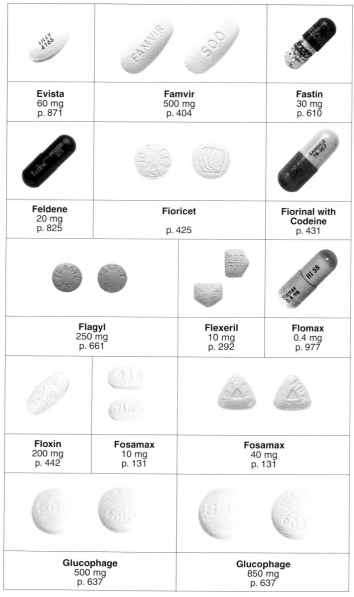

Evista 60 mg p. 871	**Famvir** 500 mg p. 404	**Fastin** 30 mg p. 610
Feldene 20 mg p. 825	**Fioricet** p. 425	**Fiorinal with Codeine** p. 431
Flagyl 250 mg p. 661	**Flexeril** 10 mg p. 292	**Flomax** 0.4 mg p. 977
Floxin 200 mg p. 442	**Fosamax** 10 mg p. 131	**Fosamax** 40 mg p. 131
Glucophage 500 mg p. 637		**Glucophage** 850 mg p. 637

K

Glucotrol 5 mg p. 957	**Glucotrol XL** 5 mg p. 957	**Glucotrol XL** 10 mg p. 957	**Glynase PresTab** 3 mg p. 957
Halcion 0.125 mg p. 1047	**Halcion** 0.25 mg p. 1047	**Haldol** 0.5 mg p. 484	**Haldol** 2 mg p. 484
Haldol 10 mg p. 484		**Halotestin** 5 mg p. 451	**Hivid** 0.375 mg p. 1095
Hivid 0.75 mg p. 1095		**Hytrin** 1 mg p. 976	**Hytrin** 5 mg p. 976
Hyzaar p. 73		**Imdur** 60 mg p. 530	

L

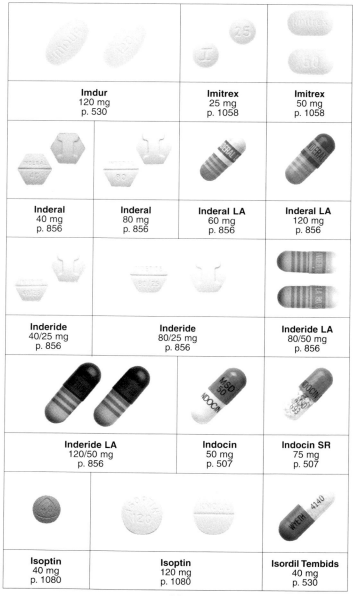

Imdur
120 mg
p. 530

Imitrex
25 mg
p. 1058

Imitrex
50 mg
p. 1058

Inderal
40 mg
p. 856

Inderal
80 mg
p. 856

Inderal LA
60 mg
p. 856

Inderal LA
120 mg
p. 856

Inderide
40/25 mg
p. 856

Inderide
80/25 mg
p. 856

Inderide LA
80/50 mg
p. 856

Inderide LA
120/50 mg
p. 856

Indocin
50 mg
p. 507

Indocin SR
75 mg
p. 507

Isoptin
40 mg
p. 1080

Isoptin
120 mg
p. 1080

Isordil Tembids
40 mg
p. 530

M

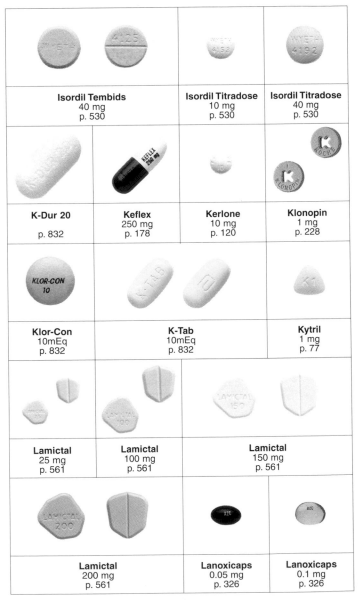

Isordil Tembids 40 mg p. 530	**Isordil Titradose** 10 mg p. 530	**Isordil Titradose** 40 mg p. 530

K-Dur 20 p. 832	**Keflex** 250 mg p. 178	**Kerlone** 10 mg p. 120	**Klonopin** 1 mg p. 228

Klor-Con 10mEq p. 832	**K-Tab** 10mEq p. 832	**Kytril** 1 mg p. 77

Lamictal 25 mg p. 561	**Lamictal** 100 mg p. 561	**Lamictal** 150 mg p. 561

Lamictal 200 mg p. 561	**Lanoxicaps** 0.05 mg p. 326	**Lanoxicaps** 0.1 mg p. 326

N

Lanoxicaps 0.2 mg p. 326	**Lanoxin** 0.125 mg p. 326	**Lanoxin** 0.25 mg p. 326	**Lanoxin** 0.5 mg p. 326
Larodopa 250 mg p. 578		**Lasix** 20 mg p. 593	**Lasix** 40 mg p. 593
Lasix 80 mg p. 593		**Lescol** 20 mg p. 942	**Lescol** 40 mg p. 942
Levaquin 500 mg p. 442		**Levatol** 20 mg p. 657	**Levoxyl** 25 mcg p. 1005
Levoxyl 50 mcg p. 1005	**Levoxyl** 100 mcg p. 1005	**Levoxyl** 125 mcg p. 1005	**Lexxel** p. 581

O

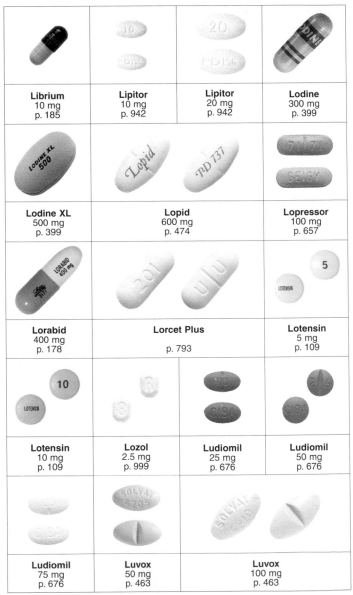

Librium 10 mg p. 185	**Lipitor** 10 mg p. 942	**Lipitor** 20 mg p. 942	**Lodine** 300 mg p. 399
Lodine XL 500 mg p. 399	**Lopid** 600 mg p. 474		**Lopressor** 100 mg p. 657
Lorabid 400 mg p. 178	**Lorcet Plus** p. 793		**Lotensin** 5 mg p. 109
Lotensin 10 mg p. 109	**Lozol** 2.5 mg p. 999	**Ludiomil** 25 mg p. 676	**Ludiomil** 50 mg p. 676
Ludiomil 75 mg p. 676	**Luvox** 50 mg p. 463	**Luvox** 100 mg p. 463	

P

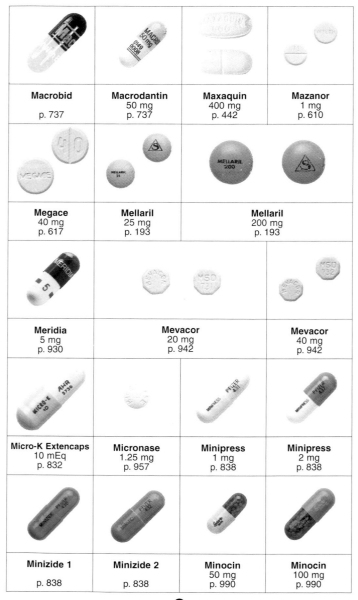

Macrobid p. 737	**Macrodantin** 50 mg p. 737	**Maxaquin** 400 mg p. 442	**Mazanor** 1 mg p. 610
Megace 40 mg p. 617	**Mellaril** 25 mg p. 193	**Mellaril** 200 mg p. 193	
Meridia 5 mg p. 930	**Mevacor** 20 mg p. 942		**Mevacor** 40 mg p. 942
Micro-K Extencaps 10 mEq p. 832	**Micronase** 1.25 mg p. 957	**Minipress** 1 mg p. 838	**Minipress** 2 mg p. 838
Minizide 1 p. 838	**Minizide 2** p. 838	**Minocin** 50 mg p. 990	**Minocin** 100 mg p. 990

Q

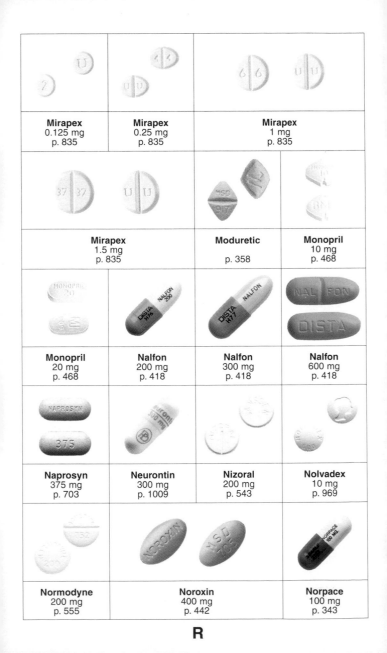

Mirapex 0.125 mg p. 835	**Mirapex** 0.25 mg p. 835	**Mirapex** 1 mg p. 835

Mirapex 1.5 mg p. 835	**Moduretic** p. 358	**Monopril** 10 mg p. 468

Monopril 20 mg p. 468	**Nalfon** 200 mg p. 418	**Nalfon** 300 mg p. 418	**Nalfon** 600 mg p. 418

Naprosyn 375 mg p. 703	**Neurontin** 300 mg p. 1009	**Nizoral** 200 mg p. 543	**Nolvadex** 10 mg p. 969

Normodyne 200 mg p. 555	**Noroxin** 400 mg p. 442	**Norpace** 100 mg p. 343

R

Norpace CR 100 mg p. 343	**Norpramin** 50 mg p. 1052	**Norvasc** 5 mg p. 61	**Novafed A** p. 82
Omnipen 250 mg p. 785	**Omnipen** 500 mg p. 785	**Orinase** 500 mg p. 957	**Orudis** 50 mg p. 546
Orudis 75 mg p. 546	**Oruvail** 200 mg p. 546	**Pamelor** 25 mg p. 1052	**Pamelor** 75 mg p. 1052
Parafon Forte DSC 500 mg p. 197		**Paxil** 20 mg p. 777	**PCE** 333 mg p. 382
PCE 500 mg p. 382	**Penetrex** 200 mg p. 442	**Penetrex** 400 mg p. 442	

S

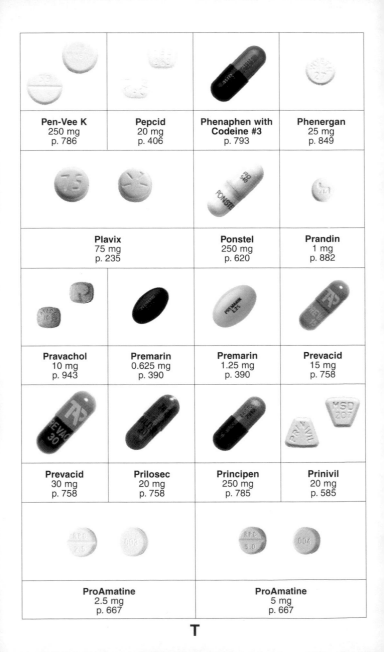

Pen-Vee K 250 mg p. 786	**Pepcid** 20 mg p. 406	**Phenaphen with Codeine #3** p. 793	**Phenergan** 25 mg p. 849
Plavix 75 mg p. 235		**Ponstel** 250 mg p. 620	**Prandin** 1 mg p. 882
Pravachol 10 mg p. 943	**Premarin** 0.625 mg p. 390	**Premarin** 1.25 mg p. 390	**Prevacid** 15 mg p. 758
Prevacid 30 mg p. 758	**Prilosec** 20 mg p. 758	**Principen** 250 mg p. 785	**Prinivil** 20 mg p. 585
ProAmatine 2.5 mg p. 667		**ProAmatine** 5 mg p. 667	

T

Procardia 10 mg p. 728	**Procardia XL** 30 mg p. 728	**Procardia XL** 60 mg p. 728	**Procardia XL** 90 mg p. 728
Prograf 1 mg p. 965	**Prograf** 5 mg p. 965	**Prolixin** 5 mg p. 193	**Prolixin** 10 mg p. 193
Pronestyl-SR 500 mg p. 842	**Propacet 100** p. 853	**Propulsid** 10 mg p. 210	**Proscar** 5 mg p. 422
Proventil 4 mg p. 35	**Proventil Repetabs** 4 mg p. 35	**Provera** 2.5 mg p. 616	**Provera** 5 mg p. 616
Prozac 10 mg p. 447	**Prozac** 20 mg p. 447	**Quinaglute Dura-Tabs** 324 mg p. 868	

U

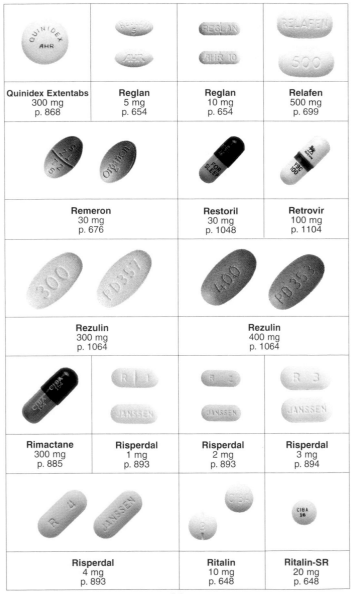

Quinidex Extentabs 300 mg p. 868	**Reglan** 5 mg p. 654	**Reglan** 10 mg p. 654	**Relafen** 500 mg p. 699

Remeron 30 mg p. 676	**Restoril** 30 mg p. 1048	**Retrovir** 100 mg p. 1104

Rezulin 300 mg p. 1064	**Rezulin** 400 mg p. 1064

Rimactane 300 mg p. 885	**Risperdal** 1 mg p. 893	**Risperdal** 2 mg p. 893	**Risperdal** 3 mg p. 894

Risperdal 4 mg p. 893	**Ritalin** 10 mg p. 648	**Ritalin-SR** 20 mg p. 648

V

Sandimmune 25 mg p. 295	**Sandimmune** 100 mg p. 295	**Sansert** 2 mg p. 650

Sectral 200 mg p. 8	**Sectral** 400 mg p. 8	**Semprex-D** p. 81	**Septra DS** p. 921
Serax 10 mg p. 307	**Serax** 30 mg p. 307	**Seroquel** 25 mg p. 860	**Seroquel** 100 mg p. 860
Seroquel 200 mg p. 860	**Serzone** 100 mg p. 707	**Serzone** 150 mg p. 707	
Serzone 200 mg p. 707		**Serzone** 250 mg p. 707	

W

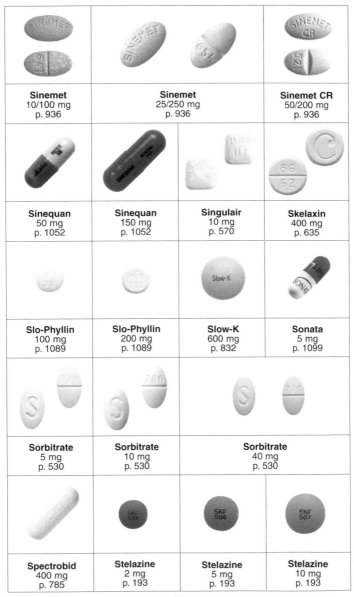

Sinemet 10/100 mg p. 936	**Sinemet** 25/250 mg p. 936	**Sinemet CR** 50/200 mg p. 936
Sinequan 50 mg p. 1052	**Sinequan** 150 mg p. 1052	**Singulair** 10 mg p. 570	**Skelaxin** 400 mg p. 635
Slo-Phyllin 100 mg p. 1089	**Slo-Phyllin** 200 mg p. 1089	**Slow-K** 600 mg p. 832	**Sonata** 5 mg p. 1099
Sorbitrate 5 mg p. 530	**Sorbitrate** 10 mg p. 530	**Sorbitrate** 40 mg p. 530	
Spectrobid 400 mg p. 785	**Stelazine** 2 mg p. 193	**Stelazine** 5 mg p. 193	**Stelazine** 10 mg p. 193

X

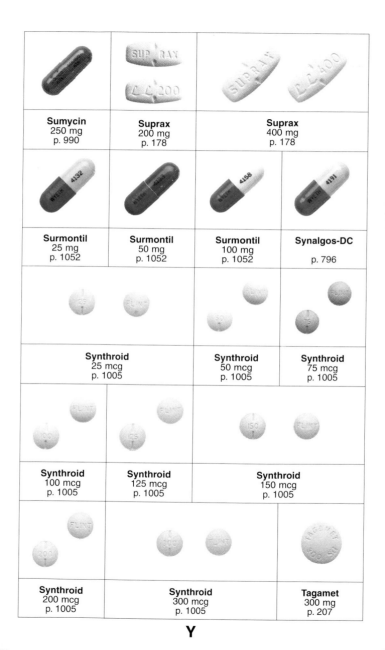

Sumycin 250 mg p. 990	**Suprax** 200 mg p. 178	**Suprax** 400 mg p. 178
Surmontil 25 mg p. 1052	**Surmontil** 50 mg p. 1052	**Surmontil** 100 mg p. 1052	**Synalgos-DC** p. 796
Synthroid 25 mcg p. 1005		**Synthroid** 50 mcg p. 1005	**Synthroid** 75 mcg p. 1005
Synthroid 100 mcg p. 1005	**Synthroid** 125 mcg p. 1005	**Synthroid** 150 mcg p. 1005	
Synthroid 200 mcg p. 1005	**Synthroid** 300 mcg p. 1005		**Tagamet** 300 mg p. 207

Y

Tagamet 400 mg p. 207	**Tagamet** 800 mg p. 207	**Talwin NX** p. 796	
Tavist 2.68 mg p. 220		**Tegretol** 200 mg p. 157	
Tegretol Chewable 100 mg p. 157		**Tenuate** 25 mg p. 611	**Tenuate Dospan** 75 mg p. 611
Theo-Dur 200 mg p. 1089	**Theo-Dur** 300 mg p. 1089	**Theo-Dur** 450 mg p. 1089	**Thorazine** 25 mg p. 193
Thorazine 50 mg p. 193	**Thorazine** 100 mg p. 193	**Thorazine Spansule** 75 mg p. 193	**Thorazine Spansule** 150 mg p. 193

Z

Tiazac 180 mg p. 330	**Tiazac** 240 mg p. 330	**Ticlid** 250 mg p. 1012
Tolectin 200 mg p. 703		**Tolectin** 600 mg p. 703	**Tolectin DS** 400 mg p. 703
Tolinase 100 mg p. 957	**Tolinase** 500 mg p. 957	**Tonocard** 400 mg p. 1022
Tonocard 600 mg p. 1022		**Topamax** 25 mg p. 1029
Toprol-XL 50 mg p. 657	**Toprol-XL** 100 mg p. 657	**Tranxene T-Tab** 7.5 mg p. 238

AA

Tranxene T-Tab 15 mg p. 238	**Triavil 2-10** p. 1051
Triavil 2-25 p. 1051	**Triavil 4-10** p. 1051
Triavil 4-25 p. 1051	**Tricor** 67 mg p. 415 — **Trimox** 250 mg p. 785
Trimox 500 mg p. 785 — **Tritec** 400 mg p. 877	**Tylenol with Codeine #2** p. 793
Tylenol with Codeine #3 p. 793	**Tylox** p. 792

BB

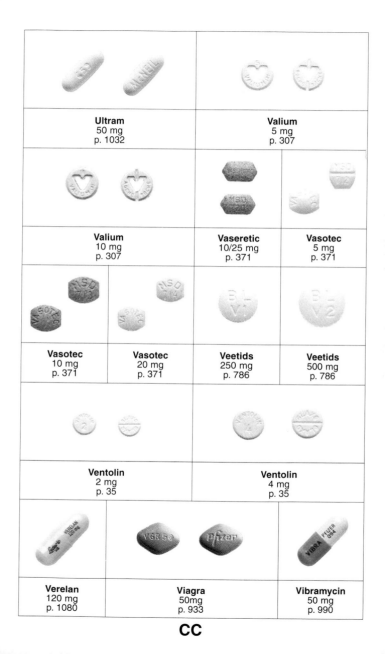

Ultram
50 mg
p. 1032

Valium
5 mg
p. 307

Valium
10 mg
p. 307

Vaseretic
10/25 mg
p. 371

Vasotec
5 mg
p. 371

Vasotec
10 mg
p. 371

Vasotec
20 mg
p. 371

Veetids
250 mg
p. 786

Veetids
500 mg
p. 786

Ventolin
2 mg
p. 35

Ventolin
4 mg
p. 35

Verelan
120 mg
p. 1080

Viagra
50mg
p. 933

Vibramycin
50 mg
p. 990

CC

Vibramycin 100 mg p. 990	**Vibra-Tabs** 100 mg p. 990	**Vicodin** p. 793
Vicodin ES p. 793	**Vioxx** 25 mg p. 901	**Visken** 5 mg p. 818

Visken 10 mg p. 818	**Vivactil** 5 mg p. 1052

Vivactil 10 mg p. 1052	**Wellbutrin** 75 mg p. 140	**Wellbutrin** 100 mg p. 140
Wellbutrin SR 100 mg p. 140	**Wymox** 250 mg p. 785	**Xanax** 0.25 mg p. 44 **Xanax** 0.5 mg p. 44

DD

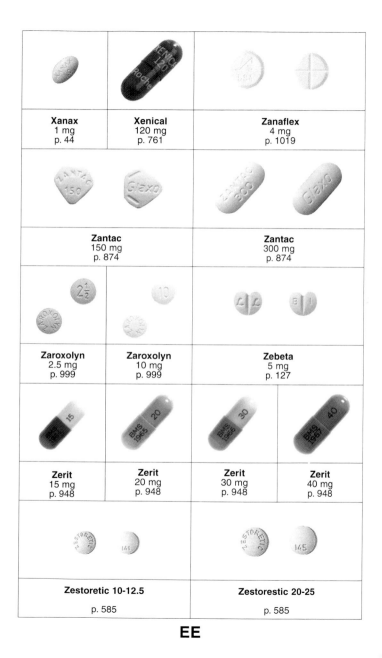

Xanax 1 mg p. 44	**Xenical** 120 mg p. 761	**Zanaflex** 4 mg p. 1019

Zantac 150 mg p. 874	**Zantac** 300 mg p. 874

Zaroxolyn 2.5 mg p. 999	**Zaroxolyn** 10 mg p. 999	**Zebeta** 5 mg p. 127

Zerit 15 mg p. 948	**Zerit** 20 mg p. 948	**Zerit** 30 mg p. 948	**Zerit** 40 mg p. 948

Zestoretic 10-12.5 p. 585	**Zestorestic 20-25** p. 585

EE

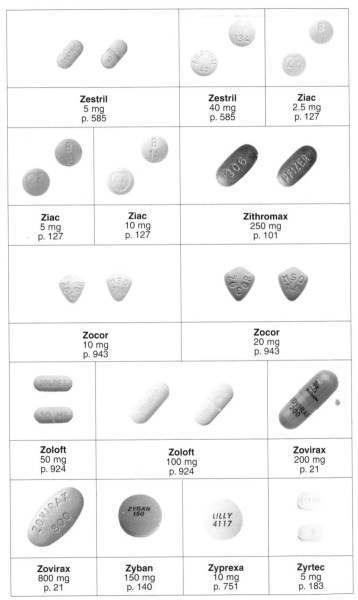

Zestril 5 mg p. 585	**Zestril** 40 mg p. 585	**Ziac** 2.5 mg p. 127
Ziac 5 mg p. 127	**Ziac** 10 mg p. 127	**Zithromax** 250 mg p. 101
Zocor 10 mg p. 943	**Zocor** 20 mg p. 943	
Zoloft 50 mg p. 924	**Zoloft** 100 mg p. 924	**Zovirax** 200 mg p. 21
Zovirax 800 mg p. 21	**Zyban** 150 mg p. 140	**Zyprexa** 10 mg p. 751	**Zyrtec** 5 mg p. 183

FF

Cautions and Warnings

People **allergic** to ketoprofen or any other NSAID and those with a history of **asthma** attacks brought on by an NSAID, iodides, or aspirin should not take ketoprofen.

Ketoprofen may cause **gastrointestinal (GI) bleeding, ulcers,** and **stomach perforation**. This can occur at any time, with or without warning, in people who take ketoprofen regularly. People with a history of active GI bleeding should be cautious about taking any NSAID. People who develop bleeding or ulcers and continue taking ketoprofen should be aware of the chances of developing more serious side effects.

Ketoprofen may affect platelets and **blood clotting** at high doses, and should be avoided by people with clotting problems and those taking warfarin.

People with **heart problems** who use ketoprofen may experience swelling in their arms, legs, or feet.

Ketoprofen may cause severe toxic effects to the **kidney**. Report any unusual side effects to your doctor, who might need to periodically test your kidney function.

Ketoprofen may make you unusually **sensitive to the effects of the sun**.

Possible Side Effects

▼ Most common: diarrhea, nausea, vomiting, constipation, minor stomach upset or distress, gas, and appetite loss, especially during the first few days of treatment.

▼ Less common: stomach ulcers, GI bleeding, hepatitis, gallbladder attacks, painful urination, poor kidney function, kidney inflammation, blood and protein in the urine, dizziness, fainting, nervousness, depression, hallucinations, confusion, disorientation, light-headedness, tingling in the hands or feet, itching, increased sweating, dry nose and mouth, heart palpitations, chest pain, breathing difficulties, and muscle cramps.

▼ Rare: severe allergic reactions including closing of the throat and fever and chills; changes in liver function; jaundice (yellowing of the skin or whites of the eyes); and kidney failure. People who experience such effects must be promptly treated in a hospital emergency room or doctor's office. NSAIDs have caused severe skin reactions; if this happens to you, see your doctor immediately.

Drug Interactions

• Ketoprofen may increase the effects of oral anticoagulant (blood-thinning) drugs such as warfarin. Your anticoagulant dose may need to be reduced.

• Mixing ketoprofen with cyclosporine may increase the kidney-related side effects of both drugs. Methotrexate side effects may be increased in people also taking ketoprofen.

• Ketoprofen may reduce the blood-pressure-lowering effect of beta blockers and loop diuretics.

• Ketoprofen may increase phenytoin side effects. Lithium blood levels may be increased by ketoprofen.

• Ketoprofen blood levels may be affected by cimetidine.

• Probenecid may increase the risk of ketoprofen side effects.

• Aspirin and other salicylates should never be combined with ketoprofen.

Food Interactions

Take ketoprofen with food or a magnesium/aluminum antacid if it upsets your stomach.

Usual Dose

Capsules
  Adult: 50–75 mg 3–4 times a day. Do not exceed 300 mg a day. Seniors and people with kidney problems should start with ⅓–½ of the usual dose.

Controlled-Release Capsules
  Adult and Senior: 200 mg once a day.

Overdosage

People have died from NSAID overdoses. Common signs of overdose are drowsiness, nausea, vomiting, diarrhea, abdominal pain, rapid breathing, rapid heartbeat, increased sweating, ringing or buzzing in the ears, confusion, disorientation, stupor, and coma. Take the victim to a hospital emergency room at once. ALWAYS bring the prescription bottle or container.

Special Information

Take each dose with a full glass of water and do not lie down for 15 to 30 minutes afterward.

Ketoprofen can make you drowsy or tired: Be careful when driving or operating hazardous equipment. Do not take any over-the-counter products containing acetaminophen or aspirin while taking ketoprofen. Avoid alcohol.

Contact your doctor if you develop rash or itching, visual disturbances, weight gain, breathing difficulties, fluid retention, hallucinations, black or tarry stools, persistent headache, or any unusual or intolerable side effect.

If you forget a dose of ketoprofen, take it as soon as you remember. If you take ketoprofen once a day and it is within 8 hours of your next dose, or if you take several doses a day and it is within 4 hours of your next dose, skip the dose you forgot and continue with your regular schedule. Never take a double dose.

Special Populations

Pregnancy/Breast-feeding

NSAIDs may affect the fetal heart during the second half of pregnancy. Pregnant women should not take ketoprofen without their doctor's approval. When this drug is considered crucial by your doctor, its potential benefits must be carefully weighed against its risks.

NSAIDs may pass into breast milk. Nursing mothers who must take this drug should bottle-feed.

Seniors

Seniors may be more susceptible to side effects, especially ulcer disease.

Generic Name

Ketorolac (kee-TOE-roe-lak) G

Brand Names

Acular Eyedrops   Toradol

Type of Drug

Nonsteroidal anti-inflammatory drug (NSAID).

Prescribed for

Moderately severe pain. The eyedrops are prescribed for eye redness and inflammation caused by seasonal allergies and for inflammation following cataract surgery.

General Information

Ketorolac tromethamine and other NSAIDs are used to relieve pain and inflammation. We do not know exactly how NSAIDs work, but they may achieve their effects by blocking the body's production of a hormone called prostaglandin and the action of other body chemicals. Pain relief comes within 1 hour after taking the first dose of ketorolac. Unlike other NSAIDs, ketorolac is a potent drug with serious risks. Taking more ketorolac than is prescribed only increases risk; it does not offer better results. People who have first been treated with ketorolac injection should only take ketorolac tablets. Total treatment with injectable and oral ketorolac should not exceed 5 days.

NSAID eyedrops may be used during eye surgery to prevent movement of the eye muscles.

Cautions and Warnings

People **allergic** to ketorolac or any other NSAID and those with a history of **asthma** attacks brought on by an NSAID, iodides, or aspirin should not take ketorolac.

Ketorolac may cause **gastrointestinal (GI) bleeding**, **ulcers**, and **stomach perforation**. This can occur at any time, with or without warning, in people who take ketorolac regularly. People with a history of active GI bleeding should be cautious about taking any NSAID. People who develop bleeding or ulcers and continue NSAID treatment should be aware of the possibility of developing more serious side effects.

Ketorolac may affect platelets and **blood clotting** at high doses and should be avoided by people with clotting problems and those who take warfarin.

People with **heart problems** who use ketorolac may experience swelling in their arms, legs, or feet.

Ketorolac may actually cause **headaches**. If this happens, you might have to stop taking this drug or switch to another NSAID.

Ketorolac may cause severe toxic effects to the **kidney**. Report any unusual side effects to your doctor, who might need to periodically test your kidney function.

People taking ketorolac on a regular basis should have their **liver function** checked periodically.

Ketorolac may make you **unusually sensitive to the effects of the sun**.

Possible Side Effects

Injection and Tablets

▼ Most common: diarrhea, nausea, vomiting, constipation, minor stomach upset or distress, gas, and appetite loss, especially during the first few days of treatment.

▼ Less common: stomach ulcers, GI bleeding, hepatitis, gallbladder attacks, painful urination, poor kidney function, kidney inflammation, blood and protein in the urine, dizziness, fainting, nervousness, depression, hallucinations, confusion, disorientation, tingling in the hands or feet, light-headedness, itching, increased sweating, dry nose and mouth, heart palpitations, chest pain, breathing difficulties, and muscle cramps.

▼ Rare: severe allergic reactions including closing of the throat, fever and chills, changes in liver function, jaundice (yellowing of the skin or whites of the eyes), and kidney failure. People who experience such effects must be promptly treated in a hospital emergency room or doctor's office. NSAIDs have caused severe skin reactions; if this happens to you, see your doctor immediately.

Eyedrops

▼ Most common: temporary burning, stinging, or other minor eye irritation.

▼ Less common: nausea, vomiting, viral infections, and eye reactions including persistent redness, burning, itching, or tearing. The risk of developing bleeding problems or other systemic (whole-body) side effects with ketorolac eyedrops is low because only a small amount of the drug is absorbed into the blood.

Drug Interactions

Injection and Tablets

• Ketorolac may increase the effects of oral anticoagulant (blood-thinning) drugs such as warfarin. Your anticoagulant dose may need to be reduced.

• Taking ketorolac with cyclosporine may increase the kidney-related side effects of both drugs. Methotrexate side effects may be increased in people also taking ketorolac.

• Ketorolac may reduce the blood-pressure-lowering effect of beta blockers and loop diuretics.

• Ketorolac may increase phenytoin side effects. Lithium blood levels may be raised by ketorolac.

• Ketorolac blood levels may be affected by cimetidine.

• Probenecid may increase the risk of ketorolac side effects.

• Aspirin and other salicylates should never be combined with ketorolac.

Eyedrops
None known.

Food Interactions

Take ketorolac with food or a magnesium/aluminum antacid if it upsets your stomach.

Usual Dose

Tablets: Up to 40 mg a day for no more than 5 consecutive days.

Eyedrops: 1 drop 4 times a day for itching and irritation due to seasonal allergies.

Overdosage

People have died from NSAID overdoses. Common signs of overdose are drowsiness, nausea, vomiting, diarrhea, abdominal pain, rapid breathing, rapid heartbeat, increased sweating, ringing or buzzing in the ears, confusion, disorientation, stupor, and coma. Take the victim to a hospital emergency room at once. ALWAYS bring the prescription bottle or container.

Special Information

Injection and Tablets: Take each dose with a full glass of water and do not lie down for 15 to 30 minutes afterward.

Ketorolac can make you drowsy or tired: Be careful when driving or operating hazardous equipment. Do not take any over-the-counter products containing acetaminophen or aspirin while taking ketorolac. Avoid alcoholic beverages.

Contact your doctor if you develop rash or itching, visual disturbances, weight gain, breathing difficulties, fluid retention, hallucinations, black or tarry stools, persistent headache, or any unusual or intolerable side effect.

If you forget a dose of ketorolac tablets, take it as soon as you remember. If you take ketorolac once a day and it is within 8 hours of your next dose, or if you take several doses a day and it is within 4 hours of your next dose, skip the dose you forgot and continue with your regular schedule. Never take a double dose.

Eyedrops: To prevent possible infection, do not allow the dropper to touch your fingers, eyelids, or any surface. Wait at least 5 minutes before using any other eyedrops.

If you forget to administer a dose of ketorolac eyedrops, do so as soon as you remember. If it is almost time for your next dose, skip the dose you forgot and continue with your regular schedule. Do not take a double dose.

Special Populations

Pregnancy/Breast-feeding

Ketorolac should not be taken by pregnant women because it may affect fetal blood circulation and prevent normal labor.

Ketorolac may pass into breast milk. There is a possibility that a nursing mother taking ketorolac could affect her baby's heart or cardiovascular system. Nursing mothers who must take this drug should bottle-feed.

Seniors

Seniors may be more susceptible to side effects, especially ulcer disease.

Generic Name

Ketotifen (kee-toe-TIH-fen)

Brand Name

Zaditor Eyedrops

The information in this profile also applies to the following drug:

Generic Ingredient: Lodoxamide
Alomide Eyedrops

Type of Drug

Antihistamine.

Prescribed for

Conjunctivitis (pinkeye) caused by allergies.

General Information

Ketotifen relieves and prevents eye itchiness and irritation associated with seasonal allergies. Lodoxamide only prevents itchiness and allergies. They achieve their effects by stabilizing mast cells in the eye, which prevents the release of chemicals such as histamine that cause redness and irritation during an allergic reaction. Ketotifen starts working within minutes after administering the drops. This drug has not been studied in children under age 3. Lodoxamide may be used in children age 2 and over.

Cautions and Warnings

Do not use this drug if you are **sensitive** or **allergic** to it.

Possible Side Effects

▼ Most common: eye redness, headache, and runny nose.

▼ Less common: a burning or stinging sensation in the eye, eye discharge, tearing, increased sensitivity to bright light, dilation of the pupil, allergic reactions, rash, flu-like symptoms, and sore throat.

Drug Interactions

• If you use more than 1 eyedrop medication, separate doses of these drugs by at least 1 hour.

Usual Dose

Ketotifen: Adults and children age 3 and over—1 drop in affected eye every 8–12 hours.

Lodoxamide: Adults and children age 2 and over—1 drop in affected eye 4 times a day.

Overdosage

Accidental ingestion of an entire bottle of ketotifen is unlikely to cause side effects since it contains less than 2 mg of medicine. Call your local poison control center or a hospital emergency room for more information. If you seek treatment, ALWAYS bring the prescription bottle or container.

Special Information

Do not wear contact lenses if your eyes are red because they may worsen the irritation.

Ketotifen does not alleviate eye irritation caused by contact lenses.

Remove your soft contact lenses before using ketotifen eyedrops; you may replace them 10 minutes after a dose.

To prevent infection, do not allow the eyedropper to touch your fingers, eyelids, or any surface.

If you forget to administer a dose, do so as soon as you remember. If it is almost time for your next dose, skip the dose you forgot and continue with your regular schedule. Do not take a double dose.

Special Populations

Pregnancy/Breast-feeding

In animal studies, very large dosages of ketotifen caused bone malformations in the fetus. When this drug is considered crucial by your doctor, its potential benefits must be carefully weighed against its risks.

Though unlikely, ketotifen may pass into breast milk. Nursing mothers who must use this drug should consider bottle-feeding.

Seniors

Seniors may use this drug without special precaution.

Generic Name

Labetalol (luh-BET-uh-lol) G

Brand Names

Normodyne   Trandate

Type of Drug

Adrenergic blocker and antihypertensive.

Prescribed for

Hypertension (high blood pressure).

General Information

Labetalol hydrochloride is unique because it selectively blocks both alpha- and beta-adrenergic impulses. This combination of actions contributes to its ability to reduce blood pressure. Other drugs can increase or decrease heart rate; labetalol has an advantage over other beta blockers because it rarely affects heart rate.

Cautions and Warnings

People with **asthma,** severe **heart failure, reduced heart rate,** and **heart block** (disruption of the electrical impulses that control heart rate) should not take labetalol. People with **angina** who take labetalol for hypertension risk aggravating their angina if they suddenly stop taking the drug. These people should have their dosage reduced gradually over 1 to 2 weeks. Labetalol should be used with caution if you have **liver disease**.

Possible Side Effects

Side effects develop early and increase with dosage.

▼ Most common: dizziness, tingling of the scalp, nausea, vomiting, upset stomach, distortion in the sense of taste, fatigue, sweating, impotence, urinary difficulties, diarrhea, bile-duct blockage, bronchial spasm, breathing difficulties, muscle weakness, cramps, dry eyes, blurred vision, rash, facial swelling, and hair loss.

▼ Less common: aggravation of lupus erythematosus (chronic condition affecting the body's connective tissue), stuffy nose, depression, confusion, disorientation, loss of short-term memory, emotional instability, colitis, drug allergy (symptoms include fever, sore throat, and breathing difficulties), and a reduction in levels of white blood cells and blood platelets.

Drug Interactions

• Labetalol may suppress normal signs of low blood sugar and interfere with the action of oral antidiabetes drugs.

• Combining labetalol and a tricyclic antidepressant may cause tremor.

• Labetalol may interfere with the effect of some antiasthma drugs, especially ephedrine, isoproterenol, and other beta stimulants.

• Cimetidine increases the amount of labetalol absorbed into the bloodstream from oral tablets.

• Glutethimide decreases the amount of labetalol in the blood.

• Labetalol may increase the blood-pressure-lowering effect of nitroglycerin.

Food Interactions

This drug may be taken with food if it upsets your stomach. In fact, food increases the amount of labetalol absorbed into the blood.

Usual Dose

Starting dosage—100 mg twice a day; may be increased gradually to as much as 1200 mg twice a day. Maintenance dosage—200–400 mg twice a day.

Overdosage

Overdose slows heart rate and causes an excessive drop in blood pressure. The possible consequences of these effects can be treated only in a hospital emergency room. ALWAYS bring the prescription bottle or container.

Special Information

You may experience scalp tingling, especially when you first start taking labetalol.

Labetalol is meant to be taken on a continuing basis. Do not stop this drug unless instructed to do so by your doctor.

Weakness; swelling of your ankles, feet, or legs; breathing difficulties; or other side effects should be reported to your doctor as soon as possible. Most side effects are not serious, but about 7% of people have to switch to another drug because of them.

If you forget a dose, take it as soon as possible. If it is within 8 hours of your next dose, skip the dose you forgot and go back to your regular schedule. Do not take a double dose.

Special Populations

Pregnancy/Breast-feeding

Labetalol enters the fetal circulation. Women who are or might be pregnant should not take this drug without their doctor's approval. When the drug is considered crucial by your doctor, its possible benefits must be carefully weighed against its risks.

This drug passes into breast milk. Nursing mothers who must take labetalol should consider bottle-feeding.

Seniors

Seniors may be more sensitive to the effects of labetalol. Your dosage must be individually adjusted by your doctor, especially if you have liver disease. Seniors may be more likely to suffer from cold hands and feet, reduced body temperature, chest pain, feeling unwell, sudden breathing difficulties, sweating, or changes in heartbeat.

Generic Name

Lamivudine (lam-IV-ue-dene)

Brand Name

Epivir

Combination Products

Generic Ingredients: Lamivudine + Zidovudine
Combivir

Type of Drug

Antiviral.

Prescribed for

Human immunodeficiency virus (HIV) infection, in combination with other anti-HIV drugs.

General Information

Lamivudine, also known as 3-TC, is a nucleoside-type antiviral that works on the HIV virus in the same way as zalcitibine, zidovudine (AZT), stavudine, and other drugs of this type. It is generally given in combination with AZT and a protease inhibitor to people who do not respond to single-drug treatment. Lamivudine is eliminated primarily through the kidneys.

Cautions and Warnings

Do not take lamivudine if you are **sensitive** or **allergic** to it.

People with **kidney disease** need less lamivudine than people with normal kidney function.

Possible Side Effects

Because this drug is always taken with AZT, the listed side effects are those of the drugs in combination. The long-term effects of lamivudine are not known.

▼ Most common: headache, not feeling well, fever, chills, rash, nausea, vomiting, diarrhea, appetite loss, abdominal pain or cramps, nervous system problems including tingling and poor coordination, sleeplessness, dizziness, depression, stuffy or runny nose, cough, and muscle pain.

▼ Common: upset stomach, joint pain, and tingling in the hands or feet in children. Lamivudine may affect the results of a variety of blood tests.

▼ Rare: pancreas irritation, more often seen in children than adults.

Drug Interactions

• Lamivudine increases maximum blood levels of AZT by 39%, which is helpful in fighting the HIV virus.

• Trimethoprim-sulfamethoxazole, taken for opportunistic AIDS-related infections, increases the amount of lamivudine in the blood.

Food Interactions

Lamivudine is absorbed more slowly when taken with food, but not enough to affect the total amount of drug that reaches the blood.

Usual Dose

Lamivudine
   Adult and Child (age 12 and over): 150 mg twice a day. Adults who weigh less than 110 lbs. should receive about 1 mg per lb. of body weight twice a day. Dosage is reduced as kidney function decreases.
   Child (age 3 months–12 years): about 2 mg per lb. of body weight twice a day, no more than 150 mg per dose.

Lamivudine-Zidovudine
   Adult and Child: 1 tablet—lamivudine 150 mg plus zidovu-

dine 300 mg—twice a day. Poor kidney function requires reducing the dosage of both drugs. In this situation, it is preferable to take the individual drugs separately so that you retain maximum dosage flexibility.

Overdosage

Little is known about the effects of lamivudine overdose. Call your local poison control center for more information.

Special Information

Lamivudine does not cure AIDS. It will not prevent you from transmitting the HIV virus to another person; you must still practice safe sex. People taking this drug will still develop opportunistic infections and other complications of AIDS.

It is very important to take lamivudine exactly as prescribed. If you forget a dose, take it as soon as you remember. If it is almost time for your next dose, skip the dose you forgot and continue with your regular schedule. Call your doctor if you forget 2 or more doses in a row.

Call your doctor at once if your child develops signs of pancreas inflammation while taking lamivudine. Symptoms include very severe abdominal pain, tense abdominal muscles, sweating, feeling very ill, shallow and rapid breathing, fever, and possible fainting.

Special Populations

Pregnancy/Breast-feeding

Lamivudine passes into the blood circulation of the fetus. Some animal studies of lamivudine indicate that it may be dangerous to the fetus, but others showed no effect. There is no information about the effect of lamivudine in pregnant women. Like all drugs, lamivudine should be taken during pregnancy only if absolutely necessary.

It is not known if lamivudine passes into breast milk. Nursing mothers who must take lamivudine should bottle-feed. In any case, nursing mothers who are HIV positive should bottle-feed to avoid transmitting the virus through their milk.

Seniors

Seniors may require a smaller dose of lamivudine, depending on their kidney function. Otherwise, seniors may take this drug without special restriction.

Generic Name

Lamotrigine (lam-OE-trih-jene)

Brand Names

Lamictal   Lamictal CD

Type of Drug

Anticonvulsant.

Prescribed for

Adult epilepsy and partial seizure; also prescribed for tonic-clonic, absence, and myoclonic seizures, and for infants and children with Lennox-Gastaut syndrome.

General Information

Much like phenytoin and carbamazepine, lamotrigine stabilizes voltage-dependent channels in the brain. This prevents the release of chemicals that would stimulate the nervous system and lead to seizure. Lamotrigine is one of the first new anti-seizure drugs available in more than 10 years. It reaches maximum blood concentration in 1½ to 5 hours. Lamotrigine is eliminated from the body by the liver.

Cautions and Warnings

Lamotrigine may cause severe and possibly **life-threatening rashes,** nearly always within 2 to 8 weeks of use. Minor rashes also occur, but it is not possible to tell which ones may become life threatening. If you develop a rash while taking this drug, call your doctor at once.

Twenty sudden and **unexplained deaths** occurred in people taking lamotrigine before it was approved for general use. These deaths are thought to be unrelated to lamotrigine.

Five people taking lamotrigine died from acute **liver failure** or **multi-organ failure** before the drug was approved for general use. It is not known if the drug played a role in these deaths.

Lamotrigine is not recommended for general use in **children under age 16**.

Lamotrigine binds to melanin, a body hormone found in the skin and eyes. The long-term effects of lamotrigine on the eyes are not known.

When you stop taking lamotrigine, the dose should be reduced gradually over a period of 2 weeks or more to prevent **withdrawal seizures**.

Status epilepticus, a severe seizure disorder, and **worsening of existing seizure disorders** may develop in a small number of people taking lamotrigine.

People with **heart disease** or severe **kidney or liver disease** should use this drug with caution.

Lamotrigine may cause unusual **sensitivity to the sun**. Wear protective clothing and use sunscreen.

Possible Side Effects

▼ Most common: headache, dizziness, nausea, weakness, tiredness, runny nose, double vision, and blurred vision.

▼ Common: accidental injury, flu-like symptoms, abdominal pain, vomiting, infection, neck pain, feeling unwell, worsening of seizure, diarrhea, upset stomach, constipation, dental problems, loss of coordination, sleeplessness, tremors, depression, anxiety, convulsions, irritability, itching, visual difficulties, painful menstruation, and vaginal irritation.

▼ Less common: chills, hot flashes, heart palpitations, appetite loss, dry mouth, joint ache, muscle weakness, speech disorders, sore throat, coughing, speech problems involving the tongue, memory loss, confusion, loss of concentration, sleep disorders, emotional upset, fainting, racing thoughts, rolling of the eyes, muscle spasm, breathing difficulties, hair loss, acne, ear pain, ringing or buzzing in the ears, and missed periods.

▼ Rare: Rare side effects can occur in almost any part of the body. Contact your doctor if you experience any side effect not listed above.

Drug Interactions

• Combining lamotrigine and sodium valproate doubles lamotrigine concentrations in the blood and reduces those of valproate by ¼. Dosage adjustments are necessary. Combining these drugs also increases the risk of rash.

• Combining carbamazepine and lamotrigine increases carbamazepine blood levels, possibly leading to side effects, and reduces the amount of lamotrigine in the blood by 40%.

• Combining acetaminophen and lamotrigine can slightly increase the rate at which lamotrigine is broken down, but occasional use of the two drugs together is not likely to be a problem. Regular acetaminophen users may require more lamotrigine.

• Anti-folate drugs—often used in cancer treatment—can increase the effects of lamotrigine.

• Phenobarbital and primidone may reduce the effects of lamotrigine.

• Phenytoin reduces the amount of lamotrigine in the blood by about ¼.

Food Interactions

None known.

Usual Dose

Adult and Child (age 16 and over): starting dosage—25 or 50 mg a day. Increase gradually to a maximum daily dosage of 500 mg. Lamotrigine is usually taken twice a day; be sure to take your doses 12 hours apart.

Child (under age 16): not recommended.

Overdosage

Symptoms include dizziness, headache, sleepiness, and coma. Take the victim to a hospital emergency room at once. ALWAYS bring the prescription bottle or container.

Special Information

Dosage increases may be required if your liver starts breaking down the drug faster over time. Periodic monitoring of lamotrigine blood levels is necessary to determine this.

Call your doctor at once if you develop a rash, but do not change your lamotrigine dosage or stop taking it.

Lamotrigine may cause drowsiness, dizziness, or blurred vision, effects that are increased by alcohol. Be careful while driving or engaging in any activity requiring concentration, alertness, and coordination.

If you take acetaminophen while you are taking lamotrigine, especially for a lamotrigine headache, do not take more acetaminophen than is recommended on the package.

If you take lamotrigine once a day and forget a dose, take it as soon as you remember. If it is within 8 hours of your next dose, skip the one you forgot and continue with your regular schedule. Do not take a double dose.

After the first 2 weeks of treatment, most people take lamotrigine twice a day. If you take it twice a day, be sure to take your medication every 12 hours. If you forget a dose, take it as soon as you remember. If it is within 4 hours of your next dose, take 1 dose as soon as you remember and another in 5 or 6 hours, then go back to your regular schedule.

Special Populations

Pregnancy/Breast-feeding
Animal studies suggest that lamotrigine causes fetal injury. It reduces the amount of folate in the fetus, an effect that is associated with birth defects. Seizure disorder itself also increases the risk of birth defects. Pregnant women should take lamotrigine only after discussing with their doctors its potential benefits and risks.

Lamotrigine passes into breast milk. Nursing mothers who must take it should bottle-feed.

Seniors
Seniors may take lamotrigine without special restriction.

Lanoxin   *see Digitalis Glycosides, page 326*

Generic Name

Latanoprost (lah-TAN-oe-prost)

Brand Name
Xalatan

Type of Drug
Anti-glaucoma.

Prescribed for
Open-angle glaucoma and ocular hypertension (high pressure inside the eye).

General Information

Latanoprost is believed to reduce pressure inside the eye by increasing the outflow of eye fluid. Latanoprost is absorbed through the cornea, where it is transformed into its active form. Maximum pressure-lowering occurs in 8 to 12 hours. Studies show that the 0.005% concentration of latanoprost is equivalent to 0.5% of timolol in its ability to reduce eye pressure.

Cautions and Warnings

Do not use latanoprost if you are **allergic** or **sensitive** to it.

Latanoprost may **change your eye color** because it increases the number of pigment granules in the cornea, which in turn increases the brown pigment in the iris. This color change occurs gradually over a period of months or years. Typically, the brown color around the pupil spreads slowly to the outer part of the iris. This change is more noticeable in people with green-brown, blue/gray-brown, or yellow-brown eye color. The long-term effect of latanoprost on eye pigment granules is not known; your doctor may tell you to stop using these eyedrops if the color change persists or is especially noticeable.

The effect of latanoprost on the cornea is not known.

Possible Side Effects

▼ Most common: blurred vision; stinging, burning, and redness of the eyes; a sensation of something in the eye; itching; and brownish eye coloration.

▼ Less common: dry eye, excessive tearing, swelling or redness of the eyelid, eyelid discomfort or pain, and increased sensitivity to bright light.

▼ Rare: blood clot in the artery supplying the retina, detachment of the retina, and bleeding inside the eye. General side effects from traces of latanoprost passing into the blood can include colds, flu, or other respiratory infections; muscle, joint, or back pain; chest pain; angina pain; and rash or allergic reactions.

Drug Interactions

• If you use other eyedrops that contain a thimerosal preservative, separate the administration of each eyedrop by at least 5 minutes.

Usual Dose

Adult: 1 drop (1.5 mcg) in the affected eye once a day in the evening.

Child: not recommended.

Overdosage

Symptoms include eye irritation and redness. Severe overdosage may also cause abdominal pain, dizziness, fatigue, flushing, nausea, and sweating. Overdose victims may require emergency room care. Call your local poison control center or a hospital emergency room for more information.

Special Information

Call your doctor if you develop eye irritation or any other side effect.

If you use any eyedrops in addition to latanoprost, wait 5 minutes between each application.

To prevent infection, keep the eyedropper from touching your fingers, eyelids, or any surface.

If you wear contact lenses, take them out before using latanoprost eyedrops. Latanoprost contains a benzalkonium preservative that can be absorbed by the contacts.

Store unopened bottles of latanoprost in the refrigerator. Once opened, the eyedrops can be kept at room temperature—up to 77°F—for 6 weeks.

Do not take more latanoprost than prescribed. Taking it more often may actually reduce its effectiveness. If you forget to administer a dose, do so as soon as you remember. If it is almost time for your next dose, skip the one you forgot and continue with your regular schedule. Do not take a double dose.

Special Populations

Pregnancy/Breast-feeding

Animal studies have shown that latanoprost can be harmful to the fetus at extremely high dosages. When this drug is considered crucial by your doctor, its potential benefits must be carefully weighed against its risks.

It is not known if latanoprost passes into breast milk. Nursing mothers who must use this drug should consider bottle-feeding.

Seniors

Seniors may use latanoprost without special precaution.

Generic Name

Leflunomide (leh-FLUE-noe-mide)

Brand Name

Arava

Type of Drug

Anti-inflammatory and antiproliferative (cell growth slower).

Prescribed for

Rheumatoid arthritis.

General Information

Leflunomide can help relieve symptoms of rheumatoid arthritis and slow the structural damage and erosion of tissues in affected joints. In studies, it was found to be as effective as methotrexate and sulfasalazine. It takes about a month for leflunomide to begin working and it reaches maximum effect in 3 to 6 months. The maximum effect is retained for as long as you take this medicine. Leflunomide is broken down in the liver.

Cautions and Warnings

Leflunomide should not be taken during pregnancy.

People who are **sensitive** or **allergic** to leflunomide should not take it.

Leflunomide causes **liver irritation** and an increase in certain liver enzymes. Your dosage may have to be reduced or the drug discontinued if the effect is severe. People with **hepatitis B or C** should not take this drug. People with **kidney problems** should use it with caution.

Leflunomide is not recommended for people with severely **depressed immune systems, abnormal bone marrow,** or severe and uncontrolled **infection**.

Use of **live-virus vaccines** is not recommended while taking leflunomide

---

Possible Side Effects

▼ Most common: diarrhea, high blood pressure, hair loss, rash, and respiratory infection.

Possible Side Effects *(continued)*

▼ Common: headache, upset stomach, stomach or abdominal pain, abnormal liver function, nausea, bronchitis, generalized pain, back pain, urinary infection, and accidents or injuries.

▼ Less common: chest pain, dizziness, tingling in the hands or feet, eczema, mouth ulcer, itching, dry skin, appetite loss, vomiting, low blood potassium, weight loss, muscle pain, leg cramps, inflamed tendons, arthritis, cough, sore throat, pneumonia, runny nose, sinus irritation, allergic reaction, weakness, flu-like symptoms, and infections.

▼ Rare: Rare side effects can occur in almost any part of the body. Contact your doctor if you experience any side effect not listed above.

Drug Interactions

• Cholestyramine and charcoal rapidly reduce leflunomide blood levels.

• Rifampin increases the amount of leflunomide in the blood by 40%.

• Leflunomide can increase the liver toxicity of other drugs that are toxic to the liver, such as methotrexate.

• Leflunomide increases blood levels of nonsteroidal anti-inflammatory drugs (NSAIDs). The importance of this effect is unclear.

• Leflunomide increases the amount of tolbutamide (an antidiabetes drug) in the blood by up to 50%. The importance of this effect is unclear.

Food Interactions

Leflunomide may be taken without regard to food or meals.

Usual Dose

Adult: 100 mg a day for 3 days, then 20 mg once a day.
Child: not recommended.

When you stop taking leflunomide, it is recommended that you follow a drug elimination procedure: Take 8 g of

cholestyramine (ordinarily used to help lower blood cholesterol) 3 times a day for 11 days. Without this procedure, it
may take up to 2 years to eliminate the drug and its breakdown products from your body.

Overdosage

Symptoms are likely to include drug side effects. Take the victim to a hospital emergency room at once. ALWAYS bring the
prescription bottle or container.

Special Information

Your liver function must be monitored regularly while you
take this drug.

If you forget a dose, take it as soon as you remember. If it is
almost time for your next dose, skip the one you forgot and
continue with your regular schedule.

Special Populations

Pregnancy/Breast-feeding

Leflunomide causes birth defects and should not be used
during pregnancy. Women of childbearing age must be
tested for pregnancy before taking leflunomide and use effective contraception during treatment. Women who plan to
become pregnant after discontinuing the drug must follow
the drug elimination procedure (see "Usual Dose").

Leflunomide may pass into breast milk. Nursing mothers
who must take it should bottle-feed.

Seniors

Seniors may take this drug without special precaution.

Lescol   *see Statin Cholesterol-Lowering Agents, page 942*

Type of Drug

Leukotriene Antagonist/Inhibitor

(LUE-koe-treen)

Brand Names

Generic Ingredient: Montelukast
Singulair

Generic Ingredient: Zafirlukast
Accolate

Generic Ingredient: Zileuton
Zyflo Filmtab

Prescribed for

Asthma.

General Information

Leukotrienes play an important role in the body's allergic response. They are associated with the swelling of tissues and tightening of muscles in the throat that cause the throat to close during an asthma attack. Leukotriene receptor antagonists (montelukast and zafirlukast) help to prevent attacks by blocking leukotriene from binding to special tissue receptors. Zileuton interferes with the formation of leukotriene and has no effect on the receptor. When taken on a regular basis, these drugs can reduce the number of asthma attacks you experience but do not treat them once they occur; other drugs must be used to treat attacks.

Cautions and Warnings

Do not take any of these drugs if you are **allergic** or **sensitive** to them. It may be possible to be sensitive to one drug and tolerate another.

Avoid aspirin and other nonsteroidal anti-inflammatory drugs (NSAIDs) if they have triggered an asthma attack in the past. These drugs may not offer protection against **NSAID-related asthma attacks**.

Keep your regular inhalants and other asthma drugs handy at all times in case you have an asthma attack. These drugs do not prevent all attacks.

People age 56 and older taking zafirlukast reported more mild to moderate **respiratory infections** than those taking a placebo (sugar pill). Infections were more common in people taking larger dosages of zafirlukast and among those who took zafirlukast with an inhaled corticosteroid.

People with **cirrhosis of the liver** may require lower dosages of zafirlukast.

Possible Side Effects

Montelukast

▼ Most common: headache.

▼ Less common: flu, dizziness, upset stomach, gastroenteritis (inflammation of the mucous lining of the stomach and intestine), cough, stuffy nose, and abdominal pain.

▼ Rare: dental pain, rash, fever, injuries, weakness, and tiredness.

Zafirlukast

▼ Most common: headache.

▼ Less common: nausea, diarrhea, and infections.

▼ Rare: dizziness, abdominal pain, vomiting, generalized pain, weakness, accidental injury, muscle aches, fever, back pain, liver inflammation, and upset stomach.

Zileuton

▼ Most common: headache.

▼ Common: general pains, upset stomach, nausea, and liver inflammation.

▼ Less common: abdominal pain, weakness, accidental injury, and muscle aches.

▼ Rare: joint pain, chest pain, eye redness, constipation, dizziness, fever, gas, muscle stiffness, sleeplessness, swollen lymph glands, feeling unwell, neck pain or rigidity, nervousness, itching, tiredness, urinary infections, vaginal inflammation, and vomiting.

Drug Interactions

Montelukast

• Phenobarbital and rifampin may increase montelukast dosage requirements.

Zafirlukast
- Aspirin increases the amount of zafirlukast in the blood by almost 50%.
- Zafirlukast may increase the effects of other drugs broken down in the liver.
- Erythromycin, terfenadine, and theophylline may reduce zafirlukast's effectiveness.
- Zafirlukast increases the effects of astemizole, carbamazepine, cisapride, cyclosporine, felodipine, isradipine, nicardipine, nifedipine, nimodipine, phenytoin, tolbutamide, and warfarin.

Zileuton
- Zileuton increases the effects of astemizole, beta-blockers, cisapride, cyclosporine, felodipine, isradipine, nicardipine, nifedipine, nimodipine, theophylline, and warfarin. Dosage adjustments are necessary.

Food Interactions

Zileuton and montelukast may be taken with or without food. For optimal effectiveness, take each dose of zafirlukast at least 1 hour before or 2 hours after meals.

Usual Dose

Montelukast
   Adult and Child (age 15 and over): 10 mg every evening.
   Child (age 6–14): 5-mg chewable tablet every evening.

Zafirlukast
   Adult and Child (age 12 and over): 20 mg 2 times a day.
   Child (under age 12): not recommended.

Zileuton
   Adult and Child (age 12 and over): 600 mg 4 times a day.
   Child (under age 12): not recommended.

Overdosage

Little is known about the effects of overdose. Call your local poison control center or a hospital emergency room for more information. If you seek treatment, ALWAYS bring the prescription bottle or container.

Special Information

These drugs must be taken on a regular basis to prevent asthma attacks. You should continue taking them even if you are having an asthma attack, unless instructed by your doctor to stop.

Your dosage of inhaled corticosteroids, commonly used for asthma prevention, may be gradually reduced if you take these drugs. This reduction should be gradual and occur only under your doctor's supervision. Do not stop using your corticosteroid inhaler without your doctor's knowledge.

Call your doctor if, after starting on leukotriene antagonist/inhibitor, your need for your regular asthma drug increases.

If you forget a dose, take it as soon as you remember. If it is almost time for your next dose, skip the one you forgot and continue with your regular schedule. Do not take a double dose.

Special Populations

Pregnancy/Breast-feeding
Montelukast passes into fetal circulation. Zafirlukast and zileuton have harmed the fetus in animal studies. When any of these drugs is considered crucial by your doctor, its potential benefits must be carefully weighed against its risks.

These drugs may pass into breast milk. Nursing mothers who must take any of these drugs should bottle-feed.

Seniors
In studies, people age 55 and older who took zafirlukast reported more infections (see "Cautions and Warnings"). Seniors taking this drug may require reduced dosage.

Generic Name

Levamisole (lee-VAM-ih-sole)

Brand Name

Ergamisol

Type of Drug

Immune-system modulator.

Prescribed for

Duke's stage-C colon cancer, together with fluorouracil; also prescribed for malignant melanoma after surgery in people in whom the disease has not metastasized (spread).

General Information

Levamisole hydrochloride can restore depressed immune function. It stimulates the formation of antibodies to various agents, enhances T-cell response by stimulating and activating these important immune-system cells, and stimulates the infection-fighting and other functions of white blood cells. The exact way that it works in concert with fluorouracil is not known. In a clinical study of levamisole and Duke's stage-C colon cancer, survival rates were improved by 27% for levamisole plus fluorouracil and 28% for levamisole alone. The reduced recurrence rate for the disease was 36% for the drug combination and 28% for levamisole alone. Another study showed 33% improved survival and 41% reduction in disease recurrence for the 2 drugs. Levamisole is broken down in the liver.

Cautions and Warnings

Do not take levamisole if you are **allergic** to it.

People taking levamisole may develop **agranulocytosis** (a drastic reduction in the number of white blood cells) suddenly and without warning. Common symptoms of agranulocytosis are fever, chills, and flu-like symptoms. Regular blood monitoring is necessary while you are on levamisole: Your doctor may suddenly stop treatment if blood tests indicate the development of this problem, which may go away when you stop the drug.

Possible Side Effects

Virtually everyone taking fluorouracil and levamisole experiences side effects, which are due to either or both drugs. Some people decide to stop drug treatment because of side effects such as rash, joint and muscle aches, fever, white-blood-cell reduction, urinary infection, and cough.

▼ Most common: nausea, vomiting, diarrhea, mouth sores, appetite loss, abdominal pain, constipation, a metallic taste, joint and muscle aches, dizziness, headache, tingling in the hands or feet, white-blood-cell reduction, rash, hair loss, fatigue, sleepiness, fever, chills, and infection.

Possible Side Effects (continued)

▼ Less common: reduced platelet levels, itching, upset stomach, gas, changes in sense of smell, depression, nervousness, sleeplessness, anxiety, blurred vision, and eye redness.

▼ Rare: peeling rash, swelling around the eyes, vaginal bleeding, severe allergic reaction (symptoms include breathing difficulties, rash, intense itching, and elevated pulse), confusion, convulsions, hallucinations, loss of concentration, and kidney failure.

Drug Interactions

• Combining levamisole and alcohol may cause severe side effects.

• Combining phenytoin with fluorouracil and levamisole may increase phenytoin blood levels and the risk of side effects.

Food Interactions

None known.

Usual Dose

Colon Cancer: 50 mg every 8 hours for 3 days starting 7–30 days after surgery; then 50 mg every 8 hours for 3 days every 2 weeks.

Malignant Melanoma: 2.5 mg once daily for 2 consecutive days each week.

Overdosage

Levamisole overdose is potentially fatal. The most likely symptoms are severe side effects including those that affect the blood system, stomach, and intestines. Take the victim to a hospital emergency room at once. ALWAYS bring the prescription bottle or container.

Special Information

Call your doctor if you develop any side effects, especially fever, chills, or flu-like symptoms.

Taking more than the recommended dosage of levamisole increases side-effect risk without improving the drug's effectiveness. Carefully follow your doctor's directions.

If you forget a dose, call your doctor. Do not take the dose you forgot and do not take a double dose.

Special Populations

Pregnancy/Breast-feeding
Animal studies indicate that levamisole may injure the fetus. When this drug is considered crucial by your doctor, its potential benefits must be carefully weighed against its risks. Use effective contraceptive measures to be sure that you do not become pregnant while taking levamisole and fluorouracil.

Levamisole may pass into breast milk. Nursing mothers who must take levamisole should bottle-feed.

Seniors
Seniors may take this drug without special restriction.

Levaquin   *see Fluoroquinolone Anti-Infectives, page 442*

Generic Name

Levetiracetam (leh-veh-tir-ASS-eh-tam)

Brand Name
Keppra

Type of Drug
Antiepileptic.

Prescribed for
Partial onset seizures.

General Information
Levetiracetam works differently than other antiepileptic drugs. While it does not affect any pathway known to either block or stimulate nerve transmissions, research shows that it can help prevent seizures in adults with epilepsy. Levetiracetam is always prescribed in combination with other antiepileptics.

Cautions and Warnings

Do not take this drug if you are **sensitive** or **allergic** to it. People with **kidney problems** require reduced dosage.

Levetiracetam is a **nervous system depressant** and can cause **fatigue, poor coordination,** and **behavioral changes**.

Levetiracetam can cause **reductions in white- and red-blood-cell counts**. Your doctor will evaluate your blood components periodically.

Possible Side Effects

▼ Most common: tiredness, weakness, dizziness, and infection.

▼ Common: pain and sore throat.

▼ Less common: appetite loss, memory loss, anxiety, poor muscle coordination, depression, emotional upset, hostility, nervousness, tingling in the hands or feet, fainting, cough, runny nose, sinus irritation, and double vision.

▼ Rare: muscle aches, diarrhea, constipation, stomach problems, chest pain, black and blue marks, fever, flu-like symptoms, convulsions, sleeplessness, rash, middle ear infection, tremors, swollen gums, and weight gain.

Food and Drug Interactions

None known.

Usual Dose

Adult: 500–1500 mg twice a day.

Overdosage

Symptoms may include drowsiness. Call your local poison control center or a hospital emergency room for more information. If you seek treatment, ALWAYS bring the prescription bottle or container.

Special Information

Levetiracetam must be discontinued gradually. Stopping the drug too suddenly can lead to "withdrawal seizures."

Levetiracetam causes dizziness and tiredness. Be careful when driving or performing any task that requires concentration.

Call your doctor if you become pregnant or are planning on becoming pregnant while taking this medication.

If you forget a dose, take it as soon as you remember. If it is almost time for your next dose, skip the one you forgot and continue with your regular schedule. Do not take a double dose.

Special Populations

Pregnancy/Breast-feeding

Animal studies show that levetiracetam can cause birth defects. When this drug is considered crucial by your doctor, its potential benefits must be carefully weighed against its risks.

This drug may pass into breast milk. Nursing mothers who must take it should bottle-feed.

Seniors

Seniors should receive lower dosages.

Generic Name

Levodopa (lee-voe-DOE-puh) [G]

Brand Names

Dopar   Larodopa

Type of Drug

Antiparkinsonian.

Prescribed for

Parkinson's disease, restless leg syndrome, and herpes zoster (shingles).

General Information

When levodopa—also known as L-dopa—enters the brain, it is converted to dopamine, a chemical found in the central nervous system and deficient in people with Parkinson's disease. Some people who take levodopa develop the "on-off" phenomenon, in which they suddenly lose all drug effect and then regain it minutes or hours later. About 15% to 40% of people with Parkinson's disease develop this phenomenon after 2 to 3 years of levodopa treatment. The on-off effect becomes more frequent after 5 years and may result in a gradual decline in drug effect.

Cautions and Warnings

People with a history of **heart attacks,** severe **heart or lung disease, glaucoma, asthma,** or **kidney, liver, or hormone disease** should be cautious about using this drug. Do not take it if you have a history of stomach **ulcer.** People with a **psychotic history** must be treated with extreme care; this drug can cause depression with suicidal tendencies. Levodopa may activate an existing **malignant melanoma:** People with a family history of melanoma or suspicious skin lesions should not take this drug.

Possible Side Effects

▼ Most common: muscle spasms or inability to control arm, leg, or facial muscles; appetite loss; nausea; vomiting, with or without stomach pain; dry mouth; drooling; difficulty eating due to poor muscle control; tiredness; hand tremors; headache; dizziness; numbness; weakness or a faint feeling; confusion; sleeplessness; grinding of the teeth; nightmares; euphoria (feeling "high"); hallucinations; delusions; agitation; anxiousness; and feeling unwell.

▼ Less common: heart irregularities or palpitations; dizziness when standing or rising, particularly in the morning; changes in mental state, including depression with or without suicidal tendencies, paranoia, and loss of intellectual function; difficulty urinating; muscle twitching; burning sensation on the tongue; bitter taste in the mouth; diarrhea; constipation; unusual breathing patterns; blurred or double vision; hot flashes; weight gain or loss; darkening of the urine; and increased perspiration.

▼ Rare: stomach bleeding, ulcer, high blood pressure, convulsions, adverse effects on the blood, difficulty controlling eye muscles, stimulation, hiccups, hair loss, hoarseness, decreasing size of male genitalia, and fluid retention.

Drug Interactions

• Anticholinergic drugs such as trihexyphenidyl decrease levodopa's effects. Other drugs that may interfere with levodopa are benzodiazepine-type tranquilizers and sedatives, phenothiazine antipsychotic medication, phenytoin, methionine, papaverine, pyridoxine, and tricyclic antidepressants.

• Antacids may increase levodopa's effects.

• Metoclopramide may increase levodopa blood levels, levodopa may reduce metoclopramide's effects on the stomach. Levodopa may interact with drugs for high blood pressure to further reduce pressure. Dosage adjustments in the high-blood-pressure medication may be required. Methyldopa (an antihypertensive) may increase levodopa's effects.

• People taking monoamine oxidase inhibitor (MAOI) antidepressants should stop taking them at least 2 weeks before starting on levodopa.

Food Interactions

Take each dose with food to avoid upset stomach. A low-protein diet may help to minimize variations in drug response that occur in some people. Do not take vitamin preparations that contain vitamin B_6 (pyridoxine), which decreases the effectiveness of levodopa.

Usual Dose

0.5–8 g a day.

Overdosage

Take the victim to a hospital emergency room immediately. ALWAYS bring the prescription bottle or container.

Special Information

Be careful when driving or performing any task that requires concentration.

Call your doctor immediately if you experience: fainting, dizziness, or light-headedness; abnormal results in diabetic urine tests; uncontrollable movements of the face, eyelids, mouth, tongue, neck, arms, hands, or legs; mood changes; palpitations or irregular heartbeats; difficulty urinating; or severe nausea or vomiting.

If you forget a dose, take it as soon as possible. If it is within 2 hours of your next dose, skip the dose you forgot and go back to your regular schedule. Do not take a double dose.

Special Populations

Pregnancy/Breast-feeding
Animal studies indicate that levodopa may interfere with fetal development. Pregnant women should take levodopa only when it is absolutely necessary.

Levodopa may pass into breast milk. Nursing mothers who must take it should bottle-feed.

Seniors
Seniors may require smaller dosages and are more likely to experience abnormal heart rhythms and other cardiac effects, especially if they have heart disease.

Levoxyl see Thyroid Hormone Replacements, page 1005

Brand Name

Lexxel

Generic Ingredients

Enalapril + Felodipine

Type of Drug

Antihypertensive combination.

Prescribed for

Hypertension (high blood pressure).

General Information

Lexxel contains 5 mg of felodipine, a calcium channel blocker, and 5 mg of enalapril, an angiotensin-converting enzyme (ACE) inhibitor. The two drugs in this combination belong to widely prescribed groups of hypertension medication. Lexxel is not meant for the initial treatment of hypertension. Most people taking this product have taken one of the ingredients as an individual pill and need more medication to control their blood pressure.

Felodipine works by blocking the passage of calcium into heart and smooth-muscle tissue, especially the smooth muscle found in arteries. Since calcium is an essential factor in muscle contraction, any drug that affects calcium in this way will interfere with the contraction of these muscles. This causes the veins to dilate (widen), reducing blood pressure. Also, the amount of oxygen used by these muscles is reduced.

ACE inhibitors such as enalapril work by preventing the conversion of a hormone called angiotensin I to another hormone called angiotensin II, a potent blood-vessel constrictor. Preventing this conversion relaxes blood vessels and helps to reduce blood pressure and relieve the symptoms of heart failure. Enalapril's effect on other hormones may also help to promote blood-vessel dilation. It begins working about 1 hour after you take it and continues to work for 24 hours.

Cautions and Warnings

Do not take Lexxel if you are **sensitive** or **allergic** to either ingredient. Rarely, it causes **very low blood pressure**. It may also affect your **kidneys,** especially if you have **congestive heart failure (CHF)**. Your doctor should check your urine for protein content during the first few months of treatment.

Enalapril may affect **white-blood-cell counts,** possibly increasing your susceptibility to **infection**. Your doctor should monitor your blood counts periodically.

People taking a beta-blocking drug who begin taking felodipine may develop **heart failure** or increased **angina pain**. Angina pain may also increase if your felodipine dosage is increased. People with severe **liver disease** break down felodipine much more slowly than those with less severe disease or normal livers.

A sudden, painless **swelling** in the hands, face, feet, lips, tongue, or throat may develop while you are taking any ACE inhibitor. If this happens, you must call your doctor and stop taking the medication at once. This condition usually goes away on its own, though antihistamines may also prove helpful.

Possible Side Effects

Calcium-channel-blocker side effects are generally mild. Side effects are more common with higher dosages and increasing age.

Possible Side Effects *(continued)*

▼ Most common: swelling in the ankles, feet, and legs; dizziness; light-headedness; muscle weakness or cramps; facial flushing; headache; fatigue; nausea; and chronic (long-term) cough. The cough usually goes away a few days after you stop taking the medication.

▼ Less common: respiratory infection, cough, tingling in the hands or feet, upset stomach, abdominal pain, chest pain, nausea, constipation, diarrhea, heart palpitations, sore throat, runny nose, back pain, rash, angina (condition characterized by brief attacks of chest pain), dizziness when rising from a sitting or lying position, fainting, vomiting, bronchitis, urinary tract infection, breathing difficulties, and weakness.

▼ Rare: Rare side effects can affect your heart, muscles and joints, stomach and intestines, sexual function, kidney or liver, and other body parts. Contact your doctor if you experience any side effect not listed above.

Drug Interactions

• The blood-pressure-lowering effect of Lexxel adds to that of diuretic (agent that increases urination) drugs or beta blockers. Any other drug that causes a rapid blood-pressure drop should be used with caution if you are taking Lexxel.

• Lexxel may raise blood-potassium levels, especially when taken with Dyazide or other potassium-sparing diuretics.

• Lexxel may increase the effects of lithium; this combination should be used with caution.

• Capsaicin may cause or aggravate the cough associated with Lexxel therapy.

• Indomethacin may reduce the blood-pressure-lowering effect of Lexxel.

• Phenothiazine tranquilizers and antiemetics may increase the effects of Lexxel.

• Rifampin may reduce the effects of Lexxel.

• Combining allopurinol with Lexxel increases the risk of an adverse drug reaction.

• Cimetidine and ranitidine increase the amount of felodipine in the blood, causing a slight increase in the drug's effect.

• Phenytoin and other hydantoin anti-seizure drugs, carbamazepine, and barbiturate sleeping pills and sedatives may decrease the amount of felodipine in the blood, reducing its effect.

• Erythromycin may increase the side effects of felodipine.

• Felodipine may increase the effects of theophylline (a drug used to treat asthma and other respiratory problems) and oral anticoagulant (blood-thinning) drugs.

• Felodipine may interact with quinidine (an antiarrhythmic) to produce low blood pressure, very slow heart rate, abnormal heart rhythms, and swelling in the arms or legs.

Food Interactions

Lexxel may be taken without regard to food or meals; you may take it with food if it upsets your stomach. Avoid grapefruit juice while you are on Lexxel.

Usual Dose

1 tablet a day.

Overdosage

Overdose may cause low blood pressure. In case of overdose, call your doctor or go to a hospital emergency room. ALWAYS bring the prescription bottle or container.

Special Information

Call your doctor if you develop a sore throat, mouth sores, abnormal heartbeat, chest pain, a persistent rash, loss of taste perception, constipation, nausea, very low blood pressure, breathing difficulties, increased heart pain, dizziness, lightheadedness, or any bothersome or persistent side effect.

Continue taking your medication and follow any instructions for diet restriction or other treatments to help maintain lower blood pressure, even if you feel well. Hypertension may be present without symptoms.

Do not break or crush Lexxel tablets.

Maintain good dental hygiene while taking Lexxel and use extra care when brushing or flossing because of the increased risk of oral infection associated with Lexxel.

Avoid over-the-counter diet pills, decongestants, and stimulants while taking Lexxel; they may raise blood pressure.

If you forget a dose, take it as soon as you remember. If it is almost time for your next dose, skip the dose you forgot and continue with your regular schedule. Do not take a double dose.

Special Populations

Pregnancy/Breast-feeding

Women who are or might be pregnant should not take Lexxel. ACE inhibitors have caused low blood pressure, kidney failure, slow skull formation, and death in the fetus when taken during the last 6 months of pregnancy. Women of childbearing age who must take Lexxel must use an effective contraceptive method. If you become pregnant, stop taking the medication and call your doctor immediately.

Small amounts of enalapril and felodipine pass into breast milk. Nursing mothers who must take Lexxel should consider bottle-feeding.

Seniors

Seniors, especially those with liver disease, may be more sensitive to the drug's effects.

Lipitor *see Statin Cholesterol-Lowering Agents, page 942*

Generic Name

Lisinopril (lih-SIN-oe-pril)

Brand Names

Prinivil   Zestril

Combination Products

Generic Ingredients: Lisinopril + Hydrochlorothiazide
Prinzide   Zestoretic

Type of Drug

Angiotensin-converting enzyme (ACE) inhibitor.

Prescribed for

Hypertension (high blood pressure), congestive heart failure, kidney protection in people with diabetes, and improving survival after a heart attack.

General Information

Lisinopril and other ACE inhibitors work by preventing the conversion of a hormone called angiotensin I to another hormone called angiotensin II, a potent blood-vessel constrictor. Preventing this conversion relaxes blood vessels, thus reducing blood pressure and relieving the symptoms of heart failure. Lisinopril also affects the production of other hormones and enzymes that participate in the regulation of blood vessel dilation. Lisinopril begins working about 1 hour after you take it and lasts for 24 hours.

Some people who start taking an ACE inhibitor after they are already on a diuretic (an agent that increases urination) experience a rapid drop in blood pressure after their first doses or when the dosage is increased. To prevent this from happening, you may be told to stop taking the diuretic 2 or 3 days before starting the ACE inhibitor or to increase your salt intake during that time. The diuretic may then be restarted gradually.

Cautions and Warnings

Do not take lisinopril if you have had an **allergic reaction** to it. Occasionally, severe allergic reactions have occurred in people undergoing desensitization treatments or certain kinds of kidney dialysis.

Lisinopril occasionally causes **very low blood pressure**.

Lisinopril can affect your **kidneys,** especially if you have congestive **heart failure**. Your doctor should check your urine for changes during the first few months of treatment. Dosage adjustment is required if you have reduced kidney function.

ACE inhibitors can affect white-blood-cell count, possibly increasing your susceptibility to **infection**. Blood counts should be monitored periodically.

Possible Side Effects

▼ Most common: headache, dizziness, fatigue, nausea, diarrhea, and chronic cough. The cough is more common in women and usually goes away a few days after the medication is stopped.

▼ Less common: chest pain, low blood pressure, vomiting, upset stomach, breathing difficulties, rash, and muscle weakness.

Possible Side Effects *(continued)*

▼ Rare: Rare side effects can affect your muscles and joints, sex drive, liver, mental status, and respiratory tract. Contact your doctor if you experience any side effect not listed above.

Drug Interactions

• The blood-pressure-lowering effect of lisinopril is additive with diuretic drugs and beta blockers. Any other drug that can reduce blood pressure should be used with caution if you are taking an ACE inhibitor.

• Lisinopril may increase your blood potassium levels, especially when taken with Dyazide or other potassium-sparing diuretics.

• Lisinopril may increase the effects of lithium; this combination should be used with caution.

• Antacids and lisinopril should be taken at least 2 hours apart.

• Capsaicin may trigger or aggravate lisinopril cough.

• Indomethacin may reduce the blood-pressure-lowering effect of lisinopril.

• Phenothiazine tranquilizers and antiemetics may increase the effects of lisinopril.

• The combination of allopurinol and lisinopril increases the chance of side effects.

• Lisinopril increases blood levels of digoxin, possibly increasing the chance of digoxin-related side effects.

Food Interactions

None known.

Usual Dose

5–40 mg a day. People with severe kidney disease should begin with 2.5 mg a day; dosage may then be increased up to 5–20 mg a day.

Overdosage

The principal effect of lisinopril overdose is a rapid drop in blood pressure, as evidenced by dizziness or fainting. Take the overdose victim to a hospital emergency room immediately. ALWAYS remember to bring the prescription bottle or container.

Special Information

Unexplained swelling of the face, lips, hands, and feet can also affect the larynx (throat) and tongue and interfere with breathing. If this happens, the victim should be taken to a hospital emergency room at once for treatment. Also, call your doctor if you develop a sore throat, mouth sores, abnormal heartbeat, chest pain, persistent rash, or loss of taste perception.

You may get dizzy if you rise quickly from a sitting or lying position.

Avoid strenuous exercise and very hot weather because heavy sweating or dehydration can cause a rapid drop in blood pressure.

Avoid over-the-counter diet pills, decongestants, and other stimulants that can raise blood pressure.

If you forget to take a dose of lisinopril, take it as soon as you remember. If it is within 8 hours of your next dose, skip the one you forgot and continue with your regular schedule. Do not take a double dose.

Special Populations

Pregnancy/Breast-feeding

ACE inhibitors can cause fetal injury or death. Women who are or might be pregnant should not take lisinopril. Stop taking the medication and contact your doctor if you become pregnant.

It is not known if lisinopril passes into breast milk. Nursing mothers who must take this drug should consider bottle-feeding.

Seniors

Seniors may be more sensitive to the effects of lisinopril due to age-related kidney impairment.

Generic Name

Lithium Carbonate

(LITH-ee-um CAR-buh-nate) Ⓖ

Brand Names

Eskalith	Lithonate
Lithobid	Lithotabs

The information in this profile also applies to the following drug:

Generic Ingredient: Lithium Citrate [G]
Only available in generic form.

Type of Drug

Antipsychotic and antimanic.

Prescribed for

Bipolar (manic-depressive) disorder, especially suppression of manic attacks or reduction in their number and intensity; also prescribed for cancer and acquired immunodeficiency syndrome (AIDS), premenstrual tension, bulimia, postpartum depression, overactive thyroid, and alcoholism, especially in people who are also depressed. Lithium lotion has been used for genital herpes and dandruff.

General Information

Lithium carbonate and lithium citrate are the only effective antimanic drugs. They reduce the levels of manic episodes and may produce normal activity within the first 3 weeks of treatment. Typical manic symptoms include rapid speech, elation, hyperactive movements, little need for sleep, grandiose ideas, poor judgment, aggressiveness, and hostility.

Cautions and Warnings

Lithium should not be taken by people with **heart or kidney disease, dehydration, low blood sodium,** or those taking **diuretic drugs**. If such people require lithium carbonate, they must be very carefully monitored by their doctors, and hospitalization may be needed until the lithium carbonate dose is stabilized.

A few people treated with both lithium carbonate and haloperidol or another antipsychotic have developed **encephalopathic syndrome** (symptoms include weakness, tiredness, fever, confusion, tremulousness, and uncontrollable muscle spasms). In addition, your doctor may find laboratory indicators of liver or kidney disease. Rarely, this combination of symptoms is followed by irreversible brain damage.

Up to 20% of people on long-term lithium carbonate treatment develop **structural changes in their kidneys** and **reduced kidney function**.

Long-term use of this drug may lead to **reduced thyroid activity, enlargement of the thyroid gland,** and **increased blood levels of thyroid-stimulating hormone**. All of these conditions may be treated with thyroid hormone replacement therapy. **Overactive thyroid** has occasionally occurred.

Frequent urination and thirst associated with lithium carbonate may be a sign of a condition known as diabetes insipidus, in which the kidney stops responding to a hormone called vasopressin. This causes the kidney to reabsorb water and make concentrated urine. Lithium carbonate may reverse the kidneys' ability to perform this function, but things usually go back to normal when lithium carbonate treatment is stopped, dosage is reduced, or small doses of a thiazide diuretic are taken.

Your lithium carbonate dosage may have to be temporarily reduced if you develop an infection or fever.

Some lithium carbonate products contain tartrazine dyes for coloring purposes. Tartrazine can stimulate allergic responses in some people, including asthma.

Possible Side Effects

Side effects of lithium carbonate are directly related to the amount of drug in the bloodstream.

▼ Most common: fine hand tremor, thirst, and excessive urination, especially when treatment is first started; mild nausea and discomfort during the first few days of treatment.

▼ Less common: diarrhea, vomiting, drowsiness, muscle weakness, poor coordination, giddiness, ringing or buzzing in the ears, and blurred vision.

▼ Rare: Rare side effects can affect muscles and nerves (blackouts, seizures, and dizziness), stomach and intestines, kidneys and urinary tract, skin, and thyroid function. Contact your doctor if you experience any side effect not listed above. Lithium carbonate can also affect tests used to monitor heart and brain function.

Drug Interactions

• When lithium carbonate is combined with haloperidol, weakness, tiredness, fever, or confusion may result. In some people, these symptoms have been followed by permanent brain damage. Also, haloperidol may increase the effect of lithium carbonate.

• Combining lithium carbonate and chlorpromazine may reduce the effect of chlorpromazine and increase the lithium carbonate effect.

• Lithium carbonate is counteracted by sodium bicarbonate, acetazolamide, urea, mannitol, and theophylline drugs. Verapamil can lower blood levels of lithium carbonate and reduce the risk of toxicity.

• Lithium's effect may be increased by methyldopa, fluoxetine and other SSRIs, carbamazepine, thiazide and loop diuretics, and nonsteroidal anti-inflammatory drugs (NSAIDs).

• Lithium carbonate may increase the effects of tricyclic antidepressant medications.

Food Interactions

Lithium carbonate should be taken immediately after meals or with food or milk.

Usual Dose

Dosage must be individualized. Most people respond to 1800 mg a day at first. Once the person has responded, daily lithium dosage is reduced to the lowest effective level, usually 300 mg 3–4 times a day.

Overdosage

Toxic blood levels of lithium carbonate are only slightly above the levels required for treatment. Signs of drug toxicity may be diarrhea, vomiting, nausea, tremors, drowsiness, poor coordination, giddiness, weakness, blurred vision, ringing or buzzing in the ears, dizziness, fainting, confusion, muscle twitching, uncontrollable muscle movements, loss of bladder control, worsening of manic symptoms, overactive reflexes, and painful muscles or joints. If any of these symptoms occur, stop taking the medication and call your doctor immediately. ALWAYS bring the prescription bottle or container with you when you go to an emergency room.

Special Information

Lithium carbonate may cause drowsiness. Be cautious while driving or operating hazardous machinery.

Lithium carbonate causes your body to lose sodium (salt). You must maintain a well-balanced diet and drink 8 to 12 glasses of water a day while taking this drug. Excessive sweating or diarrhea may make you more sensitive to side effects.

Call your doctor if you develop diarrhea, vomiting, unsteady walking, tremors, drowsiness, or muscle weakness.

To avoid side effects, your doctor may need to reduce your dosage once manic symptoms decline.

If you forget to take a dose of lithium carbonate, take it as soon as possible. However, if it is within 2 hours of your next dose, or 6 hours if you take the long-acting form, skip the missed dose and go back to your regular schedule. Do not take a double dose. Call your doctor if you miss more than 1 dose.

Special Populations

Pregnancy/Breast-feeding
Lithium can cause heart and thyroid birth defects, especially if taken during the first 3 months of pregnancy. Talk with your doctor about the risks of taking lithium during pregnancy.

Lithium carbonate passes into breast milk. It may cause weak muscle tone, low body temperature, bluish discoloration of the skin, and abnormal heart rhythm in an infant. You should bottle-feed your baby while taking this medication.

Seniors
Seniors are more sensitive to the effects of lithium carbonate. It is potentially toxic to the central nervous system in older adults, even when lithium carbonate blood levels are in the desired range. Seniors are also more likely to develop an underactive thyroid.

Type of Drug
Loop Diuretics

Brand Names

Generic Ingredient: Bumetanide G
Bumex

Generic Ingredient: Ethacrynic Acid
Edecrin

Generic Ingredient: Furosemide Ⓖ
Lasix

Generic Ingredient: Torsemide
Demadex

Prescribed for

Congestive heart failure (CHF), cirrhosis of the liver, fluid accumulation in the lungs, kidney dysfunction, high blood pressure, and other conditions where it may be desirable to rid the body of excess fluid. Bumetanide can be used to treat people who urinate frequently at night.

General Information

Stronger than thiazide diuretics, loop diuretics work in a similar fashion. Not only do they affect the same part of the kidney as thiazide diuretics, they also act in another portion called the "loop of Henle." This dual action is what makes loop diuretics so potent. All 4 loop diuretics can be used for the same purposes, but their dosages vary.

Cautions and Warnings

Do not take these drugs if you are **sensitive** or **allergic** to them. People allergic to sulfa drugs may also be allergic to furosemide, torsemide, or bumetanide.

Loop diuretics can cause **depletion of water and electrolytes**. They should not be taken without constant medical supervision. Frequent lab evaluations of electrolytes should be performed during therapy and periodically thereafter. You should not take these drugs if your urine production has been decreased abnormally by kidney disease.

Excessive use of loop diuretics results in **dehydration** or **reduction in blood volume,** and may cause **circulatory collapse** or other related problems, particularly in older adults.

Ringing or buzzing in the ears, hearing loss, deafness, fainting, and a **sensation of fullness in the ears** can occur with these drugs. Hearing usually returns within 24 hours, but some loss may be permanent.

These drugs may worsen systemic **lupus erythematosus**. **Diarrhea** may occur with ethacrynic acid or furosemide solution. Rarely people taking bumetanide develop **thrombocytopenia** (low blood-platelet count).

People taking a loop diuretic may develop increased levels of total **cholesterol,** low-density lipoprotein (LDL) cholesterol, and triglycerides.

Possible Side Effects

▼ Common: Changes may occur in blood levels of potassium or other electrolytes. Hypokalemia (low blood potassium), may cause dry mouth, excessive thirst, weakness, lethargy, drowsiness, restlessness, muscle pain or cramps, muscular tiredness, low blood pressure, decreased frequency of urination and urine volume, abnormal heart rate, and upset stomach, including nausea and vomiting. Loop diuretics may alter sugar metabolism. If you have diabetes mellitus, you may develop high blood sugar or sugar in the urine. To treat this problem, the dosage of your antidiabetes drugs must be increased.

▼ Less common: abdominal discomfort, nausea, vomiting, diarrhea, rash, dizziness, light-headedness, headache, blurred vision, fatigue, weakness, jaundice (symptoms include yellowing of the skin or whites of the eyes), acute gout attacks, dermatitis and other skin reactions, tingling in the extremities, dizziness upon rising quickly from a sitting or lying position, and anemia.

▼ Rare: a sweet taste in the mouth, a burning sensation in the stomach or mouth, excessive thirst, increased perspiration, and frequent urination.

Drug Interactions

• Loop diuretics increase the effects of other blood-pressure-lowering drugs. This is beneficial and is frequently used to help lower blood pressure in people with hypertension.

• Combining a loop diuretic and digitalis drugs or adrenal corticosteroids increases the risk of developing electrolyte imbalances. Potassium loss caused by loop diuretics significantly increases the toxicity of digitalis.

• Loop diuretics may increase the effect of oral anticoagulants (blood thinners); a dosage adjustment may be needed.

• The dosage of an oral antidiabetes drug—except metformin—may need to be altered if you start taking a loop diuretic.

• The effect of theophylline may be altered by any loop diuretic. Your doctor should check your theophylline levels after you have started on a loop diuretic.

• If you are taking lithium carbonate, you should probably not take a diuretic, which greatly increases the risk of lithium side effects.

• People taking chloral hydrate as a nighttime sedative may, in rare cases, experience hot flashes, high blood pressure, sweating, abnormal heart rhythms, weakness, and nausea when they also take a loop diuretic.

• Periodic hearing loss or ringing or buzzing in the ears may occur if a loop diuretic is taken with cisplatin (an anticancer drug) or an aminoglycoside antibiotic. Make sure your doctor knows you are taking a loop diuretic before giving you an injection of either of these.

• Clofibrate and thiazide diuretics increase the effect of loop diuretics.

Charcoal tablets, phenytoin, probenecid, and aspirin and other salicylate drugs, or nonsteroidal anti-inflammatory drugs (NSAIDs) may decrease the effectiveness of loop diuretics.

• If you are taking a loop diuretic for high blood pressure or CHF, avoid over-the-counter (OTC) cough, cold, and allergy products, which often contain stimulant drugs that can raise your blood pressure. Check with your pharmacist before taking any OTC drug if you are taking a loop diuretic.

Food Interactions

Furosemide should be taken on an empty stomach at least 1 hour before or 2 hours after meals. The other loop diuretics may be taken with food if they upset your stomach.

Usual Dose

Bumetanide
0.5–2 mg a day. It may also be taken every other day for 3–4 consecutive days followed by 1–2 days off the drug.

Ethacrynic Acid
   Adult: 50–200 mg taken every day or every other day.
   Child: starting dose—25 mg; increase slowly.

Furosemide
   Adult: 20–80 mg a day. Dosages of 600 mg or more a day have been prescribed.

Child: 0.9 mg per lb. of body weight in a single daily dose. If therapy is not successful, the dosage may be increased in small steps up to 2.7 mg per lb. a day.

Torsemide
   Adult: 5–20 mg once a day. Dosages up to 200 mg may be prescribed.
   Child: not recommended.

Maintenance dosages for all of the loop diuretics are adjusted to individual needs.

Overdosage

Symptoms include dehydration, reduced blood volume, high urine volume, weakness, dizziness, confusion, appetite loss, tiredness, vomiting, and cramps. Take the victim to a hospital emergency room. ALWAYS bring the prescription bottle or container.

Special Information

If the amount of urine you produce each day is dropping, or if you suffer from cramps, significant appetite loss, muscle weakness, tiredness, or nausea, contact your doctor immediately.
   Loop diuretics are usually taken once a day after breakfast. If a second dose is needed, it should be taken no later than 2 p.m. to avoid nighttime urination.
   To avoid the dizziness associated with these drugs, rise slowly and carefully from a sitting or lying position.
   Loop diuretics can increase blood sugar. People with diabetes may need their medication adjusted.
   Loop diuretics rob your body of potassium. To counteract this effect, be sure to eat high-potassium foods such as bananas, citrus fruits, melons, and tomatoes.
   Loop diuretics can increase your sensitivity to the sun. Use sunscreen and wear protective clothing.
   If you forget a dose, take it as soon as you remember. If it is almost time for your next dose, skip the one you forgot and continue with your regular schedule. Do not take a double dose.

Special Populations

Pregnancy/Breast-feeding
Loop diuretics have been used to treat specific conditions in

pregnancy, but they should be used only when absolutely necessary.

Furosemide passes into breast milk, and the other loop diuretics may pass into breast milk. Nursing mothers who must take any of these drugs should bottle-feed.

Seniors

Seniors are more sensitive to the effects of these drugs.

Lo/Ovral see **Contraceptives**, page 254

Generic Name

Loperamide (loe-PER-uh-mide) G

Brand Name

Imodium

Type of Drug

Antidiarrheal.

Prescribed for

Acute and chronic diarrhea; also prescribed to reduce the amount of discharge in an ileostomy (surgical procedure in which a hole is made in the small intestine, usually through the abdominal wall).

General Information

Loperamide hydrochloride, which relieves diarrhea but does not address the underlying cause, should be used only for short periods. It works by slowing intestinal movement and affecting the movement of water and salts in the intestines. In some cases antidiarrheals should not be used at all; these drugs may harm people with bowel, stomach, or other diseases. Loperamide is available over-the-counter (OTC) under a variety of brand names. OTC loperamide products are used to treat acute diarrhea and traveler's diarrhea.

Cautions and Warnings

Do not use loperamide if you are **allergic** or **sensitive** to it, if you suffer from diarrhea associated with **colitis,** or if you have an **intestinal infection** of *Escherichia coli, Salmonella,* or *Shigella.*

If you have **ulcerative colitis** and start taking loperamide, stop the drug at once and call your doctor if you develop abdominal problems of any kind.

Possible Side Effects

Incidence of side effects is low. They are most likely to occur when loperamide is taken over longer periods to treat chronic diarrhea.

▼ Most common: stomach and abdominal pain, bloating or other discomfort, constipation, dry mouth, dizziness, tiredness, nausea and vomiting, and drug-sensitivity reactions, including rash.

Drug Interactions

• Loperamide increases the sedative effects of sleeping pills, tranquilizers, and alcohol. Avoid these combinations.

• Loperamide should not be taken with clindamycin or lincomycin, agents that can cause severe and possibly fatal colitis.

Food Interactions

Loperamide should be taken on an empty stomach.

Usual Dose

Acute Diarrhea

Adult and Child (age 12 and over): 4 mg to start, followed by 2 mg after each loose stool, up to 16 mg a day maximum. Improvement should be seen in 2 days.

Child (age 9–12): 2 mg 3 times a day to start, followed by 1 mg per 22 lbs. of body weight after each loose stool, up to 6 mg a day maximum.

Child (age 6–8): 2 mg twice a day to start, followed by 1 mg per 22 lbs. of body weight after each loose stool, up to 4 mg a day maximum.

Child (age 2–5): 1 mg 3 times a day to start, followed by 1 mg per 22 lbs. of body weight after each loose stool, up to 3 mg a day maximum.

Chronic Diarrhea

Adult and Child (age 12 and over): 4 mg to start, followed by 2 mg after each loose stool, until symptoms are controlled. Then dosage should be tailored to individual needs—usually 4–8 mg a day. Loperamide is usually effective within 10 days or not at all.

Overdosage

Symptoms include constipation, irritation of the stomach, and tiredness. Large doses usually cause vomiting. Take the victim to a hospital emergency room immediately. ALWAYS bring the prescription bottle or container.

Special Information

Loperamide depresses the central nervous system (CNS), which may cause drowsiness: Be careful when driving or performing any task that requires concentration.

Loperamide may cause dry mouth. Drink plenty of water or other clear fluids to prevent dehydration due to diarrhea. It is important to maintain a proper diet and drink plenty of fluids to restore normal bowel function.

Call your doctor if diarrhea persists after a few days of loperamide treatment or if you develop abdominal discomfort or pain, fever, or any bothersome or persistent side effect.

If you forget a dose, skip it and go back to your regular schedule. Do not take a double dose.

Special Populations

Pregnancy/Breast-feeding

Loperamide has not been found to cause birth defects; however, women who are or might be pregnant should not take this drug without their doctor's approval. When loperamide is considered crucial by your doctor, its potential benefits must be carefully weighed against its risks.

It is not known if loperamide passes into breast milk. Nursing mothers who must take this drug should consider bottle-feeding.

Seniors

Seniors may be more sensitive to the constipating effects of loperamide.

Generic Name

Loratadine (lor-AH-tuh-dene)

Brand Names

Claritin   Claritin Reditabs

Type of Drug

Antihistamine.

Prescribed for

Stuffy and runny nose, itchy eyes, and scratchy throat caused by seasonal allergy and for other symptoms of allergy such as rash, itching, and hives; also prescribed for asthma.

General Information

Antihistamines generally work by blocking the release of histamine (chemical released by body tissue during an allergic reaction) from cells at the H_1 histamine receptor site, drying up secretions of the nose, throat, and eyes. Loratadine causes less sedation than most antihistamines and appears to be just as effective.

Cautions and Warnings

Do not take loratadine if you are **allergic** to it.

People with **liver disease** require reduced dosage.

Possible Side Effects

▼ Most common: headache, dry mouth, drowsiness, and fatigue.

▼ Less common: sweating, tearing, impotence, thirst, flushing, blurred vision, conjunctivitis (pinkeye), earache, eye pain, ringing or buzzing in the ears, weight gain, back pain, leg cramps, chest pain, fever, chills, not feeling well, weakness, worsening of allergic symptoms, respiratory infection, breathing difficulties, blood-pressure changes, dizziness, fainting, heart palpitations, rapid heartbeat, hyperactivity, tingling in the hands or feet, eye-muscle spasms, migraine, tremors, nausea, vomiting, gas, abdominal distress, stomach irritation or upset,

---

Possible Side Effects (continued)

constipation, diarrhea, changes in sense of taste, changes in appetite, toothache, joint or muscle aches or pains, anxiety, depression, agitation, sleeplessness, memory lapse, loss of concentration, paranoia, confusion, nervousness, loss of sex drive, breast pain, vaginal irritation, menstrual changes, dry nose, stuffy nose, runny nose, nosebleeds, sore throat, coughing, sneezing, vomiting blood, bronchitis, bronchial spasm, laryngitis, itching, rash, dry hair or skin, unusual sensitivity to the sun, black-and-blue marks, altered urination, and urine discoloration.

▼ Rare: swelling in the legs, ankles, or feet; yellowing of the skin or whites of the eyes; hepatitis; hair loss; seizures; breast enlargement; and erythema multiforme (skin reaction).

Drug Interactions

• Loratadine may interact with ketoconazole, erythromycin, cimetidine, ranitidine, and theophylline, but the evidence for this interaction is inconclusive.

Food Interactions

Loratadine is best taken on an empty stomach 1 hour before or 2 hours after eating; it may be taken with food or milk if it upsets your stomach.

Usual Dose

Adult and Child (over age 12): 10 mg once a day. People with liver disease should take 10 mg every other day.

Overdosage

Overdose is likely to cause drowsiness, headache, rapid heartbeat, or severe side effects. Overdose victims should be given ipecac syrup—available at any pharmacy—to make them vomit and should be taken to a hospital emergency room for treatment. Call your local poison control center or hospital emergency room for instructions. ALWAYS bring the prescription bottle or container.

Special Information

Dizziness or fainting may be the first sign of a serious side effect. Call your doctor at once if this happens to you. Also report sore throat; unusual bleeding, bruising, tiredness, or weakness; or any other unusual side effect.

If you forget to take a dose of loratadine, take it as soon as you remember. If it is almost time for your next dose, skip the one you forgot and continue with your regular schedule. Do not take a double dose.

Special Populations

Pregnancy/Breast-feeding
Do not take any antihistamine without your doctor's knowledge if you are or might be pregnant—especially during the last 3 months of pregnancy—because newborns may have severe reactions to antihistamines.

Loratadine passes into breast milk. Nursing mothers who must take loratadine should bottle-feed.

Seniors
Seniors are unlikely to experience nervous-system effects with loratadine as opposed to the older, more sedating antihistamines. However, seniors, especially those with liver disease, are more likely to experience side effects than are younger adults.

Lotensin   see Benazepril, page 109

Brand Name

Lotrel

Generic Ingredients
Amlodipine + Benazepril Hydrochloride

Type of Drug
Antihypertensive.

Prescribed for

Hypertension (high blood pressure).

General Information

Lotrel combines the calcium channel blocker amlodipine with an angiotensin-converting enzyme (ACE) inhibitor—benazepril. Both drugs are often prescribed individually for hypertension. Lotrel is not intended as a first treatment for hypertension. You should take Lotrel only after you have tried an ACE inhibitor or calcium channel blocker alone and your doctor feels you need an additional drug to control your blood pressure. (See the "Amlodipine" and "Benazepril" profiles for more information.)

Cautions and Warnings

Do not take Lotrel if you are **sensitive** or **allergic** to any of its ingredients. People taking any ACE inhibitor may experience severe **drug reactions,** including swelling of the face, throat, lips, tongue, hands, and feet—this reaction occurs in about 5 in 1000 people.

In rare instances, people taking a calcium channel blocker who have severe **heart disease** develop increased **angina pain** or a **heart attack.**

In people with **heart failure,** ACE inhibitors may cause **very low blood pressure,** rare **kidney failure,** and **death.** People with heart failure who start Lotrel must be under a doctor's care.

Another ACE inhibitor has caused **depression of bone marrow** and **reduced white-blood-cell counts,** especially in people with **kidney failure.** Fever and chills can be a sign of this problem.

Lotrel should be used with caution by people with **kidney failure.**

In rare instances, people taking ACE inhibitors have developed **liver failure.**

All ACE inhibitors may cause a persistent cough.

Possible Side Effects

Side effects are generally mild and temporary.

▼ Most common: cough, headache, dizziness, and swelling.

Possible Side Effects *(continued)*

▼ Less common: allergic reactions, weakness, fatigue, dry mouth, nausea, abdominal pain, constipation, diarrhea, upset stomach, throat irritation, low blood-potassium levels, back pain, muscle cramps and pain, sleeplessness, nervousness, anxiety, tremors, reduced sex drive, sore throat, flushing, hot flashes, rash, impotence, and frequent urination.

▼ Rare: inflammation of the pancreas, hemolytic anemia, chest pain, abnormal heart rhythms, gout, neuritis, and ringing or buzzing in the ears.

Drug Interactions

• Combining a diuretic with Lotrel lowers blood pressure, possibly excessively.

• Combining a potassium-sparing diuretic such as spironolactone, amiloride, or triamterene with benazepril increases the risk of high blood potassium. High blood-potassium levels may lead to abnormal heart rhythms.

• Combining lithium with benazepril may increase blood-lithium levels and lithium side effects.

Food Interactions

Food does not affect individual tablets of amlodipine and benazepril, but the effects of food on Lotrel have not been studied. Until more information is available, take Lotrel on an empty stomach at least 1 hour before or 2 hours after meals.

Usual Dose

Adult: Daily doses range from 2.5 mg of amlodipine and 10 mg of benazepril to 5 mg of amlodipine and 20 mg of benazepril. Dosage depends on your need for each of the 2 ingredients. Small or frail people or those with liver failure should follow dosage recommendations for seniors.

Senior: Start with 2.5 mg of amlodipine and 10 mg of benazepril a day and increase gradually. You may need to take amlodipine and benazepril in separate pills until your daily needs are established.

Overdosage

Little is known about the effects of Lotrel overdose. Call your local poison control center for more information. Overdose victims should be taken to a hospital emergency room for treatment. ALWAYS bring the prescription bottle or container.

Special Information

Continue taking your medication and follow all instructions including diet restriction and other treatments, even if you feel well. Hypertension may be present without symptoms.

Call your doctor if you develop swelling in the hands, feet, face, or throat; sudden breathing difficulties; a sore throat; mouth sores; abnormal heartbeat; increased chest pain; persistent rash; constipation; nausea; weakness; dizziness; loss of the sense of taste; or any bothersome or persistent side effect.

You may get dizzy if you rise to your feet quickly from a sitting or lying position.

Avoid strenuous exercise and very hot weather because heavy sweating or dehydration may lead to a rapid drop in blood pressure.

Avoid over-the-counter stimulants that can raise blood pressure, including diet pills and decongestants.

Maintain good dental hygiene while taking Lotrel and use extra care when brushing or flossing because of the increased risk of oral infection associated with Lotrel.

If you forget a dose, take it as soon as you remember. If it is within 8 hours of your next dose, skip the one you forgot and continue with your regular schedule. Do not take a double dose.

Special Populations

Pregnancy/Breast-feeding

ACE inhibitors may cause fetal damage or death. Lotrel should not be taken by pregnant women. If you are taking Lotrel and become pregnant, see your doctor at once about changing drugs.

Small amounts of both active ingredients pass into breast milk. Nursing mothers who must take Lotrel should bottle-feed.

Seniors

Seniors should begin with the lowest strength of Lotrel available—2.5 mg of amlodipine and 10 mg of benazepril.

Brand Name

Lotrisone

Generic Ingredients

Betamethasone Dipropionate + Clotrimazole

Type of Drug

Steroid and antifungal combination.

Prescribed for

Severe fungal infection or rash.

General Information

The steroid in Lotrisone is betamethasone dipropionate; the antifungal is clotrimazole. Lotrisone is used to relieve the symptoms of itching, rash, or skin inflammation associated with a severe fungal infection. It may also treat the underlying cause of the skin problem by killing the fungus. Improvement usually occurs within the first week of treatment. Creams that contain only clotrimazole or only betamethasone—as betamethasone diproprionate or in a slightly different form called betamethasone valerate—may be more effective than a combination product for certain skin conditions.

Cautions and Warnings

Do not use Lotrisone if you are **sensitive** or **allergic** to either of its ingredients.

Do not apply Lotrisone near or in your **eyes**. Avoid using this product on the **ear** if the eardrum is perforated, unless specifically directed to do so by your doctor.

Do not use an old tube of Lotrisone for a new skin problem without your doctor's knowledge.

Possible Side Effects

▼ Most common: itching, stinging, burning, peeling skin, and swelling.

Drug Interactions

None known.

Usual Dose

Gently rub a thin film onto the affected area and surrounding skin.

Overdosage

Accidental ingestion of Lotrisone may cause nausea and vomiting. Call your local poison control center or a hospital emergency room for more information. If you seek treatment, ALWAYS bring the prescription container.

Special Information

Washing or soaking the skin before applying the medication may increase the amount that penetrates into your skin.

Applying this drug to the face, underarms, groin, genitals or genital areas, abdomen, or between the toes for more than a few days may result in stretch marks.

Do not wear tight clothing after applying Lotrisone, especially when applied to the genitals or genital areas.

Stop using the medication and call your doctor if Lotrisone causes itching, burning, or skin irritation.

If you do not see results after 4 weeks, your doctor may need to prescribe a different medication.

If you forget a dose, apply it as soon as you remember. If it is almost time for your next application, skip the dose you forgot and continue with your regular schedule.

Special Populations

Pregnancy/Breast-feeding

Lotrisone can adversely affect fetal development. Women should not apply Lotrisone over large areas of skin during the first 3 months of pregnancy.

The ingredients in Lotrisone may pass into breast milk when applied to the breast. Nursing mothers who must apply it there should bottle-feed.

Seniors

Seniors may use Lotrisone without special restriction.

Macrobid   *see **Nitrofurantoin**, page 737*

Generic Name

Malathion   (MAL-uh-thye-on)

Brand Name

Ovide

Type of Drug

Scabicide.

Prescribed for

Head lice.

General Information

Originally used as an agricultural insecticide, malathion is effective against common lice and the eggs they leave behind in the scalp. Malathion works by interfering with the breakdown of acetylcholine, a neurohormone that carries nervous-system impulses. The excess acetylcholine produced by malathion kills lice and their eggs. Once applied to the hair, malathion binds with the hair shaft within 6 to 12 hours, providing some protection against future infestations.

Cautions and Warnings

Malathion is extremely toxic if swallowed (see "Overdosage").

People with malathion **sensitivity** should not use it. Normally, about 89% of the malathion applied to the skin is absorbed into the bloodstream; more may be absorbed if it is applied to **broken skin or open sores**—this may cause a toxic reaction.

Malathion **lotion is flammable**. Do not expose the lotion or hair that is still wet with the lotion to an open flame or an electric dryer because of the risk of fire. Allow hair to dry naturally after application.

Malathion can severely **damage the eyes**. If it gets into your eyes, flush them with water immediately and then go to a hospital emergency room.

People who have had a recent **heart attack** or who have any of the following conditions should be cautious when using malathion because it can precipitate an attack or worsen your condition: **asthma,** very **slow heartbeat, low blood pressure, stomach spasms or ulcer,** or **Parkinson's disease.**

Malathion can worsen the following conditions: **severe anemia, dehydration, insecticide exposure effects, liver disease** or **cirrhosis, malnutrition, myasthenia or other neuromuscular diseases,** and **seizure** disorders.

People with recent **brain surgery** should be cautious about using this product because it can initiate toxic nervous-system effects, including seizures.

Possible Side Effects

▼ Common: scalp irritation.

▼ Rare: Convulsions and other side effects can occur if too much of the drug is absorbed into the blood through the scalp (see "Overdosage").

Drug Interactions

• Large dosages of malathion may interact with aminoglycosides (injectable antibiotics) to cause breathing problems, with local anesthetics to cause systemic side effects, and with glaucoma eyedrops—physostigmine, echothiophate, demecarium, and isoflurophate—to cause side effects.

Usual Dose

Adult and Child (age 2 and over): Apply to the hair and scalp and repeat after 7–9 days, if necessary.

Overdosage

Accidental ingestion or absorbing too much drug through the skin is serious and potentially fatal. Symptoms of malathion toxicity include abdominal cramps; anxiety; restlessness; clumsiness or unsteadiness; confusion; depression; diarrhea; dizziness; drowsiness; increased sweating; watery eyes or mouth; loss of bowel or bladder control; muscle twitching in the eyelids, face, or neck; pinpointed pupils; difficulty breathing; seizures; slow heartbeat; trembling; and weakness. People who swallow this drug may not experience toxic effects for up to 12 hours. In case of accidental ingestion induce vomiting with ipecac syrup—available at any pharmacy. Take the victim to a hospital emergency room. ALWAYS bring the prescription bottle or container.

Special Information

Follow your prescription exactly.

Sprinkle the lotion onto dry hair and rub it in until the hair and scalp are wet. Pay special attention to the back of your head and neck. Avoid contact with the eyes. Immediately after applying the lotion, wash your hands. Allow the treated hair to dry naturally; do not cover it or use an electric dryer or other heat source. After 8 to 12 hours, wash your hair with a plain shampoo. Remove dead lice and eggs from the scalp with a fine-toothed comb.

Pregnant women should not handle this medication or apply it to others.

Avoid exposure to other insecticides while being treated with malathion.

Special Populations

Pregnancy/Breast-feeding

Malathion may enter the fetal bloodstream and affect the fetus. Pregnant women should not use it or apply it to others.

Malathion may pass into breast milk. Nursing mothers who must use it should bottle-feed.

Seniors

Seniors may use this drug without special restriction.

Generic Name

Mazindol (MAH-zin-dol)

Brand Names

Mazanor   Sanorex

The information in this profile also applies to the following drugs:

Generic Ingredient: Phentermine Hydrochloride
Adipex-P   Obe-Nix
Fastin   Obephen
Ionamin

Generic Ingredient: Phendimetrazine

Anorex   Obalan
Bontril PDM   Wehless

Generic Ingredient: Sustained-Release Phendimetrazine

Bontril Slow Release   Prelu-2
Dyrexan-OD   Wehless Timecelles
Melfiat-105

Generic Ingredient: Diethylpropion

Tenuate   Tepanil
Tenuate Dospan   Tepanil Ten-Tab

Type of Drug

Appetite suppressant.

Prescribed for

Obesity; also prescribed for Duchenne's muscular dystrophy.

General Information

While this appetite suppressant is not an amphetamine, it works in a similar fashion by affecting specific areas in the brain. Each dose of mazindol works for 8 to 15 hours. This drug should only be used for 2 to 3 months.

Cautions and Warnings

Do not take mazindol if you have **heart disease, high blood pressure, thyroid disease,** or **glaucoma,** or if you are **sensitive** or **allergic** to it or any other appetite suppressant. Do not use mazindol if you are prone to **emotional agitation** or **substance abuse,** since appetite suppressants can be easily abused.

Possible Side Effects

▼ Common: a false sense of well-being, nervousness, euphoria (feeling "high"), overstimulation, restlessness, and trouble sleeping.

▼ Less common: palpitations, high blood pressure, drowsiness or sedation, weakness, dizziness, tremors, headache, dry mouth, nausea, vomiting, diarrhea or other intestinal disturbances, rash, itching, changes in sex drive, hair loss, muscle pain, difficulty urinating, sweating, chills, blurred vision, and fever.

Drug Interactions

• Combining other stimulants—including decongestants, asthma drugs, and over-the-counter cold remedies—with mazindol may result in excessive stimulation.

• Taking this medication within 2 weeks of taking any monoamine oxidase inhibitor (MAOI) may result in very high blood pressure.

• Appetite suppressants may reduce the effects of drugs used to treat high blood pressure.

• One case of lithium toxicity occurred after combining lithium with mazindol.

Food Interactions

Mazindol may be taken with food to reduce upset stomach.

Usual Dose

1 mg 3 times a day, 1 hour before meals; or 2 mg once a day, before lunch.

Overdosage

Symptoms include restlessness, tremors, shallow breathing, confusion, hallucinations, and fever. Fatigue and depression may follow. Additional symptoms are changes in blood pressure, cold and clammy skin, nausea, vomiting, diarrhea, and stomach cramps. Take the victim to a hospital emergency room immediately. ALWAYS bring the prescription bottle or container.

Special Information

Do not take any appetite suppressant as part of a weight-control program for more than 12 weeks, and take it only under a doctor's supervision. This drug will not reduce body weight by itself. You must limit or modify your diet and follow your exercise regimen, if applicable.

Studies have shown that appetite suppressants are more effective when combined with behavior therapy.

Maintain good dental hygiene while taking this drug. Appetite suppressants often cause dry mouth, which increases the risk of an oral infection. Dry mouth usually can be relieved with sugarless candy, gum, or ice chips.

Do not crush or chew Mazindol.

If you forget a dose, skip it and continue with your regular schedule. Do not take a double dose.

Special Populations

Pregnancy/Breast-feeding

Studies have shown that large dosages of mazindol may damage the fetus. When this drug is considered crucial by your doctor, its potential benefits must be carefully weighed against its risks.

It is not known if mazindol passes into breast milk. Nursing mothers who must take it should consider bottle-feeding.

Seniors

Mazindol can aggravate diabetes or high blood pressure, conditions common in older adults.

Generic Name

Meclofenamate (mec-loe-FEN-uh-mate) G

Brand Name

Meclomen

Type of Drug

Nonsteroidal anti-inflammatory drug (NSAID).

Prescribed for

Rheumatoid arthritis, osteoarthritis, mild to moderate pain, sunburn, migraine, menstrual headache, and discomfort associated with excessive menstrual bleeding.

General Information

Meclofenamate and other NSAIDs are used to relieve pain and inflammation. We do not know exactly how NSAIDs work, but they may achieve their effects by blocking the body's production of a hormone called prostaglandin and the action of other body chemicals. Pain relief comes within 1 hour after taking the first dose of meclofenamate, but its anti-inflammatory effect generally takes several days to become apparent and may take 2 to 3 weeks to reach maximum effect. Meclofenamate is broken down in the liver.

Cautions and Warnings

People who are **allergic** to meclofenamate or any other NSAID and those with a history of **asthma** attacks brought on by an NSAID, iodides, or aspirin should not take meclofena-mate.

Meclofenamate can cause **gastrointestinal (GI) bleeding, ulcers,** and **stomach perforation**. This can occur at any time, with or without warning, in people who take meclofenamate regularly. People with a history of active GI bleeding should be cautious about taking any NSAID. People who develop bleeding or ulcers and continue NSAID treatment should be aware of the possibility of developing more serious drug toxicity.

Meclofenamate can affect platelets and **blood clotting** at high doses and should be avoided by people with clotting problems and those taking warfarin.

People with **heart problems** who use meclofenamate may experience swelling in their arms, legs, or feet.

Meclofenamate can cause severe toxic effects to the **kidney**. Report any unusual side effects to your doctor, who may need to periodically test your kidney function.

Meclofenamate can make you **unusually sensitive to the effects of the sun**.

Possible Side Effects

▼ Most common: diarrhea, nausea, vomiting, constipation, stomach gas, stomach upset or irritation, and appetite loss—especially during the first few days of treatment.

▼ Less common: stomach ulcers, GI bleeding, hepatitis, gallbladder attacks, painful urination, poor kidney function, kidney inflammation, blood and protein in the urine, dizziness, fainting, nervousness, depression, hallucinations, confusion, disorientation, tingling in the hands or feet, light-headedness, itching, increased sweating, dry nose and mouth, heart palpitations, chest pain, difficulty breathing, and muscle cramps.

▼ Rare: severe allergic reactions including closing of the throat, fever and chills, changes in liver function, jaundice (yellowing of the skin or whites of the eyes), and kidney failure. People who experience such effects must be promptly treated in a hospital emergency room or doctor's office. NSAIDs have caused severe skin reactions; if this happens to you, see your doctor immediately.

Drug Interactions

• Meclofenamate can increase the effects of oral anticoagulant (blood-thinning) drugs such as warfarin. Your anticoagulant dose may need to be reduced.

• Taking meclofenamate with cyclosporine may increase the toxic kidney effects of both drugs.

• Methotrexate toxicity may be increased in people also taking meclofenamate.

• Meclofenamate may reduce the blood-pressure-lowering effect of beta blockers and loop diuretics.

• Meclofenamate may increase phenytoin side effects. Lithium blood levels may be increased by meclofenamate.

• Meclofenamate blood levels may be affected by cimetidine.

• Probenecid may increase the risk of meclofenamate side effects.

• Aspirin and other salicylates should never be combined with meclofenamate.

Food Interactions

Take meclofenamate with food or a magnesium/aluminum antacid if it upsets your stomach.

Usual Dose

Adult and Child (age 14 and over): 200–400 mg a day.
Child (under age 14): not recommended.

Overdosage

People have died from NSAID overdoses. Common signs of overdose are drowsiness, nausea, vomiting, diarrhea, abdominal pain, rapid breathing, rapid heartbeat, increased sweating, ringing or buzzing in the ears, confusion, disorientation, stupor, and coma. Take the victim to a hospital emergency room at once. ALWAYS bring the prescription bottle or container.

Special Information

Take each dose with a full glass of water and do not lie down for 15 to 30 minutes afterward. Meclofenamate can make you drowsy or tired: Be careful when driving or operating hazardous equipment. Do not take any over-the-counter products containing acetaminophen or aspirin while taking meclofenamate. Avoid alcohol.

Contact your doctor if you develop rash or itching, visual disturbances, weight gain, breathing difficulties, fluid retention, hallucinations, black or tarry stools, persistent headache, or any unusual or intolerable side effect.

If you forget a dose of meclofenamate, take it as soon as you remember. If you take meclofenamate once a day and it is within 8 hours of your next dose, or if you take several doses a day and it is within 4 hours of your next dose, skip the dose you forgot and continue with your regular schedule. Never take a double dose.

Special Populations

Pregnancy/Breast-feeding

NSAIDs may affect the fetal heart during the second half of pregnancy. When this drug is considered crucial by your doctor, its potential benefits must be carefully weighed against its risks.

NSAIDs may pass into breast milk. There is a risk that a nursing mother taking meclofenamate could affect her baby's heart or cardiovascular system. Nursing mothers who must take this drug should bottle-feed.

Seniors

Seniors may be more susceptible to side effects, especially ulcers.

Generic Name

Medroxyprogesterone Acetate

(med-rok-see-proe-JES-ter-one) Ⓖ

Brand Names

Amen	Cycrin
Curretab	Provera

The information in this profile also applies to the following drugs:

Generic Ingredient: Norethindrone Acetate
Aygestin

Generic Ingredient: Progesterone
Crinone

Type of Drug

Progestin.

Prescribed for

Irregular menstrual bleeding, endometrial or kidney cancer, and menopause—in conjunction with estrogen replacement therapy (ERT); also prescribed to stimulate breathing in people who suffer from sleep apnea and for other conditions in which breathing rate is abnormally slow or stops completely for short periods of time. Norethindrone acetate may be used for endometriosis. Progesterone has been used to treat premenstrual syndrome (PMS), prevent spontaneous abortion or premature labor, and support embryo implantation and help maintain pregnancy in some assisted reproductive technology (ART) procedures.

General Information

Progesterone is the principal hormone involved in the process of pregnancy. It helps to prepare the womb to accept the fertilized egg and maintain the growth and development of the fetus. The decision to take medroxyprogesterone acetate on a regular basis should be made carefully by you and your doctor because of this drug's risks.

Another progestin called megestrol (Megace) is used in breast and endometrial cancer (40–320 mg a day) and for weight loss and decreased appetite in people living with AIDS (800 mg 4 times a day).

Cautions and Warnings

Do not take this drug if you are **sensitive** or **allergic** to it or any progestin or have a history of **blood clotting or similar disorders, convulsions, liver disease,** known or suspected **breast cancer,** undiagnosed **vaginal bleeding,** or **miscarriage.** Medroxyprogesterone and other progestins should not be used regularly to avoid weight loss.

Progestins have been used to prevent spontaneous abortion. Such treatment can harm a fetus if given during the first 4 months of pregnancy.

Medroxyprogesterone acetate use should be carefully considered if you have had **asthma, cardiac insufficiency, epilepsy, migraine, kidney problems, diabetes, ectopic pregnancy, high blood-fat levels,** or **depression.**

Possible Side Effects

There is a strong relationship between the use of progestin drugs and the development of blood clots in the veins, lungs, or brain.

Medroxyprogesterone Acetate and Norethindrone Acetate

▼ Most common: breakthrough bleeding, spotting, changes in or loss of menstrual flow, water retention, weight loss or gain, breast tenderness, jaundice, acne, rash with or without itching, and depression.

▼ Common: changes in sex drive, changes in appetite and mood, headache, nervousness, dizziness, tiredness, backache, loss of scalp hair, hair growth in unusual quantities or places, itching, symptoms similar to those of a urinary infection, and unusual rashes.

▼ Rare: allergy, fatigue, fever, flu-like symptoms, bloating, asthma, back or leg pain, sinus inflammation, respiratory infection, upset stomach, stomach gas or noise, emotional instability, sleeplessness, acne, itching, painful urination, and urinary infections.

Progesterone Gel

Side effects are less common if you use this drug once a day.

▼ Most common: pelvic or abdominal pain or cramps, tiredness, headache, nervousness, depression, reduced sex drive, constipation, nausea, breast enlargement, and nighttime urination.

▼ Common: bloating, dizziness, diarrhea, vomiting, painful intercourse, joint pain, itching, and vaginal infection or discharge.

Drug Interactions

• Rifampin and aminoglutethimide reduce medroxyprogesterone acetate's effectiveness.

• People with diabetes may experience a decrease in glucose tolerance, worsening their condition.

Food Interactions

You may take this drug with food if it upsets your stomach.

Usual Dose

Medroxyprogesterone Acetate: 5–10 mg a day for 5–10 days, beginning on day 16–21 of the menstrual cycle.

Norethindrone Acetate: For endometriosis—5 mg a day for 14 days, then increased gradually up to 15 mg a day; treatment may continue for 6–9 months. For abnormal periodic bleeding or no period—2.5–10 mg a day for 5–10 days during the second half of the menstrual cycle.

Progesterone Gel: Apply a single-use disposable unit once or twice a day.

Overdosage

Symptoms may include severe side effects, though small overdoses generally do not cause unusual symptoms. Call your local poison control center or a hospital emergency room for more information. If you seek treatment, ALWAYS bring the prescription bottle or container.

Special Information

Your need for this drug should be evaluated at least every 6 months.

Stop taking this drug immediately and call your doctor if you experience sudden, partial, or complete loss of vision; double vision; sudden falling; calf pain, swelling, and redness; numbness in an arm or leg; leg cramp; water retention; unusual vaginal bleeding; migraine or a sudden and severe headache; depression; or if you think you have become pregnant.

Medroxyprogesterone acetate may increase your sensitivity to the sun. Use sunscreen and wear protective clothing.

Medroxyprogesterone acetate may mask symptoms of menopause.

If you forget a dose, take it as soon as you remember. If it is almost time for your next dose, skip the one you forgot and continue with your regular schedule. Do not take a double dose.

Special Populations

Pregnancy/Breast-feeding

Medroxyprogesterone acetate and norethindrone may cause birth defects or interfere with fetal development; it can double the rate of certain birth defects if used during the first 4 months of pregnancy. It is not considered safe for use during pregnancy, except under very specific circumstances. Progesterone gel is used to support embryo implantation and help maintain pregnancies in some ART procedures.

Medroxyprogesterone acetate passes into breast milk. It may also increase the amount of milk produced and the duration of milk production when taken after childbirth. Nursing mothers who must use this drug should consider bottle-feeding.

Seniors
Seniors with severe liver disease are more sensitive to the effects of this drug.

Generic Name

Mefenamic Acid (MEF-eh-NAM-ik)

Brand Name
Ponstel

Type of Drug
Nonsteroidal anti-inflammatory drug (NSAID).

Prescribed for
Sunburn, migraine, menstrual pain and headache, and premenstrual syndrome (PMS).

General Information
Mefenamic acid and other NSAIDs are used to relieve pain and inflammation. We do not know exactly how NSAIDs work, but they may achieve their effects by blocking the body's production of a hormone called prostaglandin and the action of other body chemicals. Pain relief comes within 1 hour after taking the first dose of mefenamic acid, but its anti-inflammatory effect generally takes several days to 2 weeks to become apparent and may take a month or more to reach maximum effect. Mefenamic acid is broken down in the liver and eliminated through the kidneys. It should only be used for less than 1 week.

Cautions and Warnings

People who are **allergic** to mefenamic acid or any other NSAID and those with a history of **asthma** attacks brought on by an NSAID, iodides, or aspirin should not take mefenamic acid.

Mefenamic acid can cause **gastrointestinal (GI) bleeding, ulcers,** and **stomach perforation**. This can occur at any time, with or without warning, in people who take mefenamic acid regularly. People with a history of active GI bleeding should be cautious about taking any NSAID. People who develop bleeding or ulcers and continue NSAID treatment should be aware of the possibility of developing more serious drug toxicity.

Mefenamic acid can affect platelets and **blood clotting** at high doses and should be avoided by people with clotting problems and those taking warfarin.

People with **heart problems** who use mefenamic acid may experience swelling in their arms, legs, or feet.

Mefenamic acid can cause severe toxic effects to the **kidney**. Report any unusual side effects to your doctor, who may need to periodically test your kidney function.

Mefenamic acid can make you **unusually sensitive to the effects of the sun**.

Possible Side Effects

▼ Most common: diarrhea, nausea, vomiting, constipation, gas, stomach upset or irritation, and appetite loss—especially during the first few days of treatment.

▼ Less common: stomach ulcers, GI bleeding, hepatitis, gallbladder attacks, painful urination, poor kidney function, kidney inflammation, blood and protein in the urine, dizziness, fainting, nervousness, depression, hallucinations, confusion, disorientation, tingling in the hands or feet, light-headedness, itching, increased sweating, dry nose and mouth, heart palpitations, chest pain, breathing difficulties, and muscle cramps.

▼ Rare: severe allergic reactions including closing of the throat, fever and chills, changes in liver function, jaundice (yellowing of the skin or whites of the eyes), and kidney failure. People who experience such effects must be promptly treated in a hospital emergency room or doctor's office. NSAIDs have caused severe skin reactions; if this happens to you, see your doctor immediately.

Drug Interactions

• Mefenamic acid can increase the effects of oral anticoagulant (blood-thinning) drugs such as warfarin. Your anticoagulant dose may need to be reduced.

• Taking mefenamic acid with cyclosporine may increase the toxic kidney effects of both drugs.

• Methotrexate toxicity may be increased in people also taking mefenamic acid.

• Mefenamic acid may reduce the blood-pressure-lowering effect of beta blockers and loop diuretics.

• Mefenamic acid may increase phenytoin side effects. Lithium blood levels may be increased by mefenamic acid.

• Mefenamic acid blood levels may be affected by cimetidine.

• Probenecid may increase the risk of mefenamic acid toxic reactions.

• Aspirin and other salicylates should never be combined with mefenamic acid.

Food Interactions

Take mefenamic acid with food or a magnesium/aluminum antacid if it upsets your stomach.

Usual Dose

Adult and Child (age 14 and over): 500 mg to start, then 250 mg every 6 hours.

Child (under age 14): not recommended.

Overdosage

People have died from NSAID overdoses. Common signs of overdose are drowsiness, nausea, vomiting, diarrhea, abdominal pain, rapid breathing, rapid heartbeat, increased sweating, ringing or buzzing in the ears, confusion, disorientation, stupor, and coma. Take the victim to a hospital emergency room at once. ALWAYS bring the prescription bottle or container.

Special Information

Take each dose with a full glass of water and do not lie down for 15 to 30 minutes afterward. Mefenamic acid can make you drowsy or tired: Be careful when driving or operating hazardous equipment. Do not take any over-the-counter products containing acetaminophen or aspirin while taking mefenamic acid. Avoid alcohol.

Contact your doctor if you develop rash or itching, visual disturbances, weight gain, breathing difficulties, fluid retention, hallucinations, black or tarry stools, persistent headache, or any unusual or intolerable side effect.

If you forget a dose of mefenamic acid, take it as soon as you remember. If you take mefenamic acid once a day and it is within 8 hours of your next dose, or if you take several doses a day and it is within 4 hours of your next dose, skip the dose you forgot and continue with your regular schedule. Never take a double dose.

Special Populations

Pregnancy/Breast-feeding
NSAIDs may affect the fetal heart during the second half of pregnancy. When this drug is considered crucial by your doctor, its potential benefits must be carefully weighed against its risks.

NSAIDs may pass into breast milk. There is a risk that a nursing mother taking mefenamic acid could affect her baby's heart or cardiovascular system. Nursing mothers who must take this drug should bottle-feed.

Seniors
Seniors may be more susceptible to side effects, especially ulcer disease.

Generic Name

Meperidine (muh-PER-ih-dine) Ⓖ

Brand Name
Demerol

Type of Drug
Narcotic analgesic (pain reliever).

Prescribed for
Moderate to severe pain.

General Information
Meperidine hydrochloride is a potent narcotic analgesic and cough suppressant. It is also used before surgery to reduce

anxiety and help bring the patient into early stages of anesthesia. Meperidine is probably the most widely used narcotic in American hospitals. It compares favorably with morphine sulfate, the standard for narcotic analgesics.

It is useful for mild to moderate pain; 25 to 50 mg of meperidine are approximately equal in pain-relieving effect to 2 325-mg aspirin tablets. Meperidine may be less effective than aspirin for pain associated with inflammation because aspirin reduces inflammation but meperidine does not. Meperidine suppresses the cough reflex but does not cure the underlying cause of the cough.

Cautions and Warnings

Do not take meperidine if you are **allergic** or **sensitive** to it. Use this drug with extreme caution if you suffer from **asthma or other breathing problems.** Chronic (long-term) use of meperidine may cause drug dependence or **addiction.** Narcotic side effects are more severe in the presence of a **head injury, brain tumor,** or **increased pressure within the skull.** Narcotics may also hide the symptoms of head injury.

Possible Side Effects

▼ Most common: light-headedness, dizziness, sleepiness, nausea, vomiting, appetite loss, and increased sweating. These side effects usually disappear if you lie down. More serious side effects of meperidine are shallow breathing or breathing difficulties.

▼ Less common: euphoria (feeling "high"), weakness, headache, agitation, uncoordinated muscle movement, minor hallucinations, disorientation, visual disturbances, dry mouth, constipation, flushing of the face, rapid heartbeat, palpitations, faintness, urinary difficulties or hesitancy, reduced sex drive or potency, itching, rash, anemia, lowered blood sugar, and yellowing of the skin or whites of the eyes. Narcotic analgesics may aggravate convulsions in those who have had them.

Drug Interactions

• Because of its depressant effect and potential effect on breathing, meperidine should be taken with extreme caution in combination with alcohol, sleeping medication, tranquilizers, or other depressant drugs.

• People taking cimetidine and a narcotic analgesic may experience confusion, disorientation, nervous-system depression, seizure, or breathing difficulties.

• Combining meperidine and a monoamine oxidase inhibitor (MAOI) antidepressant may lead to breathing difficulties; blood pressure changes; bluish discoloration of the lips, fingernails, or skin; coma; or death. Do not take meperidine within 2 weeks of your last dose of an MAOI.

Food Interactions

Meperidine may be taken with food to reduce upset stomach.

Usual Dose

Adult: 50–150 mg every 3–4 hours as needed.

Child: 0.5–0.8 mg per lb. of body weight every 3–4 hours as needed, up to the adult dosage.

Overdosage

Symptoms include slow breathing, extreme tiredness progressing to stupor and then coma, pinpointed pupils, no response to pain stimulation, cold or clammy skin, slow heartbeat, low blood pressure, convulsions, and cardiac arrest. The victim should be taken to a hospital emergency room immediately. ALWAYS bring the prescription bottle or container.

Special Information

Be extremely careful when driving or doing any task that requires concentration. Avoid alcohol.

Call your doctor if you develop nausea, constipation, breathing difficulties, or any bothersome or persistent side effect.

Ask your doctor to consider lowering your meperidine dosage if you experience light-headedness, dizziness, sleepiness, nausea, vomiting, appetite loss, or increased sweating.

If you forget a dose, take it as soon as you remember. If it is almost time for your next dose, skip the one you forgot and continue with your regular schedule. Do not take a double dose.

Special Populations

Pregnancy/Breast-feeding

Large amounts of meperidine taken during pregnancy may

cause addiction in newborns. Narcotics may also cause breathing difficulties in newborns if taken just before delivery. When this drug is considered crucial by your doctor, its potential benefits must be carefully weighed against its risks.

Meperidine passes into breast milk. Nursing mothers who must take this drug should bottle-feed.

Seniors

Seniors are more likely to experience side effects and should take the smallest effective dosage.

Generic Name

Meprobamate (meh-proe-BUH-mate) Ⓖ

Brand Names

Equanil   Neuramate
Miltown

Type of Drug

Antianxiety agent.

Prescribed for

Short-term anxiety and tension.

General Information

Meprobamate works by directly affecting several areas of the brain. It can relax you, relieve anxiety, and act as a muscle relaxant, anticonvulsant, or sleeping pill. This drug should be used for less than 4 months.

Cautions and Warnings

Do not take meprobamate if you are **allergic** to it or a related drug such as carbromal, carisoprodol, felbamate, or mebutamate. Meprobamate may cause **seizures** in epileptic patients.

Long-term meprobamate users have developed severe physical and psychological **drug dependence**. It can produce chronic intoxication after prolonged use or if used in greater than recommended doses: Symptoms include slurred speech, dizziness, general sleepiness, and depression. Suddenly stopping meprobamate after prolonged and excessive use may result in drug withdrawal symptoms, including severe anxiety, vomiting, appetite loss, sleeplessness, tremors, muscle twitching, severe sleepiness, confusion, hallucinations, and convulsions. Withdrawal symptoms usually begin 12 to 48 hours after meprobamate has been stopped and may last 1 to 4 days. When stopping treatment with meprobamate, the drug should be reduced gradually over 1 or 2 weeks.

People with **kidney or liver disease** need to take lower doses.

Possible Side Effects

▼ Most common: drowsiness, sleepiness, dizziness, slurred speech, poor muscle coordination, headache, weakness, tingling in the arms and legs, and euphoria (feeling high).

▼ Less common: nausea, vomiting, diarrhea, abnormal heart rhythm, excitement or overstimulation, low blood pressure, itching, rash, and changes in blood components.

▼ Rare: allergic reactions, including high fever, chills, bronchospasm (closing of the throat), and reduced urinary function.

Drug Interactions

• Combining meprobamate with nervous-system depressants, including alcohol, other tranquilizers, narcotics, barbiturates, sleeping pills, or antihistamines, can cause excess tranquilization, depression, sleepiness, or fatigue.

Food Interactions

Take this drug with food if it upsets your stomach.

Usual Dose

Adult and Child (age 13 and over): 1200–1600 mg a day in divided doses; maximum daily dose, 2400 mg.
Child (age 6–12): 100–200 mg 2–3 times a day.
Child (under age 6): not recommended.

Overdosage

Overdose symptoms are extreme drowsiness, lethargy, stupor, and coma, with possible shock and respiratory collapse.

If alcohol or another depressant has also been taken, small overdoses can be fatal. After a large overdose, the victim will go to sleep very quickly, and blood pressure, pulse, and breathing levels will drop rapidly. The overdose victim must immediately be taken to a hospital emergency room. ALWAYS bring the prescription bottle or container.

Special Information

Take this drug according to your doctor's direction. Do not change your dose without your doctor's approval.

This drug causes drowsiness and poor concentration. Be careful when driving or performing complex activities. Avoid alcohol and other nervous-system depressants because they increase these effects.

Call your doctor if you develop fever, sore throat, rash, mouth sores, nosebleeds, unexplained black-and-blue marks, or easy bruising or bleeding, or if you become pregnant.

If you forget a dose and remember within about 1 hour of your regular time, take it right away. If you do not remember until later, skip the dose you forgot and go back to your regular schedule. Do not take a double dose.

Special Populations

Pregnancy/Breast-feeding

Meprobamate increases the risk of birth defects, particularly during the first 3 months of pregnancy. Inform your doctor immediately if you are or might be pregnant. There are few good reasons for pregnant women to take meprobamate.

Large amounts of meprobamate pass into breast milk. Nursing mothers who must take this drug should bottle-feed.

Seniors

Seniors are more sensitive to the sedative and other effects of this drug and should take the lowest effective dosage.

Generic Name

Mesalamine (meh-SAL-uh-meen)

Brand Names

Asacol
Pentasa

Rowasa

Type of Drug

Bowel anti-inflammatory.

Prescribed for

Oral Products: ulcerative colitis.

Rectal Products: distal ulcerative colitis, proctitis, and proctosigmoiditis.

General Information

A chemical cousin of aspirin, mesalamine is used to treat symptoms of bowel inflammation. No one knows exactly how mesalamine works, but it is believed to have a local effect on the bowel. Mesalamine tablets are coated with an acrylic resin that delays drug release until they reach the colon. Little of the drug is absorbed into the blood; 70% to 90% remains in the colon.

Cautions and Warnings

Mesalamine may **worsen colitis** or cause **cramping,** sudden **abdominal pain,** bloody **diarrhea, fever, headache,** or **rash.** Stop taking this drug at once and call your doctor if any of these symptoms develop.

People who are **allergic** to mesalamine or aspirin should not use this drug. Although people who are sensitive or allergic to sulfasalazine have generally been able to tolerate mesalamine—which is an active agent in sulfasalazine—they should be cautious.

Some people taking mesalamine have developed kidney problems. People who have or have had **kidney disease** should be cautious about using this drug. All people taking mesalamine should have kidney function tests before and during drug therapy.

Possible Side Effects

Mesalamine is generally well tolerated. Mesalamine tablets have the most side effects, suppositories the least.

Tablets

▼ Most common: abdominal pain, cramps, or discomfort; stomach rumbling; and generalized pain.

Possible Side Effects *(continued)*

▼ Common: constipation, diarrhea, upset stomach, vomiting, muscle weakness, dizziness, fever, runny nose, rash, skin spots, achy joints, back pain, and stiff muscles.

▼ Less common: worsening of colitis, gas, chills, sweating, feeling unwell, tiredness, acne, itching, arthritis, muscle aches, chest pain, pinkeye, painful menstruation, swelling, and flu-like symptoms.

▼ Rare: sleeplessness, hair loss, and urinary burning or infection. Other rare side effects can occur in almost any part of the body. Contact your doctor if you experience any side effect not listed above.

Capsules

▼ Less common: abdominal pain, cramps, or discomfort; diarrhea; nausea; headache; rash; and skin spots.

▼ Rare: worsening of colitis, constipation, gas, vomiting, dizziness, fever, sleeplessness, sweating, feeling unwell, tiredness, itching, acne, achy joints, leg or joint pain, muscle aches, pinkeye, swelling, and hair loss. Other rare side effects can occur in almost any part of the body. Contact your doctor if you experience any side effect not listed.

Suppositories

▼ Common: headache.

▼ Less common: abdominal pain, cramps, or discomfort; diarrhea; worsening of colitis; gas; nausea; rectal pain, soreness, or burning; muscle weakness; dizziness; fever; sore throat; cold symptoms; acne; rash; skin spots; and swelling.

Rectal Suspension

▼ Common: abdominal pain, cramps, or discomfort; gas; nausea; headache; and flu-like symptoms.

▼ Less common: bloating; diarrhea; hemorrhoids; pain on enema insertion; rectal pain, soreness, or burning; dizziness; fever; feeling unwell; tiredness; cold symptoms; sore throat; itching; rash; skin spots; back pain; leg pain; and joint pain.

▼ Rare: constipation, muscle weakness, sleeplessness, swelling, hair loss, and urinary burning or infection.

Drug Interactions

None known.

Food Interactions

Take this drug with food if it upsets your stomach.

Usual Dose

Tablets: 800 mg 3 times a day for 6 weeks.

Capsules: 1000 mg 4 times a day for up to 8 weeks.

Suppositories: 1 suppository 2 times a day for 3–6 weeks. Retain the suppository for 1–3 hours for maximum benefit.

Rectal Suspension: 1 bottle of suspension taken as an enema at bedtime every night for 3–6 weeks. The enema liquid should be retained for about 8 hours.

Overdosage

Symptoms are likely to include: ringing or buzzing in the ears, fainting or dizziness, headache, confusion, drowsiness, sweating, rapid breathing, vomiting, and diarrhea. In case of overdose, call your local poison control center or hospital emergency room. You may be told to induce vomiting with ipecac syrup—available at any pharmacy—before taking the victim to the emergency room. If you seek treatment, ALWAYS bring the prescription bottle or container.

Special Information

The tablets must be swallowed whole. Call your doctor if they are visible in your stool.

When using suppositories, handle them as little as possible to prevent melting.

When administering rectal suspension, lie on your left side with your lower leg extended and your upper leg flexed to maintain balance.

Call your doctor if you develop chest pain, breathing or urinary difficulties, worsening of colitis, or any bothersome or persistent side effect.

If you forget to administer a dose, do so as soon as you remember. If you take mesalamine tablets or capsules and it is within 4 hours of your next dose, skip the dose you forgot and continue with your regular schedule. If you take the suppositories or rectal solution and you do not remember until it is almost time for the next dose, skip the one you forgot and continue with your regular schedule. Never take a double dose.

Special Populations

Pregnancy/Breast-feeding
Mesalamine passes into the fetal circulation. When this drug is considered crucial by your doctor, its potential benefits must be carefully weighed against its risks.

Small amounts of mesalamine pass into breast milk. Nursing mothers who must take this drug should consider bottle-feeding.

Seniors
Seniors may use this drug without special restriction.

Generic Name

Metaprerenol (meh-tuh-proe-TER-uh-nol) Ⓖ

Brand Name
Alupent

Type of Drug
Bronchodilator.

Prescribed for
Asthma and bronchospasm.

General Information
Metaproterenol sulfate can be taken both by mouth as a tablet or syrup and by inhalation. This drug may be used with other drugs to produce relief from asthma symptoms. Oral metaproterenol begins working 15 to 30 minutes after a dose; its effects may last for up to 4 hours. Metaproterenol inhalation begins working in 5 to 30 minutes and lasts for 2 to 6 hours.

Cautions and Warnings
This drug should be used with caution by people with a history of **angina pectoris, heart disease, high blood pressure,**

**stroke, seizures, diabetes, thyroid disease, prostate disease,
or glaucoma**. Excessive use of metaproterenol could lead to
worsening of your condition. Using excessive amounts of
metaproterenol can lead to increased breathing difficulties
rather than relief. In the most extreme cases, people have
had heart attacks after using excessive amounts of inhalant.

Possible Side Effects

▼ Common: heart palpitations, rapid heartbeat,
tremors, convulsions, shakiness, nervous tension, dizziness, fainting, headache, heartburn, upset stomach, nausea and vomiting, cough, dry or sore and irritated throat,
muscle cramps, and urinary difficulties.

▼ Less common: high blood pressure, abnormal heart
rhythms, and angina. Metaproterenol inhalation is less
likely to cause these effects than some of the older
asthma drugs. It can also cause diarrhea, unusual tastes
or smells, dry mouth, drowsiness, hoarseness, stuffy
nose, worsening of asthma, backache, fatigue, and rash.

Drug Interactions

• The effect of this drug may be increased by antidepressant drugs, some antihistamines, levothyroxine, and
monoamine oxidase inhibitors (MAOIs).

• The risk of cardiac toxicity may be increased in people
combining metaproterenol and theophylline.

• Beta-blocking drugs such as propanolol antagonize
metaproterenol. Metaproterenol may antagonize the effects
of blood-pressure-lowering drugs, especially reserpine,
methyldopa, and guanethidine.

Food Interactions

If the tablets upset your stomach, they may be taken with
food.

Usual Dose

Tablets or Syrup
  Adult and Child (age 10 and over or 60 lbs.): 60–80 mg a
day.
  Child (age 6–9 or under 60 lbs.): 30–40 mg a day.

Child (under age 6): 0.6–1.2 mg per lb. of body weight a day. Children this age should be treated only with metaproterenol syrup.

Inhalation
Adult and Child (age 12 and over): 2–3 puffs every 3–4 hours. Each canister contains about 300 inhalations. Do not use more than 12 puffs a day.
Child (under age 12): not recommended.

Overdosage

Symptoms include palpitations, abnormal heart rhythm, rapid or slow heartbeat, chest pain, high blood pressure, fever, chills, cold sweat, blanching of the skin, nausea, vomiting, sleeplessness, delirium, tremor, pinpoint pupils, convulsions, coma, and collapse. The victim should see a doctor or be taken to a hospital emergency room. ALWAYS bring the prescription bottle or container.

Special Information

Be sure to follow your doctor's instructions for using metaproterenol. Using more than the amount prescribed can lead to drug tolerance and actually worsen your symptoms. If your condition worsens rather than improves after taking metaproterenol, stop taking it and call your doctor.

Metaproterenol inhalation should be breathed in during the second half of your inward breath, since this allows it to reach more deeply into your lungs.

Call your doctor immediately if you develop chest pain, palpitations, rapid heartbeat, muscle tremors, dizziness, headache, facial flushing, or urinary difficulty, or if you still have trouble breathing after using this medication.

If you miss a dose of metaproterenol, take it as soon as possible. Take the rest of that day's dose at regularly spaced time intervals. Go back to your regular schedule the next day.

Special Populations

Pregnancy/Breast-feeding
Metaproterenol has caused birth defects when given in large amounts to pregnant animals. When this drug is considered crucial by your doctor, its potential benefits must be carefully weighed against its risks.

It is not known if metaproterenol passes into breast milk. Nursing mothers who must use it should consider bottle-feeding.

Seniors
Seniors are more sensitive to the effects of this drug.

Generic Name

Metaxalone (meh-TAX-uh-lone)

Brand Name
Skelaxin

Type of Drug
Skeletal muscle relaxant.

Prescribed for
Muscle spasms.

General Information
Metaxalone is prescribed as part of a coordinated program of rest, physical therapy, and other measures for the relief of acute, painful spasm conditions. Exactly how metaxalone works is unknown.

Cautions and Warnings
Metaxalone should be taken with caution if you have had a **reaction** to it, have a tendency toward **anemia,** or have **poor kidney or liver function**.

Possible Side Effects

▼ Most common: nausea, vomiting, upset stomach, stomach cramps, drowsiness, dizziness, headache, nervousness, and irritability.

Possible Side Effects *(continued)*

▼ Less common: rapid or pounding heartbeat, fainting, convulsions, hallucinations, depression, clumsiness or unsteadiness, constipation, diarrhea, heartburn, hiccups, black or tarry bowel movements, vomiting of material that resembles coffee grounds, agranulocytosis (symptoms include fever with or without chills, sore throat, and sores or white spots on the lips or mouth), uncontrolled eye movement, stuffy nose, stinging or burning eyes, bloodshot eyes, weakness, unusual tiredness, chest tightness, swollen glands, unusual bleeding or bruising, and breathing difficulties.

▼ Rare: liver inflammation, yellowing of the skin or whites of the eyes, and drug-sensitivity reactions (symptoms include rash, hives, itching, changes in facial color, and breathing difficulties.

Drug Interactions

• Tranquilizers, alcohol, and other nervous system depressants may increase the depressant effects of metaxalone.

Food Interactions

Metaxalone may be taken with food or meals if it upsets your stomach.

Usual Dose

Adult and Child (age 13 and over): 800 mg 3 or 4 times a day.

Child (under age 13): not recommended.

Overdosage

Symptoms are likely to be severe side effects but may include some less common reactions as well. Overdose victims should be taken to a hospital emergency room. ALWAYS bring the prescription bottle or container.

Special Information

Long-term metaxalone treatment may cause liver toxicity or damage. If you are using this medicine for an extended period, your doctor should check your liver function about every 1 to 2 months.

Metaxalone may cause tiredness, dizziness, and lightheadedness. Be careful when driving or performing tasks that require concentration and coordination.

Call your doctor if you develop breathing difficulties, unusual tiredness or weakness, fever, chills, cough or hoarseness, lower back or side pain, painful urination, yellowing of the skin or whites of the eyes, rash, hives, itching, redness, or any other bothersome or persistent symptom.

If you miss a dose of metaxalone, take it as soon as you remember. If it is almost time for your next dose, take 1 dose as soon as you remember, another in 3 or 4 hours, and then go back to your regular schedule. Do not take a double dose.

Special Populations

Pregnancy/Breast-feeding
As with all drugs, pregnant women should not use metaxalone unless its benefits have been carefully weighed against its risks.

It is not known if metaxalone passes into breast milk. Nursing mothers who must take it should consider bottle-feeding.

Seniors
Seniors with reduced kidney or liver function may require less medicine.

Generic Name

Metformin (met-FOR-min)

Brand Name

Glucophage

Type of Drug

Biguanide antihyperglycemic.

Prescribed for

Type II diabetes.

General Information

Metformin lowers the amount of glucose produced by the liver, reduces the amount of glucose you absorb from food,

and helps cells use glucose. Generally, metformin is not prescribed until a sulfonylurea has been tried without a satisfactory response. If neither drug works alone, combining metformin with another antidiabetic drug may control your
diabetes. Metformin can also moderately lower blood fats.

Cautions and Warnings

Do not take metformin if you are **allergic** to it or have **heart
failure**. Metformin should not be taken by people with **kidney
disease**. If you are having surgery or an x-ray that requires
the injection of an iodine-based contrast material, you should
temporarily stop taking metformin because the combination
could result in acute kidney problems.

Metformin is related to an older antidiabetes drug that was
removed from the market because of the risk of a very rare
but serious complication known as **lactic acidosis**. Lactic acidosis is fatal about half of the time. It may also occur in association with a number of conditions, including diabetes mellitus. The risk of lactic acidosis increases with age, the
presence of heart failure, and worsening kidney function.
Regular monitoring of kidney function minimizes the risk of
developing lactic acidosis, as does using the minimum effective dosage of metformin. Metformin should not be taken by
people with acidosis, including those with diabetic ketoacidosis. Diabetic ketoacidosis should be treated with insulin.

People with **liver disease** should not take metformin
because of the increased risk of lactic acidosis.

People taking oral antidiabetes drugs are generally more
likely to develop **heart disease** compared with people taking
insulin or those treated by diet alone.

Possible Side Effects

People who have been stabilized on metformin should
not consider gastrointestinal (GI) symptoms to be related
to the drug unless other causes or lactic acidosis have
been excluded.

▼ Most common: diarrhea, nausea, vomiting, abdominal bloating, gas, and appetite loss. These symptoms
tend to occur when you first start taking metformin but
are generally transient and resolve on their own. Occasionally, temporary dosage reduction is useful.

Possible Side Effects *(continued)*

▼ Rare: An unpleasant or metallic taste in the mouth (this usually resolves on its own) and low blood levels of vitamin B_{12}. Blood levels of vitamin B_{12} should be periodically checked, or you may take a B_{12} supplement.

Drug Interactions

• Metformin may reduce the effect of glyburide (a sulfonylurea) but this interaction is highly variable from one person to another.

• Alcohol increases the risk of developing lactic acidosis while taking metformin.

• Metformin may interfere with amiloride, digoxin, morphine, procainamide, quinine, quinidine, ranitidine, triamterene, trimethoprim, and vancomycin. Careful monitoring is necessary.

• Cimetidine, nifedipine, and furosemide can cause a large increase in metformin blood levels and possible side effects. Furosemide levels are reduced by metformin.

Food Interactions

Metformin may be taken with food to reduce upset stomach.

Usual Dose

Adult: 500 mg twice daily, increased gradually to a maximum daily dosage of 2550 mg. Starting dosage can be 850 mg in the morning. Older adults should start with the regular dosage but generally are not given the maximum.

Child: not recommended.

Overdosage

Lactic acidosis has occurred in some cases. Take the victim to a hospital emergency room at once. ALWAYS bring the prescription bottle or container.

Special Information

Diet and exercise are the mainstays of diabetes treatment. Be sure to follow your doctor's directions in these areas while taking your medication.

Alcohol increases the risk of developing lactic acidosis while taking metformin.

Lactic acidosis is a medical emergency. Metformin treatment must be stopped immediately if you develop it. This disease is often subtle and is accompanied only by nonspecific symptoms such as feeling unwell, muscle aches, breathing difficulties, tiredness, and nonspecific upset stomach. Low body temperature, low blood pressure, and slow heartbeat can develop with more severe acidosis. Call your doctor at once if you develop these symptoms.

Stomach and intestinal side effects may be reduced by gradually increasing your dosage and by taking metformin with meals.

Metformin should be temporarily stopped if you have severe diarrhea or vomiting. However, do not stop taking your medication without first consulting your doctor.

If you forget a dose, take it as soon as you remember. If it is almost time for your next dose, skip the dose you forgot and continue with your regular schedule. Do not take a double dose.

Special Populations

Pregnancy/Breast-feeding
The safety of using metformin during pregnancy is not known. Pregnant women with diabetes should take insulin.

Metformin passes into breast milk. Nursing mothers who must take it should consider bottle-feeding.

Seniors
Seniors may require reduced dosage.

Generic Name

Methotrexate (meth-oe-TREK-sate) G

Brand Name

Rheumatrex

Type of Drug

Antimetabolite, antiarthritic, anti-inflammatory agent.

Prescribed for

Cancer chemotherapy; psoriasis; psoriatic arthritis; adult and juvenile rheumatoid arthritis; mycosis fungoides; Reiter's disease; and severe asthma.

General Information

Used effectively in cancer treatment since the late 1940s, methotrexate sodium is also prescribed for other conditions that respond to immune-system suppressants. Dosage varies widely depending on the disease being treated. Even relatively low dosages, such as those prescribed for rheumatoid arthritis, can be extremely toxic. Because of the risks associated with methotrexate, it should be used in noncancerous conditions only when the disease is severe or other treatments have failed. Methotrexate should be prescribed only by doctors who are familiar with the drug and its risks.

Cautions and Warnings

Methotrexate can trigger a unique and dangerous form of **lung disease** at any time during your course of therapy. It can occur at dosages as low as 7.5 mg per week—the antiarthritis dosage. Symptoms of this condition are cough, respiratory infection, difficulty breathing, abnormal chest x-ray, and low blood-oxygen levels. Report any changes in breathing or lung status to your doctor.

Methotrexate can cause severe **liver damage**; this usually occurs only after taking it over a long period. Changes in liver enzymes—as measured by a blood test—are common.

People with **kidney disease** should use this drug with caution and receive reduced dosage.

Methotrexate can severely lower **red- and white-blood-cell and blood-platelet counts**. Your doctor should periodically evaluate your kidney and liver function and blood components.

Methotrexate can cause severe **diarrhea, stomach irritation,** and **mouth or gum sores**. Death can result from intestinal perforation caused by methotrexate.

Aspirin and other nonsteroidal anti-inflammatory drugs (NSAIDs), as well as low-dose corticosteroid treatment, may be continued while you are taking methotrexate for rheumatoid arthritis, though an increase in drug toxicity is possible. In studies of methotrexate and rheumatoid arthritis, study participants also took NSAIDs.

Methotrexate has been studied as an **abortion drug** in combination with misoprostol (see "Misoprostol").

Possible Side Effects

▼ Most common: liver irritation, loss of kidney function, reduced blood platelet count, nausea, vomiting, diarrhea, stomach upset and irritation, itchiness, rash, hair loss, dizziness, and risk of infection.

▼ Less common: reduced red-blood-cell count, unusual sensitivity to the sun, acne, headache, drowsiness, blurred vision, respiratory infection and breathing problems, appetite loss, muscle aches, chest pain, coughing, painful urination, eye discomfort, nosebleeds, fever, infection, blood in the urine, sweating, ringing or buzzing in the ears, defective sperm production, reduced sperm count, menstrual dysfunction, vaginal discharge, convulsions, and slight paralysis.

Drug Interactions

• Fatal reactions have developed in 4 people taking methotrexate with an NSAID—3 with ketoprofen, 1 with naproxen. Do not combine methotrexate and an anti-inflammatory or antiarthritic drug—even over-the-counter drugs such as ibuprofen or naproxen—without your doctor's knowledge.

• Combining phenylbutazone and methotrexate increases the risk of severe white-blood-cell count reductions, but may be medically necessary. In these cases, your doctor should monitor your health for signs of drug toxicity (see "Cautions and Warnings").

• Aspirin and other salicylates, anticancer drugs, etretinate, procarbazine, probenecid, and sulfa drugs can increase the therapeutic and toxic effects of methotrexate.

• Folic acid counteracts the effects of methotrexate.

• Methotrexate may lower phenytoin blood levels, possibly reducing phenytoin's effectiveness.

Food Interactions

For optimal effectiveness, take this drug on an empty stomach at least 1 hour before or 2 hours after meals. It may be taken with food if it upsets your stomach.

Usual Dose

Cancer: Dosage varies. Some cancers can be treated with 10–30 mg a day, while others require hundreds or thousands of mg given intravenously.

Rheumatoid Arthritis: starting dosage—7.5 mg a week by mouth, either as a single dose or in 3 separate doses of 2.5 mg taken every 12 hours. Weekly dosage may be increased gradually up to 20 mg. Dosages above 20 mg a week are more likely to cause severe side effects.

Psoriasis: 2.5–6.5 mg a day by mouth, not to exceed 30 mg a week. In severe cases, dosage may be increased to 50 mg a week.

Overdosage

Overdose can be serious and life-threatening. Victims should be taken to a hospital emergency room immediately. A specific antidote to the effects of methotrexate—calcium leucovorin—is available in every hospital. ALWAYS bring the prescription bottle or container.

Special Information

If you vomit after taking a dose of methotrexate, do not take a replacement dose unless instructed to do so by your doctor.

Women taking this drug must use effective birth control.

To avoid birth defects, men should not attempt to father a child during treatment or for 3 months after treatment has been completed.

Call your doctor immediately if you develop diarrhea, fever or chills, skin reddening, mouth or lip sores, stomach pain, unusual bleeding or bruising, blurred vision, seizures, cough, or breathing difficulties. The following symptoms are less severe but should still be reported to your doctor: back pain, darkened urine, dizziness, drowsiness, headache, unusual tiredness or sickness, and yellowing of the skin or whites of the eyes.

If you forget a dose, skip it and continue with your regular schedule. Call your doctor at once. Do not take a double dose.

Special Populations

Pregnancy/Breast-feeding

Methotrexate can cause spontaneous abortion, stillbirth, and severe birth defects. Do not attempt to achieve pregnancy during methotrexate treatment or for at least 1 menstrual cycle after the treatment is completed. Use effective birth control while taking this drug. To avoid birth defects, men should not attempt to father a child during treatment or for 3 months after treatment has been completed. Methotrexate reduces sperm counts and may compromise sperm health.

This drug passes into breast milk. Nursing mothers who must take methotrexate should bottle-feed.

Seniors

Seniors may be more susceptible to side effects and obtain maximum benefit with smaller dosages.

Generic Name

Methyldopa (meth-ul-DOPE-uh) Ⓖ

Brand Name

Aldomet

Type of Drug

Antihypertensive.

Prescribed for

Hypertension (high blood pressure).

General Information

How methyldopa works is not well understood. It may lower blood pressure by stimulating receptors in the central nervous system and by inhibiting or reducing levels of important pressure-regulating hormones such as norepinephrine and serotonin. It takes about 2 days for methyldopa to reach its maximal antihypertensive (blood-pressure-lowering) effect. It is usually prescribed with one or more other antihypertensive drugs or a diuretic.

Cautions and Warnings

Do not take methyldopa if you have had a **reaction** to it. You should not take methyldopa if you have **hepatitis** or active **cirrhosis of the liver**. People taking this drug may develop a fever with **changes in liver function** within the first 3 weeks of treatment. Some people develop **jaundice** (symptoms include yellowing of the skin or whites of the eyes) during the first 2 or 3 months of treatment. Your doctor should periodically evaluate your liver function during the first 3 months of methyldopa treatment, or if you develop an unexplained fever.

Methyldopa should be used with caution in people with severe **kidney disease,** who may need reduced dosage.

Possible Side Effects

Most people have little trouble with methyldopa, but it can cause temporary sedation in the first few weeks of treatment or when the dose is increased. Passing headache and weakness are other possible early side effects.

▼ Less common: dizziness; light-headedness; tingling in the extremities; muscle spasms or weakness; decreased mental acuity; psychological disturbances including nightmares, mild psychosis, and depression; changes in heart rate; increased angina pain; water retention, resulting in weight gain; dizziness when rising suddenly from a sitting or lying position; nausea; vomiting; constipation; diarrhea; mild dry mouth; sore or black tongue; stuffy nose; male breast enlargement or pain; lactation in females; impotence or decreased sex drive in males; mild arthritis symptoms; and skin reactions.

▼ Rare: Methyldopa may affect white blood cells or blood platelets. It may also cause involuntary jerky movements, twitching, restlessness, and slow, continuous, wormlike movements of the fingers, toes, hands, or other body parts.

Drug Interactions

• Methyldopa increases the effect of other blood-pressure-lowering drugs. This is a desirable interaction for people with hypertension. However, the combination of methyldopa and propranolol or nadolol—two beta blockers often prescribed for hypertension—has, rarely, caused an increase in blood pressure.

• Avoid over-the-counter (OTC) cough, cold, and allergy products containing stimulant drugs that may aggravate your hypertension.

• Methyldopa may increase the blood-sugar-lowering effect of tolbutamide or other sulfonylurea-type oral antidiabetic drugs.

• If methyldopa is combined with phenoxybenzamine, urinary incontinence (inability to control the bladder) may result.

• The effect of methyldopa may be reduced by barbiturates and tricyclic antidepressants.

• The combination of methyldopa and lithium may cause symptoms of lithium overdose—upset stomach, frequent urination, muscle weakness, tiredness, and tremors—even though blood levels of lithium have not changed.

• Methyldopa in combination with haloperidol may produce irritability, aggressiveness, assaultive behavior, or other psychiatric symptoms.

• Combining methyldopa and levodopa may increase the effects of both drugs.

• Combining methyldopa and a monoamine oxidase inhibitor (MAOI) antidepressant may cause excessive stimulation.

• Combining methyldopa with stimulants or a phenothiazine-type drug may lead to a serious increase in blood pressure.

Food Interactions

Methyldopa is best taken on an empty stomach, but you may take it with food if it upsets your stomach.

Usual Dose

Adult: starting dosage—250-mg tablet 2–3 times a day for the first 2 days. Dosage may then be increased until lower blood pressure is achieved. Maintenance dose—500–3000 mg a day in 2–4 divided doses, depending on individual need. Seniors may require lower dosages.

Child: 5 mg per lb. of body weight a day in 2–4 divided doses, depending on individual need. Do not exceed 30 mg per lb. of body weight a day, or 3000 mg a day.

Overdosage

Symptoms include sedation, very low blood pressure, weakness, dizziness, light-headedness, fainting, slow heartbeat, constipation, abdominal gas or bulging, nausea, vomiting, and coma. Overdose victims should be made to vomit if they are still conscious by using ipecac syrup—available at any pharmacy—and then taken to a hospital emergency room. If some time has passed since the overdose was taken, take the victim directly to an emergency room. ALWAYS bring the prescription bottle or container.

Special Information

Take methyldopa exactly as prescribed to maintain maximum control of your hypertension. Do not stop taking this drug unless you are told to do so by your doctor.

A mild sedative effect is to be expected from methyldopa and will resolve within several days.

Your urine may darken if left exposed to air. This is normal and not a cause for alarm.

Call your doctor if you develop fever, prolonged general tiredness, or dizziness. If you develop involuntary muscle movements, fever, or jaundice, stop taking the drug and contact your doctor immediately. If these reactions are due to methyldopa, your temperature or liver abnormalities will begin to normalize as soon as you stop taking it.

If you forget a dose, take it as soon as you remember. If it is almost time for your next dose, skip the one you forgot and continue with your regular schedule. Do not take a double dose.

Special Populations

Pregnancy/Breast-feeding
Methyldopa crosses into the fetal circulation. When this drug is considered crucial by your doctor, its potential benefits must be carefully weighed against its risks.

Small amounts of methyldopa pass into breast milk. Nursing mothers who must take this drug should consider bottle-feeding.

Seniors
Seniors are more sensitive to the sedating and blood-pressure-lowering effects of methyldopa and may experience dizziness or fainting. Older adults should receive reduced dosage.

Generic Name

Methylphenidate (meth-ul-FEN-ih-date) Ⓖ

Brand Names

Ritalin   Ritalin-SR

Type of Drug

Mild central-nervous-system stimulant.

Prescribed for

Attention-deficit hyperactivity disorder (ADHD); also prescribed for psychological, educational, or social disorders and for narcolepsy and mild depression in the elderly. Methylphenidate is also used in cancer treatment and stroke recovery and for treating hiccups after anesthesia.

General Information

Methylphenidate hydrochloride is prescribed for the treatment of ADHD in children. It should be used only after conducting a complete evaluation of the child. Frequency and severity of symptoms and their appropriateness for the age of the child—not solely the presence of certain behavioral characteristics—determine whether drug therapy is required. Many experts believe that methylphenidate offers only a temporary solution because it does not permanently change behavioral patterns. Psychological measures must also be taken to ensure successful treatment in the long term.

Cautions and Warnings

Chronic or abusive use of methylphenidate can lead to drug dependence or **addiction**. This drug can also cause severe psychotic episodes.

Take methylphenidate with caution if you have **glaucoma or other visual problems, high blood pressure,** a **seizure** disorder, if you are extremely **tense or agitated,** or if you are **allergic** to this drug.

Stimulants like methylphenidate are not effective in children whose symptoms are related to environmental factors or to primary psychiatric conditions, including psychosis. Methylphenidate should not be used to treat a primary stress reaction.

Possible Side Effects

Adults

▼ Most common: nervousness and inability to sleep, which doctors generally control by reducing or eliminating the afternoon or evening dose.

▼ Rare: rash, itching, fever, symptoms resembling those of arthritis, appetite loss, nausea, dizziness, abnormal heart rhythm, headache, drowsiness, changes in blood pressure or pulse, chest pain, stomach pain, psychotic reactions, changes in blood components, and loss of some scalp hair.

Children

▼ Most common: appetite loss; stomach pain; weight loss, especially during prolonged therapy; sleeping difficulties; and abnormal heart rhythm.

Drug Interactions

• Methylphenidate reduces the effectiveness of guanethidine (an antihypertensive drug).

• Monoamine oxidase inhibitors (MAOIs) may significantly increase the effect of methylphenidate, which may lead to adverse reactions.

• Methylphenidate may increase tricyclic antidepressant blood levels and the risk of side effects.

• If you take methylphenidate regularly, avoid alcohol: This combination increases drowsiness.

Food Interactions

This medication is best taken 30 to 45 minutes before meals.

Usual Dose

Adult: Doses range from 20–30 mg a day but can be as high as 60 mg. The drug is taken 2–3 times a day.

Child (age 6 and over): starting dosage—5 mg before breakfast and lunch. Increase by 5–10 mg each week as required, not to exceed 60 mg a day.

SR-tablets are designed to last for 8 hours and may be used in place of more frequent doses during the same period of time.

Overdosage

Symptoms include vomiting, agitation, uncontrollable twitching of the muscles, convulsions followed by coma, euphoria (feeling "high"), confusion, hallucinations, delirium, sweating, flushing, headache, high fever, abnormal heart rate, high blood pressure, and dryness of the mouth and nose. Take the victim to a hospital emergency room immediately. ALWAYS bring the prescription bottle or container.

Special Information

Methylphenidate can mask the signs of temporary drowsiness or fatigue: Be careful when driving or doing any task that requires concentration. Take your last daily dose no later than 6 p.m. to avoid sleeping difficulties.

Call your doctor if you develop any persistent or bothersome side effect. Do not increase your dosage without your doctor's knowledge.

SR-tablets must be swallowed whole, never crushed or chewed.

If you miss a dose, take it as soon as possible. Space the remaining daily dosage evenly throughout the day. Go back to your regular schedule the next day.

Special Populations

Pregnancy/Breast-feeding

Methylphenidate crosses into the fetal circulation. When this drug is considered crucial by your doctor, its potential benefits must be carefully weighed against its risks.

Small amounts of methylphenidate may pass into breast milk. Nursing mothers who must take this drug should consider bottle-feeding.

Seniors

Seniors may take this drug without special restriction.

Generic Name

Methysergide (meth-ih-SER-jide)

Brand Name

Sansert

Type of Drug

Migraine preventive.

Prescribed for

Migraine.

General Information

Methysergide maleate can prevent migraine attacks or reduce their number and intensity in people who suffer at least 1 migraine a week or whose headaches are severe. Methysergide is derived from ergot, a natural plant fungus. Exactly how it works is unknown, though it may achieve its effects by blocking the actions of the hormone serotonin. Methysergide must be taken for 1 to 2 days before you notice its effects, which persist for 1 to 2 days after you stop taking it.

Cautions and Warnings

This drug should be used only by people whose headaches are severe and uncontrollable and who are under close medical supervision.

Do not take this drug if you are **sensitive** or **allergic** to it or any other ergot-derived medication. Use methysergide with caution if you have severe **hardening of the arteries,** very **high blood pressure, angina, or other signs of coronary artery disease,** a serious **infection or illness, phlebitis,** or **heart valve, vascular (blood vessel), pulmonary, liver, kidney, or connective tissue disease (such as lupus).**

People taking methysergide for long periods of time may develop **thickening of tissues surrounding the lung,** making it more difficult to breathe; **thickening of the heart valves,** which may interfere with heart function; and **fibrous tissues in the abdomen**. To prevent these effects, you should stop taking this drug for 3 to 4 consecutive weeks every 6 months during therapy with methysergide.

Methysergide tablets contain **tartrazine** dye, which should be avoided by people with asthma or an aspirin or tartrazine allergy. Tartrazine-free methysergide is available.

Possible Side Effects

Side effects are experienced by 30% to 50% of people.

Possible Side Effects *(continued)*

▼ Most common: nausea, vomiting, constipation, diarrhea, heartburn, and abdominal pain usually develop early in drug treatment; they can be avoided by increasing dosage gradually and taking the drug with food.

▼ Less common: sleeplessness, drowsiness, mild euphoria (feeling "high"), light-headedness, dizziness, weakness, feelings of disassociation or hallucinations, flushing, raised red spots, temporary hair loss, swelling, changes in blood components, muscle and joint aches, and weight gain.

▼ Rare: lung fibrosis (symptoms include chest or abdominal pain and cold, numb, or painful hands or feet with possible tingling and loss of pulse in the arms or legs), changes in vision, clumsiness, rash, and depression.

Drug Interactions

• Alcohol, tranquilizers, and other nervous-system depressants increase the depressant effects of this drug.

• Combining beta blockers and methysergide may cause reduced blood flow to the hands and feet, leading to cold hands or feet and possibly gangrene.

Food Interactions

Take this drug with food or milk to avoid upset stomach.

Usual Dose

4–8 mg daily, taken with food.

Overdosage

Symptoms include cold and pale hands or feet, severe dizziness, excitement, and convulsions. Take the victim to a hospital emergency room. ALWAYS bring the prescription bottle or container.

Special Information

Do not take methysergide for more than 6 months at a time without a 3- to 4-week drug-free period. Do not stop taking it without your doctor's knowledge. Withdrawal headaches can occur if the drug is stopped suddenly. It should be gradually discontinued over 2 to 3 weeks.

If you do not show improvement within the first 3 weeks of use, it is unlikely that the drug will be effective for you.

Heavy smokers experience blood-vessel constriction while taking methysergide, leading to cold hands or feet, chest and abdominal pain, itching, numbness, and tingling of the toes, fingers, or face. Contact your doctor if any of these symptoms develops, especially if you do not smoke.

Contact your doctor if you experience changes in vision, clumsiness, stimulation, swelling, changes in heart rate, fever, chills, cough, hoarseness, lower back or side pain, urinary difficulties, depression, rash, redness or darkening of the face, red spots, leg cramps, appetite loss, breathing difficulties, or swelling of the hands, legs, ankles, or feet.

Call your doctor if any infection develops; infections can increase your sensitivity to the effects of methysergide.

This drug can cause tiredness, dizziness, or light-headedness. Be careful when driving or doing any task that requires concentration.

Exposure to extremely cold weather may worsen feelings of coldness, tingling, or pain caused by methysergide. Protect yourself from cold winter weather.

If you take methysergide on a regular schedule and forget a dose, take it as soon as you remember. If you take it 2 times a day and it is almost time for your next dose, take 1 dose as soon as you remember and another in 5 or 6 hours, then go back to your regular schedule. If you take it 3 times a day and it is almost time for your next dose, take 1 dose as soon as you remember and another in 3 or 4 hours, then go back to your regular schedule. Never take a double dose.

Special Populations

Pregnancy/Breast-feeding
Methysergide must not be taken by pregnant women because the drug can cause miscarriage.

Methysergide passes into breast milk. It may cause vomiting, diarrhea, or seizures in an infant. Nursing mothers who must take it should bottle-feed.

Seniors
Seniors may require reduced dosage and are more likely to develop hypothermia (low body temperature) and other side effects.

Generic Name

Metoclopramide (met-oe-KLOE-pruh-mide) G

Brand Names

Clopra   Reclomide
Maxolon   Reglan*
Octamide

Some products in this brand-name group are alcohol- or sugar- free. Consult your pharmacist.

Type of Drug

Antiemetic and gastrointestinal (GI) stimulant.

Prescribed for

Nausea and vomiting; also prescribed for diabetic gastroparesis (stomach paralysis associated with diabetes), gastroesophageal reflux disease (GERD), stomach ulcer, anorexia nervosa, and bleeding from blood vessels in the esophagus—often associated with severe liver disease. It also facilitates diagnostic x-ray procedures and improves the absorption of anti-migraine medication and narcotic pain relievers. Nursing mothers are occasionally given metoclopramide to increase milk production.

General Information

Metoclopramide stimulates movement of the upper GI tract without producing excess stomach acids or other secretions. Doctors believe that it prevents nausea and vomiting primarily by affecting dopamine receptors in the brain. Metoclopramide also affects the secretion of a variety of hormones and may improve the absorption of other drugs into the bloodstream.

Cautions and Warnings

People with **high blood pressure, Parkinson's disease, asthma, liver or kidney failure,** or **seizure disorders** should use metoclopramide with caution. Do not take this drug if you are **allergic** to it. Metoclopramide should not be used if you have a **bleeding ulcer** or any condition that makes stimulation of the GI tract dangerous.

Mild to severe **depression** has occurred with metoclopramide.

Uncontrollable motions similar to those associated with Parkinson's disease have developed as a side effect of this drug. These generally occur within 6 months after starting metoclopramide and subside within 2 to 3 months.

This drug may cause **extrapyramidal side effects** similar to those associated with phenothiazine drugs. These effects, which occur in 0.2% of the people taking the drug, include restlessness and involuntary movements of the arms and legs, face, tongue, lips, and other parts of the body. Do not combine metoclopramide with a phenothiazine drug because this may increase the risk of extrapyramidal effects.

Women taking this drug develop chronic elevations of the hormone prolactin. About 33% of breast tumors are prolactin-dependent, a factor that you should consider before taking metoclopramide.

Possible Side Effects

Mild side effects occur in 20% to 30% of people. Side effects increase with dosage or prolonged use.

▼ Most common: restlessness, drowsiness, fatigue, sleeplessness, dizziness, anxiety, loss of muscle control, headache, muscle spasm, confusion, severe depression, convulsions, and hallucinations.

▼ Less common: rash, diarrhea, blood-pressure changes, abnormal heart rhythms, slow heartbeat, oozing from the nipples, tender nipples, loss of regular menstrual periods, breast swelling and tenderness, impotence, reduced white-blood-cell counts, frequent urination, loss of urinary control, visual disturbances, and worsening of bronchial spasm.

▼ Rare: People taking this drug may develop a group of possibly fatal symptoms collectively called neuroleptic malignant syndrome. These symptoms include very high fever, semi-consciousness, rigid muscles, flushing of the face and upper body, and liver toxicity after high doses.

Drug Interactions

• Narcotics and anticholinergic drugs interfere with metoclopramide's effect on stomach acid.

• Metoclopramide may increase the effects of alcohol and cyclosporine.

• Metoclopramide may increase the sedative effects of nervous-system depressants including tranquilizers and sleeping pills.

• Metoclopramide and levodopa interfere with each other.

• Metoclopramide may reduce the effects of digitalis drugs and cimetidine.

• Combining metoclopramide and a monoamine oxidase inhibitor (MAOI) antidepressant may cause very high blood pressure.

Food Interactions

Take this drug 30 minutes before meals and at bedtime.

Usual Dose

Adult and Child (age 15 and over): 5–15 mg before meals and at bedtime. Single doses of 10–20 mg are used before x-ray diagnostic procedures.

Senior: starting dosage—5 mg.

Child (age 6–14): ¼–½ the adult dosage.

Child (under age 6): 0.05 mg per lb. of body weight per dose.

Overdosage

Symptoms of overdose include drowsiness, disorientation, restlessness, or uncontrollable muscle movement. These usually disappear within 24 hours after the drug has been stopped. Anticholinergic drugs help control overdose symptoms. Call your local poison control center or a hospital emergency room for more information.

Special Information

Call your doctor if you develop chills; fever; sore throat; dizziness; severe or persistent headache; feeling unwell; rapid or irregular heartbeat; difficulty speaking or swallowing; loss of balance; stiffness of the arms or legs; a shuffling walk; a mask-like face; lip-smacking or puckering; puffing of the cheeks; rapid, worm-like tongue movement; uncontrollable chewing movement; uncontrolled arm and leg movement; or any persistent or intolerable side effect.

Metoclopramide may cause dizziness, confusion, and drowsiness. Be careful when driving or doing any task that requires concentration. Avoid alcohol and be cautious about taking tranquilizers or sleeping pills.

If you forget a dose, take it as soon as you remember. If it is almost time for your next dose, skip the dose you forgot and continue with your regular schedule. Do not take a double dose.

Special Populations

Pregnancy/Breast-feeding

Metoclopramide enters the fetal circulation. When this drug is considered crucial by your doctor, its potential benefits must be carefully weighed against its risks.

This drug passes into breast milk. Nursing mothers occasionally receive metoclopramide to increase milk production. There appears to be no risk for the infant whose nursing mother takes 45 mg or less a day. Always consider possible effects on the nursing infant if breast-feeding while taking this drug.

Seniors

Seniors, especially women, are more sensitive to side effects (see "Cautions and Warnings").

Generic Name

Metoprolol (meh-TOPE-roe-lol) Ⓖ

Brand Names

Lopressor   Toprol XL

The information in this profile also applies to the following drug:

Generic Ingredient: Penbutolol
Levatol

Type of Drug

Beta-adrenergic blocking agent.

Prescribed for

High blood pressure, angina pectoris, abnormal heart rhythms, prevention of second heart attack, migraine, tremors, aggressive behavior, side effects of antipsychotic drugs, improving cognitive performance, congestive heart failure, and bleeding from the esophagus.

General Information

Metoprolol is one of 15 beta-adrenergic-blocking drugs, or beta blockers, that interfere with the action of a specific part of the nervous system. Beta receptors are found all over the body and affect many body functions. Each beta blocker has particular characteristics that make it more suitable for certain conditions or people. Metoprolol is available in a sustained-release formulation, taken only once a day, that maintains a steady blood level of the drug for a full 24 hours.

Cautions and Warnings

You should be cautious about taking metoprolol if you have **asthma**, a **very slow heart rate,** or **heart block** (disruption of the electrical impulses that control heart rate) because the drug may aggravate these conditions.

People with **angina** who take metoprolol for high blood pressure risk aggravating their angina if they suddenly stop taking the drug. These people should have their drug dosage reduced gradually over 1 to 2 weeks.

Metoprolol should be used with caution if you have **liver or kidney disease** because your ability to eliminate the drug from your body may be impaired.

Metoprolol reduces the amount of blood pumped by the heart with each beat. This reduction in blood flow may aggravate the condition of people with **poor circulation or circulatory disease**.

If you are undergoing **major surgery,** your doctor may want you to stop taking metoprolol at least 2 days before.

Possible Side Effects

Metoprolol side effects are relatively uncommon and usually mild.

▼ Most common: impotence.

▼ Less common: unusual tiredness or weakness, slow heartbeat, heart failure, dizziness, breathing difficulties, bronchospasm, depression, confusion, anxiety, nervousness, sleeplessness, disorientation, short-term memory

Possible Side Effects *(continued)*

loss, emotional instability, cold hands and feet, constipation, diarrhea, nausea, vomiting, upset stomach, increased sweating, urinary difficulties, cramps, blurred vision, rash, hair loss, stuffy nose, facial swelling, aggravation of lupus erythematosus, itching, chest pain, back or joint pain, colitis, drug allergy (symptoms include fever and sore throat), and liver toxicity.

Drug Interactions

• Metoprolol may interact with surgical anesthetics to increase the risk of heart problems during surgery. Some anesthesiologists recommend gradually stopping the drug by 2 days before surgery.

• Metoprolol may interfere with the normal signs of low blood sugar and with the action of oral antidiabetes medications.

• Metoprolol increases the blood-pressure-lowering effect of other blood-pressure-reducing agents, including clonidine, guanabenz, and reserpine, as well as calcium-channel blockers such as nifedipine.

• Aspirin-containing drugs, indomethacin, sulfinpyrazone, and estrogen drugs may interfere with the blood-pressure-lowering effect of metoprolol.

• Cocaine may reduce the effectiveness of all beta blockers.

• Metoprolol may worsen the problem of cold hands and feet associated with taking ergot alkaloids, which are used to treat migraine. Gangrene is a possibility in people taking both an ergot and metoprolol.

• The effect of benzodiazepine antianxiety drugs may be increased by metoprolol.

• Metoprolol will counteract thyroid hormone replacements.

• Calcium channel blockers, flecainide, hydralazine, oral contraceptives, propafenone, haloperidol, phenothiazine tranquilizers (molindone and others) quinolone antibacterials, and quinidine may increase the amount of metoprolol in the bloodstream and lead to increased metoprolol effects.

• Metoprolol should not be taken within 2 weeks of taking a monoamine oxidase inhibitor (MAOI) antidepressant.

• Cimetidine increases the amount of metoprolol absorbed into the bloodstream from oral tablets.

• Metoprolol may interfere with the effectiveness of some asthma medications, including theophylline and aminophylline, and especially ephedrine and isoproterenol.

• Combining metoprolol with phenytoin or digitalis drugs may result in excessive slowing of the heart, possibly causing heart block.

• If you stop smoking while taking metoprolol, your dose may have to be reduced because your liver will break down the drug more slowly afterward.

Food Interactions

Sustained-release metoprolol—Toprol XL—may be taken with food if it upsets your stomach. Because food increases the amount of short-acting metoprolol—Lopressor—absorbed into the blood, take the short-acting form without food.

Usual Dose

Metoprolol: 100–450 mg a day; dosage must be tailored to your specific needs.

Penbutolol: 20 mg once a day. Seniors may require more or less medication and must be carefully monitored by their doctors. People with liver problems may require lower dosage.

Overdosage

Symptoms include changes in heartbeat—unusually slow, unusually fast, or irregular—severe dizziness or fainting, breathing difficulties, bluish-colored fingernails or palms, and seizures. The victim should be taken to a hospital emergency room. ALWAYS bring the prescription bottle or container.

Special Information

Metoprolol should be taken continuously. When ending metoprolol treatments, dosage should be lowered gradually over a period of about 2 weeks. Do not stop taking this drug unless directed to do so by your doctor: Abrupt withdrawal may cause chest pain, breathing difficulties, increased sweating, and unusually fast or irregular heartbeat.

Call your doctor at once if you develop back or joint pain, breathing difficulties, cold hands or feet, depression, rash, or changes in heartbeat. This drug may produce an undesirable lowering of blood pressure, leading to dizziness or fainting; call your doctor if this happens to you. Call your doctor if you experience persistent or bothersome nausea or vomiting, upset stomach, diarrhea, constipation, impotence, headache, itching, anxiety, nightmares or vivid dreams, trouble sleeping, stuffy nose, frequent urination, unusual tiredness, or weakness.

Metoprolol can cause drowsiness, light-headedness, dizziness, or blurred vision. Be careful when driving or performing complex tasks.

It is best to take metoprolol at the same time each day. If you forget a dose, take it as soon as you remember. If you take metoprolol once a day and it is within 8 hours of your next dose, skip the dose you forgot and continue with your regular schedule. If you take it twice a day and it is within 4 hours of your next dose, skip the dose you forgot and continue with your regular schedule. Never take a double dose.

Special Populations

Pregnancy/Breast-feeding

Infants born to women who took a beta blocker while pregnant had lower birth weights, low blood pressure, and reduced heart rates. Metoprolol should be avoided by women who are or might be pregnant.

Small amounts of metoprolol pass into breast milk. Nursing mothers taking metoprolol should bottle-feed.

Seniors

Seniors require less of the drug to achieve results. Seniors taking metoprolol may be more likely to suffer from cold hands and feet, reduced body temperature, chest pain, general feelings of ill health, sudden breathing difficulties, increased sweating, or changes in heartbeat.

Generic Name

Metronidazole (meh-troe-NYE-duh-zole) Ⓖ

Brand Names

Flagyl
MetroCream
MetroGel

Noritate
Protostat

Type of Drug

Amoebicide and antibiotic.

Prescribed for

Acute amoebic dysentery and infections of the vagina, bone, brain, nervous system, urinary tract, abdomen, and skin; also prescribed for pneumonia, ulcers caused by *Helicobacter pylori,* inflammatory bowel disease, colitis caused by other antibiotics, periodontal (gum) infection, and complications of severe liver disease. The gel may be used to treat acne, severe skin ulcers, and inflammation of the skin around the mouth. Metronidazole may be given by intravenous injection to prevent infectious complications of bowel surgery.

General Information

Metronidazole is effective against infections caused by a variety of fungi and some bacteria. Metronidazole kills these microorganisms by disrupting their DNA after they enter body cells. Metronidazole may be prescribed for symptomless diseases when the doctor feels that an underlying infection may be involved. For example, asymptomatic women may be treated with this drug when vaginal examination shows evidence of *Trichomonas.* Because vaginal trichomonal infection is a sexually transmitted disease, asymptomatic sexual partners should also be treated if the organism has been found in the woman's genital tract.

Cautions and Warnings

You should not use this drug if you have a history of **blood disease** or are **sensitive** or **allergic** to metronidazole.

People taking this medication have experienced **seizures** and **numbness or tingling in the hands or feet**. This effect is rare with low dosages but may be more common in people taking larger dosages for long periods, such as in Crohn's disease. If this occurs, stop taking the drug and call your doctor at once. Metronidazole should be taken with caution if you have active **nervous system disease,** including **epilepsy,** or severe **liver problems**.

Possible Side Effects

▼ Most common: gastrointestinal (GI) symptoms, including nausea that is sometimes accompanied by headache, dizziness, appetite loss, vomiting, diarrhea, upset stomach, abdominal cramping, and constipation. A sharp, unpleasant metallic taste is also associated with the use of this drug.

▼ Less common: numbness or tingling in the extremities, joint pain, confusion, irritability, depression, difficulty sleeping, and weakness. Itching and a sensation of pelvic pressure also have been reported.

▼ Rare: clumsiness or poor coordination, fever, increased urination, seizure, incontinence, and reduced sex drive.

Drug Interactions

• Avoid alcohol: Interaction with metronidazole may cause abdominal cramps, nausea, vomiting, headaches, and flushing. Modification of the taste of alcohol has also been reported. Metronidazole should not be used if you are taking disulfiram (a drug used to maintain alcohol abstinence) because the combination may cause confusion and psychotic reactions.

• Dosages of oral anticoagulants (blood-thinners) such as warfarin must be reduced because metronidazole increases their effect.

• Metronidazole increases lithium blood levels, effects, and side effects.

• Cimetidine may increase metronidazole blood levels. Metronidazole dosage may have to be reduced.

• Phenobarbital and other barbiturates may reduce metronidazole's effectiveness.

• Drugs that cause nervous system toxicity—such as mexiletine, ethambutol, isoniazid, lindane, lincomycin, lithium, pemoline, quinacrine, and long-term high-dose pyridoxine (vitamin B_6) should not be taken with metronidazole because nervous-system side effects may be increased.

• Metronidazole may increase blood levels of phenytoin and the risk of phenytoin side effects. Your doctor may need to adjust your phenytoin dosage.

Food Interactions

Take this drug with food to avoid upset stomach.

Usual Dose

Adult: amoebic dysentery—500–750 mg 3 times a day for 5–10 days. Trichomonal infection—250 mg 3 times a day for 7 days; or 2 g in 1 dose. Reduced dosage may be necessary for seniors.

Child: amoebic dysentery—16–23 mg per lb. of body weight daily, divided in 3 equal doses for 10 days.

Overdosage

Symptoms include nausea, vomiting, clumsiness, unsteadiness, seizures, and pain or tingling in the hands or feet. Call your local poison control center or a hospital emergency room for more information. If you seek treatment, ALWAYS bring the prescription bottle or container.

Special Information

Call your doctor if you become dizzy or light-headed while taking this drug, or if you develop numbness, tingling, pain, or weakness in your hands or feet; seizures; clumsiness or unsteadiness; mood changes; unusual vaginal irritation, discharge, or dryness; rash, hives, or itching; severe pain of the back or abdomen accompanied by vomiting, appetite loss, or nausea; or any bothersome or persistent side effect.

Metronidazole may cause darkening of your urine; this is probably not important, but inform your doctor if it happens.

Follow your doctor's dosage instructions exactly. Complete the full course of drug therapy.

Metronidazole may cause dry mouth, which usually can be relieved with ice, hard candy, or gum. Call your doctor or dentist if dry mouth persists for more than 2 weeks.

If you forget a dose, take it as soon as you remember. If it is almost time for your next dose, skip the dose you forgot and continue with your regular schedule. Do not take a double dose.

Special Populations

Pregnancy/Breast-feeding

Metronidazole passes into the fetal circulation. This drug should not be taken during the first 3 months of pregnancy and should be used with caution during the last 6 months.

Metronidazole passes into breast milk. Nursing mothers who must take it should bottle-feed. After you have finished metronidazole treatment, express any milk produced while you were taking the drug and discard it along with any pumped breast milk you might have saved. Nursing can be resumed 1 or 2 days after stopping metronidazole.

Seniors
Seniors, particularly those with advanced liver disease, are more sensitive to the effects of this drug and may require lower dosages.

Miacalcin see *Calcitonin*, page 148

Generic Name

Miconazole (mye-KON-uh-zole) Ⓖ

Brand Name
Monistat

The information in this profile also applies to the following drugs:

Generic Ingredient: Tioconazole
Vagistat-1

Generic Ingredient: Butoconazole
Femstat

Type of Drug
Antifungal.

Prescribed for
Fungal infections of the vagina, skin, and blood.

General Information
Miconazole nitrate is used to treat a variety of fungal infections. Monistat-Derm Cream is applied directly to the skin to

treat common fungal infections of the skin, including ring-worm, athlete's foot, and jock itch. Monistat 3 is used to treat vaginal infections. Hospitalized patients may receive this drug by intravenous injection to ward off serious fungal infections. When used for vaginal or topical infections, it is also effective against several nonfungal organisms.

Cautions and Warnings

Do not use miconazole if you are **allergic** to it. Proper diagnosis is essential for effective treatment. Do not use this product without first consulting your doctor.

Possible Side Effects

Intravenous Injection
▼ Common: vein irritation, itching, rash, nausea, vomiting, fever, drowsiness, diarrhea, loss of appetite, and flushing.

Vaginal Administration
▼ Common: itching, burning, and irritation.
▼ Less common: pelvic cramps, hives, rash, and headache.

Topical Application
▼ Less common: skin irritation or burning.

Food and Drug Interactions

None known.

Usual Dose

Vaginal Suppositories and Cream: 1 applicatorful or suppository into the vagina at bedtime for 3–7 days.

Topical Cream, Lotions, and Powder: Apply to affected areas 2 times a day for up to 1 month.

Overdosage

Accidental ingestion may cause upset stomach. Call your local poison control center or hospital emergency room for more information.

Special Information

When using the vaginal cream, insert the whole applicator of cream high into the vagina and be sure to complete the full course of treatment. Call your doctor if you develop burning or itching.

If you forget to administer a dose of miconazole, do so as soon as you remember. If it is almost time for your next dose, skip the dose you forgot and continue with your regular schedule. Do not take a double dose.

Special Populations

Pregnancy/Breast-feeding

Pregnant women should avoid using vaginal creams during pregnancy. It may be used if needed, but usage should begin during the first 3 months, and continue during the next 6 months only if absolutely necessary. Your doctor may want you to avoid using a vaginal applicator during pregnancy. Vaginal suppositories may be inserted by hand instead.

Miconazole has not been shown to cause problems in breast-fed infants.

Seniors

Seniors may take this medication without special restriction.

Generic Name

Midodrine (MYE-doe-dreen)

Brand Name

ProAmatine

Type of Drug

Alpha stimulant.

Prescribed for

Dizziness or fainting when rising from a sitting position. Midodrine is also used for poor urinary control.

General Information

Midodrine is recommended only if other treatments for dizziness or fainting have failed and symptoms are interfering with your daily routine. It stimulates nerve endings in small veins and arteries, "tightening" them slightly to raise blood pressure. This helps control dizziness and fainting caused by poor blood flow to the brain. Systolic blood pressure increases by 15 to 30 points 1 hour after taking 10 mg of midodrine. The effect lasts about 2 to 3 hours.

Cautions and Warnings

Do not take this drug if you **retain urine** or have severe **heart disease, kidney disease, diabetes, pheochromocytoma** (adrenal gland tumor), a severely **overactive thyroid gland, visual problems,** or excessive and persistent **high blood pressure** when lying down.

High blood pressure—especially when lying down—can be the most serious side effect of midodrine. This problem may be prevented by not completely reclining, or raising the head of your bed, when you sleep.

People with **kidney disease** require reduced dosage. People with **liver disease** should be cautious about using midodrine because it may be partially broken down in the liver. Your doctor should evaluate your kidney and liver function periodically.

Heart rate may decrease while taking midodrine.

Possible Side Effects

▼ Most common: tingling in the hands or feet, pain, itching, goosebumps, painful urination, high blood pressure when lying down, and chills.

▼ Less common: headache, sensation of pressure in the head, facial flushing, confusion, abnormal thinking, dry mouth, nervousness, anxiety, and rash.

▼ Rare: visual problems, dizziness, sensitive skin, sleeplessness, tiredness, canker sores, dry skin, urinary difficulties, weakness, backache, nausea, upset stomach, gas, heartburn, and leg cramps.

Drug Interactions

• Midodrine increases the effects of digoxin or digitoxin and similar drugs, psychoactive medications, beta blockers, and other stimulants. Be very cautious when combining any of these drugs and midodrine.

• People taking fludrocortisone must have their dosage reduced or salt intake lowered before starting midodrine.

• Alpha blockers such as prazosin, terazosin, and doxazosin can block midodrine's effects.

Food Interactions

None known.

Usual Dose

Dizziness or Fainting
   Adult: 10 mg 3 times a day. People with kidney failure should start with 2.5 mg.
   Child: not recommended.

Urinary Incontinence
   Adult: 2.5–5 mg 2–3 times a day.
   Child: not recommended.

Overdosage

Symptoms include high blood pressure, goosebumps, feeling cold, and difficulty urinating. Take the victim to a hospital emergency room. ALWAYS bring the prescription bottle or container.

Special Information

Your doctor may suggest that you take the medication about every 4 hours: when you get up, around noon, and in the late afternoon—no later than 6 p.m. The drug may also be taken every 3 hours to control symptoms. Do not take midodrine after dinner or less than 4 hours before you go to bed.

Continue taking midodrine only if it works for you. If you forget a dose, take it as soon as you remember. If it is almost time for your next dose, skip the dose you forgot and continue with your regular schedule. Call your doctor if you miss 2 or more doses in a row.

Special Populations

Pregnancy/Breast-feeding

Midodrine may pass into fetal circulation. When this drug is considered crucial by your doctor, its potential benefits must be carefully weighed against its risks.

It is not known if midodrine passes into breast milk. Nursing mothers who must take it should consider bottle-feeding.

Seniors
Seniors may take midodrine without special precaution.

Generic Name
Miglitol (mig-LIH-tol)

Brand Name
Glyset

Type of Drug
Antidiabetic.

Prescribed for
Non-insulin-dependent diabetes.

General Information

Miglitol works differently from other oral antidiabetes drugs, which control blood sugar levels by increasing the production of insulin or helping the body to use the hormone more efficiently. Miglitol delays the digestion of carbohydrates (sugars) by acting in the cells that line the small intestine, where sugar is absorbed. This results in less sugar being absorbed into the blood and, therefore, a lower blood-sugar level. Miglitol also has some effect against the enzyme lactase, but usually does not cause lactose intolerance. Hypoglycemia (very low blood sugar) is unlikely with miglitol because of the way the drug works in diabetes.

People taking miglitol should have their blood sugar checked periodically to see how well the drug is working. (Home glucose monitors are available.) Migitol may be prescribed with another antidiabetic drug if single-drug therapy is not enough to adequately control blood sugar levels.

Cautions and Warnings

Do not take miglitol if you are **sensitive** or **allergic** to it. Miglitol should be used with caution if you have **diabetic ketoacidosis, inflammatory bowel disease, ulcers in the colon, partial obstruction of your intestine,** or **absorption or digestion disease.**

People with kidney disease retain higher levels of miglitol in the blood, but this does not affect the drug's action because it acts locally in cells lining the small intestine. Those with severe **kidney disease** should not take this drug because of drug retention in the blood.

Miglitol may increase the risk of **hypoglycemia** if taken with a sulfonylurea-type antidiabetes drug.

Possible Side Effects

Most side effects of miglitol go away with continued use of the drug.
▼ Most common: gas, diarrhea, and abdominal pain.
▼ Common: rash and low blood iron.

Drug Interactions

• Miglitol interferes with the absorption of several drugs into the blood, including propranolol and ranitidine. Your doctor may need to adjust your dose of these drugs.
• Digestive enzymes, charcoal, and kaolin (an ingredient in Kaopectate) reduce the effects of miglitol.

Food Interactions

Miglitol must be taken with the first bite of each main meal.

Usual Dose

Adult: 25–100 mg with breakfast, lunch, and dinner.
Child: not recommended.

Overdosage

Unlike other antidiabetic medicines, a miglitol overdose does not cause hypoglycemia. Overdose symptoms are likely to include gas, diarrhea, and pain. Call your local poison control center or hospital emergency room for more information.

Special Information

Take your dose with the first bite of each meal. The drug has to be present in your intestine to prevent the absorption of sugar into your blood.

If you forget to take a dose of miglitol with your meal, skip the dose you forgot, since it cannot work unless there is food in your stomach. Continue with your regular dose at the beginning of your next meal.

Special Populations

Pregnancy/Breast-feeding
The safety of using miglitol during pregnancy is not known. When this drug is considered crucial by your doctor, its potential benefits must be carefully weighed against its risks. Diabetes that develops during pregnancy is usually treated with insulin.

Small amounts of miglitol pass into breast milk. Nursing mothers who must take this drug should bottle-feed.

Seniors
Seniors may take this drug without special precautions.

Generic Name

Minoxidil (mih-NOX-ih-dil) Ⓖ

Brand Names

Loniten   Rogaine

Type of Drug

Antihypertensive and hair-growth stimulant.

Prescribed for

Hypertension (high blood pressure), male-pattern baldness, and alopecia areata.

General Information

Minoxidil is prescribed for severe hypertension that has not responded to other drugs. It reduces blood pressure by dilating (widening) peripheral blood vessels, allowing more blood to flow through the arms and legs. This increased blood flow reduces resistance levels in central blood vessels—for example, in the heart, lungs, and kidneys—and therefore reduces blood pressure. Minoxidil's effect on blood pressure is seen 30 minutes after a dose is taken and lasts up to 3 days. Minoxidil, which is usually taken once or twice a day, reaches maximum effect in as little as 3 days if the dose is large enough—40 mg a day.

Minoxidil stimulates hair growth in men and women with hereditary hair loss. It is also used to treat alopecia areata, a condition in which patches of hair fall out all over the body. No one knows exactly how minoxidil produces this effect and it does not work for everyone. The ideal candidate is a man who has just started to lose hair. The drug is not effective unless hair in the balding area is at least ½ in. long, and it takes 4 to 6 months of applications before any effect can be expected. The application regimen must be followed carefully; stopping the drug will nullify its effects and new growth will be lost. In some men who used minoxidil for a year, hair loss was only slowed.

Cautions and Warnings

Oral minoxidil may cause severe **adverse effects on the heart,** including angina pain and fluid around the heart, which affects cardiac function. It is usually prescribed with a beta-blocking drug to prevent rapid heartbeat and a diuretic to prevent fluid accumulation. Hospitalization may be recommended for some people when they start minoxidil to avoid a rapid drop in blood pressure.

People with **pheochromocytoma** (adrenal gland tumor) should not use this drug.

This drug has not been carefully studied in people who have suffered a **heart attack** within a month of beginning minoxidil; cardiac side effects may be particularly serious in people with a history of **heart disease**. People who use minoxidil for hair growth must have a healthy scalp and no heart disease.

Possible Side Effects

Tablets
Water and sodium retention may develop (which can worsen heart failure) as well as fluid in the sacs surrounding the heart.

▼ Most common: 80% of people experience thickening, elongation, and darkening of body hair within 3 to 6 weeks, first noticed on the temples, between the eyebrows, on the forehead, or on the upper cheek. Later it may extend to the back, arms, legs, and scalp. This effect stops when the drug is stopped, and symptoms usually disappear in 1 to 6 months. Heart rhythm changes occur

Possible Side Effects *(continued)*

in 60% of people, but cause no symptoms. Some laboratory tests, such as blood, liver, and kidney tests, may be affected by minoxidil.

▼ Less common: bronchitis or other respiratory infections, sinus inflammation, rash, eczema, fungal infection, itching, redness, dry skin or scalp, flaking, worsening of hair loss, hair loss where none was present, diarrhea, nausea, vomiting, headache, dizziness, light-headedness, fainting, back pain, broken bones, tendinitis, aches and pains, swelling of the arms or legs, chest pain, blood-pressure changes, heart palpitations, pulse-rate changes, allergic reactions (symptoms include breathing difficulties, rash, and itching), hives, runny nose, facial swelling, conjunctivitis (pinkeye), ear infection, visual disturbances, weight gain, urinary infection, inflammation of the prostate or urethra, vaginal discharge, pain during sex, anxiety, depression, fatigue, menstrual changes, nonspecific breast symptoms, and pain, inflammation, or redness of the testes, vagina, or vulva.

Lotion
People using 2% minoxidil lotion may experience irritation or itching. Not enough minoxidil is absorbed into the blood to affect blood pressure or cause serious side effects.

Drug Interactions

• Minoxidil may interact with guanethidine to produce severe dizziness when rising from a sitting or lying position. These drugs should not be taken together.

• Do not take over-the-counter (OTC) products that contain stimulants.

Food Interactions

None known.

Usual Dose

Tablets
   Adult and Child (age 12 and over): 5 mg a day to start; may be increased to 40 mg a day. Do not exceed 100 mg a day.

Child (under age 12): 0.1 mg per lb. of body weight a day to start; may be increased to 0.5 mg per lb. of body weight a day. Do not exceed 50 mg a day.

Minoxidil is usually taken with a diuretic—such as 100 mg of hydrochlorothiazide, 50–100 mg of chlorthalidone, or 80 mg of furosemide daily; and a beta blocker—such as 80–160 mg a day of propranolol. People who cannot take beta blockers may take 500–1500 mg of methyldopa or 0.2–0.4 mg of clonidine daily.

Lotion
Apply to scalp twice a day.

Overdosage

Symptoms include dizziness, fainting, and rapid heartbeat. Call your local poison control center or a hospital emergency room for instructions. ALWAYS bring the prescription bottle or container if you seek treatment.

Special Information

Oral minoxidil is usually prescribed with 2 other drugs—a beta blocker and a diuretic; do not discontinue any of these drugs unless told to do so by your doctor. Take all medication exactly as prescribed.

The effect of this drug on body hair (see "Possible Side Effects") is more of a nuisance than a risk and is not a reason to stop taking it.

Call your doctor if you experience an increase in your pulse of 20 or more beats per minute; weight gain of more than 5 lbs.; swelling of your arms, legs, face, or stomach; chest pain; breathing difficulties; dizziness; or fainting spells.

If you forget a dose of oral minoxidil, take it as soon as you remember. If it is almost time for your next dose, skip the dose you forgot and continue with your regular schedule. Do not take a double dose.

Special Populations

Pregnancy/Breast-feeding

Oral minoxidil crosses into the fetal circulation. Women should avoid either form of minoxidil during pregnancy. When this drug is considered crucial by your doctor, its potential benefits must be carefully weighed against its risks.

Oral minoxidil passes into breast milk, as may the lotion. Nursing mothers who must take either form of minoxidil should bottle-feed.

Seniors

Seniors may be more sensitive to the blood-pressure-lowering effect of the drug due to loss of kidney function.

Generic Name

Mirtazapine (mur-TAZ-uh-pene)

Brand Name

Remeron

The information in this profile also applies to the following drug:

Generic Ingredient: Maprotiline [G]
Ludiomil

Type of Drug

Antidepressant.

Prescribed for

Depression, tremors, and panic disorder.

General Information

Mirtazapine blocks the passage of stimulant chemicals in and out of nerve endings and has a sedative effect. It also moderately counteracts the effects of the neurohormone acetylcholine. Recent theory maintains that antidepressants work by causing long-term changes in the way nerve endings function. Mirtazapine can elevate mood, increase physical activity and mental alertness, and improve appetite and sleep patterns 2 to 4 weeks after you start taking it. Mirtazapine is useful in treating mild forms of depression associated with anxiety. It can also significantly reduce tremors associated with Parkinson's disease and other causes, though the effect is lost soon after drug treatment is stopped. Mirtazapine is broken down in the liver. Women clear the drug more slowly than men.

Cautions and Warnings

Do not take mirtazapine if you are **allergic** or **sensitive** to it.

Mirtazapine should be taken with care if you are recovering from a **heart attack**.

Take this drug with caution if you have a history of **epilepsy or other convulsive disorders, urinary difficulties, glaucoma, heart disease, liver disease,** or **hyperthyroidism.** Antidepressants may aggravate the condition of people who are **schizophrenic** or **paranoid** and may cause people with **bipolar (manic-depressive) disorder** to switch phase. These reactions are also possible when changing or stopping antidepressants.

Suicide is always a risk in severely depressed people, who should only be allowed to have minimal quantities of medication in their possession.

Seizures are rare and can be minimized by starting with a low mirtazapine dose and staying with the lowest effective dose. Dosage should be increased gradually and only after at least 2 weeks on the starting dose.

People taking mirtazapine may develop very **low white-blood-cell counts** leading to infections, fever, and related problems. Call your doctor at once if you develop a sore throat, fever, infection, or mouth sores while taking this drug.

Mirtazapine should be taken with care if you have severe **kidney or liver disease.**

Possible Side Effects

▼ Most common: tiredness, dizziness, dry mouth, constipation, increased appetite, weight gain, large increases in blood cholesterol or triglyceride levels, weakness, and flu symptoms.

▼ Less common: back pain, nausea, vomiting, muscle ache, abnormal dreaming or thinking, anxiety, agitation, confusion, tremors, itching, rash, breathing difficulties, and frequent urination.

▼ Rare: blood-pressure changes, weakness, hair loss, uncontrollable muscle spasms or movements, hallucinations, manic reactions, and liver function changes. Other rare side effects can occur in almost any part of the body. Contact your doctor if you experience any side effect not listed above.

Drug Interactions

Mirtazapine and Maprotiline
• Combining mirtazapine or maprotiline with a mono-amine oxidase inhibitor (MAOI) antidepressant may cause high fevers, convulsions, or death. Do not take an MAOI until at least 2 weeks after mirtazapine or maprotiline has been stopped. People who take either of these drugs and an MAOI require close medical observation.
• Mirtazapine and maprotiline increase the effects of alcohol, tranquilizers, and other sedative drugs.

Maprotiline
• Maprotiline interacts with guanethidine and clonidine (drugs used to treat high blood pressure). Tell your doctor if you are taking any drug for high blood pressure.
• Barbiturates may decrease the effectiveness of maprotiline. Combining maprotiline and thyroid medication enhances the effects of both drugs and may cause abnormal heart rhythms.
• Combining maprotiline and reserpine may cause overstimulation.
• Oral contraceptives ("the pill") may reduce the effect of maprotiline, as may smoking. Charcoal tablets may block the absorption of maprotiline. Estrogen may increase or decrease the effect of maprotiline.
• Bicarbonate of soda, acetazolamide, quinidine, and procainamide increase the effect of maprotiline. Combining this drug and cimetidine, methylphenidate, or phenothiazine drugs such as thorazine and compazine may cause severe side effects.

Food Interactions

You may take mirtazapine with food if it upsets your stomach.

Usual Dose

Maprotiline
    Adult: 75–225 mg a day. Hospitalized patients may need up to 300 mg a day.
    Senior: usually 50–75 mg a day.

Mirtazapine
    Adult: 15 mg at bedtime. Dosage must be tailored to your needs.

Overdosage

Symptoms of mirtazapine overdose include disorientation, drowsiness, memory loss, and rapid heartbeat. Symptoms of maprotiline overdose include confusion, inability to concentrate, hallucinations, drowsiness, lowered body temperature, abnormal heart rate, heart failure, enlarged pupils, seizures, convulsions, very low blood pressure, stupor, and coma; agitation, stiffening of muscles, vomiting, and high fever may also develop. The victim should be taken to a hospital emergency room immediately. ALWAYS bring the prescription bottle or container.

Special Information

Do not stop taking this drug without your doctor's knowledge. Abruptly stopping mirtazapine may cause nausea, headache, and feelings of ill health.

Mirtazapine may cause drowsiness and dizziness. Be careful when driving or doing any task that requires concentration. Avoid alcohol and other depressant drugs. Avoid prolonged exposure to the sun.

Be careful when taking over-the-counter (OTC) medications because mirtazapine may interact with sedative ingredients in OTC products.

Call your doctor at once if you develop chills, difficult or rapid breathing, fever, sweating, blood-pressure changes, muscle stiffness, loss of bladder control, or unusual tiredness or weakness.

If your symptoms are unchanged after 6 to 8 weeks of treatment with an antidepressant, contact your doctor.

If you forget a dose, skip it and go back to your regular schedule. Do not take a double dose.

Special Populations

Pregnancy/Breast-feeding

Mirtazapine crosses into the fetal circulation and may cause birth defects. When this drug is considered crucial by your doctor, its potential benefits must be carefully weighed against its risks.

It is not known if mirtazapine passes into breast milk. Nursing mothers who must take this drug should consider bottle-feeding.

Seniors

Seniors are more sensitive to side effects and may require reduced dosage. Older men may need less of the drug than women of the same age.

Generic Name

Misoprostol (mye-soe-PROS-tol)

Brand Name

Cytotec

Type of Drug

Anti-ulcer.

Prescribed for

Stomach ulcer, duodenal (intestinal) ulcer, and prevention of kidney rejection after transplant.

General Information

Like most anti-ulcer drugs, misoprostol suppresses stomach acid. It has a demonstrated ability to protect the stomach lining from damage, though the exact way misoprostol works is not known. It may increase production of stomach lining and the thickness of the protective gel layer lining the stomach. Misoprostol may also increase blood flow in and subsequent healing of the stomach lining in addition to increasing production of bicarbonate, a natural antacid found in the stomach.

Misoprostol is intended to prevent severe stomach irritation and ulcers in people taking a nonsteroidal anti-inflammatory drug (NSAID). It is helpful for seniors and others with a history of ulcer or stomach disease who require NSAID treatment for arthritis. Misoprostol is also used to treat duodenal ulcers, though it does not prevent them. It is often an effective ulcer treatment for people who do not respond to or cannot tolerate cimetidine, ranitidine, famotidine, or nizatidine. Misoprostol has also been studied as a vaginal abortion drug. It is as effective as the drug RU-486 and works in the same way.

Cautions and Warnings

Misoprostol may reduce **fertility**. Do not take this drug if you are **allergic** to it or any prostaglandin agent.

People with **kidney disease** may require reduced dosages.

People with **epilepsy** or **blood-vessel disease** in the heart or brain should be cautious about taking misoprostol.

Possible Side Effects

▼ Most common: diarrhea and abdominal pain. Most cases of diarrhea are mild and last no more than 2 to 3 days.

▼ Less common: headache, nausea, vomiting, and stomach upset or gas.

▼ Rare: spotting, cramps, excessive menstrual bleeding, painful menstruation or other menstrual disorders, and vaginal bleeding.

Drug Interactions

• Misoprostol may interfere with the absorption of diazepam and theophylline.

• Rarely, antacids interfere with misoprostol's effectiveness. Magnesium-containing antacids may worsen misoprostol-induced diarrhea.

Food Interactions

Though food interferes with the absorption of this drug, it should be taken with or after meals (and at bedtime) to minimize gastrointestinal (GI) side effects.

Usual Dose

Adult: 200 mcg 4 times a day.

Overdosage

Symptoms include sedation; tremors; convulsions; breathing difficulties; stomach pain; diarrhea; fever; changes in heart rate—either very fast or very slow; and low blood pressure. Take the victim to a hospital emergency room. ALWAYS bring the prescription bottle or container.

Special Information

Do not stop taking misoprostol, or take it for more than 4 weeks, without your doctor's knowledge.

Call your doctor if side effects, especially diarrhea or abdominal or stomach pain, become severe or intolerable.

Women who experience menstrual problems and post-menopausal women who experience vaginal bleeding should discuss these side effects with their doctors.

If you forget a dose, take it as soon as you remember. If it is almost time for your next dose, skip the dose you forgot and continue with your regular schedule. Do not take a double dose.

Special Populations

Pregnancy/Breast-feeding
PREGNANT WOMEN SHOULD NOT TAKE THIS DRUG. Women of childbearing age should take misoprostol only if they absolutely must take an NSAID and already have, or are at high risk of developing, stomach ulcers. Misoprostol causes spontaneous miscarriage. Within 2 weeks of starting treatment, you must receive a negative BLOOD test result for pregnancy—an over-the-counter urine test is not sufficient. Start taking misoprostol on day 2 or 3 of your period and use effective contraception throughout drug therapy.

It is not known if misoprostol passes into breast milk, though it is unlikely. Nursing mothers who must take this drug should bottle-feed.

Seniors
Seniors should receive lower dosages if intolerable side effects develop.

Generic Name

Modafinil (moe-DAF-ih-nil)

Brand Name
Provigil

Type of Drug
Stimulant.

Prescribed for
Narcolepsy (uncontrollable desire to sleep).

General Information

Modafinil promotes wakefulness. While some of its actions are similar to those of amphetamine and methylphenidate, it is not known exactly how modafinil achieves its effects. People being treated with this drug may experience euphoria (feeling "high"), anxiety, and changes in mood, mental state, and behavior.

Cautions and Warnings

Do not take modafinil if you are **allergic** or **sensitive** to it.

People with a history of **heart failure,** an **enlarged heart ventricle, angina, chest pain, abnormal heart rhythms,** or **mitral valve prolapse** should not take modafinil.

Modafinil has not been studied in people with **high blood pressure**. People with high blood pressure who take this drug must be closely monitored.

People with **cirrhosis of the liver** or **liver failure** may require reduced dosages.

People who regularly take large dosages (more than 400 mg a day) of modafinil may develop some **resistance** to its effects.

Possible Side Effects

▼ Most common: headache, nausea, and runny nose.

▼ Common: nervousness, dizziness, diarrhea, dry mouth, appetite loss, and sore throat.

▼ Less common: depression, anxiety, cataplexy (extreme muscle weakness, often precipitated by laughter, a surprised feeling, or emotions of fear or anger), sleeplessness, tingling in the hands or feet, unusual facial or mouth movements, muscle stiffness, blood pressure changes, liver function problems, vomiting, lung problems, breathing difficulties, vision problems, chest pain, neck pain, chills, and high-white-blood-cell counts.

▼ Rare: confusion; memory loss; emotional instability; euphoria, changes in mood, marital state and behavior; flushing, fainting; dry skin; herpes infections; mouth sores; gum sores; thirst; difficulty urinating; abnormal urination; abnormal ejaculation; high blood sugar; nosebleeds; asthma; rigid neck; fever with chills; and joint problems.

Drug Interactions

• Combining modafinil and a monoamine oxidase inhibitor (MAOI) drug may increase the effects of both drugs. Use this combination with caution and only under your doctor's supervision.

• Methylphenidate can delay modafinil's effects.

• Carbamazepine, phenobarbital, rifampin, ketoconazole, and itraconazole may reduce modafinil's effects.

• Modafinil may reduce the effects of oral contraceptives ("the pill"), theophylline, clomipramine, and cyclosporine.

• Modafinil may elevate blood levels of phenytoin, diazepam, propranolol, tricyclic antidepressants, and warfarin, increasing the risk of side effects—some of these can be very serious.

• Stimulants in over-the-counter (OTC) decongestants, diet pills, and asthma drugs may cause excessive stimulation when combined with modafinil.

Food Interactions

Food can slow the rate at which modafinil is absorbed into the blood but is unlikely to change its effect on your body.

Usual Dose

Adult: 200 mg every morning; 100 mg daily for people with cirrhosis or liver failure.

Senior: start with 100 mg daily and increase if needed.

Child (under age 17): not recommended.

Overdosage

Symptoms include excitation, sleeplessness, sleep disturbances, anxiety, irritability, aggressiveness, confusion, nervousness, tremors, heart palpitations, nausea, diarrhea, and bleeding. Take the victim to a hospital emergency room. ALWAYS bring the prescription bottle or container.

Special Information

Call your doctor if you develop a rash, hives, or other signs of a drug allergy.

Modafinil's beneficial effects on mood, thought, and perception may produce psychological dependence, though drug withdrawal symptoms have not been reported.

The stimulants in OTC decongestants, diet pills, and asthma drugs may cause excessive stimulation when combined with modafinil.

Be careful when driving or doing any task that requires concentration. Avoid alcohol.

Special Populations

Pregnancy/Breast-feeding
Modafinil causes fetal malformation in animal studies. When this drug is considered crucial by your doctor, its potential benefits must be carefully weighed against its risks.

This drug may pass into breast milk. Nursing mothers who must take it should consider bottle-feeding.

Seniors
Seniors with kidney or liver problems may require reduced dosage.

Generic Name

Moexipril (moe-EX-uh-pril)

Brand Name

Univasc

Type of Drug

Angiotensin-converting enzyme (ACE) inhibitor.

Prescribed for

Hypertension (high blood pressure).

General Information

Moexipril hydrochloride and other ACE inhibitors work by preventing the conversion of a hormone called angiotensin I to another hormone called angiotensin II, a potent blood-vessel constrictor. Preventing this conversion relaxes blood vessels, thus reducing blood pressure and relieving the symptoms of heart failure. Moexipril also affects production of other hormones and enzymes that participate in the regulation of blood vessel dilation. Moexipril begins working about 1 hour after you take it and continues to work for 24 hours.

Some people who start taking an ACE inhibitor after they are already on a diuretic (an agent that increases urination) experience a rapid drop in blood pressure after their first doses or when the dosage is increased. To prevent this from happening, you may be told to stop taking the diuretic 2 or 3 days before starting the ACE inhibitor, or to increase your salt intake during that time. The diuretic may then be restarted gradually.

Cautions and Warnings

Do not take moexipril if you have had an **allergic reaction** to it.

Moexipril occasionally causes **very low blood pressure**.

Moexipril may cause a decline in **kidney function,** especially if you have congestive **heart failure**. Your doctor should check your urine for changes during the first few months of treatment. Dosage adjustment may be necessary.

Moexipril can occasionally affect white-blood-cell count, possibly increasing your susceptibility to **infection**. Blood counts should be monitored periodically.

Possible Side Effects

▼ Most common: dizziness, tiredness, headache, nausea, low blood pressure, chest pain, and chronic cough. The cough usually goes away a few days after you stop taking the medicine.

▼ Less common: chest pain, angina, dizziness when rising from a sitting or lying position, fainting, abdominal pain, nausea, vomiting, diarrhea, bronchitis, urinary tract infection, breathing difficulties, weakness, and rash.

▼ Rare: Rare side effects can occur in almost any part of the body. Contact your doctor if you experience any side effect not listed above.

Drug Interactions

• The blood-pressure-lowering effect of moexipril is increased by taking diuretic drugs and beta blockers. Any other drug that causes a rapid drop in blood pressure should be used with caution if you are taking an ACE inhibitor.

• Moexipril may increase potassium levels in your blood, especially when taken with Dyazide or other potassium-sparing diuretics.

• Moexipril may increase the effects of lithium; this combination should be used with caution.

• Antacids and moexipril should be taken at least 2 hours apart.

• Capsaicin may trigger or aggravate the cough associated with moexipril therapy.

• Indomethacin may reduce the blood-pressure-lowering effect of moexipril.

• Phenothiazine tranquilizers and antiemetics may increase the effects of moexipril.

• The combination of allopurinol and moexipril increases the chance of side effects.

• Moexipril increases the levels of digoxin in the blood, possibly increasing the chance of digoxin-related side effects.

Food Interactions

Moexipril should be taken 1 hour before or 2 hours after meals.

Usual Dose

7.5–30 mg once a day. Some people may divide their daily dosage into 2 doses. People with poor kidney function should take half the usual dose.

Overdosage

The principal effect of moexipril overdose is a rapid drop in blood pressure, as evidenced by dizziness or fainting. Take the victim to a hospital emergency room immediately. ALWAYS bring the prescription bottle or container.

Special Information

Call your doctor if you develop swelling of the face or throat, if you have sudden difficulty in breathing, a sore throat, mouth sores, abnormal heartbeat, chest pain, a persistent rash, or loss of taste perception. Unexplained swelling of the face, lips, hands, and feet can also affect the larynx (throat) and tongue and interfere with breathing. If this happens, the victim should be taken to a hospital emergency room at once for treatment.

You may get dizzy if you rise to your feet quickly from a sitting or lying position.

Avoid strenuous exercise and very hot weather because heavy sweating or dehydration can cause a rapid blood pressure drop.

Avoid over-the-counter diet pills, decongestants, and other stimulants that can raise blood pressure.

If you take moexipril on a regular schedule and forget a dose, take it as soon as you remember. If you take it once a day and it is within 8 hours of your next dose, skip the one you forgot and continue with your regular schedule. If you take moexipril twice a day and it is within 4 hours of your next dose, take 1 dose as soon as you remember and another in 5 or 6 hours, then go back to your regular schedule. Never take a double dose.

Special Populations

Pregnancy/Breast-feeding
ACE inhibitors can cause fetal injury or death. Women who are or might be pregnant should not take moexipril. Stop taking the medication and contact your doctor if you become pregnant.

Small amounts of moexipril pass into breast milk. Nursing mothers who must take this drug should consider bottle-feeding.

Seniors
Seniors may be more sensitive to the effects of moexipril due to kidney impairment.

Monopril   *see Fosinopril, page 468*

Brand Name

Motofen

Generic Ingredients

Difenoxin + Atropine Sulfate

Type of Drug

Antidiarrheal.

Prescribed for

Acute and chronic diarrhea.

General Information

Difenoxin is an antidiarrheal agent related to meperidine, a narcotic analgesic (pain reliever) used in Demerol. Difenoxin, which can be addictive, works by slowing the contractions of intestinal-wall muscles. The atropine sulfate ingredient in Motofen guards against drug overdose or abuse by producing undesirable effects at small dosages, thus deterring users from taking larger amounts of Motofen. This drug, which relieves diarrhea but does not address the underlying cause, should only be used for short periods and in cases that do not respond to other treatment. Some people should not use this drug even if diarrhea is present. Antidiarrheal drugs may harm people with stomach, bowel, or other conditions.

Cautions and Warnings

Do not take Motofen if you are **allergic** to any of its ingredients or to Lomotil. Avoid Motofen if you have advanced **liver disease** or have **jaundice** (symptoms include yellowing of the skin or whites of the eyes), or if your diarrhea was caused by taking clindamycin or another antibiotic.

Possible Side Effects

▼ Most common: nausea, vomiting, dry mouth, dizziness, light-headedness, drowsiness, and headache.

▼ Less common: constipation, upset stomach, confusion, and tiredness or sleeplessness.

▼ Rare: a burning sensation in the eyes, blurred vision, dry skin, rapid heartbeat, elevated temperature, and urinary difficulties.

Drug Interactions

• Motofen may increase the effects of alcohol, tranquilizers, pain relievers, and other nervous-system depressants. Avoid these combinations.

• Monoamine oxidase inhibitor (MAOI) antidepressants may, in theory, produce a high-blood-pressure crisis in combination with Motofen. Do not use Motofen if you are taking an MAOI unless you are under a doctor's care.

Food Interactions

None known.

Usual Dose

Adult and Child (age 12 and over): 2 tablets to start, then 1 after each loose stool or every 3–4 hours, as needed; up to 8 tablets a day. Treatment for more than 2 consecutive days is usually not needed.

Child (under age 12): not recommended.

Overdosage

Symptoms include dry skin, mouth, and nose; flushing; fever; and rapid heartbeat. These symptoms may be followed by loss of reflexes, pinpointed pupils, droopy eyelids, breathing difficulty, and lethargy or coma. Take the victim to a hospital emergency room immediately. ALWAYS bring the prescription bottle or container.

Special Information

Motofen can make you tired, dizzy, or light-headed. Be careful when driving or doing any task that requires concentration. Alcohol, tranquilizers, and other nervous-system depressants increase the depressant effects of this drug.

Your doctor may prescribe fluid and salt mixtures to replace the body fluids you lose while taking Motofen.

Call your doctor if you develop heart palpitations or your symptoms do not clear up in 2 days. You may need a different dosage or drug.

If you forget a dose, take it as soon as you remember. If it is almost time for your next dose, skip the one you forgot and continue with your regular schedule. Do not take a double dose.

Special Populations

Pregnancy/Breast-feeding

Animal studies with very large dosages of Motofen showed an increase in stillbirths. When this drug is considered crucial by your doctor, its potential benefits must be carefully weighed against its risks.

The ingredients in Motofen may pass into breast milk. Nursing mothers taking Motofen should bottle-feed.

Seniors

Seniors with severe kidney or liver disease require reduced dosage.

Generic Name

Mupirocin (mue-PYE-roe-sin)

Brand Name

Bactroban

Type of Drug

Topical antibiotic.

Prescribed for

Impetigo (streptococcal skin infections), eczema, inflammation of the hair follicles, and minor bacterial skin infections. Mupirocin nasal is used to prevent resistant *Staphylococcus aureus* infections from spreading during outbreaks of the infection.

General Information

Mupirocin is a unique, non-penicillin drug that works against the common microorganisms that cause impetigo in children. It is used to supplement other treatments for impetigo, although many doctors prefer oral medication. Mupirocin works by interfering with bacteria's ability to make the proteins it needs for survival. Large amounts of mupirocin kill bacteria and smaller amounts stop the bacteria from growing. It may be effective against antibiotic-resistant bacteria.

Cautions and Warnings

Do not use a mupirocin product if you are **allergic** to any of its components. Mupirocin ointment is **not for use in the eye**.

Mupirocin nasal should be used only to treat *Staphylococcus aureus* infections, not to prevent them.

Large quantities of mupirocin ointment should **not be applied to an open wound** because polyethylene glycol—used as a base in mupirocin ointment—may be absorbed through the wound and damage the kidneys.

Possible Side Effects

Ointment

▼ Less common: burning, itching, rash, stinging or pain where the ointment is applied, nausea, skin redness, dry skin, tenderness, swelling, and increased oozing from impetigo lesions.

Possible Side Effects *(continued)*

Nasal Ointment

▼ Most common: headache and runny nose.

▼ Less common: respiratory congestion, sore throat, changes in sense of taste, burning or stinging, cough, and itching.

▼ Rare: eyelid inflammation, diarrhea, dry mouth, ear pain, nosebleeds, nausea, and rash.

Drug Interactions

• Do not use mupirocin nasal at the same time as any other prescription or over-the-counter nasal drug product.

• Taking antibiotics while using mupirocin can lead to the development of resistant bacteria.

Usual Dose

Ointment: Apply a small amount to the affected area 3 times a day. Cover with gauze if desired.

Nasal Ointment: Put half the ointment from a single-use tube in each nostril morning and evening for 5 days. After the ointment is applied, gently squeeze your nostrils closed and allow them to open again. Repeat this continuously for about 1 minute.

Overdosage

Little is known about the effects of accidental ingestion. Call your local poison control center or a hospital emergency room for more information.

Special Information

Call your doctor if this medication does not work within 3 to 5 days or if any of the following symptoms develop: dry skin or redness, rash, itching, stinging, pain, or other possible drug reactions.

If you forget a dose, apply it as you remember. If it is almost time for your next dose, skip the one you forgot and continue with your regular schedule. Do not apply a double dose.

Special Populations

Pregnancy/Breast-feeding

While animal studies of mupirocin reveal no damage to the fetus, this drug should only be used during pregnancy after carefully weighing its potential benefits against its risks.

It is not known if mupirocin passes into breast milk. Nursing mothers who must take this drug should bottle-feed.

Seniors

Seniors may use mupirocin without special restriction.

Generic Name

Muromonab-CD3 (muh-ROE-moe-nab)

Brand Name

Orthoclone OKT3

Type of Drug

Immunosuppressant.

Prescribed for

Kidney, heart, and liver transplantation.

General Information

Muromonab-CD3 is an important alternative to cyclosporine in preventing organ transplant rejection. By blocking the activity of T-cells, which protect the body against invading microorganisms or foreign substances, this drug suppresses the immune system and prevents organ rejection. The drug starts working in minutes and continues working for as long as it is used. T-cells rapidly return to normal within 1 week after the medication is stopped.

Cautions and Warnings

This drug should not be used by people with untreated **heart failure, fluid overload,** or a history of **seizures**.

Muromonab-CD3 is made in cells from mouse tissue and causes the development of **anti-mouse antibodies** in humans. People who have received other drugs made in this way may already have high levels of this kind of anti-body in their blood and, if they do, should not be treated with muromonab-CD3. Your doctor will test for antibody levels.

People who receive this drug usually develop **cytokine release syndrome (CRS)** from 30 minutes to 2 days after the first dose is given. CRS symptoms range from mild, flu-like symptoms such as fever, chills, joint aches, weakness, and headaches, to a less common, life-threatening shock-like reaction that involves the heart and nervous system. Some of the more severe symptoms of CRS are shortness of breath; high fever—up to 107°F; wheezing; rapid heartbeat; chest pain; respiratory collapse or failure; heart attack; severe drug reactions; seizures; confusion; hallucinations; stiff neck; brain swelling; and headache. People who are at risk for more severe forms of CRS include those with a recent heart attack or uncontrolled angina pectoris, heart failure, fluid in the lungs, serious lung disease, and a history of seizure or shock. CRS may be prevented or minimized by giving methylpred-nisolone 1 to 4 hours before the first dose of muromonab-CD3.

People receiving this drug are more likely to develop **infection**. Preventive antibiotic therapy is sometimes used to reduce the risk of infection.

Possible Side Effects

More than 90% of people receiving muromonab-CD3 experience some form of CRS, though it is usually mild (see "Cautions and Warnings").

▼ Rare: Rare side effects can occur in almost any part of the body. Contact your doctor if you experience any bothersome or persistent side effect.

Drug Interactions

• Other immunosuppressants (corticosteroids, cyclospor-ine, and azathioprine) and indomethacin increase the effect of muromonab-CD3, in turn increasing the risk of CRS.

Food Interactions

Muromonab-CD3 may be taken without regard to food.

Usual Dose

Adult and Child (age 12 and over): 5 mg intravenously a day for 10–14 days.

Child (under age 12): 0.1 mg intravenously for every 2.2 lbs. of body weight a day for 10–14 days.

Overdosage

Little is known about the effects of muromonab-CD 3 overdose. Call your local poison control center or a hospital emergency room for information.

Special Information

Call your doctor at the first sign of rash, itching, rapid heartbeat, difficulty swallowing, breathing difficulties, unusual swelling, allergic reaction, or if you experience any bothersome or persistent side effect. It is essential to maintain close contact with your doctor while taking muromonab-CD3.

Mild reactions due to CRS may be treated by taking acetaminophen or antihistamines. Your body temperature should be no higher than 100°F when each dose is given.

Avoid exposure to bacterial infection and immunizations while you are taking this drug. If an infection develops, your doctor will have to stop muromonab-CD3 therapy and treat the infection.

Maintain good dental hygiene while taking muromonab-CD3 and use extra care when brushing and flossing because this drug increases your risk of oral infection. See your dentist regularly.

This drug may cause confusion or interfere with your alertness, dexterity, or coordination. Be careful when driving or doing any task that requires concentration.

It is essential to complete the full course of treatment. This medication should not be stopped unless an infection or other severe side effect develops. If you miss a dose, take it as soon as you remember and call your doctor.

Special Populations

Pregnancy/Breast-feeding

Muromonab-CD3 may cross into the fetal circulation. When this drug is considered crucial by your doctor, its potential benefits must be carefully weighed against its risks.

It is not known if muromonab-CD3 passes into breast milk. Nursing mothers who must take this drug should bottle-feed.

Seniors
Seniors may use this drug without special restriction.

Generic Name

Mycophenolate (mye-coe-FEN-oe-late)

Brand Name

CellCept

Type of Drug

Immunosuppressant.

Prescribed for

Kidney transplantation.

General Information

Mycophenolate mofetil is used with corticosteroids and cyclosporine to prevent the rejection of transplanted kidneys. In the body, the drug is metabolized into MPA, the active form of mycophenolate. MPA blocks the activity of T and B lymphocytes, which protect the body against invading microorganisms or foreign substances. MPA also suppresses antibody formation and may act directly on inflammation and organ rejection sites to prevent tissue rejection.

Cautions and Warnings

As with other immunosuppressants, people taking mycophenolate are at increased risk of developing a **lymphoma or other malignancy**. The risk increases with the degree of immune suppression and the length of time that the drug is taken.

About 2 in 100 people receiving mycophenolate develop a severe **reduction in white-blood-cell count**. Call your doctor if you develop symptoms of viral infection or other unusual symptoms.

About 3 in 100 people who take this drug develop **stomach or intestinal bleeding,** though many of these people are also taking other drugs that may affect the gastrointestinal (GI) tract. People with stomach or intestinal disease should take this drug with caution.

People with **kidney disease** should receive lower dosages. People who experience post-transplant reduction in liver function may develop kidney damage.

Mild to moderate **hypertension** (high blood pressure) is a common side effect of mycophenolate and may be a sign of kidney damage. People taking this drug should measure their blood pressure regularly.

Possible Side Effects

▼ Most common: general pain, abdominal pain, fever, headache, infection, blood infection, weakness, chest pain, back pain, hypertension, anemia, reduced white-blood-cell and platelet counts, urinary infection, blood in the urine, swelling of the arms or legs, diarrhea, constipation, nausea, vomiting, upset stomach, oral fungus infection, respiratory infection, cough, breathing difficulties, and tremors.

▼ Common: kidney damage, urinary tract problems, high blood cholesterol, low blood-phosphate levels, fluid retention, changes in blood-potassium levels, high blood sugar, sore throat, pneumonia, bronchitis, acne, rash, sleeplessness, and dizziness.

▼ Less common: painful urination, impotence, frequent urination, pyelonephritis, urinary disorder, angina pain, heart palpitations, low blood pressure, dizziness when rising from a sitting or lying position, cardiovascular disorders, appetite loss, gas, stomach irritation or bleeding, gum irritation or enlargement, liver irritation, mouth ulcer, asthma, lung disorder, stuffy or runny nose, sinus irritation, hair loss, itching, sweating, skin ulcer, anxiety, depression, stiff muscles, tingling in the hands or feet, joint or muscle pain, leg cramps, double vision, cataracts, conjunctivitis (pinkeye), chills and fever, abdominal enlargement, facial swelling, cysts, flu-like symptoms, bleeding, hernia, feeling sick, pelvic pain, and black-and-blue marks.

▼ Rare: lymphoma, skin cancer—not melanomas—and other malignancies, herpes, chickenpox or shingles, fungus infection, and pneumocystis and other opportunistic infections that usually only develop in people with suppressed immune systems.

Drug Interactions

• Combining mycophenolate and acyclovir (an antiviral drug) increases blood levels of both drugs.

• Cholestyramine and aluminum/magnesium antacids decrease mycophenolate blood levels and should be separated from mycophenolate by at least 1 hour.

• Azathioprine (an immune-system suppressant) should not be combined with mycophenolate because of the risk of excess immune-system suppression.

• Probenecid may double or triple mycophenolate blood levels. Aspirin also increases mycophenolate blood levels.

• Mycophenolate may moderately reduce phenytoin and theophylline blood levels.

Food Interactions

Mycophenolate should be taken at least 1 hour before or 2 hours after meals.

Usual Dose

Adult: 2–3 g a day divided into 2 doses.
Child: not recommended.

Overdosage

Overdose is likely to cause side effects—especially those relating to the stomach and intestines—and blood abnormalities. Take the victim to a hospital emergency room. ALWAYS bring the prescription bottle or container.

Special Information

It is extremely important to take this drug exactly as prescribed. If you forget a dose, take it as soon as you remember. If it is almost time for your next dose, skip the dose you forgot and continue with your regular schedule. Do not take a double dose. Call your doctor if you forget 2 or more doses in a row.

Because this drug causes birth defects in animals, take extra caution when handling the capsules. Do not open or crush them. Avoid inhaling the powder or allowing it to touch your skin or the inside of your mouth or nose. If such contact does occur, wash thoroughly with soap and water. If the powder gets into your eyes, rinse them thoroughly with plain water.

People taking mycophenolate require regular testing to monitor their progress.

Call your doctor at the first sign of fever; sore throat; tiredness; weakness; nervousness; unusual bleeding or bruising; tender or swollen gums; convulsions; irregular heartbeat; confusion; numbness or tingling of your hands, feet, or lips; breathing difficulties; severe stomach pain with nausea; or blood in the urine. Other side effects are less serious but should be brought to your doctor's attention, particularly if they are bothersome or persistent.

Maintain good dental hygiene while taking mycophenolate and use extra care when brushing or flossing because this drug increases your risk of oral infection. See your dentist regularly.

This drug should be continued for as long as prescribed by your doctor. Do not stop taking it because of side effects or other problems without your doctor's knowledge.

Special Populations

Pregnancy/Breast-feeding

Animal studies show that mycophenolate may be highly toxic to the fetus. Women of childbearing age should have a negative pregnancy test at least 1 week before treatment is started. They should either use 2 effective contraceptive methods before treatment is started and continue until 6 weeks after mycophenolate is discontinued, or they should practice abstinence during this period. Should you accidentally become pregnant during mycophenolate treatment, discuss with your doctor the advisability of continuing the pregnancy. When this drug is considered crucial by your doctor, its potential benefits must be carefully weighed against its risks.

Mycophenolate passes into breast milk. Nursing mothers who must take this drug should bottle-feed.

Seniors

Seniors may require reduced dosage due to loss of kidney function.

Generic Name

Nabumetone (nah-BUE-meh-tone)

Brand Name

Relafen

Type of Drug

Nonsteroidal anti-inflammatory drug (NSAID).

Prescribed for

Rheumatoid arthritis and osteoarthritis.

General Information

Nabumetone and other NSAIDs are used to relieve pain and inflammation. They may achieve their effects by blocking the body's production of a hormone called prostaglandin and the action of other body chemicals. Pain relief generally comes within 1 hour after taking the first dose of nabumetone, but its anti-inflammatory effect takes several days to 2 weeks to become apparent and may take a month or more to reach maximum effect. Nabumetone is broken down in the liver.

Cautions and Warnings

People who are **allergic** to nabumetone or any other NSAID and those with a history of **asthma** attacks brought on by an NSAID, iodides, or aspirin should not take nabumetone.

Nabumetone can cause **gastrointestinal (GI) bleeding, ulcers,** and **stomach perforation**. This can occur at any time, with or without warning, in people who take nabumetone regularly. People with a history of active GI bleeding should be cautious about taking any NSAID. People who develop bleeding or ulcers and continue NSAID treatment should be aware of the possibility of developing more serious side effects.

Nabumetone can affect platelets and **blood clotting** at high doses and should be avoided by people with clotting problems and those taking warfarin.

People with **heart problems** who use nabumetone may experience swelling in their arms, legs, or feet.

Nabumetone can cause severe toxic effects to the **kidney**. Report any unusual side effects to your doctor, who may need to periodically test your kidney function.

Nabumetone can make you **unusually sensitive to the effects of the sun**.

Possible Side Effects

▼ Most common: diarrhea, nausea, vomiting, constipation, gas, stomach upset or irritation, and appetite loss, especially during the first few days of treatment.

▼ Less common: stomach ulcers, GI bleeding, hepatitis, gallbladder attacks, painful urination, poor kidney function, kidney inflammation, blood and protein in the urine, dizziness, fainting, nervousness, depression, hallucinations, confusion, disorientation, tingling in the hands or feet, light-headedness, itching, increased sweating, dry nose and mouth, heart palpitations, chest pain, breathing difficulties, and muscle cramps.

▼ Rare: severe allergic reactions including closing of the throat, fever and chills, changes in liver function, jaundice (yellowing of the skin or whites of the eyes), and kidney failure. People who experience such effects must be promptly treated in a hospital emergency room or doctor's office. NSAIDs have caused severe skin reactions; if this happens to you, see your doctor immediately.

Drug Interactions

• Nabumetone can increase the effects of oral anticoagulant (blood-thinning) drugs such as warfarin. Your anticoagulant dose may need to be reduced.

• Combining nabumetone with cyclosporine may increase the toxic kidney effects of both drugs.

• Methotrexate toxicity may be increased in people also taking nabumetone.

• Nabumetone may reduce the blood-pressure-lowering effect of beta blockers and loop diuretics.

• Nabumetone may increase phenytoin side effects. Lithium blood levels may be increased by nabumetone.

• Nabumetone blood levels may be affected by cimetidine.

• Probenecid may increase the risk of nabumetone side effects.

• Aspirin and other salicylates should never be combined with nabumetone.

Food Interactions

Take nabumetone with food or a magnesium-aluminum antacid if it upsets your stomach.

Usual Dose

1000–2000 mg a day, taken in 1 or 2 doses.

Overdosage

People have died from NSAID overdoses. Common signs of overdose are drowsiness, nausea, vomiting, diarrhea, abdominal pain, rapid breathing, rapid heartbeat, increased sweating, ringing or buzzing in the ears, confusion, disorientation, stupor, and coma. Take the victim to a hospital emergency room at once. ALWAYS bring the prescription bottle or container.

Special Information

Take each dose with a full glass of water and do not lie down for 15 to 30 minutes afterward.

Nabumetone can make you drowsy or tired: Be careful when driving or operating hazardous equipment. Do not take any over-the-counter products containing acetaminophen or aspirin while taking nabumetone. Avoid alcohol.

Contact your doctor if you develop rash or itching, visual disturbances, weight gain, breathing difficulties, fluid retention, hallucinations, black or tarry stools, persistent headache, or any unusual or intolerable side effect.

If you forget a dose of nabumetone, take it as soon as you remember. If you take nabumetone once a day and it is within 8 hours of your next dose, or if you take several doses a day and it is within 4 hours of your next dose, skip the dose you forgot and continue with your regular schedule. Never take a double dose.

Special Populations

Pregnancy/Breast-feeding

NSAIDs may affect a fetal heart during the second half of pregnancy. Pregnant women should not take nabumetone without their doctor's approval. When this drug is considered crucial by your doctor, its potential benefits must be carefully weighed against its risks.

NSAIDs may pass into breast milk. There is a possibility that a nursing mother taking nabumetone could affect her baby's heart or cardiovascular system. Nursing mothers who must take this drug should bottle-feed.

Seniors

Seniors may be more susceptible to side effects, especially ulcer disease.

Generic Name

Naproxen/Naproxen Sodium

(nah-PROX-en) Ⓖ

Brand Names

Aleve	Naprelan
Anaprox	Napron X
EC-Naprosyn	Naprosyn

The information in this profile also applies to the following drug:

Generic Ingredient: Tolmetin Sodium

Tolectin	Tolectin DS

Type of Drug

Nonsteroidal anti-inflammatory drug (NSAID).

Prescribed for

Rheumatoid arthritis, osteoarthritis, ankylosing spondylitis, mild to moderate pain, tendinitis, bursitis, gout, fever, sunburn, migraine, and menstrual pain and headache. Only naproxen is prescribed for juvenile rheumatoid arthritis, only naproxen sodium for migraine and premenstrual syndrome (PMS).

General Information

Naproxen and other NSAIDs are used to relieve pain and inflammation. They may achieve their effects by blocking the body's production of a hormone called prostaglandin and the action of other body chemicals. Pain relief comes within 1 hour after taking the first dose of naproxen and lasts for about 7 hours, but its anti-inflammatory effect takes several days to 2 weeks to become apparent and may take a month to reach maximum effect.

Cautions and Warnings

People who are **allergic** to naproxen or any other NSAID and those with a history of **asthma** attacks brought on by an NSAID, iodides, or aspirin should not take naproxen.

Naproxen can cause **gastrointestinal (GI) bleeding, ulcers,** and **stomach perforation.** This can occur at any time, with or without warning, in people who take naproxen regularly. People with a history of active GI bleeding should be cautious about taking any NSAID. People who develop bleeding or ulcers and continue NSAID treatment should be aware of the possibility of developing more serious side effects.

Naproxen can affect platelets and **blood clotting** at high doses, and should be avoided by people with clotting problems and those taking warfarin.

People with **heart problems** who use naproxen may experience swelling in their arms, legs, or feet.

Naproxen dosage should be reduced in people with severe **liver disease.**

Naproxen can cause severe toxic effects to the **kidney.** Report any unusual side effects to your doctor, who may need to periodically test your kidney function.

Naproxen can make you **unusually sensitive to the effects of the sun.**

Possible Side Effects

▼ Most common: diarrhea, nausea, vomiting, constipation, gas, stomach upset or irritation, and appetite loss, especially during the first few days of treatment.

▼ Less common: stomach ulcers, GI bleeding, hepatitis, gallbladder attacks, painful urination, poor kidney function, kidney inflammation, blood and protein in the urine, dizziness, fainting, nervousness, depression, hallucinations, confusion, disorientation, tingling in the hands or feet, light-headedness, itching, increased sweating, dry nose and mouth, heart palpitations, chest pain, difficulty breathing, and muscle cramps.

Possible Side Effects *(continued)*

▼ Rare: severe allergic reactions including closing of the throat, fever and chills, changes in liver function, jaundice (yellowing of the skin or whites of the eyes), and kidney failure. People who experience such effects must be promptly treated in a hospital emergency room or doctor's office. NSAIDs have caused severe skin reactions; if this happens to you, see your doctor immediately.

Drug Interactions

• Naproxen can increase the effects of oral anticoagulant (blood-thinning) drugs such as warfarin. Your anticoagulant dose may need to be reduced.

• Naproxen may reduce the effect of thiazide diuretics.

• Taking naproxen with cyclosporine may increase the toxic kidney effects of both drugs.

• Methotrexate toxicity may be increased in people also taking naproxen.

• Naproxen may reduce the blood-pressure-lowering effect of beta blockers—except atenolol—and loop diuretics.

• Naproxen may increase phenytoin side effects. Lithium blood levels may be increased by naproxen.

• Naproxen blood levels may be affected by cimetidine.

• Probenecid may increase the risk of naproxen side effects.

• Aspirin and other salicylates should never be combined with naproxen.

Food Interactions

Take naproxen with a full glass of water. Take it with food or a magnesium-aluminum antacid if it upsets your stomach.

Usual Dose

Naproxen

Adult: starting dose—250–375 mg morning and evening; up to 1250 mg a day if needed. For mild to moderate pain, take 250–275 mg every 6–8 hours.

Child (age 2 and over): 4.5 mg per lb. of body weight divided into 2 doses a day.

Child (under age 2): not recommended.

Overdosage

People have died from NSAID overdoses. Common signs of overdose are drowsiness, nausea, vomiting, diarrhea, abdominal pain, rapid breathing, rapid heartbeat, increased sweating, ringing or buzzing in the ears, confusion, disorientation, stupor, and coma. Take the victim to a hospital emergency room at once. ALWAYS bring the prescription bottle or container.

Special Information

Take each dose with a full glass of water and do not lie down for 15 to 30 minutes afterward.

Naproxen can make you drowsy or tired: Be careful when driving or operating hazardous equipment. Do not take any over-the-counter products containing acetaminophen or aspirin while taking naproxen. Avoid alcohol.

Contact your doctor if you develop rash or itching, visual disturbances, weight gain, breathing difficulties, fluid retention, hallucinations, black or tarry stools, persistent headache, or any unusual or intolerable side effect.

If you forget a dose of naproxen, take it as soon as you remember. If you take naproxen once a day and it is within 8 hours of your next dose, or if you take several doses a day and it is within 4 hours of your next dose, skip the dose you forgot and continue with your regular schedule. Never take a double dose.

Special Populations

Pregnancy/Breast-feeding

NSAIDs may affect fetal heart development during the second half of pregnancy. Pregnant women should not take naproxen without their doctor's approval. When the drug is considered crucial by your doctor, its potential benefits must be carefully weighed against its risks.

NSAIDs may pass into breast milk. There is a possibility that a nursing mother taking naproxen could affect her baby's heart or cardiovascular system. Nursing mothers who must take this drug should bottle-feed.

Seniors

Seniors may be more susceptible to side effects, especially ulcer disease.

Nasonex *see Corticosteroids, Nasal, page 274*

Generic Name

Nefazodone (neh-FAZ-oe-don)

Brand Name

Serzone

Type of Drug

Antidepressant.

Prescribed for

Depression.

General Information

A unique compound, nefazodone is chemically unrelated to other antidepressants. It interferes with the ability of nerve endings in the brain to absorb serotonin and norepinephrine, two key neurohormones. Nefazodone is broken down in the liver; severe liver disease may increase nefazodone blood levels by 25%. Very little of the drug is released through the kidneys.

Cautions and Warnings

Suicide is always a risk in severely depressed people, who should only be allowed to have minimal quantities of medication in their possession.

People with a history of **seizure disorders** may experience seizures while taking nefazodone.

People who have recently had a **heart attack** should use this drug with caution because it can substantially reduce heart rate.

Possible Side Effects

▼ Most common: weakness, dry mouth, nausea, constipation, blurred or abnormal vision, tiredness, dizziness, light-headedness, and confusion.

Possible Side Effects *(continued)*

▼ Common: upset stomach, increased appetite, cough, memory loss, tingling in the hands or feet, flushing or feelings of warmth, poor muscle coordination, and dizziness when rising from a lying or sitting position.

▼ Less common: low blood pressure, fever, chills, flu-like symptoms, joint pain, stiff neck, itching, rash, diarrhea, nausea, vomiting, thirst, sore throat, changes in sense of taste, ringing or buzzing in the ear, unusual dreams, poor coordination, tremors, muscle stiffness, reduced sex drive, urinary difficulties including infection, vaginitis, and breast pain.

▼ Rare: Rare side effects can affect your liver, gastrointestinal tract, joints, sexual function, and skin. Severe nefazodone allergy is rare. Contact your doctor if you experience any side effect not listed above.

Drug Interactions

• People who take nefazodone within 2 weeks of taking a monoamine oxidase inhibitor (MAOI) antidepressant may experience severe reactions including high fever, muscle rigidity or spasm, changes in mental state, and fluctuations in pulse, temperature, and breathing rate. People stopping nefazodone should wait at least 1 week before starting an MAOI.

• Nefazodone increases blood levels of astemizole and terfenadine (nonsedating antihistamines), which may lead to cardiac side effects associated with those drugs. Nefazodone may increase blood levels of alprazolam and triazolam (benzodiazepine anti-anxiety drugs). Do not combine these drugs with nefazodone.

• Blood levels of digoxin may be substantially increased by nefazodone. People taking these drugs together should have their digoxin blood levels checked periodically.

• The clearance of haloperidol (an antipsychotic drug) may be drastically reduced by nefazodone; the implications of this are not clear.

• Combining nefazodone and propranolol may cause substantial reductions in propranolol blood levels and substantial increases in blood levels of nefazodone. Do not take these drugs together.

- Drinking alcohol while taking nefazodone may make you very tired; avoid this combination.

Food Interactions

Take this drug on an empty stomach at least 1 hour before or 2 hours after meals.

Usual Dose

Adult: 100 mg twice a day to start. Dosage may be increased by 100 mg a week to a maximum daily dose of approximately 600 mg.

Senior: Start at half the regular adult dose and increase as needed up to 600 mg a day.

Child (under age 18): not recommended.

Overdosage

Symptoms of overdose include nausea, vomiting, and sleepiness. Overdose victims should be taken to a hospital emergency room. ALWAYS bring the prescription bottle or container.

Special Information

Several weeks of nefazodone treatment may be necessary before you notice any effect. Continue taking the medication during this period.

Call your doctor at once if you develop hives, rash, or other allergic side effects while taking nefazodone.

Nefazodone may make you drowsy. Be careful when driving or doing any task that requires concentration. Avoid alcohol.

Check with your pharmacist or doctor before taking any over-the-counter medication because of the risk of drug interactions.

Special Populations

Pregnancy/Breast-feeding

Animal studies of nefazodone suggest decreased fertility and a risk of fetal damage. When this drug is considered crucial by your doctor, its potential benefits must be carefully weighed against its risks.

It is not known if nefazodone passes into breast milk. Nursing mothers who must take this drug should consider bottle-feeding.

Seniors

Seniors, especially women, should start treatment at half the usual dose. Dosage may be gradually increased as needed, up to the maximum recommended dosage.

Generic Name

Nelfinavir (nel-FIN-uh-vere)

Brand Name

Viracept

Type of Drug

Protease inhibitor.

Prescribed for

Human immunodeficiency virus (HIV) infection.

General Information

Part of the triple-drug cocktail responsible for the most important gains in the fight against acquired immunodeficiency syndrome (AIDS), nelfinavir belongs to a group of anti-HIV drugs called protease inhibitors. Triple-drug cocktails are considered responsible for the first overall reduction in the AIDS death rate, recorded in 1996. When the HIV virus attacks a cell, it must be converted into viral DNA. Older drugs known as reverse transcriptase inhibitors interfered with this step but are inferior to protease inhibitors. Protease inhibitors work at the end of the process of HIV reproduction, at the point when proteins are "cut" into strands of exactly the right size to duplicate HIV; these proteins are cut by protease enzymes. Protease inhibitors prevent the mature HIV virus from being formed by interfering with this cutting process. Proteins that are cut to the wrong length or remain uncut are inactive. Protease inhibitors are not a cure for HIV infection or AIDS.

Protease inhibitors are always taken with 1 or 2 nucleoside antiviral drugs such as AZT, ddI, ddC, or 3TC. Protease inhibitors revolutionized HIV treatment because, when taken in combination with other drugs, they reduce the amount of HIV virus in the bloodstream to levels that are often undetectable by current methods such as CD_4 cell counts of immune system cells and viral load (amount of virus in the blood) measurements. Multiple-drug therapy has changed the current view of HIV disease from a fatal disease to a manageable chronic (long-term) illness.

People taking a protease inhibitor may still develop infection or other conditions normally associated with HIV disease. Because of this, it is very important for you to remain under the care of a doctor or other health care provider. The long-term effects of nelfinavir are not known. You may be able to spread the HIV virus to others even if you are on triple-drug therapy.

Cautions and Warnings

Do not take nelfinavir if you are **allergic** to it. People with **liver disease** or **cirrhosis** break down nelfinavir more slowly than do those with normal liver function.

Nelfinavir may raise **blood sugar,** worsen **diabetes,** or bring out latent diabetes.

Possible Side Effects

▼ Most common: diarrhea.

▼ Common: liver inflammation.

▼ Less common: nausea, abdominal pain, gas, weakness, and rash.

▼ Rare: Rare side effects can occur in almost any part of the body including your blood, muscles and joints, gastrointestinal tract, kidneys, and eyes, and can affect your mental state and sexual function. Contact your doctor if you experience any side effect not listed above.

Drug Interactions

• Anticonvulsant medication such as carbamazepine, phenytoin, or phenobarbital may reduce the amount of nelfinavir in the blood.

• Combining nelfinavir with indinavir or saquinavir, other protease inhibitors, results in large increases in the amounts of both drugs in the blood. Other drugs that increase the amount of nelfinavir in the blood are ketoconazole and ritonavir.

• Combining rifabutin with nelfinavir lowers the amount of nelfinavir in the blood and raises the amount of rifabutin.

Rifabutin dosage should be cut in half when this combination is used.

• Do not combine rifampin and nelfinavir.

• Avoid combining nelfinavir with terfenadine or astemizole or severe side effects may result.

• Nelfinavir reduces the amount of oral contraceptive hormones in your bloodstream (see "Special Information").

• If you combine nelfinavir, lamivudine, and zidovudine (an AIDS drug—also known as AZT), your AZT dosage may have to be increased.

Food Interactions

Take nelfinavir with food.

Usual Dose

Adult and Child (age 14 and over): 250 mg every 8 hours around the clock.

Child (age 2–13): 9–13 mg per lb. of body weight.

Overdosage

Little is known about the effects of nelfinavir overdose except that it may cause severe side effects. Take overdose victims to a hospital emergency room for treatment. ALWAYS bring the prescription bottle or container.

Special Information

It is imperative for you to take your HIV medication exactly as prescribed. Missing or skipping doses of nelfinavir increases your risk of becoming resistant to the drug and losing the benefits of nelfinavir therapy.

Nelfinavir does not cure AIDS. It will not prevent you from transmitting the HIV virus to another person; you must still practice safe sex.

Diarrhea associated with nelfinavir may be controlled by using loperamide, an over-the-counter remedy.

Do not depend on oral contraceptives while taking nelfinavir. Use another contraceptive method.

Report anything unusual to your doctor.

If you forget a dose, take it as soon as you remember. If it is almost time for your next dose, skip the dose you forgot and continue with your regular schedule. Do not take a double dose.

Special Populations

Pregnancy/Breast-feeding

The safety of using nelfinavir during pregnancy is not known. When this drug is considered crucial by your doctor, its potential benefits must be carefully weighed against its risks.

Nursing mothers with HIV should always bottle-feed, regardless of whether they take this drug, to avoid transmitting the virus.

Seniors

Seniors may take nelfinavir without special restriction.

Brand Name

Neosporin Ophthalmic

Generic Ingredients

Gramicidin + Neomycin Sulfate + Polymyxin B Sulfate Ⓖ

Other Brand Names

AK-Spore

Type of Drug

Ophthalmic and antibiotic combination.

Prescribed for

Superficial eye infection.

General Information

Neosporin Ophthalmic is a combination of antibiotics that is effective against the most common types of eye infection. It is most useful when the infecting organism is known to be sensitive to any of the 3 antibiotics contained in Neosporin Ophthalmic. It may also be useful when the infecting organism is not known because of the drug's broad range of coverage. This product is also available as an eye ointment with a minor formula change—bacitracin is substituted for gramicidin. Both the eyedrops and eye ointment are used for the same kinds of eye infection.

Cautions and Warnings

Do not use Neosporin Ophthalmic if you are **allergic** or **sensitive** to any of its ingredients.

Prolonged use of any antibiotic product in the eye should be avoided because of the risk of becoming sensitive to it and because other organisms such as fungi may grow. If the infection does not clear up within a few days, call your doctor.

Possible Side Effects

▼ Less common: occasional eye irritation, itching, or burning.

Drug Interactions

None known.

Usual Dose

1–2 drops in the affected eye 2–4 times a day or more frequently if the infection is severe.

Overdosage

There is not enough medicine in this product to cause serious problems. Call your local poison control center or a hospital emergency room for more information. If you seek treatment, ALWAYS bring the prescription bottle or container.

Special Information

To avoid infection, do not touch the eyedropper tip to your finger, eyelid, or any other surface. Wait at least 5 minutes before using another eyedrop or eye ointment.

Call your doctor if the itching or burning does not go away after a few minutes, or if redness, irritation, swelling, visual disturbance, loss of vision, or eye pain persists.

In general, you should not wear contact lenses if you have an eye infection but your doctor may determine that the use of lenses is acceptable in your situation.

If you forget to administer a dose, do so as soon as you remember. If it is almost time for your next dose, skip the forgotten dose and continue with your regular schedule. Do not take a double dose.

Special Populations

Pregnancy/Breast-feeding
This drug has been found to be safe for use during pregnancy and breast-feeding. Remember to check with your doctor before taking any drug if you are pregnant.

Seniors
Seniors may take this drug without special restriction.

Neurontin see Tiagabine, page 1009

Generic Name

Nevirapine (nev-EYE-ruh-peen)

Brand Name
Viramune

Type of Drug
Antiviral.

Prescribed for
Human immunodeficiency virus (HIV) in adults whose condition has deteriorated on other anti-HIV treatments.

General Information
Nevirapine is a non-nucleoside reverse transcriptase inhibitor (NNRTI). It inhibits the reverse transcriptase (RT) enzyme, necessary for reproduction of the HIV virus in body cells, by binding directly to it. The duration of benefit from taking this drug may be limited because HIV can become resistant to nevirapine. In one study of nevirapine plus zidovudine (AZT), resistance began to develop in some people as soon as 2 weeks after treatment began. For this reason, nevirapine is generally prescribed as part of a triple therapy anti-HIV "cocktail."

Cautions and Warnings
People who are **allergic** or **sensitive** to nevirapine should avoid it.

Severe and **potentially fatal skin reactions** may develop in people taking this drug, including Stevens-Johnson syndrome (symptoms include fever, skin blisters, mouth sores, eye irritation, swelling, muscle or joint aches, and not feeling well). Call your doctor at once if any of these symptoms or any other skin reactions develop. Most rashes occur within the first 6 weeks of nevirapine treatment.

Possible Side Effects

▼ Most common: rash, fever, nausea, headache, and changes in liver function tests.

▼ Less common: abdominal pain, mouth or throat sores, tingling in the hands or feet, muscle aches, and liver inflammation.

▼ Rare: diarrhea, pain, and changes of sensation in the arms or legs.

Drug Interactions

• Rifampin and rifabutin may stimulate liver enzymes that break down nevirapine, reducing the amount of nevirapine in the blood. Neither of these drugs should be combined with nevirapine.

• The enzyme systems that break down protease inhibitors are stimulated by nevirapine. Combining nevirapine and a protease inhibitor may reduce the amount of protease inhibitor in the blood, reducing its effectiveness and increasing the risk of protease inhibitor resistance.

• Combining nevirapine with an oral contraceptive may reduce the effectiveness of the contraceptive by lowering the amount of hormone in the blood.

Food Interactions

None known.

Usual Dose

Adult: starting dose—200 mg a day for 2 weeks. Maintenance dose—200 mg twice a day in combination with a nucleoside-type antiviral such as didanosine or AZT.

Child: not recommended.

Overdosage

Little is known about the effects of nevirapine overdose. Call your local emergency room or poison control center for more information. If you seek treatment, ALWAYS bring the prescription bottle or container.

Special Information

Call your doctor at once if you develop any rash or other skin side effect (see "Cautions and Warnings").

Nevirapine does not cure AIDS. It will not prevent you from transmitting HIV to another person; you must still practice safe sex.

Take nevirapine according to your doctor's direction; this is very important in preventing the development of drug-resistant HIV. If you do forget a dose of nevirapine, take it as soon as you remember. If it almost time for your next dose, skip the dose you forgot and continue with your regular schedule. If you forget your nevirapine for a week, you will have to start the treatment program all over again, beginning with 200 mg a day for 2 weeks.

Special Populations

Pregnancy/Breast-feeding

Animal studies have shown no effect on the developing fetus but nothing is known about the safety of using nevirapine during human pregnancy. When this drug is considered crucial by your doctor, its potential benefits must be carefully weighed against its risks.

Nevirapine passes into breast milk. Nursing mothers with HIV should always bottle-feed, regardless of whether they take this drug, to avoid transmitting the virus.

Seniors

Seniors may take nevirapine without special restriction.

Generic Name

Niacin (NYE-uh-sin) G

Brand Names

Niacor   Nicolar
Niaspan

Type of Drug

Vitamin.

Prescribed for

Pellagra (niacin deficiency); also prescribed for high blood levels of cholesterol and triglycerides and to dilate (widen) blood vessels.

General Information

Niacin, also known as vitamin B_3 and nicotinic acid, is essential to maintaining health through the role it plays in enzyme activity. It is effective in lowering blood fat levels and helps to dilate blood vessels, but we do not know exactly how it works. The effect of niacin on blood fats is seen as early as 1 week after treatment is started.

Cautions and Warnings

Do not take niacin if you are **sensitive** or **allergic** to it or related drugs or have **liver disease,** stomach **ulcer,** severely **low blood pressure, gout,** or **hemorrhage** (bleeding).

When you are taking niacin in therapeutic dosages, your doctor should periodically check your liver function and blood-sugar level. People with **diabetes** may experience an increase in blood sugar. Blood levels of uric acid may rise; people who are prone to gout may experience an attack.

Possible Side Effects

▼ Most common: flushing, which may occur within 2 hours of taking the first dose of niacin.

▼ Less common: decreased sugar tolerance in people with diabetes, activation of stomach ulcer, jaundice (symptoms include yellowing of the skin or whites of the eyes), upset stomach, oily or dry skin, aggravation of skin conditions such as acne, itching, high blood levels of uric acid, low blood pressure, headache, tingling in the hands or feet, rash, abnormal heartbeats, and dizziness.

Drug Interactions

• Niacin may increase the effect of blood-pressure-lowering drugs, causing dizziness when rising quickly from a sitting or lying position.

• Niacin may interfere with sulfinpyrazone (a gout medication).

• Combining lovastatin and niacin may lead to the destruction of skeletal muscle. One case of this has been reported.

Food Interactions

Take niacin with or after meals to reduce the risk of upset stomach.

Usual Dose

Vitamin Supplement: 25 mg a day.

Niacin Deficiency: not more than 100 mg a day.

Pellagra: not more than 500 mg a day.

High Blood-Fat Levels: 1–2 g 3 times a day to start; take with a glass of cold water to help you swallow; dosage should be increased slowly.

Overdosage

Symptoms may include drug side effects. Take the victim to a hospital emergency room. ALWAYS bring the prescription bottle or container.

Special Information

Skin reactions may occur within 2 hours of the first dose and include flushing and warmth, especially in the face, ears, or neck; tingling; itching; and headache. Call your doctor if these effects do not disappear as you continue taking niacin.

If you forget a dose, take it as soon as you remember. If it is almost time for your next dose, skip the missed dose and continue with your regular schedule. Do not take a double dose.

Special Populations

Pregnancy/Breast-feeding

When used in normal dosages, niacin may and should be taken during pregnancy as part of a prenatal vitamin formulation. Dosages larger than 25 mg a day are not recommended during pregnancy.

Niacin passes into breast milk. Usual doses (up to 25 mg a day) will not affect a nursing infant. Larger doses used for lowering blood fats may affect a nursing infant.

Seniors
Seniors may take this drug without special restriction.

Generic Name

Nicardipine (nye-KAR-dih-pene)

Brand Name

Cardene   Cardene SR

Type of Drug

Calcium channel blocker.

Prescribed for

Angina pectoris, high blood pressure, and congestive heart failure.

General Information

Nicardipine hydrochloride is one of many calcium channel blockers available in the U.S. These drugs block the passage of calcium, an essential factor in muscle contraction, into the heart and smooth muscles. Such blockage of calcium interferes with the contraction of these muscles, which in turn dilates (widens) the veins and vessels that supply blood to them. This dilating effect reduces blood pressure, the amount of oxygen used by the heart muscle, and the risk of blood vessel spasm. Nicardipine is therefore useful in treating not only high blood pressure but also angina pectoris (brief attacks of chest pain), a condition related to poor oxygen supply to the heart muscle.

Nicardipine affects the movement of calcium only into muscle cells; it has no effect on calcium in the blood.

Cautions and Warnings

Nicardipine can **slow your heart rate** and interfere with normal electrical conduction in heart muscle. For some people, this action can result in temporary heart stoppage, but such a reaction will not occur in people whose hearts are otherwise healthy.

You should not use nicardipine if you have had a **stroke** or bleeding in the brain or if you have advanced **hardening of**

the arteries—particularly the aorta—because the drug can cause heart failure.

People who take nicardipine for congestive **heart failure** should be aware that the drug may aggravate the condition.

If you are also taking a **beta blocker,** its dosage should be reduced gradually rather than stopped abruptly when starting on nicardipine.

Nicardipine dosage should be adjusted in the presence of **kidney or liver disease.**

Nicardipine may cause **angina** when treatment is first started, when dosage is increased, or if the drug is rapidly withdrawn. This can be avoided by reducing dosage gradually.

Studies of calcium channel blockers—usually those taken several times a day, not those taken only once daily—have shown that people taking them are more likely to have a **heart attack** than are people taking beta blockers or other medication for the same purposes. Discuss this with your doctor to be sure you are receiving the best possible treatment.

Possible Side Effects

▼ Most common: dizziness or light-headedness; fluid accumulation in the hands, legs, or feet; headache; weakness or fatigue; heart palpitations; angina; and facial flushing.

▼ Less common: low blood pressure; abnormal heart rhythms; fainting; increase or decrease in heart rate; heart failure; nausea; rash; nervousness; tingling in the hands or feet; hallucinations; temporary memory loss; difficulty sleeping; weakness; diarrhea; vomiting; constipation; upset stomach; itching; unusual sensitivity to the sun; painful or stiff joints; liver inflammation; increased urination, especially at night; infection; allergic reactions; sore throat; and hyperactivity.

Drug Interactions

• Combining nicardipine with a beta-blocking drug in order to treat high blood pressure is usually well tolerated but may lead to heart failure in susceptible people.

• Blood levels of cyclosporine may be increased by nicardipine, increasing the chance for cyclosporine-related kidney damage.

• The effect of quinidine (an antiarrhythmic) may be altered by nicardipine.

• Cimetidine and ranitidine may increase the amount of nicardipine in the bloodstream.

• Combining nicardipine with fentanyl (a narcotic pain reliever) may cause very low blood pressure.

Food Interactions

Nicardipine is best taken on an empty stomach at least 1 hour before or 2 hours after meals, but it may be taken with food or milk if it upsets your stomach. Avoid high-fat meals and grapefruit juice while on this drug.

Usual Dose

Immediate-Release: 20–40 mg 3 times a day. People with kidney disease should take 20 mg 3 times a day. People with liver disease should take 20 mg 2 times a day. Seniors should start with 20 mg 2–3 times a day and increase dosage gradually.

Sustained-Release: 30–60 mg 2 times a day. People with kidney disease should take 30 mg 2 times a day.

Overdosage

Symptoms of nicardipine overdose are very low blood pressure and reduced heart rate. Nicardipine can be removed from the victim's stomach by inducing vomiting with ipecac syrup—available at any pharmacy. This must be done within 30 minutes of the actual overdose, before the drug can be absorbed into the blood. Once symptoms develop or if more than 30 minutes have passed since the overdose, the victim must be taken to an emergency room. ALWAYS bring the prescription bottle or container.

Special Information

Call your doctor if you develop any of the following symptoms: worsening angina pain; swelling of the hands, legs, or feet; severe dizziness; constipation or nausea; or very low blood pressure.

Some people may experience a slight increase in blood pressure just before their next dose is due. You will be able to see this effect only if you use a home blood-pressure-monitoring device. If this happens, contact your doctor.

If you take nicardipine 3 times a day and forget a dose, take it as soon as you remember. If it is almost time for your next dose, take it and space the remaining doses evenly throughout the rest of the day. If you take nicardipine 2 times a day and forget a dose, take it as soon as you remember. If it is almost time for your next dose, skip the dose you forgot and continue with your regular schedule. Never take a double dose.

Special Populations

Pregnancy/Breast-feeding

In animal studies, large doses of nicardipine have been shown to harm the fetus. Nicardipine should be avoided by women who are or might be pregnant. When your doctor considers this drug crucial, its potential benefits must be carefully weighed against its risks.

Nicardipine passes into breast milk; nursing mothers who must take this drug should consider bottle-feeding.

Seniors

Seniors may be more sensitive to the side effects of nicardipine and require reduced dosage.

Generic Name

Nicotine (NIK-uh-teen) G

Brand Names

Habitrol	Nicotrol
Nicoderm	Nicotrol Inhaler
Nicorette	Nicotrol NS
Nicorette DS	ProStep

Type of Drug

Smoking deterrent.

Prescribed for

Addiction to cigarettes. Nicotine gum has been prescribed with haloperidol for children with Tourette's syndrome.

General Information

Nicotine replacement products are prescribed for short-term treatment and make cigarette withdrawal easier for many people. Because nicotine addiction also has a psychological component, counseling or other psychological support is necessary in order for a smoking cessation program to be successful.

The major advantage of patches over chewing gum or nasal spray is their convenience and ease of use. There are differences among the various patch products in terms of how much nicotine is absorbed into the bloodstream. All of the products are labeled according to the amount of nicotine absorbed. Obese men absorb significantly less nicotine.

Cautions and Warnings

Do not use nicotine if you are **sensitive** or **allergic** to it.

Nicotine should be used only by people addicted to nicotine. It should not be used during the period immediately following a **heart attack** or if you have severe **abnormal heart rhythms** or **angina pains**.

People with severe **temporomandibular joint (TMJ) disease** should not chew nicotine gum.

People with **heart conditions** must be evaluated by a cardiologist before starting treatment.

Nicotine should be used with caution by people with **diabetes** who take insulin and by people with an **overactive thyroid, kidney or liver disease, pheochromocytoma, hypertension** (high blood pressure), stomach **ulcer**, or chronic **dental problems** that might be worsened by nicotine chewing gum.

The nasal spray should not be used by people with **asthma, bronchospasm, allergic rhinitis, sinusitis**, or **nasal polyps**.

It is possible to become addicted to nicotine replacement products. Your nicotine addiction may worsen while using this product.

Possible Side Effects

Chewing Gum

▼ Most common: injury to the gums, jaw, or teeth; sore mouth or throat; stomach growling due to swallowing air while chewing.

▼ Common: nausea, vomiting, upset stomach, and hiccups.

Possible Side Effects *(continued)*

▼ Less common: excessive salivation, dizziness, light-headedness, irritability, headache, more frequent bowel movements, diarrhea, constipation, gas pain, dry mouth, hoarseness, flushing, sneezing, coughing, sleeplessness, swelling of the arms or legs, hypertension, heart palpitations, rapid and abnormal heartbeat, confusion, convulsions, depression, euphoria (feeling "high"), numbness, tingling in the hands or feet, ringing or buzzing in the ears, fainting, weakness, redness, itching, and rash.

Transdermal Patch
▼ Most common: feeling tired and irritation at the patch site. Transdermal systems may be more irritating to people with eczema or other skin conditions.
▼ Common: weakness, back pain, body ache, diarrhea, upset stomach, headache, sleeplessness, dizziness, nervousness, unusual dreams, increased cough or sore throat, muscle and joint pain, changes in sense of taste, and painful menstruation.
▼ Less common: chest pain, allergic reaction (symptoms include hives, breathing difficulties, and peeling skin), dry mouth, abdominal pain, vomiting, poor concentration, tingling in the hands or feet, sinus irritation or inflammation, increased sweating, and hypertension.

Nasal Spray
▼ Most common: nose, throat, and eye irritation.

Drug Interactions

• Heavy smokers who suddenly stop smoking may experience an increase in the effects of drugs whose breakdown is stimulated by cigarettes, including: acetaminophen, theophylline, imipramine, pentazocine, furosemide, oxazepam, propranolol, and propoxyphene hydrochloride.

• Stopping nicotine may make you more sensitive to the effects of caffeine.

• Any drug that affects the nervous system—either blockers or stimulants—may be affected by nicotine. Your doctor may need to make dosage adjustments.

• Smoking may reduce the effects of furosemide (a diuretic). Once you stop smoking, the drug's effect may increase and your dosage may need adjustment.

• The absorption of glutethimide (a sleeping pill) may be increased when you stop smoking. Also, more insulin may be absorbed into the blood after each injection. Your doctor may have to reevaluate your insulin dosage.

• More propoxyphene (a pain reliever) may be absorbed after you stop smoking, increasing the risk of side effects.

Food Interactions

Do not eat or drink anything while or immediately after you chew nicotine gum. Caffeine, juice, wine, and soft drinks may interfere with its effects.

Usual Dose

Chewing Gum: 1 piece of gum whenever you feel the urge for a cigarette; do not use more than 30 pieces a day. Gradually reduce the number of pieces you chew and the time you chew each piece every 4–7 days. Substituting sugarless gum for nicotine gum may help in the process of gradual dosage reduction. Each piece contains 2–4 mg of nicotine.

Transdermal Patch: Apply the patch to the skin as soon as you remove it from the package. Nicotrol patches should be applied when you get up in the morning and removed at bedtime. Prescription nicotine patches should be left on for 24 hours at a time. Use a different skin site when applying a new patch. The dosage of the patch will be gradually reduced by your doctor.

Nasal Spray: 1–2 sprays in each nostril up to 5 times an hour. The spray should be used at least 8 times a day to ease symptoms of nicotine withdrawal. Do not use more than 40 doses a day.

Overdosage

Overdose may be deadly. Symptoms include excessive salivation, nausea, vomiting, diarrhea, abdominal pain, headache, cold sweats, dizziness, hearing and visual disturbances, weakness, and confusion. These symptoms may be followed by fainting; very low blood pressure; a pulse that is weak, rapid, and irregular; convulsions; and death by paralysis of the muscles that control breathing.

Nicotine stimulates the brain's vomiting center, making this reaction common but not automatic; spontaneous vomiting may be sufficient to remove the poison from the victim's system. In case of overdose, call your local poison control center or a hospital emergency room. If the victim has not already vomited, you may be told to induce vomiting with ipecac syrup—available at any pharmacy—before taking the victim to an emergency room. If you seek treatment, ALWAYS bring the nicotine package.

Special Information

When using the gum, follow the product instructions. Chew each piece slowly and intermittently for about 30 minutes. Rapid chewing releases the nicotine too quickly and may lead to side effects including nausea, hiccups, and throat irritation. Do not chew more than 30 pieces a day. The amount of gum chewed should be gradually reduced and stopped after 3 months of successful treatment.

When administering the nasal spray, tilt your head back slightly and do not sniff or inhale through your nose. A dose consists of 1 spray in each nostril. Administering less than 8 doses a day may not be effective. Do not exceed 40 doses a day. The spray should not be used for longer than 6 months.

Do not store nicotine patches in an area that is warmer than 86°F. Slight discoloration is not a sign of loss of potency, but do not store a patch after you have removed it from its pouch. Nicotine patches should not be used for more than 3 consecutive months.

Keep nicotine patches and nasal spray containers—used or unused—out of the reach of children or pets to avoid accidental poisoning.

Special Populations

Pregnancy/Breast-feeding
Nicotine is not safe for use during pregnancy. It is known to cause fetal harm when used during the last 3 months of pregnancy and is associated with breathing difficulties in newborns and miscarriage.

Nicotine passes into breast milk. Nursing mothers who use it should bottle-feed.

Seniors
Seniors may be more sensitive to side effects including weakness, dizziness, and body aches.

Generic Name

Nifedipine (nih-FED-ih-pene) Ⓖ

Brand Names

Adalat	Procardia
Adalat CC	Procardia XL

Type of Drug

Calcium channel blocker.

Prescribed for

Angina pectoris, Prinzmetal's angina, and high blood pressure; also prescribed for migraine headache prevention, asthma, heart failure, Raynaud's disease, disorders of the esophagus, gallbladder and kidney stone attacks, severe high blood pressure triggered by pregnancy, and premature labor.

General Information

Nifedipine is one of many calcium channel blockers available in the U.S. These drugs block the passage of calcium, an essential factor in muscle contractions, into the heart and smooth muscles. Such blockage of calcium interferes with the contraction of these muscles, which in turn dilates (widens) the veins and vessels that supply blood to them. This dilating effect reduces blood pressure, the amount of oxygen used by the heart muscle, and the risk of blood vessel spasm. Nifedipine is therefore useful in treating not only high blood pressure but also angina pectoris (brief attacks of chest pain), a condition related to poor oxygen supply to the heart muscle.

Nifedipine affects the movement of calcium only into muscle cells; it has no effect on calcium in the blood.

Nifedipine capsules contain liquid medication. In cases in which the drug is needed in the blood immediately, the capsules may be punctured and their content squeezed under the tongue; the medication is rapidly absorbed into the blood when taken in this manner. Thus nifedipine capsules are particularly useful when extremely high blood pressure must be lowered as quickly as possible. Some researchers assert that biting the capsule and swallowing the contents is an even faster way of absorbing the drug.

Cautions and Warnings

Nifedipine may cause unwanted **low blood pressure** in some people who take it for reasons other than hypertension.

Patients taking a beta-blocking drug who begin taking nifedipine may develop an increase in incidences of **angina** pain. Angina may also intensify when nifedipine is first started, when it is increased, or if it is stopped abruptly.

Studies have shown that people taking calcium channel blockers—usually those taken several times a day, not those that are taken only once daily—have a greater chance of having a **heart attack** than people taking beta blockers or other medications for the same purposes. Discuss this with your doctor to be sure you are receiving the best possible treatment.

Congestive **heart failure** has, on rare occasions, developed in people taking nifedipine.

Do not take this drug if you have had an **allergic reaction** to it in the past.

Nifedipine may interfere with one of the mechanisms by which **blood clots** form, especially if you are also taking aspirin. Call your doctor if you develop unusual bruises, bleeding, or black-and-blue marks.

People with kidney disease or severe **liver disease** may require dosage adjustments.

Possible Side Effects

Nifedipine side effects are generally mild and rarely cause people to stop taking the drug.

▼ Most common: swelling of the ankles, feet, and legs; dizziness or light-headedness; flushing; a feeling of warmth; and nausea.

▼ Less common: headache; weakness, shakiness, or jitteriness; giddiness; muscle cramps, inflammation, and pain; nervousness; mood changes; heart palpitations; heart failure; heart attack; breathing difficulties; coughing; fluid in the lungs; wheezing; stuffy nose; fever and chills; and sore throat.

▼ Rare: Rare side effects can occur in your heart, stomach or intestines, urinary tract, and joints and muscles and can affect your mental and sexual function, hearing, and balance. Contact your doctor if you experience any side effect not listed above.

Drug Interactions

• Nifedipine may interact with beta-blocking drugs to cause heart failure, very low blood pressure, or an increased incidence of angina pain. However, in many cases these drugs have been taken together with no problem.

• Nifedipine may cause unexpected blood pressure reduction in patients who also take other drugs to control their high blood pressure. Low blood pressure can also result from taking nifedipine with fentanyl (a narcotic pain reliever).

• Cimetidine and ranitidine increase the amount of nifedipine in the blood and may account for a slight increase in nifedipine's effect.

• The combination of quinidine (an antiarrhythmic) and nifedipine must be used with caution because it can produce low blood pressure, very slow heart rate, abnormal heart rhythm, and swelling in the arms or legs.

• On rare occasions, nifedipine may increase the effects of oral anticoagulant (blood-thinning) drugs.

• Nifedipine may intensify the effects of cyclosporine, digoxin, and theophylline products, increasing the chances of side effects from those drugs.

Food Interactions

Avoid drinking grapefruit juice if you are taking nifedipine.

Usual Dose

Immediate-Release: 10–30 mg 3 times a day. Do not exceed 180 mg a day.

Sustained-Release: 30–60 mg once a day.

Do not stop taking nifedipine abruptly. The dosage should be reduced gradually.

Overdosage

Overdose of nifedipine can cause low blood pressure. If you think you have taken an overdose of nifedipine, call your doctor or go to a hospital emergency room. ALWAYS bring the prescription bottle or container.

Special Information

Call your doctor if you develop constipation, nausea, very low blood pressure, worsening angina, swelling in the hands or feet, breathing difficulties, increased heart pain, or dizziness or light-headedness, or if other side effects are particularly bothersome or persistent.

If you are taking nifedipine for high blood pressure, be sure to continue taking your medication and follow any instructions for diet restriction or other treatments. High blood pressure is a condition with few recognizable symptoms; it may seem to you that you are taking medication for no good reason. Call your doctor or pharmacist if you have any questions.

If you take Procardia XL, be sure not to break or crush the tablets. You may notice an empty tablet in your stool. This is not a cause for alarm, because the drug is normally released without actually destroying the tablet.

It is important to maintain good dental hygiene while taking nifedipine and to use extra care when using your toothbrush or dental floss: The drug may make you more susceptible to some infections.

If you forget a dose of nifedipine and you take it 3 or more times a day, take it as soon as you remember. If it is almost time for your next dose, take the dose you forgot and space the rest evenly throughout the remainder of the day. If you take nifedipine 2 times a day and forget a dose, take it as soon as you remember. If it is almost time for your next dose, skip the dose you forgot and continue with your regular schedule. Never take a double dose.

Special Populations

Pregnancy/Breast-feeding
Nifedipine crosses into the fetal blood circulation. It has been used to treat severe high blood pressure associated with pregnancy without causing any unusual effect on the fetus. Nevertheless, women who are or might be pregnant should not take nifedipine without their doctor's approval. When this drug is considered crucial by your doctor, its potential benefits must be carefully weighed against its risks.

Small amounts of nifedipine may pass into breast milk. You must consider the potential effect on the nursing infant if breast-feeding while taking this medication.

Seniors
Seniors are more sensitive to the effects of nifedipine and may require dosage adjustments.

Generic Name

Nimodipine (nih-MOE-dih-pene)

Brand Name

Nimotop

Type of Drug

Calcium channel blocker.

Prescribed for

Functional losses following a stroke and migraine and cluster headaches.

General Information

Unlike other calcium channel blockers, nimodipine has a negligible effect on the heart. It is the only calcium channel blocker proven to improve neurological function after a stroke. Nimodipine has a greater effect on blood vessels in the brain than on those in other parts of the body.

Cautions and Warnings

Nimodipine should not be taken if you are **sensitive** or **allergic** to it.

People with **liver disease,** including cirrhosis, may require reduced dosage.

Possible Side Effects

▼ Most common: diarrhea, low blood pressure, and headache.

▼ Less common: swelling of the arms or legs, high blood pressure, heart failure, rapid heartbeat, changes in the electrocardiogram, depression, memory loss, psychosis, paranoid feelings, hallucinations, nausea, itching, acne, rash, anemia, bleeding or bruising, abnormal blood clotting, flushing, breathing difficulties, stomach bleeding, and muscle cramps.

▼ Rare: dizziness, heart attack, liver inflammation or jaundice, vomiting, and sexual difficulties.

Drug Interactions

- Calcium channel blockers may cause bleeding when taken alone or combined with aspirin.
- Combining nimodipine with a beta-blocking drug is usually tolerated well but may lead to heart failure in susceptible people.
- Calcium channel blockers, including nimodipine, may add to the effects of digoxin.

Food Interactions

Nimodipine is best taken at least 1 hour before or 2 hours after meals, but may be taken with food or milk if it upsets your stomach. Avoid drinking grapefruit juice if you are taking this drug.

Usual Dose

Stroke: 60 mg 4 times a day, beginning within 96 hours after the stroke and continuing for 21 days.

Migraine Headache: 40 mg 3 times a day.

Overdosage

Symptoms of nimodipine overdose are nausea, weakness, dizziness, drowsiness, confusion, and slurred speech. Blood pressure and heart rate may also be affected. Nimodipine can be removed from a victim's stomach by giving ipecac syrup—available at any pharmacy—to induce vomiting, but this should be done only under a doctor's supervision or direction. Once symptoms develop, the victim must be taken to a hospital emergency room for treatment. ALWAYS bring the prescription bottle or container.

Special Information

Call your doctor if you develop any of the following symptoms: swelling of the arms or legs, breathing difficulties, severe dizziness, constipation, or nausea.

Patients who are unable to swallow nimodipine capsules because of their condition may have the liquid withdrawn from the capsule with a syringe, mixed with other liquids, and given orally or through a feeding tube.

If you forget a dose of nimodipine, take it as soon as you remember. If it is almost time for your next dose, skip the dose you forgot and continue with your regular schedule. Call your doctor if you miss more than 2 consecutive doses.

Special Populations

Pregnancy/Breast-feeding
Animal studies have shown that nimodipine may cause fetal malformation. Nimodipine should be avoided by women who are or might be pregnant. When your doctor considers this drug crucial, its potential benefits must be carefully weighed against its risks.

Nimodipine passes into breast milk. Nursing mothers who must take nimodipine should bottle-feed.

Seniors
Seniors, especially those with severe liver disease, may be more sensitive to side effects.

Generic Name

Nisoldipine (nih-SOL-dih-pene)

Brand Name

Sular

Type of Drug

Calcium channel blocker.

Prescribed for

Hypertension (high blood pressure).

General Information

Nisoldipine is one of many calcium channel blockers available in the U.S. These drugs block the passage of calcium, an essential factor in muscle contraction, into the heart and smooth muscles. Such blockage of calcium interferes with the contraction of these muscles, which in turn dilates (widens) the veins and vessels that supply blood to them. This dilating effect reduces blood pressure, the amount of oxygen used by the heart muscle, and the risk of blood-vessel spasm. Nisoldipine is therefore useful in treating not only high blood pressure but also angina pectoris (brief attacks of chest pain), a condition related to poor oxygen supply to the heart muscle.

Nisoldipine affects the movement of calcium only into muscle cells; it has no effect on calcium in the blood.

Cautions and Warnings

Do not take this drug if you have had an **allergic reaction** to it or to a chemically similar calcium channel blocker. Use nisoldipine with caution if you have **heart failure,** since calcium channel blockers may worsen the condition.

On rare occasions, nisoldipine may cause very **low blood pressure**.

Nisoldipine may cause **angina** pain when treatment is first started, when dosage is increased, or if the drug is rapidly withdrawn. This can be avoided by reducing dosage gradually.

Studies of calcium channel blockers—usually those taken several times a day and not those taken only once daily—show that people taking them are more likely to have a **heart attack** than are people taking beta blockers or other medication for the same purposes.

People with severe **liver disease** may require dosage adjustments.

Possible Side Effects

▼ Most common: headache and swelling in the arms or legs.

▼ Common: sore throat, flushing, sinus irritation, and heart palpitations.

▼ Less common: chest pain, nausea, and rash.

▼ Rare: Rare side effects can occur in almost any part of the body. Contact your doctor if you experience any side effect not listed above.

Drug Interactions

• Nisoldipine may interact with beta-blocking drugs to cause heart failure, very low blood pressure, or an increased incidence of angina pain. However, in most cases these drugs can be taken together with no problem.

• When nisoldipine is combined with cimetidine, blood levels of nisoldipine increase substantially.

• Quinidine reduces the amount of nisoldipine in the blood, but maximum levels remain unaffected.

Food Interactions

Avoid fatty foods and grapefruit with your nisoldipine dose.

Usual Dose

Adult: starting dose—20 mg a day. Maintenance dose—40 or 60 mg, as needed.

Seniors and People with Liver Disease: starting dose—10 mg a day. Maintenance dose—40 or 60 mg, as needed and tolerated.

Child: not recommended.

Overdosage

Little is known about the effects of nisoldipine overdose. Overdose of chemically similar calcium channel blockers can cause very low blood pressure, nausea, dizziness, weakness, drowsiness, confusion and slurred speech, reduced heart efficiency, and unusual heart rhythms. Victims of a nisoldipine overdose should be taken to a hospital emergency room. ALWAYS bring the prescription bottle or container.

Special Information

Do not crush, chew, or divide nisoldipine tablets.

Call your doctor if you develop swelling in the arms or legs, breathing difficulties, abnormal heartbeat, increased heart pain, dizziness, constipation, nausea, light-headedness, or very low blood pressure.

If you forget to take a dose of nisoldipine, take it as soon as you remember. If it is almost time for your next regular dose, skip the dose you forgot and continue with your regular schedule. Do not take a double dose.

Special Populations

Pregnancy/Breast-feeding

At high doses, nisoldipine affected the development of animal fetuses. Women who are or might become pregnant should not take nisoldipine without their doctor's approval. When your doctor considers nisoldipine to be crucial, its potential benefits must be carefully weighed against its risks.

It is not known if nisoldipine passes into breast milk. Nursing mothers who must take it should consider bottle-feeding.

Seniors

Seniors may have more nisoldipine in their blood and require lower starting doses. Headache is less common in older adults.

Generic Name

Nitrofurantoin (NYE-troe-few-RAN-toe-in) Ⓖ

Brand Names

Furadantin
Macrobid

Macrodantin

Type of Drug

Urinary anti-infective.

Prescribed for

Urinary tract infections (UTIs), such as pyelonephritis, pyelitis, and cystitis.

General Information

Nitrofurantoin is helpful in treating UTIs because large amounts of it pass into the urine. It works by interfering with the metabolism of carbohydrates, or sugars, in the infecting bacteria. It may also interfere with the formation of the bacterial cell wall.

Cautions and Warnings

Do not take nitrofurantoin if you are **allergic** to it or have **kidney disease**.

Rarely, severe **chest pain, breathing difficulties, cough, fever,** and **chills** may develop within a few hours to 3 weeks after taking nitrofurantoin. These symptoms usually go away within 1 to 2 days after you stop taking it. Nitrofurantoin therapy may cause **cough, breathing difficulties,** and **feelings of ill health** after 1 to 6 months. Respiratory failure and death have occurred in a few cases.

Rarely, nitrofurantoin causes **hemolytic anemia**. People with a deficiency of the enzyme G-6-PD are most susceptible to this reaction and should not take nitrofurantoin.

Rarely, nitrofurantoin causes **hepatitis,** which may lead to death. It is most likely to develop during long-term treatment.

This drug is only used to treat UTIs caused by organisms susceptible to nitrofurantoin. It should not be used to treat **infections in other parts of the body**.

Possible Side Effects

Side effects are less prominent with Macrodantin than with Furadantin.

▼ Most common: loss of appetite, nausea, vomiting, stomach pain, and diarrhea. Some people develop hepatitis symptoms.

▼ Less common: fever, chills, cough, chest pain, breathing difficulties, and development of fluid in the lungs. If these reactions occur in the first week of therapy, they can generally be resolved by stopping the medication. If they develop after taking nitrofurantoin for a longer period, they are considered chronic and may be more serious.

▼ Rare: rash, itching, asthmatic attacks in people with a history of asthma, drug fever, symptoms similar to arthritis, jaundice (yellowing of the skin or whites of the eyes), effects on components of the blood, headache, dizziness, drowsiness, and temporary hair loss.

This drug is known to cause changes in white and red blood cells. It should be used only under the strict supervision of your doctor.

Drug Interactions

• Nitrofurantoin may increase other drugs' toxic effects on the liver and the risk of hemolytic anemia if you are taking another drug associated with that condition. These drugs include oral antidiabetes drugs, methyldopa, primaquine, procainamide, quinidine, quinine, and sulfa drugs.

• Nitrofurantoin interferes with nalidixic acid. Do not combine these drugs.

• Sulfinpyrazone and probenecid may reduce this drug's effectiveness and increase side effects.

• Anticholinergic drugs, including propantheline, may increase the risk of nitrofurantoin side effects.

• Magnesium, found most commonly in antacids, delays the absorption of nitrofurantoin or reduces the amount absorbed.

• Combining nitrofurantoin and metronidazole, mexiletine, ethambutol, isoniazid, lindane, lincomycin, lithium, pemoline, quinacrine, or long-term high-dose pyridoxine (vitamin B_6), may increase the risk of nervous system effects. Do not combine nitrofurantoin and any of these drugs.

Food Interactions

Nitrofurantoin should be taken with food to minimize upset stomach, loss of appetite, nausea, or other gastrointestinal symptoms. For optimal effectiveness, avoid citrus fruits or dairy products while taking nitrofurantoin.

Usual Dose

Adult: 50–100 mg 4 times a day, with meals and at bedtime.
Child (over age 1 month): 2–3 mg per lb. of body weight in 4 doses.
Child (under age 1 month): not recommended.

People with chronic urinary infections may require lower-dosage, longer-term therapy.

Overdosage

Induce vomiting with ipecac syrup—available at any pharmacy—and take the victim to a hospital emergency room for treatment. If you seek treatment, ALWAYS bring the prescription bottle or container.

Special Information

Call your doctor if you develop chest pain or breathing difficulties; sore throat; pale skin; unusual tiredness or weakness; dizziness; drowsiness; headache; rash and itching; yellow skin; achy joints; fever and chills; numbness, tingling, or burning of the face or mouth; or any persistent or bothersome side effect.

Continue to take this drug for at least 3 days after you stop experiencing symptoms of a UTI.

Nitrofurantoin may give your urine a brownish color: This is not a cause for concern.

The liquid form can stain your teeth if you do not swallow it rapidly.

If you miss a dose, take it as soon as possible. If it is almost time for your next dose and you take it 3 or more times a day, space the missed dose and your next dose by 2 to 4 hours, or double your next dose and then continue with your regular schedule.

Special Populations

Pregnancy/Breast-feeding
Nitrofurantoin should never be taken by pregnant women with G-6-PD deficiency or those who are near term because it can interfere with the immature enzyme systems of the fetus and cause hemolytic anemia. When this drug is considered crucial by your doctor, its potential benefits must be carefully weighed against its risks.

This drug passes into breast milk. Nursing mothers who must take nitrofurantoin should consider bottle-feeding, especially if the baby is G-6-PD deficient.

Seniors
Seniors with kidney disease may be more sensitive to nervous-system and lung effects. Seniors may also require reduced dosage due to reduction of kidney function.

Generic Name

Nitroglycerin (nye-troe-GLIH-ser-in) G

Brand Names

Deponit	Nitroglyn
Minitran	Nitrol
Nitrek	Nitrolingual
Nitro-Bid	Nitrong
Nitro-Derm	NitroQuick
Nitrodisc	Nitrostat
Nitro-Dur	Nitro-Time
Nitrogard	Transderm-Nitro

Type of Drug

Antianginal agent.

Prescribed for

Chest pain associated with angina pectoris; nitroglycerin injection is also used as a treatment after a heart attack, for heart failure, and for high blood pressure.

General Information

Nitroglycerin and other nitrates are used to treat pain associated with heart problems. While the exact nature of their action is not fully understood, they are believed to relax muscles in veins and arteries. Nitroglycerin is available in several forms: sublingual tablets, which are taken under the tongue and allowed to dissolve; capsules, which are swallowed; transmucosal tablets, which are placed between the lip or cheek and gum and allowed to dissolve; oral sprays, which are sprayed directly onto or under the tongue; transdermal patches, which deliver nitroglycerin through the skin over a 24-hour period; and ointment, which is usually spread over the chest or another area of the body. One or more forms of nitroglycerin are often used to prevent or alleviate chest pain associated with angina.

Cautions and Warnings

You should not take nitroglycerin if you are **allergic** to it or to another nitrate product, such as isosorbide.

Nitroglycerin should be taken with great caution if **head trauma** or **bleeding in the head** is present.

This drug may be inappropriate for you if you have had a recent **heart attack** or have severe **anemia, glaucoma,** severe **liver disease, overactive thyroid, cardiomyopathy** (loss of blood-pumping ability due to damaged heart muscle), **low blood pressure,** severe **kidney problems,** or an **overactive gastrointestinal tract.**

Possible Side Effects

▼ Most common: flushing and headache, which may be severe or persistent.

▼ Less common: dizziness and weakness. Blurred vision may occur; if it does, stop taking the drug and call your doctor. In some people, the blood-pressure-lowering effect of nitroglycerin causes severe responses, including nausea, vomiting, weakness, restlessness, pallor (loss of facial color), increased perspiration, and collapse. Rash may also occur.

Drug Interactions

• Avoid over-the-counter drugs containing stimulants, such

as cough, cold, and allergy remedies and appetite suppressants; they may aggravate heart disease.

• Do not take sildenafil (Viagra) if you are taking this or another nitrate product. The combination can result in a rapid and potentially fatal drop in blood pressure.

• Interaction with large amounts of alcohol may rapidly lower blood pressure, resulting in weakness, dizziness, and fainting.

• Aspirin and calcium channel blockers may increase nitrate blood levels and the risk of side effects.

• Nitroglycerin may interfere with heparin (an injectable anticoagulant drug).

• Nitrates increase dihydroergotamine blood levels, which may raise blood pressure or block the effects of nitroglycerin.

Food Interactions

Do not use any oral form of nitroglycerin with food or gum in your mouth. Nitroglycerin pills intended for swallowing are best taken on an empty stomach.

Usual Dose

Use only as much as is necessary to control chest pain.

Sublingual Tablets: Since this form acts within 10–15 seconds, it should be taken only when necessary.

Transmucosal Tablets: The tablets are placed between the upper lip and gum or between the cheek and gum and allowed to dissolve over a 3- to 5-hour period. The tablet releases the drug faster when touched with the tongue or when you drink a hot liquid. Insert another tablet after the previous one is dissolved. Do not sleep with a tablet in your mouth.

Sustained-Release Capsules and Tablets: Generally, the dosage is 1 capsule or tablet every 8–12 hours.

Ointment: 1–2 in. squeezed from the tube onto a specially marked piece of paper—some people may require as much as 4–5 in. The ointment is spread on the skin every 3–4 hours as needed to control chest pain. The medication is absorbed through the skin. The application sites should be rotated to prevent skin inflammation and rash.

Transdermal Patch: The patch is placed on a hairless site on the body that is not associated with excess movement. It is applied once a day and removed after 12–14 hours. Dosages start at 0.2–0.4 mg per hour and may increase to 0.8 mg. Higher dosages are preferable for once-daily patch applications.

Aerosol: 1–2 sprays (0.4–0.8 mg) under or on your tongue; repeat as needed to relieve an angina attack.

Overdosage

Overdose can result in low blood pressure; very rapid heartbeat; flushing; increased perspiration followed by cold, bluish, and clammy skin; headache; heart palpitations; blurred vision and other visual disturbances; dizziness; nausea; vomiting; slow and difficult breathing; slow pulse; confusion; moderate fever; and paralysis. Take the victim to a hospital emergency room immediately. ALWAYS bring the prescription bottle or container.

Special Information

Do not change brands of nitroglycerin without your doctor's and pharmacist's knowledge—they may not be equivalent.

Sublingual nitroglycerin should be acquired from your pharmacist only in the original, unopened bottle; the tablets must not be transferred to another bottle or container because they may lose potency. Close the bottle tightly after each use or the drug may evaporate from the tablets. Sublingual nitroglycerin should be taken while you are sitting down. This form of nitroglycerin frequently produces a burning sensation under the tongue, but this sensation does not necessarily indicate that the drug is working for you. If 1 tablet does not relieve your symptoms in 5 minutes, take another. If the second one does not work, take a third. If the pain continues or worsens, call your doctor or go to an emergency room at once.

When applying nitroglycerin ointment, do not rub or massage it into the skin. Any excess ointment should be washed from the hands after application.

People who use transdermal patches for more than 12 hours a day for an extended period can build up a tolerance to the patch and may have to use another form of nitroglycerin.

Nitroglycerin patches contain a significant amount of medication even after they have been used. They can be a hazard to children and small pets; be certain to dispose of them properly.

Orthostatic hypotension may become a problem if you take nitroglycerin over a long period of time. More blood stays in the extremities and less becomes available to the brain, resulting in light-headedness or faintness if you stand up suddenly. Avoid prolonged standing and always stand up slowly.

If you take nitroglycerin on a regular schedule and forget a dose, take it as soon as you remember. If you use immediate-release tablets and it is within 2 hours of your next dose, skip the dose you forgot and continue with your regular schedule. If you take sustained-release tablets or capsules and it is within 6 hours of your next dose, skip the dose you forgot and continue with your regular schedule.

Special Populations

Pregnancy/Breast-feeding

Nitroglycerin crosses into the fetal circulation. When this drug is considered crucial by your doctor, its potential benefits must be carefully weighed against its risks.

Nitroglycerin passes into breast milk. Nursing mothers who must take it should consider bottle-feeding.

Seniors

Seniors may take nitroglycerin without special restriction. Because saliva is necessary for the absorption of sublingual nitroglycerin, seniors with reduced saliva secretion may need to use another form of nitroglycerin or add a saliva substitute; this also applies to younger people with dry mouth.

Nitrostat   see **Nitroglycerin,** page 740

Generic Name

Nizatidine   (nih-ZAY-tih-dene)

Brand Names

Axid   Axid-AR

Type of Drug

Histamine H$_2$ antagonist.

Prescribed for

Ulcers of the stomach and duodenum (upper intestine); also used to treat gastroesophageal reflux disease (GERD).

General Information

H$_2$ antagonists work by turning off the system that produces stomach acid and other secretions. Nizatidine is effective in treating the symptoms of ulcer and preventing complications of the disease, although an ulcer that does not respond to another histamine H$_2$ antagonist will probably not respond to nizatidine. Histamine H$_2$ antagonists differ only in their potency. Cimetidine is the least potent; 1000 mg are roughly equal to 300 mg of either nizatidine or ranitidine, or 40 mg of famotidine. All these drugs have roughly equivalent success rates in treating ulcer disease and comparable risk of side effects.

Cautions and Warnings

Do not take nizatidine if you have had an **allergic reaction** to it or any histamine H$_2$ antagonist.

People with **kidney or liver disease** should take nizatidine with caution because 1/3 of each dose is broken down in the liver and the rest passes out of the body through the kidneys.

Possible Side Effects

Side effects are infrequent.
▼ Most common: tiredness and increased sweating.
▼ Rare: Rare side effects can affect the heart, liver, kidneys, stomach and intestines, blood, joints and muscles, mental status, and sexual function. Contact your doctor if you experience any side effect not listed above.

Drug Interactions

• Antacids, anticholinergics, and metoclopramide may slightly reduce the amount of nizatidine absorbed into the blood, but no precaution is needed.

• Enteric-coated tablets should not be taken with nizatidine. The change in stomach acidity produced by nizatidine causes the tablets to disintegrate prematurely in the stomach.

• Nizatidine may increase blood levels of aspirin in people taking very large doses of aspirin.

Food Interactions

You may take nizatidine without regard to food or meals.

Usual Dose

Adult: 300 mg at bedtime or 150 mg twice a day. Dosage is reduced in people with kidney disease.

Overdosage

Little is known about the effects of nizatidine overdose, but victims may experience exaggerated side effects. Your local poison control center may advise giving ipecac syrup—available at any pharmacy—to induce vomiting and remove any drug remaining in the stomach. Victims who have definite symptoms should be taken to a hospital emergency room. ALWAYS bring the prescription bottle or container.

Special Information

Take nizatidine exactly as directed and follow your doctor's instructions regarding diet and other treatments to get the maximum benefit from the drug. Antacids may be taken together with nizatidine, if needed. Cigarette smoking is associated with stomach ulcer and may reduce nizatidine's effectiveness.

Call your doctor at once if you develop any unusual side effects such as bleeding or bruising, tiredness, diarrhea, dizziness, or rash. Black or tarry stools or vomiting material that resembles coffee grounds may indicate that your ulcer is bleeding.

If you empty the nizatidine capsule and mix it with juice before taking it, you may keep it in the refrigerator. Do not store it for more than 2 days because the drug may lose potency.

If you forget a dose of nizatidine, take it as soon as you remember. If it is almost time for your next dose, skip the one you forgot and continue with your regular schedule. Do not take a double dose.

Special Populations

Pregnancy/Breast-feeding

Although animal studies revealed no damage to the fetus, nizatidine should be avoided by women who are or might be pregnant. When the drug is considered crucial by your doctor, its potential benefits must be carefully weighed against its risks.

Very small amounts of nizatidine may pass into breast milk. Nursing mothers who must take this drug should consider bottle-feeding.

Seniors

Seniors may need lower doses due to loss of kidney function and may be more susceptible to side effects.

Brand Name

Norgesic Forte

Generic Ingredients

Aspirin + Caffeine + Orphenadrine Citrate

Other Brand Names

Norgesic

Type of Drug

Analgesic combination.

Prescribed for

Pain of muscle spasms, sprains, strains, or back pain.

General Information

The main ingredient in Norgesic Forte is orphenadrine citrate, a pain reliever. The aspirin adds extra pain relief. Norgesic Forte cannot treat the cause of muscle spasm; it can only temporarily relieve the pain.

Cautions and Warnings

Do not take Norgesic Forte if you have **glaucoma, stomach ulcer, heart disease, intestinal obstruction, difficulty in passing urine,** or known **sensitivity** or **allergy** to this drug or any of its ingredients.

Orphenadrine can make you **light-headed** or dizzy. Be careful doing anything that requires concentration or alertness. Norgesic Forte should not be taken by children.

Possible Side Effects

▼ Most common: dry mouth.

▼ Less common: rapid heartbeat, palpitations, difficulty in urination, blurred vision, enlarged pupils, weakness, nausea, vomiting, headache, dizziness, constipation, drowsiness, rash or itching, runny or stuffy nose, hallucinations, agitation, tremors, and stomach upset. These side effects increase as dosage increases.

▼ Large doses or prolonged therapy with Norgesic Forte may lead to aspirin poisoning (symptoms include ringing in the ears, fever, confusion, sweating, thirst, dimness of vision, rapid breathing, increased pulse rate, and diarrhea).

Drug Interactions

• The aspirin in Norgesic Forte may interact with anticoagulant (blood-thinning) drugs, increase the effect of probenecid, and increase the blood-sugar-lowering effects of antidiabetic drugs.

• Combining Norgesic Forte with propoxyphene (Darvon) may cause confusion, anxiety, and tremors or shaking.

• Long-term users should avoid alcohol, which may worsen stomach upset, bleeding, and the depressive effects associated with this drug.

Food Interactions

Take this medication with food or at least half a glass of water to prevent stomach upset.

Usual Dose

½–1 tablet 3–4 times a day.

Overdosage

A single dose of 40 to 60 Norgesic Forte tablets is lethal to adults, and large overdoses below this level can rapidly become fatal. The victim must be taken to a hospital emergency room immediately. ALWAYS bring the prescription bottle or container.

Special Information

Norgesic Forte may make you drowsy. Be careful while driving or operating complex or hazardous equipment.

Call your doctor if you develop a rash or itching, rapid heart rate, palpitations, confusion, or if side effects are persistent or bothersome.

Avoid alcohol, which can increase the stomach irritation and depressive effects caused by this drug.

If you forget a dose of Norgesic Forte and you remember within about 1 hour of your regular time, take the dose right away. If you do not remember until later, skip the missed dose and go back to your regular schedule. Do not take a double dose.

Special Populations

Pregnancy/Breast-feeding

Taking too much aspirin late in pregnancy can decrease a newborn's weight and cause other problems. When Norgesic Forte is considered essential by your doctor, its potential benefits must be carefully weighed against its risks.

The ingredients in Norgesic Forte may pass into breast milk. Nursing mothers who must take this product should watch their infants for drug-related side effects.

Seniors

Seniors may be more sensitive to the side effects of this medication and should take the lowest effective dose of Norgesic Forte. Seniors may experience some degree of mental confusion in reaction to this medication.

Norvasc   see Amlodipine, page 61

Generic Name

Nystatin (nye-STAH-tin) G

Brand Names

Mycostatin   Nystop
Nilstat

Type of Drug

Antifungal.

Prescribed for

Fungal infections.

General Information

Nystatin comes in a number of dosage forms and can be prescribed when fungus infection is a possible complication of a disease or treatment. Generally, nystatin relieves symptoms in 1 to 3 days. Nystatin vaginal tablets effectively control symptoms such as itching, inflammation, and discharge. In most cases, 2 weeks of therapy is sufficient, but prolonged treatment may be necessary. It is important that you continue using this drug during menstruation. This drug has been used to prevent thrush or *Candida* in newborns by treating the mother for 3 to 6 weeks before her due date.

Cautions and Warnings

Do not take this drug if you know you may be **sensitive** or **allergic** to it. Proper diagnosis is essential for effective treatment. Do not use nystatin without first consulting your doctor.

Possible Side Effects

Nystatin is generally well tolerated.

Oral Form
▼ Most common: nausea, upset stomach, and diarrhea may occur with large doses.

Vaginal Form
▼ Most common: vaginal irritation; if this occurs, discontinue the drug and contact your doctor.

Food and Drug Interactions

None known.

Usual Dose

Oral Suspension or Pastilles: 200,000–600,000 units 4 or 5 times a day.

Oral Tablets: 500,000–1,000,000 units 3 times a day.

Vaginal Tablets: 1 tablet inserted high in the vagina daily for 2 weeks.

Overdosage

Nystatin overdose may cause stomach irritation or upset. Call your local poison control center for more information.

Special Information

Do not stop taking nystatin just because you begin to feel better. You must continue taking the medication as prescribed for at least 2 days after the relief of symptoms.

Some nystatin brands require storage in the refrigerator. Ask your pharmacist for specific instructions.

If you forget to administer a dose, do so as soon as you remember. If it is almost time for your next dose, skip the one you forgot and continue with your regular schedule. Do not take a double dose.

Special Populations

Pregnancy/Breast-feeding
Pregnant and breast-feeding women may use nystatin with no restrictions.

Seniors
Seniors may use nystatin without special restriction.

Generic Name

Olanzapine (oeh-LAN-zuh-pene)

Brand Name

Zyprexa

Type of Drug

Antipsychotic.

Prescribed for

Psychotic behavior. Olanzapine is only for people with a chronic condition.

General Information

Olanzapine is a potent antipsychotic that blocks several different chemical receptors in the brain. The exact way in which olanzapine works is not known, but its antipsychotic effect may be produced by its blockage of dopamine and serotonin receptors. A small portion of each dose of olanzapine is eliminated through the kidneys, but most of it is broken down in the liver.

Cautions and Warnings

Do not take olanzapine if you are **sensitive** or **allergic** to it.

Women clear olanzapine about 30% more slowly than men, but this effect is not considered a problem.

Smokers clear olanzapine from their bodies about 40% faster than non-smokers, but most people do not require dosage adjustments.

People with **liver disease** may require dosage adjustments.

A serious set of side effects known as **neuroleptic malignant syndrome (NMS)** includes high fever, convulsions, difficult or fast breathing, rapid heartbeat, and rapid pulse. This condition has been associated with antipsychotic medicines. Other symptoms of NMS include muscle rigidity, mental changes, irregular pulse or blood pressure, and increased sweating. NMS can be fatal and requires immediate medical attention.

Tardive dyskinesia (symptoms include lip smacking or puckering, puffing of the cheeks, rapid or worm-like movements of the tongue, uncontrolled chewing motions, and uncontrolled arm or leg movements) can occur and is often considered a reason to stop taking this drug. Report any of these side effects to your doctor.

Olanzapine can cause **dizziness** or **fainting** when rising from a sitting or standing position, especially when people first start taking the drug.

Avoid being exposed to **extreme heat**. Antipsychotics can upset your body's temperature-regulating mechanism.

Swallowing problems and inhaling food intended to be swallowed, have been a problem with antipsychotics, including olanzapine.

Suicide is a danger with all psychotics. People taking this drug should be limited to no more than a 30-day supply of medication at any time to reduce the chances of possible overdose.

Seizures occur in a small number of people taking olanzapine. Olanzapine should be taken with care if you have had seizures or are at increased risk.

Possible Side Effects

Olanzapine side effects are similar to those of placebo (sugar pill).

▼ Most common: headache, tiredness, agitation, sleeplessness, nervousness, hostility, dizziness, and runny nose.

▼ Less common: fever; abdominal, back, or chest pains; a rigid neck; dizziness or fainting when rising from a sitting or standing position; rapid heartbeat; low blood pressure; constipation; dry mouth; increased appetite; weight gain; swelling in the arms or legs; joint pain; arm or leg pain; twitching; anxiety; personality changes; restlessness or a feeling that you need to keep moving; muscle stiffness; tremors; memory loss; difficulty speaking or expressing thoughts; euphoria (feeling high); stuttering; cough; sore throat; double vision or other eye problems; and symptoms of premenstrual syndrome (PMS).

▼ Rare: Other side effects can occur in almost any part of the body. Contact your doctor if you experience any side effect not listed above.

Drug Interactions

• Your dosage of olanzapine must be adjusted when the drug is combined with carbamazepine.

• Olanzapine increases the effects of blood-pressure-lowering drugs and nervous system depressants. Dosage adjustments may be needed if you add olanzapine to another medicine.

Food Interactions

None known.

Usual Dose

Adult: starting dose—5–10 mg a day. Maintenance dose—increase gradually up to 20 mg a day if needed. Seniors should start with lower doses and increase gradually until maximum benefit is achieved.

Child (under age 18): not recommended.

Overdosage

Overdose symptoms are drowsiness and slurred speech. Overdose victims should be taken to a hospital emergency room for treatment. ALWAYS bring the prescription bottle or container.

Special Information

Sleepiness occurs in about 25% of people who take olanzapine; this effect may increase with larger doses. Take care when engaging in activities, such as driving, that require concentration or coordination.

Avoid alcohol and other nervous-system depressants while taking olanzapine.

Olanzapine can cause dry mouth. See your dentist regularly while you are taking this medication, since dental problems are more likely.

Be sure your doctor knows about all medication you are taking, including over-the-counter products.

If you forget to take a dose of olanzapine, take it as soon as you remember. If it is almost time for your next dose, skip the dose you forgot and continue with your regular schedule. Do not take a double dose.

Special Populations

Pregnancy/Breast-feeding

Olanzapine should only be taken by pregnant women if the potential benefits outweigh the risks. Birth defects and other problems have occurred in women taking olanzapine, but there is no definite link between the drug and these effects.

It is not known if olanzapine passes into breast milk. Nursing mothers who must take this medication should bottle-feed.

Seniors

Seniors usually need less olanzapine than younger adults.

Generic Name

Olopatadine (oe-loe-PAT-uh-dene)

Brand Name

Patanol

The information in this profile also applies to the following drug:

Generic Ingredient: Levocabastine
Livostan

Type of Drug

Antihistamine.

Prescribed for

Eye itching due to allergy.

General Information

Olopatadine hydrochloride is an antihistamine eyedrop that alleviates irritation caused by conjunctivitis (pinkeye).

Cautions and Warnings

Do not use olopatadine if you are **allergic** to it.

Possible Side Effects

▼ Common: headache.

▼ Less common: burning or stinging in the eye, dry eye, sensation that something is in your eye, eye redness, inflammation of the cornea, eyelid swelling, itching, weakness, sore throat, runny nose, common cold symptoms, sinus inflammation, and changes in sense of taste.

Drug Interactions

None known.

Usual Dose

Olopatadine
    Adult and Child (age 3 and over): 1–2 drops in each eye 2 times a day, 6–8 hours apart.
    Child (under age 3): not recommended.

Levocabastine
    Adult and Child (age 12 and over): 1 drop in the affected eye 4 times a day for up to 2 weeks.
    Child (under age 12): not recommended.

Overdosage

Little is known about the effects of olopatadine overdose, but it is likely to increase side effects. Accidental ingestion of olopatadine is not likely to be associated with side effects because each bottle contains only 5 mg of the drug. Call your local poison control center or hospital emergency room for more information.

Special Information

If you wear contact lenses, wait at least 15 minutes after using olopatadine before putting in your lenses.

To avoid infection, do not touch the dropper tip to your finger, eyelid, or any other surface. Wait at least 5 minutes before using another eyedrop or eye ointment.

If you forget a dose of olopatadine, administer it as soon as you remember. If it is almost time for your next dose, skip the one you forgot and continue with your regular schedule. Do not take a double dose.

Special Populations

Pregnancy/Breast-feeding

Since little olopatadine gets into the circulation, risk of birth defects is low. Do not take any antihistamine without your doctor's knowledge if you are or might be pregnant—especially during the last 3 months of pregnancy—because newborns may have severe reactions to antihistamines.

Olopatadine may pass into breast milk. Nursing mothers using olopatadine should consider bottle-feeding.

Seniors

Seniors may take olopatadine without special precaution.

Generic Name

Olsalazine (ol-SAL-uh-zeen)

Brand Name

Dipentum

Type of Drug

Bowel anti-inflammatory.

Prescribed for

Ulcerative colitis.

General Information

Olsalazine sodium is broken down to an anti-inflammatory compound, mesalamine, after it enters the colon. Mesalamine acts inside the bowel and is effective in treating ulcerative colitis. The amount of mesalamine absorbed into the blood is 10% to 30%; 70% to 90% of it remains in the colon, where it works on colitis. People who cannot take sulfasalazine may be able to take olsalazine.

Cautions and Warnings

Do not take this product if you are **allergic** to it, to mesalamine, or to aspirin (or aspirin-related compounds).

Possible Side Effects

Many side effects in addition to those listed below have been reported, but their link to olsalazine has not been well established.

▼ Most common: diarrhea and stomach cramps or pain.

▼ Less common: muscle aches, headache, fatigue or drowsiness, depression, nausea, vomiting, upset stomach, bloating, yellowing of the skin or whites of the eyes, dizziness, fainting, appetite loss, respiratory infections, and rash or itching.

Drug Interactions

None known.

Food Interactions

Take this drug with food to reduce upset stomach.

Usual Dose

1000 mg a day divided into 2 doses.

Overdosage

Symptoms include diarrhea, vomiting, and lethargy. In case of overdose, call your local poison control center or a hospital emergency room. You may be told to induce vomiting with ipecac syrup—available at any pharmacy—before taking the victim to an emergency room. If you seek treatment, ALWAYS bring the prescription bottle or container.

Special Information

Call your doctor if you develop fever, pale skin, sore throat, unusual bruising or bleeding, unusual tiredness or weakness, or yellowing of the skin or whites of the eyes, or if your colitis gets worse. Other symptoms, such as diarrhea, abdominal pain, upset stomach, appetite loss, nausea, and vomiting, should be reported if they become bothersome or severe.

If you forget a dose, take it as soon as you remember. If it is almost time for your next dose, take 1 dose right away and another in 5 or 6 hours, then go back to your regular schedule. Do not take a double dose.

Special Populations

Pregnancy/Breast-feeding

Olsalazine has caused birth defects in lab animals. When this drug is considered crucial by your doctor, its potential benefits must be carefully weighed against its risks.

Olsalazine and mesalamine pass into breast milk. Nursing mothers who must take olsalazine should consider bottle-feeding.

Seniors

Seniors may use this drug without special restriction.

Generic Name

Omeprazole (oe-MEP-ruh-zole)

Brand Name

Prilosec

The information in this profile also applies to the following drugs:

Generic Ingredient: Lansoprazole
Prevacid

Generic Ingredients: Lansoprazole + Amoxicillin + Clarithromycin
Prevpac

Generic Ingredient: Pantoprazole
Protonix

Generic Ingredient: Rabeprazole Sodium
AcipHex

Type of Drug

Proton-pump inhibitor.

Prescribed for

Stomach or duodenal (upper intestinal) ulcers, gastroesophageal reflux disease (GERD), and conditions in which there is an excess of stomach acid; also used to maintain healing of ulcer of the esophagus.

General Information

Omeprazole stops the production of stomach acid by interfering with the "proton pump" in the mucous lining of the stomach, at the last stage of acid production. Omeprazole can turn off stomach acid production within 1 hour. This drug is useful in treating ulcers, GERD, and other conditions in which stomach acid plays a key role. It is prescribed together with amoxicillin or clarithromycin for people with ulcers caused by *Heliobacter pylori* infections.

Cautions and Warnings

Do not take omeprazole if you are **allergic** to it.

Omeprazole should not be taken as maintenance treatment for duodenal ulcers and is not recommended for treatment of GERD beyond 8 to16 weeks.

Possible Side Effects

Generally, omeprazole causes few side effects. Those that may occur include headache, diarrhea, abdominal pain, nausea, sore throat, upper respiratory infection, fever, vomiting, dizziness, rash, constipation, muscle pain, unusual tiredness, cough, and back pain.

▼ Rare: Rare side effects can occur in almost any part of the body. Contact your doctor if you experience any side effect not listed above.

Drug Interactions

• Omeprazole may increase the effects of diazepam, phenytoin, and warfarin. It may also interact with other drugs broken down by the liver.

• Combining omeprazole and clarithromycin increases blood levels of both drugs.

• Omeprazole may interfere with the absorption of iron, ampicillin, and ketoconazole.

• Omeprazole may increase the effects of drugs that reduce the production of blood cells by bone marrow.

Food Interactions

Omeprazole should be taken immediately before a meal, preferably breakfast.

Usual Dose

Lansoprazole
   Adult: 15–30 mg a day; up to 120 mg a day. People with liver and kidney disease need reduced dosage.
   Child (under age 18): not recommended.

Omeprazole
   Adult: 20–80 mg a day; up to 120 mg a day has been used. Antacids may be taken with omeprazole.
   Child (age 3 months–13 years): 20–60 mg a day.
   Child (under age 3 months): 0.22 mg per lb. of body weight a day.

Pantoprazole
   Adult: 40 mg a day.
   Child (under age 18): not recommended.

Prevpac
2 amoxicillin (Trimox) capsules, 1 clarithromycin (Biaxin) tablet, and 1 lansoprazole (Prevacid) capsule before breakfast and dinner for 10–14 days.

Rabeprazole
   Adult: 20 mg a day.
   Child (under age 18): not recommended.

Overdosage

Omeprazole overdose symptoms are likely to resemble side effects. If you seek treatment, ALWAYS bring the prescription bottle or container.

Special Information

Call your doctor if you are unusually tired or weak, or if you develop a sore throat, fever, sores in the mouth that do not heal, unusual bleeding or bruising, bloody or cloudy urine, urinary difficulties, or any persistent or bothersome side effect.

Take the full course of treatment prescribed, even if your symptoms improve after 1 or 2 weeks.

Do not open, crush, or chew the capsule; swallow it whole.

If you forget a dose, take it as soon as you remember. If it is almost time for your next dose, skip the one you forgot and continue with your regular schedule. Do not take a double dose.

Special Populations

Pregnancy/Breast-feeding

Omeprazole may be toxic to pregnant animals. When this drug is considered crucial by your doctor, its potential benefits must be carefully weighed against its risks.

Omeprazole may pass into breast milk. Nursing mothers who use this drug should consider bottle-feeding.

Seniors

Seniors report the same side effects as younger adults.

Generic Name

Orlistat (OR-lih-stat)

Brand Name

Xenical

Type of Drug

Fat blocker.

Prescribed for

Weight reduction and maintenance.

General Information

Orlistat is the first "fat blocker" to be approved by the Food and Drug Administration (FDA). It works in the stomach and intestine by interfering with an enzyme that is key to the breakdown and absorption of one kind of fat. The unabsorbed fat, about 30% of that in your diet, passes out of the body in the stool. Since fat is the most concentrated form of calories, blocking fat absorption also reduces the number of calories you take in. People taking orlistat usually begin losing weight in a few weeks and continue to lose it for 6 months to a year. After that, weight loss is maintained. If you increase your exercise level or further reduce your caloric intake, you may lose more weight. More than 40% of people taking orlistat in clinical studies lost at least 5% of their body weight after a year of continuous treatment. About 18% lost more than 10% of body weight.

By losing weight, people taking orlistat achieved improved blood-fat profiles and lower blood pressure and blood sugar. They also reduced their waist and hip measurements—2 in. and 2.5 in., respectively—more than people taking a placebo (sugar pill) and following a weight-loss diet.

Cautions and Warnings

Do not take orlistat if you are **sensitive** or **allergic** to it. Some people may develop **kidney stones** while taking this drug, especially those prone to kidney stones.

Orlistat, like any weight-loss drug, **may be abused** or misused.

Possible Side Effects

Most side effects are mild and temporary and tend to decrease during the second year of treatment.

▼ Most common: oily underwear spotting, gas with discharge, the feeling that you have to move your bowels, an oily or fat-laden stool, releasing an oily liquid during a bowel movement, more frequent bowel movements, abdominal pain or discomfort, flu, respiratory infections, back pain, and headache.

▼ Common: an inability to control bowel movements, nausea, infectious diarrhea, rectal pain or discomfort, arthritis, dizziness, fatigue, rash, menstrual problems, and urinary infection.

▼ Less common: tooth or gum problems; vomiting; ear, nose, or throat problems; muscle pain; joint problems; tendonitis; sleep disturbances; dry skin; vaginal irritation; anxiety; depression; and swollen feet.

Possible Side Effects *(continued)*

▼ Rare: Rare side effects can occur in almost any part of the body. Contact your doctor if you experience any side effect not listed above.

Drug Interactions

• Orlistat interferes with the absorption of fat-soluble vitamins and drugs.

• The blood-fat-lowering effect of statin cholesterol-lowering drugs is increased by orlistat.

Food Interactions

Take a dose with, or within an hour of, every meal.

Usual Dose

Adult: 120 mg taken with, or within an hour of, each meal.
Child: not recommended.

Overdosage

Symptoms are likely to include severe side effects, especially those related to the stomach and intestines. Take the victim to a hospital emergency room. ALWAYS bring the prescription bottle or container.

Special Information

Orlistat should be taken as part of a program of diet and exercise. Taking more than 1 capsule with each meal does not provide extra benefit.

Daily fat intake should be distributed over 3 meals to reduce the risk of developing a stomach or gastrointestinal (GI) problem.

Orlistat can interfere with the absorption of the fat-soluble vitamins A, D, and E. Take a vitamin supplement while using this drug.

If you forget to take an orlistat capsule within an hour of any meal, skip the forgotten dose and take a capsule with your next meal. Do not take a double dose.

Special Populations

Pregnancy/Breast-feeding

While animal studies of orlistat reveal no damage to the

fetus, this drug is not recommended during pregnancy and should only be used after carefully weighing its potential benefits against its risks.

It is not known if orlistat passes into breast milk. Nursing mothers who must take this drug should bottle-feed.

Seniors
Orlistat has not been studied in older adults, who should use caution.

Ortho-Cyclen   see Contraceptives, page 254

Ortho-Novum   see Contraceptives, page 254

Ortho-Tri-Cyclen   see Contraceptives, page 254

Generic Name

Oseltamivir   (oe-sel-TAM-ih-veer)

Brand Name

Tamiflu

Type of Drug

Antiviral.

Prescribed for

Influenza type A and B.

General Information

Oseltamivir is the first pill approved to treat both type A and B influenza. It is thought to work by interfering with a virus enzyme called neuraminidase; this interference limits the spread of virus particles through the respiratory tract. In studies, people taking the drug for 5 days got better 1.3 days sooner than those taking a placebo (sugar pill). Oseltamivir is only prescribed for adults who have had flu symptoms for no more than 2 days. It is also being studied for flu prevention. This drug is broken down in the liver.

Cautions and Warnings

Do not take oseltamivir if you are **sensitive** or **allergic** to it.

People using oseltamivir to treat the flu should still get an annual **influenza vaccination**.

The effect of oseltamivir in people with chronic **heart disease, lung disease,** or any condition requiring hospitalization is not known. The safety and effectiveness of repeated oseltamivir use is not known.

Flu viruses can become resistant to oseltamivir, especially those already resistant to zanamivir (another flu medication).

People with moderate **kidney disease** require reduced dosage. People with severe kidney disease should be cautious about using oseltamivir because it has not been studied in this group.

Possible Side Effects

▼ Most common: nausea and vomiting.

▼ Common: diarrhea.

▼ Less common: bronchitis, abdominal pain, dizziness, headache, cough, sleeplessness, dizziness or fainting, and fatigue.

▼ Rare: chest pain, anemia, colitis, bone fracture, pneumonia, fever, and abscesses around the tonsils.

Food and Drug Interactions

None known.

Usual Dose

Adult: 75 mg twice daily for 5 days. Daily dosage may be reduced to a single 75-mg capsule in people with kidney disease.

Child (under age 19): not recommended.

Overdosage

Little is known about the effects of oseltamivir overdose, though symptoms may include nausea and vomiting. Call your local poison control center or a hospital emergency room for more information. If you seek treatment, ALWAYS bring the prescription bottle or container.

Special Information

Taking oseltamivir is not a substitute for an annual flu shot.

If you forget a dose, take it as soon as you remember. If it is almost time for your next dose, skip the one you forgot and continue with your regular schedule. Do not take a double dose.

Special Populations

Pregnancy/Breast-feeding

Animal studies indicate that oseltamivir may cause fetal abnormalities. When this drug is considered crucial by your doctor, its potential benefits must be carefully weighed against its risks.

This drug may pass into breast milk. Nursing mothers who must take it should bottle-feed.

Seniors

Oseltamivir may be less effective in seniors.

Generic Name

Oxaprozin (ox-uh-PROE-zin)

Brand Name

Daypro

The information in this profile also applies to the following drug:

Generic Ingredient: Sulindac Ⓖ
Clinoril

Type of Drug

Nonsteroidal anti-inflammatory drug (NSAID).

Prescribed for

Rheumatoid arthritis and osteoarthritis.

General Information

Oxaprozin and other NSAIDs are used to relieve pain and inflammation. We do not know exactly how NSAIDs work, but they may achieve their effects by blocking the body's production of a hormone called prostaglandin and the action of other body chemicals. Pain relief comes within 1 hour after taking the first dose of oxaprozin, but its anti-inflammatory effect takes up to 1 week to become apparent and may take a month or more to reach maximum effect. Oxaprozin is broken down in the liver and eliminated through the kidneys.

Cautions and Warnings

People who are **allergic** to oxaprozin or any other NSAID and those with a history of **asthma** attacks brought on by an NSAID, iodides, or aspirin should not take oxaprozin.

Oxaprozin can cause **gastrointestinal (GI) bleeding, ulcers,** and **stomach perforation**. This can occur at any time, with or without warning, in people who take oxaprozin regularly. People with a history of active GI bleeding should be cautious about taking any NSAID. People who develop bleeding or ulcers and continue NSAID treatment should be aware of the possibility of developing more serious drug toxicity.

Oxaprozin can affect platelets and **blood clotting** at high doses, and should be avoided by people with clotting problems and those taking warfarin.

People with **heart problems** who use oxaprozin may experience swelling in their arms, legs, or feet.

Oxaprozin can cause severe toxic effects to the **kidney**. Report any unusual side effects to your doctor, who may need to periodically test your kidney function.

Oxaprozin can make you **unusually sensitive to the effects of the sun**.

Possible Side Effects

▼ Most common: diarrhea, nausea, vomiting, constipation, gas, stomach upset or irritation, and appetite loss—especially during the first few days of treatment.

▼ Less common: stomach ulcers, GI bleeding, hepatitis, gallbladder attacks, painful urination, poor kidney function, kidney inflammation, blood and protein in the

---

Possible Side Effects *(continued)*

---

urine, dizziness, fainting, nervousness, depression, hallucinations, confusion, disorientation, tingling in the hands
or feet, light-headedness, itching, increased sweating,
dry nose and mouth, heart palpitations, chest pain,
breathing difficulties, and muscle cramps.

▼ Rare: severe allergic reactions including closing of
the throat, fever and chills, changes in liver function, jaundice (yellowing of the skin or whites of the eyes), and kidney failure. People who experience such effects must be
promptly treated in a hospital emergency room or doctor's office. NSAIDs have caused severe skin reactions; if
this happens to you, see your doctor immediately.

Drug Interactions

• Oxaprozin can increase the effects of oral anticoagulant
(blood-thinning) drugs such as warfarin. Your anticoagulant
dose may need to be reduced.

• Taking oxaprozin with cyclosporine may increase the
toxic kidney effects of both drugs.

• Methotrexate toxicity may be increased in people also
taking oxaprozin.

• Oxaprozin may reduce the blood-pressure-lowering
effect of beta blockers and loop diuretics.

• Oxaprozin may increase phenytoin side effects. Lithium
blood levels may be increased by oxaprozin.

• Oxaprozin blood levels may be affected by cimetidine.

• Probenecid may increase the risk of oxaprozin side
effects.

• Aspirin and other salicylates should never be combined
with oxaprozin.

Food Interactions

Take oxaprozin with food or a magnesium/aluminum antacid
if it upsets your stomach.

Usual Dose

Oxaprozin: 600–1800 mg taken once a day. Do not exceed 12
mg per lb. of body weight daily.

Sulindac: 200–300 mg twice a day.

Overdosage

People have died from NSAID overdoses. Common signs of overdose are drowsiness, nausea, vomiting, diarrhea, abdominal pain, rapid breathing, rapid heartbeat, increased sweating, ringing or buzzing in the ears, confusion, disorientation, stupor, and coma. Take the victim to a hospital emergency room at once. ALWAYS bring the prescription bottle or container.

Special Information

Take each dose with a full glass of water and do not lie down for 15 to 30 minutes afterward.

Oxaprozin can make you drowsy or tired: Be careful when driving or operating hazardous equipment. Do not take any over-the-counter products containing acetaminophen or aspirin while taking oxaprozin. Avoid alcohol.

Contact your doctor if you develop rash or itching, visual disturbances, weight gain, breathing difficulties, fluid retention, hallucinations, black or tarry stools, persistent headache, or any unusual or intolerable side effect.

If you forget a dose of oxaprozin, take it as soon as you remember. If you take oxaprozin once a day and it is within 8 hours of your next dose, or if you take several doses a day and it is within 4 hours of your next dose, skip the dose you forgot and continue with your regular schedule. Never take a double dose.

Special Populations

Pregnancy/Breast-feeding

NSAIDs may affect the fetal heart during the second half of pregnancy. Pregnant women should not take oxaprozin without their doctor's approval. When the drug is considered crucial by your doctor, its potential benefits must be carefully weighed against its risks.

NSAIDs may pass into breast milk. There is a possibility that a nursing mother taking oxaprozin could affect her baby's heart or cardiovascular system. Nursing mothers who must take this drug should bottle-feed.

Seniors

Seniors may be more susceptible to side effects, especially ulcer disease.

Generic Name

Oxiconazole (ox-ih-KON-uh-zole)

Brand Name

Oxistat

Type of Drug

Antifungal.

Prescribed for

Fungal infections of the skin.

General Information

Oxiconazole nitrate is a general-purpose antifungal drug. It works by interfering with the cell membrane (outer skin) of the fungus. Little of the drug is absorbed into the bloodstream.

Cautions and Warnings

Do not use oxiconazole if you are **allergic** to it or to any other ingredient in this product.

Possible Side Effects

Oxiconazole side effects are infrequent.
  ▼ Common: itching and burning.
  ▼ Rare: stinging, irritation, rash, scaling, tingling, pain, eczema, redness and swelling, and cracked skin.

Drug Interactions

None known.

Usual Dose

Oxiconazole should be applied to affected areas every evening for 2–4 weeks, depending on the fungus type.

Overdosage

Little is known about the effects of accidental ingestion. Victims should be taken to a hospital emergency room. ALWAYS bring the prescription bottle or container.

Special Information

Oxiconazole is meant only for application to the skin. Do not put this drug into your eyes or mouth.

Stop using the drug and call your doctor if skin irritation or redness develops.

If you forget a dose of oxiconazole, apply it as soon as you remember. If it is almost time for your next dose, skip the dose you forgot and continue with your regular schedule.

Special Populations

Pregnancy/Breast-feeding

Oxiconazole is not likely to affect your pregnancy because little is absorbed into the bloodstream. Nevertheless, you should not use this drug without your doctor's knowledge and approval.

Large amounts of oxiconazole may pass into breast milk. Nursing mothers who must use this drug should consider bottle-feeding.

Seniors

Seniors may use oxiconazole without special restriction.

Generic Name

Oxybutynin (ox-ee-BYUE-tih-nin) G

Brand Names

Ditropan   Ditropan XL

Type of Drug

Antispasmodic and anticholinergic.

Prescribed for

Bladder instability including an urgent need to urinate, frequent urination, urinary leakage, and painful urination.

General Information

Oxybutynin directly affects the smooth muscle that controls the opening and closing of the bladder. It is 4 to 10 times more potent than atropine but much less likely to cause side effects.

Cautions and Warnings

Do not take oxybutynin if you are **allergic** or **sensitive** to it.

Oxybutynin should be used with caution if you have **glaucoma, intestinal obstruction or poor intestinal function, megacolon,** severe or ulcerative **colitis, myasthenia gravis,** or unstable **heart disease** including abnormal heart rhythms, heart failure, or recent heart attack. **Heat prostration** may develop more easily while you are taking this drug because it makes you more sensitive to high temperatures.

Oxybutynin should be used with caution if you have **liver or kidney disease.** It may worsen symptoms of an **overactive thyroid gland, coronary heart disease, abnormal heart rhythms, rapid heartbeat, high blood pressure, prostate disease,** or **hiatal hernia.**

Possible Side Effects

▼ Most common: dry mouth, decreased sweating, and constipation.

▼ Less common: difficulty urinating, blurred vision, enlarging of the pupils, worsening of glaucoma, palpitations, drowsiness, sleeplessness, weakness, nausea, vomiting, bloating, impotence, reduced production of breast milk, rash, and itching.

Drug Interactions

• Atenolol (a beta blocker) may increase the effect of oxybutynin.

• Oxybutynin may reduce haloperidol blood levels, which in turn may worsen schizophrenic symptoms. Oxybutynin may increase blood levels of digoxin and nitrofurantoin, increasing the risk of side effects.

• Oxybutynin may interfere with levodopa.

• Amantadine may increase oxybutynin side effects.

• Combining oxybutynin with a phenothiazine antipsychotic drug may increase side effects and raise or lower phenothiazine blood levels.

Food Interactions

Take oxybutynin with food or milk if it upsets your stomach.

Usual Dose

Ditropan
   Adult: 10–20 mg a day in divided doses.
   Child (age 6 and over): 10–15 mg a day in divided doses.

Ditropan XL
   Adult (age 18 and over): 5–10 mg once a day.
   Child: not recommended.

Overdosage

Symptoms may include restlessness, tremors, irritability, convulsions, hallucinations, flushing, fever, nausea, vomiting, rapid heartbeat, blood-pressure changes, respiratory failure, paralysis, delirium, and coma. Take the victim to a hospital emergency room at once. ALWAYS bring the prescription bottle or container.

Special Information

Oxybutynin may interfere with your vision and ability to concentrate. Be careful while driving or doing any task that requires concentration or clear vision.

Your eyes may become more sensitive to bright light while taking oxybutynin; wearing sunglasses or protective lenses should help to alleviate this problem.

Dry mouth may be relieved with sugarless gum, candy, or ice chips. Excessive mouth dryness may lead to tooth decay and should be brought to your dentist's attention if it lasts for more than 2 weeks.

If you forget a dose, take it as soon as you remember. If it is almost time for your next dose, skip the dose you forgot and continue with your regular schedule. Do not take a double dose.

Special Populations

Pregnancy/Breast-feeding

The safety of using oxybutynin during pregnancy is not known. When this drug is considered crucial by your doctor, its potential benefits must be carefully weighed against its risks.

It is not known if oxybutynin passes into breast milk. Nursing mothers who must take this drug should consider bottle-feeding.

Seniors
Seniors may be more susceptible to side effects and should take this drug with caution.

Generic Name

Paclitaxel (PAK-lih-TAX-ul)

Brand Name

Taxol

Type of Drug

Antineoplastic.

Prescribed for

Ovarian and breast cancer; Kaposi's sarcoma related to acquired immunodeficiency syndrome (AIDS). Also prescribed for cancers of the head and neck, lung, gastrointestinal tract, prostate, and kidney and for Hodgkin's lymphoma.

General Information

Paclitaxel interferes with cell division in cancerous cells. It is recommended only after other treatments have failed. Studies in ovarian cancer indicate that 22% to 30% of women who receive paclitaxel respond to the drug; of a total of 92 women studied, there were 6 complete and 18 partial responses. In breast cancer, response rates range from 26% and 30% to 57%. People who receive paclitaxel are premedicated with other drugs to minimize side effects. Paclitaxel is also being studied as a treatment for other cancers.

Cautions and Warnings

Paclitaxel must be prescribed by a doctor who is experienced in the use of cancer chemotherapies. Management of drug complications is possible only when adequate treatment facilities are available.

Severe **drug sensitivity reactions,** including breathing difficulties; low blood pressure (symptoms include dizziness and fainting); swelling of the face, hands, feet, genitals, or internal organs; and generalized itching and rash have occurred in 2%

of people taking this drug. People who experience these reactions should not use paclitaxel.

Bone-marrow suppression is the major toxic effect of paclitaxel. People with low white-blood-cell counts should not receive paclitaxel.

Fewer than 1% of people who take paclitaxel develop severe **heart problems;** these people may require cardiac therapy while continuing to receive this drug.

Paclitaxel is broken down in the liver and should be used with caution in people with severe **liver disease**.

Possible Side Effects

In order to minimize side effects, paclitaxel should be administered before cisplatin, another antineoplastic drug.

▼ Most common: reduced blood-cell counts, anemia, infection, drug sensitivity reactions, dizziness or fainting, changes in electrocardiogram (EKG) measurements, muscle or joint pain, nausea and vomiting, diarrhea, mouth sores, liver inflammation, kidney damage, hair loss, numbness, tingling or burning in the hands or feet, and swelling or retention of fluid.

▼ Less common: bleeding, blood in the urine, bruising, black and tarry stool, severe sensitivity reactions, and slow heartbeat.

▼ Rare: severe heart problems and nail changes.

Drug Interactions

• Ketoconazole, verapamil, diazepam, quinidine, dexamethasone, cyclosporine, teniposide, etoposide, vincristine, testosterone, estradiol, and retinoic acid may increase the risk of paclitaxel side effects.

• Paclitaxel may increase the risk of doxorubicin side effects.

Food Interactions

None known.

Usual Dose

Adult: Paclitaxel is given by intravenous injection. Dosage is individualized.

Child: not recommended.

Overdosage

Little is known about the effects of paclitaxel overdose, though it is likely to cause severe side effects. Breathing difficulties, chest pain, burning eyes, sore throat, and nausea have occurred after accidental inhalation of paclitaxel. Take the overdose victim or those with symptoms of inhalation to a hospital emergency room.

Special Information

Drug therapy must be closely supervised by your doctor.

Do not receive any immunizations or vaccinations while taking paclitaxel, unless approved by your doctor.

Avoid exposure to people with bacterial or viral infections, especially when your blood counts are likely to be low. Contact your doctor at the first sign of cold or infection. Do not touch the inside of your mouth or nose unless you have first washed your hands.

Call your doctor if you experience any unusual bleeding or bruising, black or tarry stool, blood in the urine or stool, or pinpoint red spots on the skin.

Ask your doctor about the proper way to brush and floss while using this drug, since brushing and flossing may introduce bacteria into your bloodstream. Check with your doctor before you have any dental work done and inform your dentist that you are receiving chemotherapy.

Take care to avoid accidental cuts. Avoid contact sports or other situations in which bruising or injury could occur.

Special Populations

Pregnancy/Breast-feeding

Paclitaxel can harm the fetus. Women taking this drug must be sure to use an effective contraceptive during treatment. If you are pregnant and must start taking paclitaxel or if you become pregnant while taking it, discuss the possible hazards with your doctor.

It is not known if paclitaxel passes into breast milk. Nursing mothers who must use it should bottle-feed.

Seniors

Seniors may use this drug without special restriction.

Generic Name

Paroxetine (pah-ROX-eh-teen)

Brand Names

Paxil   Paxil CR

Type of Drug

Selective serotonin reuptake inhibitor (SSRI).

Prescribed for

Depression, panic disorder, social anxiety disorder, obsessive-compulsive disorder, and post-traumatic stress syndrome; also prescribed for diabetic nerve disease, headache, and premature ejaculation.

General Information

Paroxetine and other SSRIs, which are chemically unrelated to the older tricyclic and tetracyclic antidepressant drugs, work by preventing the movement of the neurohormone serotonin into nerve endings. This forces serotonin to remain in the spaces surrounding nerve endings, where it works. Paroxetine is effective in treating common symptoms of depression. It can help improve mood and mental alertness, increase physical activity, and improve sleep patterns. Resistance to paroxetine may develop over time. The drug takes between 1 and 4 weeks to start working, although you may start sleeping better within 1 to 2 weeks. Paroxetine stays in your body for several weeks after you stop taking it. This fact may be important as your doctor considers when to start or stop treatment. Unlike other SSRIs, paroxetine does not have any weight-reducing effect.

Cautions and Warnings

Do not take paroxetine if you are **allergic** to it.

Serious, **potentially fatal reactions** may occur if paroxetine and a **monoamine oxidase inhibitor (MAOI)** are taken together (see "Drug Interactions").

Paroxetine is broken down in the liver. People with severe **liver or kidney disease** should use caution with this drug and be treated with lower-than-normal dosage.

A small number of **manic** or **hypomanic** patients may experience an activation of their condition while taking paroxetine.

Paroxetine should be given with caution to people who suffer from **seizures**.

Paroxetine causes low blood levels of **uric acid,** but has not caused kidney failure.

The risk of **suicide** exists in severely depressed people and may be present until the condition is significantly improved. Depressed people should be allowed to carry only small quantities of paroxetine with them to limit the risk of overdose.

Possible Side Effects

Side effects are generally mild and often related to the size of the dose; they occur primarily during the first week of treatment. About 15% of people stop taking it because of side effects.

▼ Most common: headache, weakness, sleep disturbances, dizziness, and tremors.

▼ Common: nausea, excessive sweating, weakness, dry mouth, constipation, dizziness, decreased sex drive, abnormal ejaculation, blurred vision, dry mouth, and weight gain.

▼ Less common: flushing, pinpoint pupils, increased saliva, cold and clammy skin, dizziness when rising quickly from a sitting or lying position, blood pressure changes, swelling around the eyes and in the arms or legs, coldness in the hands or feet, fainting and dizziness, rapid heartbeat, weakness, loss of coordination, unusual walk, changes in the general level of activity, migraine, droopy eyelids, tingling in the hands or feet, acne, hair loss, dry skin, difficulty swallowing, gas, joint pain, muscle pain, cramps and weakness, aggressiveness, abnormal dreaming or thinking, memory loss, apathy, delusions, feelings of detachment, worsened depression, emotional instability, euphoria (feeling "high"), hallucinations, neurosis, paranoia, suicide attempts, teeth grinding, menstrual cramps or pain, bleeding between periods, coughing, bronchospasm, nosebleed, breathing difficulties, conjunctivitis, double vision, difficulty accommodating to bright light, eye pain, earaches, painful urination, facial swelling, frequent urination, nighttime urination, loss of urinary control, generalized swelling, not feeling well, and lymph swelling.

Possible Side Effects *(continued)*

▼ Rare: Rare side effects can occur in almost any part of the body. Contact your doctor if you experience any side effect not listed above.

Drug Interactions

• At least 5 weeks should elapse between stopping treatment and starting an MAOI antidepressant. Two weeks should elapse between stopping an MAOI and starting paroxetine. Taking these two drugs too close together or at the same time may cause serious, life-threatening reactions.

• People taking warfarin may experience an increase in its effect, and possibly a bleeding episode, if they start taking paroxetine. Your doctor should reevaluate your warfarin dosage.

• Combining paroxetine and theophylline increases the risk of side effects. Report anything unusual to your doctor.

• Paroxetine may reduce the amount of digoxin absorbed into the blood by 15%.

• Cimetidine increases blood levels of paroxetine by about 50%.

• Phenobarbital decreases the amount of paroxetine in the blood and increases the rate at which it is released from the body.

• Combining paroxetine and phenytoin (which is prescribed for seizure disorders) may decrease blood levels of both drugs and increase the rate at which both drugs are released from the body. Your doctor should adjust your dosages.

• Alcohol may increase the tiredness and other depressant effects of paroxetine.

• People who combine l-tryptophan and paroxetine may develop agitation, restlessness, and upset stomach.

• People combining paroxetine with procyclidine (used in Parkinson's disease) have experienced increased procyclidine side effects. Your doctor may reduce your procyclidine dosage.

Food Interactions

This drug can be taken with or without food.

Usual Dose

10–50 mg once a day, morning or night. Seniors, people with kidney or liver disease, and people taking several different drugs should take the lowest effective dosage.

Overdosage

Symptoms include the most common side effects. Any person suspected of having taken an overdose should be taken to a hospital emergency room, or call your local poison control center for information and instructions. If you go to an emergency room, ALWAYS bring the prescription bottle or container.

Special Information

Paroxetine can make you dizzy or drowsy. Take care when driving or doing any task that requires concentration.

Do not drink alcohol if you are taking paroxetine.

Be sure your doctor knows if you are pregnant, breast-feeding, or taking other drugs, including over-the-counter drugs, while taking paroxetine. Notify your doctor if you experience any unusual side effect.

If you forget a dose, take it as soon as you remember. If it is almost time for your next dose, skip the dose you forgot and continue with your regular schedule. Do not take a double dose.

Special Populations

Pregnancy/Breast-feeding

While animal studies of paroxetine reveal no damage to the fetus, this drug should only be used during pregnancy after carefully weighing its potential benefits against its risks.

Paroxetine passes into breast milk. Nursing mothers who must take this drug should bottle-feed.

Seniors

Seniors with liver or kidney disease should receive reduced dosage.

Paxil   *see Paroxetine, page 777*

Generic Name

Pemoline (PEM-oe-leen) Ⓖ

Brand Name

Cylert

Type of Drug

Psychotherapeutic agent.

Prescribed for

Attention-deficit hyperactivity disorder (ADHD); may also be used to treat daytime sleepiness in adults.

General Information

This drug stimulates the central nervous system (CNS), although its exact action in children with ADHD is not known. It should be prescribed only by a doctor trained to treat ADHD, and always used as part of a total therapeutic program that includes social, psychological, and educational counseling.

Cautions and Warnings

People who are **allergic** or **sensitive** to pemoline should not use it. **Children under age 6** should not take this drug. The condition of **psychotic children** who take pemoline may get worse. People taking pemoline should have periodic **liver function tests**.

Possible Side Effects

▼ Less common: sleeplessness, appetite loss, stomachache, rash, irritability, depression, nausea, dizziness, headache, drowsiness, and hallucinations.

▼ Rare: drug hypersensitivity, wandering eye, and uncontrolled movements of the lips, face, tongue, and extremities.

Drug Interactions

• Pemoline lowers the seizure threshold; anticonvulsant drug dosage may need to be increased.

• Pemoline increases the effects of other nervous-system stimulants, which may cause nervousness, irritability, sleeplessness, and other side effects.

Food Interactions

Take this drug with food if it upsets your stomach.

Usual Dose

37.5–75 mg a day. Do not exceed 112.5 mg a day.

Overdosage

Symptoms include rapid heartbeat, hallucinations, agitation, uncontrolled muscle movements, and restlessness. Take the victim to a hospital emergency room. ALWAYS bring the prescription bottle or container.

Special Information

Take your daily dose at the same time each morning. Taking pemoline too late in the day may result in trouble sleeping; call your doctor if this happens.

If you forget a dose, take it as soon as you remember. If it is almost time for your next dose, skip the dose you forgot and continue with your regular schedule. Do not take a double dose.

Special Populations

Pregnancy/Breast-feeding

Pemoline crosses into the fetal circulation. Animal studies show that large dosages of pemoline can cause stillbirth and reduce newborn survival rates. When this drug is considered crucial by your doctor, its potential benefits must be carefully weighed against its risks.

Pemoline passes into breast milk. Nursing mothers who must take this drug should consider bottle-feeding.

Seniors

Seniors should take this drug with caution.

Generic Name

Penciclovir (pen-SYE-kloe-veer)

Brand Name

Denavir

Type of Drug

Antiviral.

Prescribed for

Cold sores.

General Information

Penciclovir works against different types of herpes viruses
responsible for common cold sores. Cold sores treated with
penciclovir cream go away sooner and are less painful than
those that are not treated. Once applied to the skin, penciclovir is converted to its active form and interferes with DNA
production inside the viral particle; this inhibits the reproduction process of the herpes virus.

Cautions and Warnings

Do not use penciclovir if you are **sensitive** or **allergic** to it.

Penciclovir should **be applied only to the face or lips**. Avoid
applying it near your eyes because it may be irritating. The
effectiveness of penciclovir in people with **compromised
immune systems** is not known.

Male animals given massive doses of penciclovir intravenously suffered damage to the testicles. This effect
appears to be related to the dose of penciclovir. Men using
famciclovir—the oral form of penciclovir—for 8 to 13 weeks
experienced no changes in sperm count.

Drug resistance may develop with repeated use.

Possible Side Effects

Side effects are generally mild and infrequent. In studies,
side effects were similar in type and frequency among
people who used penciclovir and those who used an
inactive cream.

▼ Common: headache, redness, and swelling.

Possible Side Effects *(continued)*

▼ Less common: skin reactions to the cream.
▼ Rare: loss of skin sensation where the cream has been applied, changes in the sense of taste, and rash.

Drug Interactions

None known.

Usual Dose

Adult: Apply to affected areas every 2 hours, during waking hours, for 4 days.
Child: not recommended.

Overdosage

Little is known about the effects of penciclovir overdose or accidental ingestion. Call your poison control center or a hospital emergency room for more information.

Special Information

Begin cold sore treatment as early as possible. Early application of penciclovir cream will help prevent cold sores from appearing and reduce accompanying pain.

It is very important to apply penciclovir cream every 2 hours during the day for the drug to work. If you forget to apply a dose of penciclovir, apply it as soon as you remember. If you realize you forgot a dose within 30 to 45 minutes of your next dose, skip the dose you forgot and continue with your regular schedule.

Special Populations

Pregnancy/Breast-feeding

In animal studies, penciclovir had no effect on the fetus. There is no information on the effect of penciclovir in pregnant women. This drug should be used during pregnancy only if its possible benefits outweigh its risks.

It is not known if penciclovir passes into breast milk, though famciclovir—the oral form of penciclovir—passes into breast milk in concentrations larger than those found in the mother's blood. Nursing mothers who must use penciclovir should bottle-feed.

Seniors
Seniors may use this drug without special precaution.

Type of Drug
Penicillin Antibiotics (pen-ih-SIL-in)

Brand Names

Generic Ingredient: Amoxicillin [G]
Amoxil   Wymox
Trimox

Generic Ingredients: Amoxicillin + Potassium Clavulanate
Augmentin

Generic Ingredient: Ampicillin [G]
Marcillin   Principen
Omnipen   Totacillin

Generic Ingredients: Ampicillin + Probenecid
Probampacin

Generic Ingredient: Bacampicillin
Spectrobid

Generic Ingredient: Carbenicillin Indanyl Sodium
Geocillin

Generic Ingredient: Cloxacillin Sodium [G]
Cloxapen

Generic Ingredient: Dicloxacillin Sodium [G]
Dycill   Pathocil
Dynapen

Generic Ingredient: Nafcillin
Unipen

Generic Ingredient: Oxacillin [G]
Bactocill

Generic Ingredient: Penicillin G [G]
Pfizerpen

Generic Ingredient: Penicillin V [G]

Beepen-VK	Pen-Vee K
Betapen-VK	V-Cillin K
Ledercillin VK	Veetids
Penicillin VK	

Prescribed for

Bacterial and other infections.

General Information

Penicillin antibiotics kill bacteria and other microorganisms by destroying the cell wall of the invading organisms. Many infections respond to almost any kind of penicillin; some respond only to a specific penicillin antibiotic. Penicillin cannot cure a cold, the flu, or any other viral infection and should never be taken unless prescribed by a doctor for a specific condition. Always take penicillin exactly as prescribed, including the number of pills to take every day and number of days to take the drug, otherwise you will not get the drug's full effect.

Cautions and Warnings

Serious and sometimes **fatal allergic reactions** have occurred with penicillin. Though more common following penicillin injections, these reactions have also occurred with oral penicillin. Reactions are more common among people who have had a previous penicillin reaction and those who have had asthma, hay fever, or other allergies. Allergic symptoms include itching, rash, swelling, breathing difficulties, very low blood pressure, blood vessel collapse, peeling skin, chills, fever, muscle aches, arthritis-like pains, and feeling unwell. Beta-blocker drugs may worsen penicillin reactions. Sometimes, when an infection is life-threatening and can only be treated with penicillin, minor reactions may be treated with another drug while the penicillin is continued. About 1 in 20 people allergic to a penicillin antibiotic are also allergic to the cephalosporin antibiotics.

Cystic fibrosis patients are more likely to suffer from side effects of certain penicillins.

Some injectable penicillins have caused **bleeding problems**.

Possible Side Effects

The most important penicillin side effect, seen in up to 10% of people, is allergy.

About 9% of ampicillin users develop an itchy rash, which is not a true allergic reaction. This rash is more likely to occur when ampicillin is combined with allopurinol.

People who receive injectable penicillin may become lethargic, dizzy, or tired, or experience hallucinations, seizure, anxiety, depression, confusion, agitation, or hyperactivity.

▼ Common: upset stomach, abdominal pain, nausea, vomiting, diarrhea, colitis, sore mouth, coated tongue, anemia, bleeding abnormalities, low platelet and white-blood-cell counts, and oral or rectal fungal infections.

▼ Less common: vaginal irritation, appetite loss, itchy eyes, and feelings of body warmth.

▼ Rare: yellowing of the skin or whites of the eyes.

Drug Interactions

• Penicillin should not be mixed with a bacteriostatic antibiotic such as chloramphenicol, erythromycin, tetracycline, or neomycin. These drugs can interfere with each other.

• Penicillin can interfere with oral contraceptives. Use additional contraception while taking a penicillin drug. Breakthrough bleeding may occur.

• Nafcillin can interfere with cyclosporine (used to prevent rejection in people who have received an organ transplant).

• Penicillin allergies may be intensified by beta-blocking drugs.

• Ampicillin may reduce the effect of atenolol.

• Penicillin G blood levels may be increased by aspirin, phenylbutazone, sulfa drugs, indomethacin, thiazide-type diuretics, furosemide, or ethacrynic acid.

• Large doses of injectable penicillin may increase the effect of anticoagulant (blood-thinning) drugs.

Food Interactions

Do not take penicillin with fruit juice or carbonated beverages. The acid in these beverages may destroy the drug.

Most penicillins, including bacampicillin suspension, are best absorbed on an empty stomach. These medications may be taken 1 hour before or 2 hours after meals, or first thing in the morning and last thing at night with the other doses spaced evenly throughout the day.

Amoxicillin and bacampicillin tablets may be taken without regard to food.

Augmentin (amoxicillin and potassium clavulanate) is best taken right before a meal for optimum effectiveness and minimum stomach upset.

Usual Dose

Amoxicillin
   Adult: 250–500 mg every 8 hours.
   Child: 10–20 mg per lb. a day divided into 3 doses.

Amoxicillin and Potassium Clavulanate
   Adult: a "250" tablet every 8 hours; a "500" or "875" tablet every 12 hours.
   Child: 10–20 mg per lb. a day divided into 3 doses.

Different strengths of this product are not interchangeable. Take only the exact strength and product your doctor has prescribed.

Ampicillin
   Adult: 1–12 g a day divided into 4–6 doses.
   Child: 25–100 mg per lb. a day divided into 4–6 doses.

Ampicillin with Probenecid
3.5 g of ampicillin and 1 g of probenecid as a single dose for gonorrhea.

Bacampicillin
   Adult: 400–800 mg every 12 hours; 1600 mg plus 1 g of probenecid for gonorrhea.
   Child: 12–25 mg per lb. a day divided into 2 doses.

Carbenicillin Indanyl Sodium
   Adult: 382–764 mg 4 times a day.
   Child: not recommended.

Cloxacillin Sodium
   Adult: 250 mg every 6 hours.
   Child: 25 mg per lb. a day divided into 4 doses.

Dicloxacillin Sodium
  Adult: 125–250 mg every 6 hours.
  Child: 6–12 mg per lb. a day divided into 4 doses.

Nafcillin
  Adult: 250–1000 mg every 4–6 hours.
  Child: 5–25 mg per lb. every 6–8 hours.

Oxacillin
  Adult: 500–1000 mg every 4–6 hours.
  Child: 25–50 mg per lb. a day divided into 4 or 6 doses.

Penicillin G
  Adult (age 12 and over): 200,000–800,000 units, or 125–500 mg, every 6–8 hours for 10 days.
  Child (under age 12): 12,000–40,000 units per lb. a day divided into 3–6 doses.

Penicillin V
  Adult (age 12 and over): 125–500 mg 4 times a day. People with severe kidney disease should not take more than 250 mg every 6 hours.
  Child (under age 12): 12–25 mg per lb. a day divided into 3 or 4 doses.

Overdosage

Overdose is unlikely, but diarrhea or upset stomach is the primary symptom. Massive overdose may result in seizure or excitability. Call your local poison control center or a hospital emergency room for more information. ALWAYS bring the prescription bottle or container.

Special Information

Liquid penicillin should be refrigerated and must be thrown out after 14 days in the refrigerator or 7 days at room temperature.

Call your doctor if you develop black tongue, rash, itching, hives, diarrhea, breathing difficulties, sore throat, nausea, vomiting, fever, swollen joints, unusual bleeding or bruising, or if you are feeling unwell.

Penicillin eradicates most susceptible organisms in 7 to 10 days; be sure to take all the medication prescribed for the full period prescribed. It is best taken at evenly spaced intervals throughout the day.

If you miss a dose, take it as soon as possible. If it is almost time for your next dose, space the missed dose and your next dose by 2 to 4 hours and then continue with your regular schedule.

Special Populations

Pregnancy/Breast-feeding
Penicillin crosses into the fetal circulation but has not caused birth defects and is often prescribed for pregnant women. Be sure your doctor knows that you are taking a penicillin antibiotic if you are pregnant.

Penicillin is generally safe during breast-feeding; however, small amounts may pass into breast milk and cause upset stomach, diarrhea, allergic reaction, or other problems in the nursing infant.

Seniors
Seniors may take penicillin without special restriction.

Generic Name

Pentosan Polysulfate Sodium
(PEN-toe-san pol-ee-SUL-fate)

Brand Name

Elmiron

Type of Drug

Kidney analgesic.

Prescribed for

Bladder pain or discomfort due to cystitis.

General Information

Interstitial cystitis is a painful, long-term infection of the bladder. Pentosan does not affect the infectious process, but it may stick to the membranes of the bladder wall, preventing irritating substances from reaching bladder cells. About ⅓ of people who take this drug for 3 months or more have less cystitis pain.

Cautions and Warnings

Do not take this product if you are **sensitive** or **allergic** to it.

Pentosan is a weak anticoagulant and can cause **black-and-blue marks, nosebleeds,** and **bleeding gums**.

People with **liver disease** should use this drug with caution because its breakdown can be reduced in people with liver problems. Also, pentosan can cause mild liver toxicity.

Possible Side Effects

▼ Most common: patchy hair loss beginning within 4 weeks of treatment, diarrhea, and nausea.

▼ Common: headache, emotional upset or depression, dizziness, abdominal pain, and upset stomach.

▼ Rare: Rare side effects can include sleeplessness and effects on your blood, eyes, breathing, stomach and intestines, ears, and liver. Contact your doctor if you experience any side effect not listed above.

Drug Interactions

• Aspirin, clopidogrel, warfarin, and other blood-thinning drugs should be taken with caution if you are already taking pentosan. Pentosan may increase the anticoagulant effect of these drugs.

Food Interactions

Take this drug on an empty stomach, at least 1 hour before or 2 hours after a meal.

Usual Dose

Adult: 100 mg 3 times a day.

Overdosage

Symptoms include bleeding, liver problems, and upset stomach. Overdose victims should be taken to a hospital emergency room at once. ALWAYS bring the prescription bottle or container.

Special Information

Pentosan has a mild anticoagulant effect. Make sure that your pharmacist, dentist, and all of your doctors know you are taking pentosan. Check with your doctor before combining aspirin or other drugs with pentosan.

Patchy hair loss, usually starting within the first 4 weeks of taking pentosan, occurs in about 4% of people who take this medication.

Pentosan should be taken exactly as directed. If you forget to take a dose of pentosan, take it as soon as you remember. If it is almost time for your next dose, skip the dose you forgot and continue with your regular schedule. Do not take a double dose.

Special Populations

Pregnancy/Breast-feeding
While animal studies of pentosan reveal no damage to the fetus, this drug should only be used during pregnancy after carefully weighing its potential benefits against its risks.

It is not known if pentosan passes into breast milk. Nursing mothers who must take it should consider bottle-feeding.

Seniors
Seniors may use this medication without special precaution.

Pepcid   see Famotidine, page 406

Brand Name
Percocet

Generic Ingredients
Acetaminophen + Oxycodone Hydrochloride [G]

Other Brand Names
Roxicet   Roxilox
Roxicet 5/500   Tylox

The information in this profile also applies to the following drugs:

Generic Ingredients: Acetaminophen + Codeine Phosphate [G]

Aceta with Codeine
Capital with Codeine
Phenaphen with Codeine No. 3
Phenaphen with Codeine No. 4

Tylenol with Codeine No. 2
Tylenol with Codeine No. 3
Tylenol with Codeine No. 4

Generic Ingredients: Acetaminophen + Hydrocodone Bitartrate [G]

Anexsia 5/500
Anexsia 7.5/650
Anexsia 10/660
Bancap HC
Ceta-Plus
Co-Gesic
Dolacet
Duocet
Hydrocet
Hydrogesic
Hy-Phen
Lorcet-HD
Lorcet Plus
Lorcet 10/650

Lortab
Lortab 2.5/500
Lortab 5/500
Lortab 7.5/500
Lortab 10/500
Margesic H
Norco
Panacet 5/500
Stagesic
T-Gesic
Vicodin
Vicodin-ES
Vicodin-HP
Zydone

Generic Ingredient: Oxycodone

Oxycontin
Percolone

Roxicodone

Type of Drug

Narcotic and analgesic (pain reliever) combination.

Prescribed for

Mild to moderate pain.

General Information

Percocet is generally prescribed for those who require a greater analgesic effect than acetaminophen alone can deliver or for those who cannot take aspirin. Percocet is not considered effective for arthritis or other pain caused by inflammation because it does not reduce inflammation.

Cautions and Warnings

Do not take Percocet if you are **allergic** or **sensitive** to any of its ingredients. Use this drug with extreme caution if you suffer from **asthma or other breathing problems** or have **kidney or liver disease** or **viral infection of the liver**. Chronic (long-term) use of Percocet may cause drug dependence or **addiction**.

Oxycodone is a respiratory depressant and affects the central nervous system (CNS), producing **sleepiness, tiredness**, and **inability to concentrate**.

Alcohol may increase the risk of acetaminophen-related liver toxicity and oxycodone-related drowsiness.

Possible Side Effects

▼ Most common: light-headedness, dizziness, sleepiness, nausea, vomiting, appetite loss, and increased sweating. If any of these effects occur, ask your doctor to consider lowering your dosage. Most of these side effects disappear if you lie down. More serious side effects are shallow breathing or breathing difficulties.

▼ Rare: Rare side effects can occur in almost any part of the body. Contact your doctor if you experience any side effect not listed above. Narcotic pain relievers may aggravate convulsions in those who have had them.

Drug Interactions

• Because of its depressant effect and potential effect on breathing, Percocet should be taken with extreme care in combination with alcohol, sleeping medication, tranquilizers, antihistamines, or other drugs producing sedation.

Food Interactions

Percocet is best taken with food or at least half a glass of water to prevent upset stomach.

Usual Dose

Percocet
    Adult: 1–2 tablets every 4 hours.
    Child: not recommended.

Acetaminophen with Codeine
  Adult and Child (age 13 and over): 1–2 tablets every 4 hours.
  Child (age 7–12): equivalent of 5–10 mg of codeine every 4–6 hours; do not exceed 60 mg in 24 hours.
  Child (age 2–6): equivalent of 2.5–5 mg of codeine every 4–6 hours; do not exceed 30 mg in 24 hours.

Oxycodone
  Adult: 10–30 mg every 4 hours.

Vicodin
  Adult: 1 tablet every 6 hours.
  Child: not recommended.

Overdosage

Symptoms include depressed respiration, extreme tiredness progressing to stupor and then coma, pinpointed pupils, no response to pain stimulation, cold and clammy skin, slowing of heart rate, lowering of blood pressure, yellowing of the skin or whites of the eyes, bluish discoloration of the hands or feet, fever, excitement, delirium, convulsions, cardiac arrest, and liver toxicity (symptoms include nausea, vomiting, abdominal pain, and diarrhea). Induce vomiting with ipecac syrup—available at any pharmacy—and take the victim to a hospital emergency room immediately. ALWAYS bring the prescription bottle or container.

Special Information

Percocet is a respiratory depressant that affects the CNS, producing sleepiness, tiredness, and inability to concentrate. Be careful when driving or performing any task that requires concentration.
  If you forget a dose, take it as soon as you remember. If it is almost time for your next dose, skip the dose you forgot and continue with your regular schedule. Do not take a double dose.

Special Populations

Pregnancy/Breast-feeding

High doses of acetaminophen, one of the ingredients in Percocet, have caused problems when taken during pregnancy. Regular use of oxycodone, the other active ingredient in Percocet, during pregnancy may cause addiction in newborns. If used during labor, it may cause breathing problems in the infant. If you are pregnant, do not take Percocet.

The ingredients in Percocet may pass into breast milk. Nursing mothers who must take this drug should wait 4 to 6 hours after their last dose before nursing or they should consider bottle-feeding.

Seniors
Seniors may be sensitive to the depressant effects of this drug.

Brand Name
Percodan

Generic Ingredients
Aspirin + Oxycodone Hydrochloride + Oxycodone Terephthalate [G]

Other Brand Names
Percodan-Demi   Roxiprin

The information in this profile also applies to the following drugs:

Generic Ingredients: Aspirin + Codeine Phosphate [G]
Empirin with Codeine No. 3   Empirin with Codeine No. 4

Generic Ingredients: Aspirin + Caffeine + Dihydrocodeine Bitartrate
Synalgos-DC

Generic Ingredients: Pentazocine + Acetaminophen
Talacen

Generic Ingredients: Pentazocine + Aspirin
Talwin Compound

Generic Ingredients: Pentazocine + Naloxone
Talwin Nx

Type of Drug
Narcotic and aspirin combination.

Prescribed for

Mild to moderate pain.

General Information

Percodan is one of many combination products containing a narcotic and a non-narcotic analgesic (pain reliever). It is prescribed to relieve pain and reduce inflammation.

Cautions and Warnings

Do not take Percodan if you are **allergic** or **sensitive** to any of its ingredients. Do not take Percodan if you are allergic to any salicylate, including aspirin, or any nonsteroidal anti-inflammatory drug (NSAID). Use this medication with extreme caution if you suffer from **asthma or other breathing problems**. Chronic (long-term) use of this drug may cause drug dependence or **addiction**. Percodan is a respiratory depressant and affects the central nervous system (CNS), producing **sleepiness, tiredness,** and **inability to concentrate**.

This and other aspirin-containing products should not be taken by **children under age 16**.

People with **liver damage** should avoid Percodan and all products that contain either aspirin or oxycodone.

Alcohol may aggravate the stomach irritation caused by aspirin. The risk of aspirin-related ulcer is increased by alcohol. Alcohol will also increase the nervous-system depression caused by the oxycodone ingredient in this drug.

Do not use Percodan if you develop **dizziness, hearing loss,** or **ringing or buzzing in your ears**.

Percodan may interfere with **blood coagulation** and should be avoided for 1 week before **surgery**. Ask your surgeon or dentist for a recommendation before taking an aspirin-containing product for pain after surgery.

Possible Side Effects

▼ Most common: light-headedness, dizziness, sleepiness, nausea, vomiting, appetite loss, and increased sweating. If these occur, ask your doctor to consider lowering your dosage. Usually they go away if you lie down.

Possible Side Effects *(continued)*

▼ Less common: shallow breathing or serious breathing difficulties, euphoria (feeling "high"), weakness,
headache, agitation, uncoordinated muscle movement,
minor hallucinations, disorientation, visual disturbances,
dry mouth, constipation, facial flushing, rapid heartbeat,
palpitations, feeling faint, urinary difficulties or hesitancy, reduced sex drive or potency, rash, itching, anemia, low blood sugar, and yellowing of the skin or whites
of the eyes. These drugs may aggravate convulsions in
those who have had them.

Drug Interactions

• Combining Percodan and alcohol, tranquilizers, barbiturates, or sleeping pills produces sleepiness or an inability to
concentrate and significantly increases Percodan's depressive effect.

• The aspirin in Percodan may affect anticoagulant (blood-
thinning) therapy. Your doctor may recommend a dosage
adjustment.

• Combining Percodan and adrenal corticosteroids,
phenylbutazone, or alcohol may cause severe stomach irritation with possible bleeding.

• The aspirin in Percodan counteracts the uric-acid-eliminating effect of probenecid and sulfinpyrazone; may counteract the blood-pressure-lowering effect of angiotensin-
converting enzyme (ACE) inhibitors and beta-blocking
drugs and the effects of diuretics (agents that increase urination) when given to people with severe liver disease; and
may increase blood levels of methotrexate and valproic
acid when taken together, leading to increased risk of drug
toxicity.

• The aspirin in Percodan, when taken with nitroglycerin
tablets, may lead to an unexpected drop in blood pressure.

• Do not take Percodan with any NSAID. There is no benefit from the combination and the risk of side effects, especially stomach irritation, is significantly increased.

• Large dosages of aspirin—2000 mg a day or more—
may lower blood sugar, a potentially serious side effect for
people with diabetes. Percodan tablets contain 325 mg of
aspirin.

Food Interactions

Take with food or half a glass of water to prevent upset stomach.

Usual Dose

Percodan
 Adult: 1 tablet every 6 hours as needed for pain relief.
 Child: not recommended.

Empirin with Codeine
 Adult: 1–2 tablets 3–4 times a day.
 Child: not recommended.

Synalgos-DC
 Adult: 2 capsules every 4 hours.
 Child: not recommended.

Overdosage

Symptoms include breathing difficulties, extreme tiredness progressing to stupor and then coma, pinpointed pupils, no response to pain stimulation, cold and clammy skin, slowing of heartbeat, dizziness or fainting, convulsions, cardiac arrest, fever, excitement, confusion, liver or kidney failure, and bleeding. Symptoms of mild overdose include nausea, vomiting, dizziness, ringing or buzzing in the ears, flushing, increased sweating, thirst, headache, drowsiness, diarrhea, and rapid heartbeat. Take the victim to a hospital emergency room immediately. ALWAYS bring the prescription bottle or container.

Special Information

Drowsiness may occur: Be careful when driving or performing any task that requires concentration.

Contact your doctor if you develop continuous stomach pain or ringing or buzzing in the ears.

Do not use Percodan if it has a strong odor of vinegar. This is an indication that the product has started to break down in the bottle.

If you forget a dose, take it as soon as you remember. If it is almost time for your next dose, skip the one you forgot and continue with your regular schedule. Do not take a double dose.

Special Populations

Pregnancy/Breast-feeding

Aspirin, one of the ingredients in Percodan, may cause bleeding problems in the fetus, particularly during the last 2 weeks of pregnancy. Taking aspirin during the last 3 months of pregnancy may lead to a low-birth-weight infant, prolong labor, and extend the duration of pregnancy; it may also cause bleeding in the mother before, during, or after delivery. Large amounts of oxycodone, the other ingredient in Percodan, may cause addiction in newborns. It may also cause breathing problems in newborns if taken just before delivery. When Percodan is considered crucial by your doctor, its potential benefits must be carefully weighed against its risks.

The ingredients in Percodan may pass into breast milk. Nursing mothers who must take this drug should consider bottle-feeding.

Seniors
Seniors may be more sensitive to the depressant effects of this drug as well as dizziness, light-headedness, and fainting, particularly upon rising suddenly from a sitting or lying position.

Generic Name

Pergolide (PER-goe-lide)

Brand Name

Permax

Type of Drug

Antiparkinsonian.

Prescribed for

Parkinson's disease.

General Information

Pergolide mesylate is combined with levodopa or carbidopa to control Parkinson's disease. It works by stimulating a specific nerve ending in the central nervous system that is normally stimulated by the hormone dopamine. Pergolide also inhibits the production of prolactin, a hormone that is involved in the production of breast milk. Pergolide affects growth-hormone levels and the reproductive hormone called luteinizing hormone (LH).

Cautions and Warnings

Do not take pergolide if you have had a reaction to it or other drugs derived from the fungus ergot.

Pergolide causes **hallucinations** in about 14% of people. If this occurs, contact your doctor at once.

People who are prone to abnormal heart rhythms should be cautious when taking pergolide because of possible **cardiac side effects**.

Possible Side Effects

In studies, about 25% of people stopped taking pergolide because of side effects.

▼ Most common: hallucinations, confusion, twisting body movements, tiredness, difficulty sleeping, nausea, constipation, diarrhea, upset stomach, and runny nose.

▼ Less common: generalized pain; abdominal pain; neck or back pain; migraine headaches; muscle weakness; chest pain; flu-like illness; chills; facial swelling; infections; dizziness when rising from a sitting or lying position; fainting; heart palpitations; changes in blood pressure; abnormal heart rhythm; heart attack; heart failure; changes in appetite; dry mouth; vomiting; gas; yellowing of the skin or whites of the eyes; enlarged saliva glands; stomach irritation; intestinal ulcer or obstruction; gum irritation; dental cavities; colitis; loss of bowel control; blood in the stool; vomiting blood; bursitis; muscle twitching; anxiety; tremors; depression; unusual dreams; personality changes; psychosis; changes in how you walk; loss of coordination; tingling in the hands or feet; speech problems; muscle stiffness; breathing difficulties; hiccups; pneumonia; coughing; sinus irritation; bronchitis; asthma; nosebleed; rash; skin discoloration; skin ulcers; acne; fungal infections; eczema; hair growth or loss; cold sores; increased sweating; visual abnormalities such as double vision, conjunctivitis (pinkeye), cataracts, retinal detachment, blindness, and eye pain; earaches; middle-ear infection; ringing or buzzing in the ears; deafness; changes in sense of taste; frequent or painful urination; urinary infection; blood in the urine; swelling of the arms or legs; weight gain; anemia; breast pain; painful menstruation; breast oozing; underactive thyroid; thyroid tumor; diabetes; and muscle, bone, and joint pain.

Drug Interactions

* Phenothiazines, thioxanthenes, haloperidol, droperidol, loxapine, methyldopa, molindone, papaverine, reserpine, and metoclopramide counter the effects of pergolide.·

* Alcohol, tranquilizers, and other nervous-system depressants increase the depressant effects of this drug.

* Drugs that cause low blood pressure increase the blood-pressure-lowering effect of pergolide.

Food Interactions

Take pergolide with food if it upsets your stomach.

Usual Dose

Starting dosage—.05 mg a day. Dosage is increased by 0.1–0.25 mg every third day until an effect is achieved. Maximum dosage is 5 mg a day.

Overdosage

Symptoms may include nausea, vomiting, agitation, low blood pressure, hallucinations, involuntary body and muscular movements, tingling in the arms or legs, heart palpitations, abnormal heart rhythms, and nervous-system stimulation. Take the victim to a hospital emergency room. ALWAYS bring the prescription bottle or container.

Special Information

Many people taking pergolide for the first time experience dizziness and fainting caused by low blood pressure. Your doctor will need to increase your pergolide dosage gradually to reduce this effect. However, any dizziness or fainting should be reported to your doctor at once.

Contact your doctor if you experience nervous-system effects, such as confusion, uncontrolled body movements, or hallucinations; pain or burning upon urination; high blood pressure; severe headache; seizure; sudden changes in vision; severe chest pain; fainting; rapid heartbeat; severe nausea; excessive sweating; nervousness; shortness of breath; sudden weakness; or any bothersome or persistent side effect.

Do not stop taking pergolide or change your dosage without your doctor's knowledge.

This drug may make you tired, dizzy, or light-headed. Be careful when driving or doing any task that requires concentration.

Dry mouth may be relieved with sugarless gum, candy, ice, or a saliva substitute. Maintain good oral hygiene while taking pergolide because dry mouth increases the risk of oral infections.

If you forget a dose, take it as soon as you remember. If you take pergolide once a day and it is almost time for your next dose, skip the one you forgot and continue with your regular schedule. If you take pergolide 2 or 3 times a day and it is almost time for your next dose, take 1 dose as soon as you remember and another in 3 or 4 hours, then go back to your regular schedule. Never take a double dose.

Special Populations

Pregnancy/Breast-feeding
While animal studies of pergolide revealed no damage to the fetus, this drug should only be used after carefully weighing its benefits against its risks.

Pergolide may pass into breast milk and interfere with milk production. Nursing mothers who must take it should bottle-feed.

Seniors
Seniors may take pergolide without special restriction.

Generic Name

Permethrin (per-MEE-thrin) G

Brand Names

Acticin	Nix
Elimite	Rid

Type of Drug

Scabicide.

Prescribed for

Scabies and head lice.

General Information

Permethrin is a synthetic chemical that kills lice, ticks, mites, and fleas. It paralyzes the parasite by interfering with its nervous system. Only 2 or 3 in 100 people who use permethrin for head lice need to be re-treated because it kills both the parasite and its eggs. Permethrin, which remains on hair shafts after application, prevents reinfection for up to 2 weeks. Less than 2% of permethrin is absorbed through the skin into the bloodstream.

Cautions and Warnings

Do not use permethrin if you are **sensitive** or **allergic** to it or chrysanthemums. Stop using permethrin if you develop a reaction to it.

Possible Side Effects

Cream
▼ Most common: burning and stinging.
▼ Common: mild, temporary itching.
▼ Rare: tingling, numbness, mild swelling, and rash.

Liquid
▼ Common: mild, temporary itching.
▼ Less common: mild, temporary burning or stinging; tingling; numbness; discomfort; mild swelling; and rash.

Drug Interactions

• Do not apply this product with any other topical medication.

Usual Dose

Cream: For adults and children age 2 months and over—Thoroughly massage the cream into the skin from the head to the soles of the feet; 1 oz. (30 g) is usually enough for a single treatment. Infants should be treated at the hairline, neck, scalp, and forehead. Leave the cream on for 8–14 hours and then remove it by washing.

Liquid: For adults and children age 2 and over—Wash your hair with regular shampoo, rinse, and towel dry. Then, apply enough permethrin liquid to saturate the hair and scalp; leave it in for 10 minutes. Rinse off with water.

Overdosage

In case of accidental ingestion, call your local poison control center or a hospital emergency room. You may be told to induce vomiting with ipecac syrup—available at any pharmacy—before taking the victim to an emergency room. If you seek treatment, ALWAYS bring the prescription bottle or container.

Special Information

This drug should be applied only to hairy areas of the body with intact skin. It should never be swallowed.

Do not apply permethrin to areas around the eyes, nose, or mouth. Call your doctor if anything unusual develops or if irritation continues after you have stopped using the drug.

It is not necessary to comb the hair to remove parasite eggs after permethrin treatment but you may wish to do so for cosmetic reasons.

Special Populations

Pregnancy/Breast-feeding

The safety of using permethrin during pregnancy is not known. When this drug is considered crucial by your doctor, its potential benefits must be carefully weighed against its risks.

It is not known if permethrin passes into breast milk. Nursing mothers who must use it should bottle-feed.

Seniors

This drug may be used without special precaution.

Generic Name

Phenelzine (FEH-nel-zeen)

Brand Name

Nardil

The information in this profile also applies to the following drug:

Generic Ingredient: Tranylcypromine Sulfate
Parnate

Type of Drug

Monoamine oxidase inhibitor (MAOI).

Prescribed for

Atypical depression and depression that does not respond to other drugs; also prescribed for a variety of conditions including bulimia, cocaine addiction, night terrors, post-traumatic stress disorder, migraine, seasonal affective disorder, and symptoms of multiple sclerosis.

General Information

Monoamine oxidase (MAO) is a complex enzyme system found throughout the body. MAO is responsible for breaking down hormones that make the nervous system work. MAOIs such as phenelzine sulfate interfere with MAO action, causing an increase in the amount of norepinephrine and other monoamines stored throughout the nervous system. This increase is what gives phenelzine its therapeutic effect, which is long lasting and may continue for up to 2 weeks after you stop taking it.

Cautions and Warnings

Do not take phenelzine if you are **allergic** to it or have **pheochromocytoma** (adrenal-gland tumor), **heart failure, liver disease** or **abnormal liver function,** severe **kidney-function loss, heart disease,** or a history of **headaches, stroke, transient ischemic attack** (TIA)—"mini-stroke"—or **high blood pressure**. The most severe reactions to phenelzine, which can be deadly, involve very high blood pressure. **Bleeding inside the head** has occurred in people with very high blood pressure. Serious, potentially fatal reactions may occur if phenelzine and a selective serotonin reuptake inhibitor (SSRI) antidepressant are taken together (see "Drug Interactions").

Possible Side Effects

▼ Common: dizziness when rising from a sitting or lying position, dizziness, fainting, headache, tremors, muscle twitching, overly reactive reflexes, manic reactions, confusion, memory loss, sleeping difficulties,

Possible Side Effects *(continued)*

weakness, uncontrollable muscle movement, fatigue, drowsiness, restlessness, overstimulation, anxiety and agitation, constipation, nausea, diarrhea, abdominal pain, swelling, dry mouth, liver irritation, appetite loss, weight changes, and sexual difficulties.

▼ Less common: jitteriness, a need to pace the floor or change positions often, euphoria (feeling "high"), nerve irritation, chills, a need to repeat words or phrases, convulsions, tingling in the hands or feet, heart palpitations, rapid heartbeat, painful or infrequent urination, changes in blood components, glaucoma, blurred vision, uncontrolled eyeball movement, sweating, and rash.

▼ Rare: poor coordination, coma, hallucinations at high dosages, severe anxiety, schizophrenia, delirious reactions, muscle spasm, jerky movements, numbness, and yellowing of the skin or whites of the eyes.

Drug Interactions

• Phenelzine interferes with the blood-pressure-lowering effect of guanethidine. Do not combine these drugs.

• Taking an SSRI antidepressant and phenelzine at the same time or too close together may result in a serious, sometimes fatal reaction characterized by very high fever, rigidity, muscle spasms, and changes in mental state, blood pressure, pulse, and breathing rate. Two weeks should elapse between stopping phenelzine and taking an SSRI. At least 5 weeks should elapse between stopping an SSRI and taking phenelzine.

• A tricyclic antidepressant and phenelzine may be combined only under your doctor's direct supervision. If dosages are not strictly controlled, this combination can lead to seizures, sweating, coma, hyperexcitability, high fever, rapid heartbeat, rapid breathing, headache, dilated pupils, flushing, confusion, and low blood pressure. When severe, this reaction can be fatal. Generally, 2 weeks must pass between stopping phenelzine and taking a tricyclic antidepressant.

• Phenelzine increases the effects of sulfonylurea-type antidiabetic drugs, barbiturates, beta blockers, levodopa, meperidine, methyldopa, rauwolfia drugs, sulfa drugs, sumatriptan, stimulants, thiazide-type diuretics, and L-tryptophan.

The combination of any of these drugs and phenelzine can result in severe reactions.

• Combining dextromethorphan (a cough suppressant found in many over-the-counter products) and phenelzine may lead to a high fever and low blood pressure. Avoid this combination.

• Combining phenelzine with another MAOI or methylphenidate may lead to excessively high blood pressure.

• Combining tranylcypromine sulfate and disulfiram may lead to delirium, agitation, disorientation, and hallucinations.

Food Interactions

Avoid the following while taking phenelzine and for at least 2 weeks after stopping phenelzine:

Alcohol: imported beer and ale; red wine, especially Chianti; sherry; vermouth; and distilled spirits.

Cheese and Dairy: processed American cheese, blue cheese, Boursault, natural brick cheese, Brie, Camembert, cheddar, Emmenthaler, Gruyere, mozzarella, Parmesan, Romano, Roquefort, sour cream, Stilton, Swiss cheese, and yogurt.

Fruits and Vegetables: avocados, especially when overripe; yeast extracts, including marmite; canned figs; raisins; sauerkraut; soy sauce; miso soup; and bean curd.

Meat and Fish: beef or chicken liver, meats prepared with a tenderizer, summer sausage, bologna, pepperoni, salami, game, meat extracts, caviar, dried fish, salted herring, pickled and spoiled herring, and shrimp paste.

Other: fava beans, caffeine, chocolate, and ginseng.

Usual Dose

Phenelzine
    Adult and Child (age 17 and over): 15 mg 3 times a day to start, increased gradually to 90 mg a day. Maintenance dosage may be as low as 15 mg a day.
    Senior: 15 mg in the morning. Dosage is increased very gradually.
    Child (under age 17): not recommended.

Tranylcypromine Sulfate
    Adult and Child (age 17 and over): 10–60 mg a day. Usual dosage is 30 mg a day.

Senior: starting dosage—2.5–5 mg a day. Maintenance dosage—45 mg a day.

Child (under age 17): not recommended.

Overdosage

Early symptoms may include excitement; irritability; hyperactivity; anxiety; low blood pressure; vascular system collapse; sleeplessness; restlessness; dizziness; fainting; weakness; drowsiness; hallucinations; jaw-muscle spasms; flushing; sweating; rapid breathing; rapid heartbeat; movement disorders including grimacing, rigidity, muscle tremors, and large muscle spasms; and severe headache. Take the victim to a hospital emergency room at once. ALWAYS bring the prescription bottle or container.

Special Information

Serious side effects include intense headache; heart palpitations; stiff or sore neck; nausea; vomiting; sweating, sometimes accompanied by fever or cold, clammy skin; dilated pupils; and sensitivity to bright light. Report these or any bothersome or persistent side effect to your doctor.

Vivid nightmares, agitation, psychosis, and convulsions occasionally occur 1 to 3 days after phenelzine is abruptly stopped. Gradually stopping phenelzine should prevent these problems.

Phenelzine causes drowsiness and blurred vision. Be careful when driving or performing any task that requires concentration. Avoid alcohol.

People with diabetes should be cautious because this drug may lower blood-sugar readings.

Be sure your surgeon or dentist knows that you are taking phenelzine before administering any anesthetic drug.

Do not take any other prescription or over-the-counter drug without first checking with your pharmacist or the doctor who prescribed phenelzine.

If you forget a dose, take it as soon as possible. If it is less than 2 hours until your next dose, skip the dose you forgot and continue with your regular schedule. Do not take a double dose.

Special Populations

Pregnancy/Breast-feeding

Phenelzine may pass into the fetal circulation. When this drug is considered crucial by your doctor, its potential benefits must be carefully weighed against its risks.

This drug may pass into breast milk. Nursing mothers who must take it should bottle-feed.

Seniors

Seniors are more susceptible to side effects and must use caution.

Generic Name

Phenobarbital (FEEN-oe-BAR-bih-tol) Ⓖ

Brand Names

Bellatal   Solfoton

Type of Drug

Hypnotic, sedative, and anticonvulsant.

Prescribed for

Epileptic and other seizures, convulsions, daytime sedation, and sleeplessness.

General Information

Phenobarbital is a sustained-release barbiturate. It takes 30 to 60 minutes to start working and its effect lasts for 10 to 16 hours. Like other barbiturates, phenobarbital appears to act by interfering with nerve impulses to the brain. When used as an anticonvulsant, phenobarbital is not very effective by itself; when used with anticonvulsant agents such as phenytoin, the combined action is dramatic. This combination has been used very successfully to control epileptic seizure.

Cautions and Warnings

Phenobarbital may **dull your physical and mental reflexes**. Be extremely careful when driving or performing any task that requires concentration.

Phenobarbital may be **addicting** if taken for an extended period of time. It may also cause **signs of intoxication** including slurred speech, a wobbly walk, rolling of the eyes, confusion, poor judgment, irritability, and sleeplessness. Combining this drug with alcohol worsens the situation.

Barbiturates are broken down in the liver and eliminated through the kidneys; people with **liver or kidney disease** should be cautious about taking phenobarbital.

You should not take phenobarbital if you are **sensitive** or **allergic** to any barbiturate, if you have been addicted to sedatives or hypnotics, or if you have a **respiratory condition**.

People with chronic pain should be careful about taking this drug because it may mask symptoms or cause stimulation, though using phenobarbital after surgery and in people with cancer has proven effective.

People abruptly stopping this drug may develop **seizure**. Dosage should be reduced gradually.

Barbiturates may increase your need for **vitamin D**; take a vitamin supplement while using this drug.

Possible Side Effects

▼ Most common: drowsiness, lethargy, dizziness, drug "hangover," breathing difficulties, rash, and general allergic reaction (symptoms include runny nose, watery eyes, sneezing, scratchy throat, and cough).

▼ Less common: nausea, vomiting, constipation and diarrhea, slow heartbeat, low blood pressure, and fainting. Severe adverse reactions may include anemia and yellowing of the skin or whites of the eyes.

Drug Interactions

• Alcohol, monoamine oxidase inhibitor (MAOI) antidepressants, and valproic acid increase the effects of phenobarbital.

• Charcoal, chloramphenicol, and rifampin may counteract the effects of phenobarbital.

• Phenobarbital interferes with the effects of anticoagulant (blood-thinning) drugs, beta-blocker drugs, carbamazepine, chloramphenicol, oral contraceptives ("the pill"), corticosteroids, clonazepam, digitoxin, doxorubicin, doxycycline, felodipine, fenoprofen, griseofulvin, metronidazole, phenylbutazone, quinidine, theophylline, and verapamil.

• Phenobarbital enhances the toxic effects of acetaminophen and methoxyflurane (an anesthetic).

• Phenobarbital has a variable effect on phenytoin and other antiseizure medication and on narcotic drugs. Dosage adjustments are necessary.

Food Interactions

Phenobarbital is best taken on an empty stomach but may be taken with food if it upsets your stomach.

Usual Dose

Anticonvulsant
    Adult: 50–100 mg 2–3 times a day.
    Child: 1.3–2.25 mg per lb. of body weight divided into 2 or 3 doses a day.

Sleeplessness
100–320 mg at bedtime.

Daytime Sedation
30–120 mg in 2–3 divided doses.

Overdosage

Severe barbiturate overdose may be fatal. Overdose symptoms include breathing difficulties, moderate reduction in pupil size, lowered body temperature progressing to fever, fluid in the lungs, and eventually coma. Take the victim to a hospital emergency room immediately. ALWAYS bring the prescription bottle or container.

Special Information

Avoid alcohol and other drugs that depress the nervous system.
    Take this medication exactly as prescribed.
    This drug causes drowsiness. Be careful when driving or doing any task that requires concentration.
    Call your doctor at once if you develop fever, sore throat, nosebleeds, mouth sores, unexplainable black-and-blue marks, or easy bruising or bleeding.
    If you forget a dose, take it as soon as you remember. If it is almost time for your next dose, skip the one you forgot and continue with your regular schedule. Do not take a double dose.

Special Populations

Pregnancy/Breast-feeding

Barbiturate use during pregnancy may increase the risk of birth defects and cause bleeding problems, brain tumors, and breathing difficulties in newborns. Regular use of a barbiturate during the last 3 months of pregnancy may cause drug dependency in newborns. However, phenobarbital may be necessary to control major episodes of seizure during pregnancy. Talk to your doctor about the potential benefits and risks of using phenobarbital.

Barbiturates pass into breast milk. They may cause drowsiness, slow heartbeat, and breathing difficulties in infants. Nursing mothers who must take phenobarbital should bottle-feed.

Seniors
Seniors are more sensitive to the effects of barbiturates and often need less medication.

Generic Name

Phenytoin (FEN-ih-toin) G

Brand Name

Dilantin

The information in this profile also applies to the following drugs:

Generic Ingredient: Ethotoin
Peganone

Generic Ingredient: Fosphenytoin
Cerebyx

Generic Ingredient: Mephenytoin
Mesantoin

Type of Drug

Hydantoin anticonvulsant.

Prescribed for

Epileptic seizure; also prescribed for prevention of seizure following neurosurgery in nonepileptics and for abnormal heart rhythm. Phenytoin injection is used to control preeclampsia (a condition in which pregnant women experience severe increases in blood pressure during the second half of pregnancy), trigeminal neuralgia (tic douloureux), and severe skin conditions.

General Information

Phenytoin is the most widely prescribed of several hydantoin antiseizure drugs. These drugs all inhibit activity in that area of the brain responsible for grand mal seizures. People may respond to some hydantoins and not others.

Immediate-release phenytoin must be taken several times a day, while the sustained-release form can be taken either once or several times a day. Many people find the latter more convenient, but the immediate-release form allows your doctor more flexibility in designing an effective dosage schedule. Phenytoin may be used together with other anticonvulsants, such as phenobarbital.

Cautions and Warnings

Do not take phenytoin if you are **allergic** to it or any hydantoin anticonvulsant.

When discontinuing phenytoin, **dosage should be gradually reduced** over a period of about a week—otherwise, severe seizures may occur.

Phenytoin should not be used if you have **low blood pressure, myocardial insufficiency,** a very **slow heart rate,** or certain other **heart conditions**.

People with **liver disease** are more likely to experience phenytoin side effects.

Periodical blood tests are necessary to monitor **red- and white-blood-cell counts**. Sore throat, feeling unwell, fever, mucous-membrane bleeding, swollen glands, nosebleeds, black-and-blue marks, and easy bruising may be signs of blood disorders.

Rash may be a sign of a serious reaction and cause for stopping this medication. Tell your doctor at once if this happens.

Possible Side Effects

▼ Most common: rapid or unusual growth of the gums, slurred speech, mental confusion, nystagmus (rhythmic, uncontrolled movement of the eye), dizziness, insomnia, nervousness, uncontrollable twitching, double vision, tiredness, irritability, depression, tremors, headache. These side effects generally disappear as therapy continues and dosage is reduced.

Possible Side Effects *(continued)*

▼ Less common: nausea, vomiting, diarrhea, constipation, fever, rash, balding, weight gain, numbness in
the hands or feet, chest pain, water retention, sensitivity
to bright light (especially sunlight), conjunctivitis (pinkeye), joint pain and inflammation, and high blood sugar.
Phenytoin may cause coarse facial features, lip enlargement, and Peyronie's disease (in which the penis is permanently deformed or misshapen). Phenytoin rash may
be accompanied by fever and may be serious or fatal.
Some fatal blood-system side effects have occurred with
phenytoin.

▼ Rare: liver damage (including hepatitis) and
unusual body-hair growth.

Drug Interactions

• The following drugs may increase the effects of phenytoin, possibly necessitating a decrease in phenytoin dosage:
alcohol in small amounts, allopurinol, amiodarone, aspirin
and other salicylate drugs, benzodiazepine drugs, chloramphenicol, chlorpheniramine, cimetidine, disulfiram, fluconazole, ibuprofen, isoniazid, metronidazole, miconazole,
omeprazole, phenacemide, phenothiazine antipsychotic
drugs, phenylbutazone, succinimide antiseizure drugs, sulfa
drugs, tricyclic antidepressants, trimethoprim, and valproic
acid.

• The following drugs may interfere with the effects of
phenytoin, possibly necessitating an increase in phenytoin
dosage: large amounts of alcohol, antacids, anticancer drugs,
barbiturates, carbamazepine, charcoal tablets, diazoxide,
folic acid, influenza virus vaccine, loxapine succinate, nitrofurantoin, pyridoxine, rifampin, sucralfate, and theophylline
drugs.

• Calcium supplements may slow the absorption of phenytoin

• Phenytoin may reduce the effectiveness of amiodarone,
carbamazepine, digitalis drugs, corticosteroids, dicumarol,
disopyramide, doxycycline, estrogen drugs, haloperidol,
methadone, metyrapone, mexiletine, oral contraceptives
("the pill"), quinidine, theophylline drugs, and valproic acid.
Dosage increases may be necessary.

• Phenytoin may increase the risk of liver toxicity caused by acetaminophen, especially if phenytoin is taken regularly.

• Phenytoin may affect certain other drugs in an unpredictable manner. If you take phenytoin and one or more of these drugs, your doctor will have to determine if dosage adjustment is needed: cyclosporine, dopamine, furosemide, levodopa, levonorgestrel, mebendazole, phenothiazine antipsychotic drugs, and oral antidiabetes drugs.

• Combining clonazepam and phenytoin yields unpredictable results: The effect of either drug may be reduced or phenytoin side effects may occur.

• Corticosteroid drugs may mask the effects of phenytoin sensitivity reactions.

• Lithium toxicity may be increased if lithium is taken with phenytoin.

• Phenytoin may decrease meperidine's pain-relieving effects and increase the risk of meperidine side effects. This combination is not recommended.

• Long-term phenytoin therapy may result in extreme folic acid deficiency, or megaloblastic anemia. This imbalance may be corrected with folic acid supplements.

• Warfarin's effects may be increased by phenytoin; warfarin dosage must be adjusted.

Food Interactions

Take phenytoin with food to avoid stomach upset. Calcium can slow phenytoin absorption. Separate your phenytoin dose from high-calcium foods, such as milk, cheese, almonds, hazelnuts, and sesame seeds and calcium supplements, by 1 to 2 hours.

Usual Dose

Adult: starting dosage—300 mg a day. Maintenance dosage—300–400 mg a day. Dosage can be raised gradually to 600 mg a day. Sustained-release phenytoin is taken once a day; the immediate-release form must be taken throughout the day.

Child: starting dosage—2.5 mg per lb. of body weight a day, divided into 2 or 3 equal doses. Maintenance dosage—2–4 mg per lb. of body weight a day. Dosage should be adjusted according to the child's needs. Children age 6 and over may take the adult dosage, but no child should take more than 300 mg a day.

Overdosage

Symptoms include drug side effects. Take the victim to a hospital emergency room at once. ALWAYS bring the prescription bottle or container.

Special Information

Call your doctor at once if you feel unwell or develop a rash, severe nausea or vomiting, swollen glands, swollen or tender gums, yellowing of the skin or whites of the eyes, joint pain, sore throat, fever, unusual bleeding or bruising, persistent headache, infection, slurred speech, or poor coordination.

Do not stop taking phenytoin or change dosage without your doctor's knowledge.

Phenytoin may cause drowsiness, dizziness, or blurred vision, effects which are increased by alcoholic beverages. Be careful when driving or doing any task that requires concentration.

Phenytoin sometimes produces a pink-brown color in the urine, which is normal and not a cause for concern.

People with diabetes who take phenytoin must monitor their urine regularly and report any changes to their doctors.

Good oral hygiene—including gum massage, frequent brushing, and flossing—is very important because phenytoin can cause abnormal growth of your gums.

DO NOT SWITCH PHENYTOIN BRANDS without notifying your doctor. Different brands may not be equivalent.

If you use phenytoin suspension, be sure to shake the bottle vigorously just before a dose.

Do not use phenytoin capsules that have become discolored. Throw them away.

If you forget a dose, take it as soon as you remember. If you take phenytoin once a day and it is almost time for your next dose, skip the one you forgot and continue with your regular schedule. If you take phenytoin several times a day and do not remember it within 4 hours of your regular time, skip the forgotten dose and go back to your regular schedule. Never take a double dose.

Special Populations

Pregnancy/Breast-feeding

Phenytoin crosses into the fetal circulation. The great majority of mothers who take phenytoin deliver healthy babies, but some are born with cleft lip, cleft palate, or heart malformations. There is a recognized group of deformities, fetal hydantoin syndrome, which affects children of women taking phenytoin, though the drug has not been definitively established as the cause. This syndrome consists of skull and face abnormalities, reduced brain size, growth deficiency, deformed fingernails, and mental deficiency. Phenytoin increases the risk of vitamin K deficiency in newborns, which can lead to serious, life-threatening bleeding during the first 24 hours of life. Also, mothers taking phenytoin may be deficient in vitamin K, increasing the risk of bleeding during delivery.

Phenytoin passes into breast milk. Nursing mothers who must take it should bottle-feed.

Seniors
Seniors are more sensitive to side effects.

Generic Name

Pindolol (PIN-doe-lol) Ⓖ

Brand Name
Visken

Type of Drug
Beta-adrenergic blocking agent.

Prescribed for
High blood pressure, abnormal heart rhythms, side effects of antipsychotic drugs, and stage fright and other anxieties.

General Information
Pindolol is one of 15 beta-adrenergic blocking drugs, or beta blockers, that interfere with the action of a specific part of the nervous system. Beta receptors are found all over the body and affect many body functions. Each beta blocker has particular characteristics that make it more suitable for certain conditions or people. Pindolol is a mild heart stimulant, which is an advantage for some.

Cautions and Warnings
You should be cautious about taking pindolol if you have

asthma, severe heart failure, a **very slow heart rate,** or **heart block** (disruption of the electrical impulses that control heart rate) because the drug may aggravate these conditions.

People with **angina** who take pindolol for high blood pressure risk aggravating their angina if they suddenly stop taking the drug. These people should have their drug dosage reduced gradually over 1 to 2 weeks.

Pindolol should be used with caution if you have **liver or kidney disease** because your ability to eliminate the drug from your body may be impaired.

Pindolol reduces the amount of blood pumped by the heart with each beat. This reduction in blood flow may aggravate the condition of people with **poor circulation** or **circulatory disease.**

If you are undergoing **major surgery,** your doctor may want you to stop taking pindolol at least 2 days before surgery. This is a controversial practice and may not be recommended for all surgeries.

Possible Side Effects

Side effects are relatively uncommon and usually mild.

▼ Most common: impotence.

▼ Less common: unusual tiredness or weakness, slow heartbeat, heart failure, dizziness, breathing difficulties, bronchospasm, depression, confusion, anxiety, nervousness, sleeplessness, disorientation, short-term memory loss, emotional instability, cold hands and feet, constipation, diarrhea, nausea, vomiting, upset stomach, increased sweating, urinary difficulties, cramps, blurred vision, rash, hair loss, stuffy nose, facial swelling, aggravation of lupus erythematosus, itching, chest pain, back or joint pain, colitis, drug allergy (symptoms include fever and sore throat), and liver toxicity.

Drug Interactions

• Pindolol may interact with surgical anesthetics to increase the risk of heart problems during surgery. Some anesthesiologists recommend gradually stopping the drug by 2 days before surgery.

• Pindolol may interfere with the normal signs of low blood sugar and with the action of oral antidiabetes drugs.

• Pindolol increases the blood-pressure-lowering effect of other blood-pressure-reducing agents, including clonidine, guanabenz, and reserpine as well as calcium channel blockers such as nifedipine.

• Aspirin, indomethacin, sulfinpyrazone, and estrogen drugs may interfere with the blood-pressure-lowering effect of pindolol.

• Cocaine may reduce the effectiveness of all beta blockers.

• Pindolol may worsen the cold hands and feet associated with taking ergot alkaloids for migraine. Gangrene is possible in people taking both ergot and pindolol.

• Pindolol counteracts thyroid hormone replacements.

• Calcium channel blockers, flecainide, hydralazine, oral contraceptives, propafenone, haloperidol, phenothiazine tranquilizers—molindone and others—quinolone antibacterials, and quinidine may increase the amount of pindolol in the bloodstream and lead to increased pindolol effects.

• Pindolol should not be taken within 2 weeks of taking a monoamine oxidase inhibitor (MAOI) antidepressant.

• Cimetidine increases the amount of pindolol absorbed into the bloodstream from oral tablets.

• Pindolol may interfere with the effectiveness of some antiasthma drugs, including theophylline and aminophylline, and especially ephedrine and isoproterenol.

• Combining pindolol and phenytoin or digitalis drugs may result in excessive slowing of the heart, possibly causing heart block.

• If you stop smoking while taking pindolol, your dose may have to be reduced because your liver will break down the drug more slowly afterward.

Food Interactions

None known.

Usual Dose

10–60 mg a day.

Overdosage

Symptoms include changes in heartbeat—unusually slow, unusually fast, or irregular; severe dizziness or fainting; breathing difficulties; bluish-colored fingernails or palms; and seizures. The victim should be taken to a hospital emergency room. ALWAYS bring the prescription bottle or container.

Special Information

Pindolol is taken continuously. When ending pindolol treatment, dosage should be reduced gradually over a period of about 2 weeks. Do not stop taking this drug unless directed to do so by your doctor: Abrupt withdrawal may cause chest pain, breathing difficulties, increased sweating, and unusually fast or irregular heartbeat.

Call your doctor at once if you develop back or joint pain, breathing difficulties, cold hands or feet, depression, rash, or changes in heartbeat. Pindolol may produce an undesirable lowering of blood pressure, leading to dizziness or fainting; call your doctor if this happens to you. Call your doctor if you experience persistent or bothersome anxiety, diarrhea, constipation, impotence, headache, itching, nausea or vomiting, nightmares or vivid dreams, upset stomach, trouble sleeping, stuffy nose, frequent urination, unusual tiredness, or weakness.

Pindolol may cause drowsiness, blurred vision, dizziness, and light-headedness. Be careful when driving or performing complex tasks.

It is best to take pindolol at the same time each day. If you forget a dose, take it as soon as you remember. If you take pindolol once a day and it is within 8 hours of your next dose, skip the dose you forgot and continue with your regular schedule. If you take it twice a day and it is within 4 hours of your next dose, skip the one you forgot and continue with your regular schedule. Never take a double dose.

Special Populations

Pregnancy/Breast-feeding

In studies, infants born to women who took a beta blocker while pregnant had lower birth weights, low blood pressure, and reduced heart rate. Pindolol should be avoided by women who are pregnant.

Pindolol passes into breast milk. Nursing mothers who must take it should bottle-feed.

Seniors

Seniors may require less of the drug to achieve results. Seniors taking pindolol may be more likely to suffer from cold hands and feet, reduced body temperature, chest pain, general feelings of ill health, sudden breathing difficulties, increased sweating, or changes in heartbeat.

Generic Name

Pioglitazone (pee-oe-GLIT-uh-zone)

Brand Name

Actos

Type of Drug

Antidiabetic.

Prescribed for

Type II diabetes.

General Information

Pioglitazone reduces the amount of sugar produced by the liver and increases the amount used by muscle, liver, and fat cells. Pioglitazone apparently works by affecting genes responsible for the control of sugar and fat use in the body, making cells more sensitive to insulin. This drug is effective for people with type II diabetes, who generally have enough insulin but whose cells do not respond to it. Pioglitazone, which may be taken only once a day, can be used alone or with a sulfonylurea-type antidiabetes drug or metformin. Pioglitazone is broken down in the liver.

Cautions and Warnings

Do not take pioglitazone if you are **allergic** or **sensitive** to it. Pioglitazone should be taken with caution by people who have **hepatitis** or **liver disease**; it can be toxic to the liver in some people.

Pioglitazone causes **weight gain,** which generally increases with dosage.

Pioglitazone should be used with caution if you have **heart failure** or **swollen legs or arms**. Animals given pioglitazone developed enlarged hearts, a sign of heart failure. This effect has not been seen in people taking pioglitazone, but increased blood volume, another sign of heart failure, occurred in some people taking the drug. Since people with heart failure were not included in studies of pioglitazone, caution is advised.

Premenopausal women who are not ovulating may be at risk of becoming pregnant because pioglitazone can trigger **ovulation**.

Pioglitazone can worsen **anemia** by affecting red blood cells in the first 3 months of treatment.

Women may obtain maximum benefit with smaller dosages.

There is no information on how pioglitazone affects **children**.

Possible Side Effects

In studies, the side effects of pioglitazone were about the same as those for a placebo (sugar pill).

▼ Most common: respiratory infections, headaches, and sinus irritation.

▼ Common: muscle aches, tooth problems, and sore throat.

▼ Less common: anemia and swollen legs or arms.

▼ Rare: yellowing of the skin or whites of the eyes, hepatitis, liver failure, and death.

Drug Interactions

• Pioglitazone may reduce the effectiveness of oral contraceptives ("the pill") containing norethindrone and ethinyl estradiol. Higher-dose contraceptives or another contraceptive method may be needed.

• Combining pioglitazone with another oral antidiabetes drug or insulin can lead to very low blood sugar. Dosage adjustments may be needed.

• Pioglitazone may stimulate the breakdown of other drugs also metabolized in the liver.

• Erythromycin, astemizole, calcium channel blockers, cisapride corticosteroids, cyclosporine, statin-type blood-fat reducers, tacrolimus, triazolam, and trimetrexate may be affected by pioglitazone; dosage adjustments may be needed.

• Combining pioglitazone and ketoconazole or itraconazole can lead to very low blood sugar.

Food Interactions

Pioglitazone may be taken with or without food.

Usual Dose

Adult: 15–45 mg once a day.
Child (under age 19): not recommended.

Overdosage

Little is known about the effects of pioglitazone overdose. Call your local poison control center or a hospital emergency room for more information. If you seek treatment, ALWAYS bring the prescription bottle or container.

Special Information

Follow your doctor's directions for diet and exercise and have your doctor check your glycosylated hemoglobin level. It is a more sensitive indicator of blood sugar.

Your doctor should check your liver function every 2 months for the first year of pioglitazone treatment and periodically afterward.

Call your doctor if you develop nausea, vomiting, abdominal pain, appetite loss, fatigue, or dark-colored urine. These may be signs of liver disease.

Fever, infection, surgery, trauma, and the use of other drugs can increase your pioglitazone dosage requirements.

If you forget a dose, take it as soon as you remember. If it is almost time for your next dose, skip the dose you forgot and continue with your regular schedule. Do not take a double dose.

Special Populations

Pregnancy/Breast-feeding

The safety of using pioglitazone during pregnancy is not known, though it does not affect pregnant animals or their fetuses. Most experts recommend that diabetes should be controlled with insulin during pregnancy.

It is not known if pioglitazone passes into breast milk, though it does in animal studies. Nursing mothers who must take this drug should bottle-feed.

Seniors

Seniors may take pioglitazone without special precaution.

Generic Name

Piroxicam (pih-ROX-ih-kam) Ⓖ

Brand Name

Feldene

Type of Drug

Nonsteroidal anti-inflammatory drug (NSAID).

Prescribed for

Rheumatoid arthritis, juvenile rheumatoid arthritis, osteoarthritis, menstrual pain, and sunburn.

General Information

Piroxicam and other NSAIDs are used to relieve pain and inflammation. We do not know exactly how NSAIDs work, but they may achieve their effects by blocking the body's production of a hormone called prostaglandin and the action of other body chemicals. Pain relief comes within 1 hour after taking the first dose of piroxicam and lasts for 2 to 3 days, but its anti-inflammatory effect takes several days to 2 weeks to become apparent and may take 3 weeks to reach maximum effect. Piroxicam is broken down in the liver and eliminated through the kidneys.

Cautions and Warnings

People who are **allergic** to piroxicam or any other NSAID and those with a history of **asthma** attacks brought on by an NSAID, iodides, or aspirin should not take piroxicam.

Piroxicam can cause **gastrointestinal (GI) bleeding, ulcers,** and **stomach perforation**. This can occur at any time, with or without warning, in people who take piroxicam regularly. People with a history of active GI bleeding should be cautious about taking any NSAID. People who develop bleeding or ulcers and continue NSAID treatment should be aware of the possibility of developing more serious drug toxicity.

Piroxicam can affect platelets and **blood clotting** at high doses and should be avoided by people with clotting problems and those taking warfarin.

People with **heart problems** who use piroxicam may experience swelling in their arms, legs, or feet.

Piroxicam can cause severe toxic effects to the **kidney**. Report any unusual side effects to your doctor, who may need to periodically test your kidney function.

Piroxicam can make you **unusually sensitive to the effects of the sun**.

Possible Side Effects

▼ Most common: diarrhea, nausea, vomiting, constipation, gas, stomach upset or irritation, and appetite loss—especially during the first few days of treatment.

▼ Less common: stomach ulcers, GI bleeding, hepatitis, gallbladder attacks, painful urination, poor kidney function, kidney inflammation, blood and protein in the urine, dizziness, fainting, nervousness, depression, hallucinations, confusion, disorientation, tingling in the hands or feet, light-headedness, itching, increased sweating, dry nose and mouth, heart palpitations, chest pain, difficulty breathing, and muscle cramps.

▼ Rare: severe allergic reactions including closing of the throat, fever and chills, changes in liver function, jaundice (yellowing of the skin or whites of the eyes), and kidney failure. People who experience such effects must be promptly treated in a hospital emergency room or doctor's office. NSAIDs have caused severe skin reactions; if this happens to you, see your doctor immediately.

Drug Interactions

• Piroxicam can increase the effects of oral anticoagulant (blood-thinning) drugs such as warfarin. Your anticoagulant dose may need to be reduced.

• Taking piroxicam with cyclosporine may increase the toxic kidney effects of both drugs.

• Methotrexate toxicity may be increased in people who are also taking piroxicam.

• Piroxicam may reduce the blood-pressure-lowering effect of beta blockers and loop diuretics.

• Piroxicam may increase phenytoin side effects. Lithium blood levels may be increased by piroxicam.

• Piroxicam blood levels may be affected by cimetidine.

• Probenecid may increase the risk of piroxicam side effects.

• Aspirin and other salicylates should never be combined with piroxicam.

Food Interactions

Take piroxicam with food or a magnesium/aluminum antacid if it upsets your stomach.

Usual Dose

Adult: 20 mg a day.
Child: not recommended.

Overdosage

People have died from NSAID overdoses. Common signs of overdose are drowsiness, nausea, vomiting, diarrhea, abdominal pain, rapid breathing, rapid heartbeat, increased sweating, ringing or buzzing in the ears, confusion, disorientation, stupor, and coma. Take the victim to a hospital emergency room at once. ALWAYS bring the prescription bottle or container.

Special Information

Take each dose with a full glass of water and do not lie down for 15 to 30 minutes afterward.

Piroxicam can make you drowsy or tired: Be careful when driving or operating hazardous equipment. Do not take any over-the-counter products containing acetaminophen or aspirin while taking piroxicam. Avoid alcohol.

Contact your doctor if you develop rash or itching, visual disturbances, weight gain, breathing difficulties, fluid retention, hallucinations, black or tarry stools, persistent headache, or any unusual or intolerable side effect.

If you forget a dose of piroxicam, take it as soon as you remember. If you take it once a day and it is within 8 hours of your next dose, skip the missed dose and continue with your regular schedule. Do not take a double dose.

Special Populations

Pregnancy/Breast-feeding

NSAIDs may affect the fetal heart during the second half of pregnancy. When this drug is considered crucial by your doctor, its potential benefits must be carefully weighed against its risks.

NSAIDs may pass into breast milk. There is a risk that a nursing mother taking piroxicam could affect her baby's heart or cardiovascular system. Nursing mothers who must take this drug should bottle-feed.

Seniors
Seniors may be more susceptible to side effects, especially ulcer disease.

Plavix   see Clopidogrel, page 235

Generic Name
Podofilox (poe-DUH-fil-ox)

Brand Name
Condylox

Type of Drug
Antimitotic drug.

Prescribed for
External genital warts or warts around the anal area.

General Information
Podofilox, which can be either manufactured from chemicals or purified from natural sources, kills visible wart tissues. Exactly how it works is not known. Condylomas or genital warts are caused by the human papillomavirus and can appear in various places including the sex organs, anus, and abdomen. The risk of developing warts increases if your immune system is suppressed.

Cautions and Warnings
Do not use podofilox if you are **sensitive** or **allergic** to it.

Proper diagnosis of genital warts is necessary before you use this product: See your doctor before you start using podofilox. Do not use podofilox for any other purpose.

If you get podofilox in your **eyes,** wash it out at once with cool water and seek medical attention.

Possible Side Effects

▼ Most common: burning, pain, inflammation, skin erosion, itching, and bleeding.

▼ Common: pain during intercourse, sleeplessness, tingling, tenderness, chafing, bad odor, dizziness, scarring, small sores or ulcers, dryness, difficulty retracting the foreskin, blood in the urine, vomiting, headache, stinging, and redness.

▼ Less common: skin peeling, scabbing, skin discoloration, tenderness, crusting, skin cracks, soreness, swelling, rash, and blisters.

Drug Interactions

None known.

Usual Dose

Apply morning and night—every 12 hours—for 3 consecutive days, then apply nothing for 4 days. Repeat this cycle for up to 4 weeks in a row. Use the cotton-tipped applicator supplied with the solution, or your finger if you are using the gel. Try to limit the amount of podofilox that gets on intact skin. Thoroughly wash your hands before and after each application.

Overdosage

Swallowing podofilox may lead to nausea, vomiting, fever, diarrhea, mouth sores, tingling in the hands or feet, changes in mental state, lethargy, coma, rapid breathing, respiratory failure, blood in the urine, kidney failure, and seizures. Excess podofilox should be washed off the skin as soon as possible. In case of overdose or accidental ingestion, take the victim to a hospital emergency room. ALWAYS bring the prescription bottle or container.

Special Information

Thoroughly wash your hands before and after each application.

Call your doctor if you develop any bothersome or persistent side effect. If you do not see any improvement in 4 weeks, stop using the drug and call your doctor.

If you forget a dose, apply it as soon as you remember. If it is within 4 hours of your next dose, skip the dose you forgot and continue with your regular schedule.

Special Populations

Pregnancy/Breast-feeding
Podofilox is toxic to animal fetuses at very high dosages. When this drug is considered crucial by your doctor, its potential benefits must be carefully weighed against its risks.

It is not known if podofilox passes into breast milk. Nursing mothers who must use it should bottle-feed.

Seniors
Seniors may use podofilox without special precaution.

Brand Name

Poly-Vi-Flor

Generic Ingredients

Folic Acid + Sodium Fluoride + Vitamin A + Vitamin B_1 (Thiamine) + Vitamin B_2 (Riboflavin) + Vitamin B_3 (Niacin) + Vitamin B_6 (Pyridoxine) + Vitamin B_{12} (Cyanocobalamin) + Vitamin C + Vitamin D + Vitamin E [G]

Other Brand Names
Florvite*   Soluvite*
Polytabs-F   Vi-Daylin/F*

Some products in this brand-name group are alcohol- or sugar-free. Consult your pharmacist.

Type of Drug

Multivitamin supplement with fluoride.

Prescribed for

Vitamin deficiencies and prevention of dental cavities in infants and children.

General Information

Fluoride taken in small daily dosages has been effective in preventing cavities in children by strengthening the teeth.

Multivitamins with fluoride are also available in preparations with iron.

Cautions and Warnings

Too much fluoride can **damage teeth**. Because of this, Poly-Vi-Flor should not be used where the fluoride content of the water supply exceeds 0.7 parts per million (ppm)—consult your pediatrician or local water company.

> ### Possible Side Effects
>
> ▼ Common: occasional rash, itching, upset stomach, headache, and weakness.

Food and Drug Interactions

None known.

Usual Dose

1 tablet or dropperful a day.

Special Information

If you forget to give your child a dose of Poly-Vi-Flor, do so as soon as you remember. If it is almost time for the next dose, skip the dose you forgot and continue with the regular schedule. Do not give a double dose.

Type of Drug

Potassium Replacements

Brand Names

Generic Ingredient: Potassium Chloride (Liquid) 🄶

Cena-K 🅢

Kaochlor 10%

Kaochlor S-F 🅢

Kaon-Cl 20% 🅢

Kay Ciel 🅢

Klorvess

Potasalan 🅢

Rum-K 🅢

Generic Ingredient: Potassium Gluconate (Liquid) 🄶

Kaon 🅢

Kaylixir

K-G Elixir

Generic Ingredient: Potassium Salt Combination (Liquid) G

Kolyum $	Twin-K
Tri-K	

Generic Ingredient: Potassium Chloride (Powder) G

Gen-K $	Klor-Con $
K+Care	Klor-Con/25 $
Kay Ciel $	K-Lyte/Cl
K-Lor	Micro-K LS

Generic Ingredient: Potassium Salt Combination (Powder) G

Klorvess $	Kolyum $

Generic Ingredient: Potassium (Effervescent Tablets) G

Effer-K	K-Lyte
K + Care ET	K-Lyte/Cl
Klor-Con/EF $	K-Lyte/Cl 50
Klorvess $	K-Lyte DS

Generic Ingredient: Potassium Chloride (Controlled-Release) G

K + 10	Klotrix
Kaon-Cl-10	K-Norm
K-Dur 10	K-Tab
K-Dur 20	Micro-K Extencaps
K-Lease	Micro-K 10 Extencaps
Klor-Con 8	Slow-K
Klor-Con 10	Ten-K

Generic Ingredient: Potassium Gluconate (Tablets) G
Only available in generic form.

Prescribed for

Hypokalemia (low blood-potassium levels) and mild hypertension (high blood pressure).

General Information

A major component of body fluids, potassium helps to maintain electrolyte balance, kidney function, and blood pressure. Low potassium levels, which can affect the central nervous system (CNS) and heart functions, are usually caused by extended diuretic treatment, severe diarrhea, vomiting, complications of diabetes, or other medical conditions.

Potassium supplements are available in different types and forms. Potassium chloride is most often prescribed because it contains the most potassium per unit weight. Another advantage of potassium chloride is that it provides chloride ion, another important body-fluid component. Potassium gluconate provides about ⅓ as much potassium as the chloride, so you have to take 3 times as much to get an equal dose of potassium. However, it is preferable to potassium chloride in circumstances where chloride is undesirable.

Cautions and Warnings

Potassium replacement therapy should always be monitored and controlled by your doctor.

Potassium tablets have caused **ulcers** in some people with compression of the esophagus, who should use the liquid form. Potassium tablets have been reported to cause small bowel ulcer, leading to bleeding, obstruction, or perforation (formation of a hole through the bowel into the abdomen).

People with **kidney disease** who take potassium may develop **hyperkalemia** (high blood-potassium levels). Hyperkalemia can develop rapidly, without warning or symptoms, and is potentially fatal. It is often discovered through an EKG, but the following symptoms may also occur: tingling in the hands and feet, a feeling of heaviness or weakness in the muscles, listlessness, confusion, low blood pressure, extreme difficulty moving the arms and legs, abnormal heart rhythms, weak pulse, loss of consciousness, pallor, restlessness, and low urine output.

Do not take potassium if you are **dehydrated** or experiencing **muscle cramps** due to excessive sun exposure. Potassium should be used with caution in people with **kidney or heart disease**.

Possible Side Effects

▼ Most common: nausea, vomiting, diarrhea, gas, and abdominal discomfort.

▼ Less common: rash, tingling in hands or feet, weakness and heaviness in the legs, listlessness, mental confusion, decreased blood pressure, and heart-rhythm changes.

Drug Interactions

- Potassium supplements should not be taken with the

potassium-sparing diuretics spironolactone or triamterene. Potassium toxicity may occur.

• Combining potassium supplements with an angiotensin-converting enzyme (ACE) inhibitor may result in hyperkalemia.

• People taking digitalis drugs must keep their blood-potassium levels within acceptable limits. Too little potassium in the blood may increase digitalis side effects and toxic reactions.

Food Interactions

Eating excess salt contributes to the problem of potassium depletion. Salt substitutes contain large amounts of potassium; do not use them while taking a potassium supplement unless directed by your doctor. If stomach upset occurs, take potassium supplements with food.

Usual Dose

16–100 milliequivalents (meq) a day.

Overdosage

Symptoms include muscle weakness, tingling in the hands or feet, a feeling of heaviness in the legs, listlessness, confusion, breathing difficulties, low blood pressure, shock, abnormal heart rhythms, and heart attack. Call your local poison control center or a hospital emergency room for more information. If you seek treatment, ALWAYS bring the prescription bottle or container.

Special Information

Directions for taking and using any potassium supplement must be followed closely. Effervescent tablets, powders, and liquids should be properly and completely dissolved, or diluted in 3 to 8 oz. of cold water or juice and drunk slowly. Noneffervescent tablets or capsules should never be chewed or crushed; they must be swallowed whole.

Many of the controlled-release potassium supplements contain potassium distributed throughout an indigestible wax core or matrix; you may notice the depleted wax matrix in your stool several hours after swallowing a tablet. This is normal and not a cause for alarm.

Call your doctor at once if you experience tingling in your hands or feet, a feeling of heaviness in the legs, unusual tiredness or weakness, nausea, vomiting, continued abdominal pain, or black stool.

If you forget a dose, take it right away if you remember within 2 hours of your regular time. If you do not remember until later, skip the dose you forgot and go back to your regular schedule. Do not take a double dose.

Special Populations

Pregnancy/Breast-feeding
Potassium supplements are considered safe for use during pregnancy. Always consult your doctor before using any drug if you are pregnant.

Normal doses of potassium supplements add little to the potassium already in breast milk. Nursing mothers may take potassium supplements.

Seniors
Seniors may take potassium supplements without special restriction.

Generic Name

Pramipexole (pram-ih-PEX-ole)

Brand Name

Mirapex

Type of Drug

Antiparkinsonian.

Prescribed for

Parkinson's disease.

General Information

Pramipexole is thought to relieve symptoms of Parkinson's disease by stimulating dopamine receptors in the brain. Studies of pramipexole in people with early Parkinson's disease showed improvement after 4 weeks of treatment. People with advanced Parkinson's disease showed improvement after 6 months.

Cautions and Warnings

Do not take pramipexole if you are **sensitive** or **allergic** to it. Pramipexole may cause **low blood pressure** and make you **dizzy or faint** when rising from a sitting or lying position, especially during the early stages of treatment. About 1 in 10 to 15 people who take pramipexole experience hallucinations that may be serious enough to require stopping drug therapy.

One person taking pramipexole developed a disease in which **skeletal muscle** is destroyed.

People who stop taking other antiparkinsonians may develop **high fever** and **confusion**. Breathing difficulties caused by lung changes have also occurred with other antiparkinsonians. These symptoms have not been associated with pramipexole, but there is a risk that you may experience similar problems if you stop taking pramipexole.

Possible Side Effects

Early Parkinson's Disease

▼ Most common: sleepiness or tiredness and nausea.

▼ Common: sleeplessness, hallucinations, and constipation.

▼ Less common: dizziness, confusion, memory loss, reduced touch sensation, loss of muscle tone, a tendency to frequently change positions or pace the floor, odd thoughts, loss of sex drive, impotence, unusual muscle spasms, swelling in the arms or legs, generalized swelling, appetite loss, difficulty swallowing, weight loss, weakness, feeling unwell, fever, and abnormal vision.

Advanced Parkinson's Disease

▼ Most common: dizziness or fainting when rising from a sitting or lying position, abnormal movements, tremors, muscle rigidity, and hallucinations.

▼ Common: sleeplessness.

▼ Less common: accidental injury, weakness, generalized swelling, chest pain, feeling unwell, dizziness, abnormal dreaming, confusion, sleepiness, unusual muscle spasms, unusual walking, muscle stiffness, memory loss, a tendency to frequently change positions or pace the floor, odd thoughts, paranoid reactions, delusions, sleeping problems, frequent urination, urinary

> **Possible Side Effects** *(continued)*
>
> infection, loss of urinary control, swelling in the arms or legs, arthritis, twitching, bursitis, muscle weakness, breathing difficulties, runny nose, pneumonia, visual difficulties, difficulty focusing, double vision, constipation, dry mouth, and rash.

Drug Interactions

• Pramipexole increases levodopa blood levels and may worsen the uncontrolled muscle spasms that occur with levodopa. Your doctor may reduce your levodopa dosage.

• Cimetidine increases the amount of pramipexole absorbed by 50% and lengthens the time it takes for pramipexole to leave your body by 40%. Dose adjustment may be required if you take both drugs.

• Drugs that are eliminated through the kidneys—including cimetidine, ranitidine, diltiazem, triamterene, verapamil, quinidine, and quinine—reduce by 20% the ability to clear pramipexole from the body. Dosage adjustment may be required.

• Phenothiazine tranquilizers, haloperidol and similar tranquilizers, thioxanthene tranquilizers, metoclopramide, and other drugs that antagonize the effects of dopamine can reduce the effect of pramipexole.

• Pramipexole increases the sedative effect of tranquilizers, sleeping pills, and other nervous-system depressants.

Food Interactions

You may take this drug with food to prevent nausea.

Usual Dose

Adult: 0.125 mg 3 times a day to start, gradually increasing to a maximum of 4.5 mg a day. Dosage is reduced for people with kidney disease.

Overdosage

Little is known about the effects of pramipexole overdose. Symptoms are likely to include the most common side effects. Take the victim to a hospital emergency room. ALWAYS bring the prescription bottle or container.

Special Information

Take this drug exactly as prescribed.

Pramipexole causes sedation. Be careful when driving or performing any task that requires concentration. Avoid alcohol and other nervous system depressants.

Call your doctor if you develop hallucinations or any bothersome or persistent side effect.

If you forget a dose, take it as soon as you remember. Space the remaining daily dosage evenly throughout the day. Continue with your regular schedule on the next day. Do not take a double dose.

Special Populations

Pregnancy/Breast-feeding

The safety of using pramipexole during pregnancy is not known. When this drug is considered crucial by your doctor, its potential benefits must be carefully weighed against its risks.

It is not known if pramipexole passes into breast milk but this drug can interfere with milk production. Nursing mothers who must take this drug should bottle-feed.

Seniors

Seniors are more likely to experience side effects.

Pravachol   see Statin Cholesterol-Lowering Agents,

page 942

Generic Name

Prazosin (PRAY-zoe-sin) Ⓖ

Brand Name

Minipress

Combination Products

Generic Ingredients: Prazosin + Polythiazide
Minizide 1   Minizide 5
Minizide 2

Type of Drug

Antihypertensive.

Prescribed for

High blood pressure, benign prostatic hyperplasia (BPH), congestive heart failure (CHF), and Raynaud's disease. Prasozin combined with the diuretic polythiazide is used to treat high blood pressure.

General Information

Prazosin hydrochloride and other alpha-adrenergic blocking agents, or alpha blockers, reduce blood pressure by dilating (widening) blood vessels. They achieve this effect by blocking nerve endings known as $alpha_1$ receptors. The maximum blood-pressure-lowering effect of prazosin is seen between 2 and 6 hours after taking a dose. Prazosin's effect in CHF is seen within 1 hour of taking the drug. In BPH treatment, prazosin works by relaxing smooth muscles in the prostate and neck of the bladder. Despite the fact that prazosin reduces the symptoms of BPH, the drug's long-term effect on complications of BPH or the need for urinary surgery is not known. Prazosin's effect lasts between 6 and 10 hours. It is broken down in the liver.

Cautions and Warnings

Prazosin may cause **dizziness** and **fainting,** especially the first few doses. This is known as the first-dose effect, which can be minimized by limiting the first dose to 1 mg at bedtime. First-dose effects occur in about 1% of people taking an alpha blocker and may recur if the drug is stopped for a few days and then restarted.

People who are **allergic** or **sensitive** to any alpha blocker should avoid prazosin.

Prazosin may slightly reduce cholesterol levels and improve the ratio of high-density lipoprotein (HDL)/low-density lipoprotein (LDL), a positive step for people with a blood-cholesterol problem.

Possible Side Effects

Side effects occur less often with prazosin than with other alpha blockers.

▼ Most common: dizziness, drowsiness, weakness, nausea, and headache.

Possible Side Effects *(continued)*

▼ Less common: low blood pressure, dizziness when rising from a sitting or lying position, rapid heartbeat, vomiting, dry mouth, diarrhea, constipation, abdominal pain or discomfort, breathing difficulties, stuffy nose, nosebleed, joint or muscle pain, blurred vision, conjunctivitis (pinkeye), ringing or buzzing in the ears, depression, nervousness, tingling in the hands or feet, frequent urination, impotence, poor urinary control, painful erection, itching, sweating, rash, hair loss, fluid retention, and fever.

Drug Interactions

• Prazosin may interact with beta blockers to increase the risk of dizziness or fainting after the first dose of prazosin.

• The blood-pressure-lowering effect of prazosin may be reduced by indomethacin.

• When taken with other blood-pressure-lowering drugs, prazosin produces an exaggerated reduction of blood pressure.

• The blood-pressure-lowering effect of clonidine may be reduced by prazosin.

Food Interactions

None known.

Usual Dose

1 mg 2–3 times a day to start; may be increased to a total daily dose of 20 mg although 40 mg a day has been used in some cases.

Overdosage

Overdose may produce drowsiness, poor reflexes, and very low blood pressure. Overdose victims should be taken to a hospital emergency room immediately. ALWAYS bring the prescription bottle or container.

Special Information

Take prazosin exactly as prescribed. Do not stop taking prazosin unless directed to do so by your doctor. Avoid over-the-counter drugs that contain stimulants because they may increase your blood pressure.

Prazosin may cause dizziness, headache, and drowsiness, especially 2 to 6 hours after you take your first dose, although these effects can persist after the first few doses.

Call your doctor if you develop severe dizziness, heart palpitations, or any bothersome or persistent side effect.

Wait 12 to 24 hours after taking your first dose of prazosin before driving or doing anything that requires intense concentration. Take your dose at bedtime to minimize this problem.

If you forget a dose, take it as soon as you remember. If it is almost time for your next dose, skip the dose you forgot and continue with your regular schedule. Do not take a double dose.

Special Populations

Pregnancy/Breast-feeding
The safety of using prazosin during pregnancy is not known. When this drug is considered crucial by your doctor, its potential benefits must be carefully weighed against its risks.

Small amounts of prazosin pass into breast milk. Nursing mothers who must take this drug should bottle-feed.

Seniors
Seniors, especially those with liver disease, may be more sensitive to the side effects of prazosin.

Premarin   *see Estrogens, page 389*

Prempro   *see Estrogens, page 389*

Prevacid   *see Omeprazole, page 758*

Prilosec   *see Omeprazole, page 758*

Prinivil   *see Lisinopril, page 585*

___

Generic Name

Procainamide   (proe-KAY-nuh-mide) Ⓖ

___

Brand Names

Pronestyl   Procanbid
Procan

Type of Drug

Antiarrhythmic.

Prescribed for

Abnormal heart rhythms.

General Information

Procainamide hydrochloride works by slowing the response of heart muscle to nervous-system stimulation. It also slows the rate at which nervous-system impulses are carried through the heart. Procainamide begins working 30 minutes after you take it and continues working for 3 or more hours. As with other antiarrhythmic drugs, studies have not proven that people who take procainamide live longer than people who do not take it.

Sustained-release or long-acting forms of generic procainamide may not be equivalent to each other and should not be interchanged without your doctor's knowledge.

Cautions and Warnings

About 1 in 200 people taking procainamide in the usual dosage range develop bone marrow depression, a drastic drop in white-blood-cell count, low platelet count, or other **abnormalities of blood components**. Because these abnormalities happen most often during the first 3 months of taking procainamide, you should be checked with weekly blood counts during your first 3 months on this drug.

Procainamide should not be taken by people who have complete **heart block** or the arrhythmia called **"torsade de**

pointes." Long-term use may cause up to 30% of people taking procainamide to test positive for **lupus erythematosus** (long-term condition affecting the body's connective tissues).

If you have **myasthenia gravis,** tell your doctor when procainamide is first prescribed; you should be taking a drug other than procainamide. You should also tell your doctor if you are **allergic** to procainamide or to the local anesthetic **procaine**.

Procainamide may aggravate congestive **heart failure**.

This drug is eliminated from the body through the kidney and liver. If you have either **kidney or liver disease,** your dosage of procainamide may have to be adjusted.

Possible Side Effects

▼ Common: appetite loss; nausea; itching; symptoms resembling the disease lupus erythematosus (fever and chills, nausea, vomiting, muscle aches, skin lesions, arthritis, and abdominal pains; enlargement of the liver or changes in blood tests that indicate a change in the liver; soreness of the mouth or throat; unusual bleeding; rash; and fever. If any of these symptoms occur while you are taking procainamide, tell your doctor immediately.

▼ Less common: bitter taste in the mouth, vomiting, diarrhea, weakness, dizziness, mental depression, giddiness, hallucinations, and drug allergy (symptoms include rash, itching, and fever).

Drug Interactions

• Procainamide blood levels and the risk of side effects are increased by propranolol and other beta blockers; cimetidine, ranitidine, and other H_2 antagonists; lidocaine; quinidine; and trimethoprim.

• Do not take procainamide with other antiarrhythmic drugs unless specifically instructed by your doctor. These combinations can depress heart function.

• The interaction between alcohol and procainamide is variable and may alter the effects of procainamide.

• Avoid over-the-counter (OTC) cough, cold, or allergy remedies containing drugs that have a stimulating effect on the heart. Ask your pharmacist about the ingredients in OTC remedies.

Food Interactions

This medication is best taken on an empty stomach, but you may take it with food if it upsets your stomach.

Usual Dose

Starting dosage—1000 mg. Maintenance dosage—23 mg a day per lb. of body weight, in doses every 3 hours around the clock, adjusted according to individual needs. Taking a sustained-release product allows doses to be spaced 6 hours apart. Seniors and people with kidney or liver disease are treated with lower dosages or given the medication less often.

Overdosage

Symptoms include abnormal heart rhythms, slow heart rate, low blood pressure, tremors, and nervous-system depression. Overdose victims should be taken to an emergency room immediately. ALWAYS bring the prescription bottle or container.

Special Information

Call your doctor at once if you develop any sign of infection, including fever, chills, sore throat, or mouth sores, or if you develop any of the following: joint or muscle pain, dark urine, wheezing, weakness, chest or abdominal pains, heart palpitations, nausea, vomiting, diarrhea, appetite loss, dizziness, depression, hallucinations, or unusual bruising or bleeding.

Be sure you discuss with your doctor any drug sensitivity or reaction, especially to procaine or other local anesthetics or to aspirin. Also, be sure your doctor knows if you have heart failure, lupus erythematosus, liver or kidney disease, or myasthenia gravis.

Because procainamide is taken so frequently during the day, it is essential that you follow your doctor's directions about taking your medicine. Taking more medicine will not necessarily help you, and skipping doses or taking them less often than directed may lead to a loss of control over your heart problem.

If you forget to take a dose of procainamide and remember within 2 hours, or within 4 hours if you are taking long-acting procainamide, take it right away. If it is almost time for your next dose, skip the one you forgot and continue with your regular schedule. Do not take a double dose.

Special Populations

Pregnancy/Breast-feeding

Procainamide passes into the fetal circulation. When this drug is considered crucial by your doctor, its potential benefits must be carefully weighed against its risks.

This drug passes into breast milk. Nursing mothers who must take it should bottle-feed.

Seniors

Seniors are more sensitive to procainamide.

Procardia XL   *see Nifedipine, page 728*

Generic Name

Prochlorperazine   (proe-klor-PER-uh-zeen) [G]

Brand Name

Compazine

Type of Drug

Antinauseant and phenothiazine antipsychotic.

Prescribed for

Severe nausea and vomiting; also prescribed for psychotic disorders such as excessive anxiety, tension, and agitation.

General Information

Prochlorperazine and other phenothiazine drugs act on a portion of the brain called the hypothalamus. They affect areas of the hypothalamus that control metabolism, body temperature, alertness, muscle tone, hormone balance, and vomiting. The exact way that phenothiazines work is not completely understood.

Cautions and Warnings

Prochlorperazine may depress the **gag (cough) reflex**. Some people who have taken this drug have accidentally choked to death because the gag reflex failed to respond. Because it can prevent vomiting, prochlorperazine **may obscure symptoms of disease or toxicity** due to drug overdose.

Do not take prochlorperazine if you are **allergic** to it or any phenothiazine drug or have very low **blood pressure, Parkinson's disease,** or **blood, liver, kidney, or heart disease**. If you have **glaucoma, epilepsy, ulcers,** or **difficulty passing urine,** prochlorperazine should be used with caution and under the strict supervision of your doctor.

Avoid **extreme heat** because prochlorperazine can upset your body's temperature-control mechanism.

Possible Side Effects

▼ Most common: drowsiness, especially during the first or second week of therapy. If the drowsiness becomes troublesome, call your doctor. Prochlorperazine can cause jaundice (symptoms include yellowing of the skin or whites of the eyes), typically within the first 4 weeks of treatment. It usually goes away when the drug is discontinued. If you notice this effect or feel feverish or unwell, call your doctor immediately.

▼ Less common: changes in blood components including anemia (condition characterized by a reduction in the number of red blood cells or amount of hemoglobin or blood), raised or lowered blood pressure, abnormal heart rate, heart attack, feeling faint, and dizziness. Phenothiazines may produce extrapyramidal effects such as spasm of the neck muscles, rolling back of the eyes, convulsions, difficulty swallowing, and symptoms associated with Parkinson's disease. These effects look very serious but disappear after the drug is withdrawn; however, face, tongue, and jaw symptoms may persist for several years, especially in seniors with a history of brain damage. If you experience extrapyramidal effects, contact your doctor immediately.

▼ Rare: Prochlorperazine may cause an increase in psychotic symptoms or cause paranoid reactions. Other rare side effects can occur in almost any part of the body. Contact your doctor if you experience any side effect not listed above.

Drug Interactions

• Be cautious about combining prochlorperazine and barbiturates, sleeping pills, narcotics, tranquilizers, or other drugs that produce a depressive effect. Avoid alcohol.

• Aluminum antacids may reduce the effectiveness of prochlorperazine. Anticholinergic drugs may reduce the effectiveness of prochlorperazine and increase the risk of side effects.

• Prochlorperazine may reduce the effects of bromocriptine and appetite suppressants. The blood-pressure-lowering effect of guanethidine may be counteracted by this drug.

• Combining lithium and prochlorperazine may lead to disorientation, loss of consciousness, and uncontrolled muscle movements. Combining propranolol and prochlorperazine may lead to unusually low blood pressure.

• Prochlorperazine may increase blood levels of tricyclic antidepressant and the risk of their side effects.

Food Interactions

Prochlorperazine's effectiveness as an antipsychotic may be counteracted by beverages or foods containing caffeine.

Usual Dose

Adult: 15–150 mg a day. By mouth for nausea and vomiting—15–40 mg a day; rectal suppositories—25 mg twice a day.

Child (40–85 lbs.): 10–15 mg a day. The syrup form contains 5 mg of prochlorperazine per tsp.

Child (30–39 lbs.): 2.5 mg 2–3 times a day.

Child (20–29 lbs.): 2.5 mg 1–2 times a day.

Child (under age 2 or 20 lbs.): not recommended unless considered to be life-saving. Usually only 1–2 days of therapy are needed to relieve nausea and vomiting.

For psychosis, dosages of 25 mg or more a day may be required.

Overdosage

Symptoms include depression, extreme weakness, tiredness or a desire to sleep, lowered blood pressure, uncontrolled muscle spasms, agitation, restlessness, convulsions, fever, dry mouth, abnormal heart rhythms, and coma. Take the victim to a hospital emergency room immediately. ALWAYS bring the prescription bottle or container.

Special Information

Prochlorperazine is a tranquilizer and may have a depressive effect, especially during the first few days of therapy. Be careful when driving or performing any task that requires concentration.

Call your doctor if you develop sore throat, fever, rash, weakness, tremors, visual disturbances, or yellowing of the skin or whites of the eyes.

Prochlorperazine may cause increased sensitivity to the sun. It may also turn your urine reddish-brown to pink; this is not a cause for concern.

If dizziness occurs, avoid sudden changes in posture and climbing stairs. Use caution in hot weather because this medication may make you more prone to heatstroke.

The liquid form of prochlorperazine may cause skin irritation or rash; do not get it on your skin. Liquid prochlorperazine must be protected from light. Do not remove it from its opaque bottle.

If you miss a dose, take it as soon as you remember. If it is almost time for your next dose, skip the dose you forgot and go back to your regular schedule. Do not take a double dose.

Special Populations

Pregnancy/Breast-feeding
Taking prochlorperazine during pregnancy may cause jaundice and nervous-system effects in newborns. When this drug is considered crucial by your doctor, its potential benefits must be carefully weighed against its risks.

Prochlorperazine may pass into breast milk. Nursing mothers who must take it should consider bottle-feeding.

Seniors
Seniors are more sensitive to prochlorperazine's effects and usually require lower dosages to achieve desired results. Some experts feel that they should be treated with 25% to 50% of the usual adult dosage.

Generic Name

Promethazine (proe-METH-uh-zeen) G

Brand Name

Phenergan

Combination Products

Generic Ingredients: Promethazine + Codeine Phosphate G
Pentazine VC with Codeine Liquid A
Phenergan with Codeine Syrup
Pherazine with Codeine Syrup
Prometh with Codeine Syrup

Generic Ingredients: Promethazine + Dextromethorphan Hydrobromide G
Phenergan with Dextromethorphan Syrup
Phenameth DM Syrup A
Pherazine DM Syrup
Prometh with Dextromethorphan Syrup

Generic Ingredients: Promethazine + Phenylephrine Hydrochloride G
Phenergan VC Syrup
Promethazine VC Plain Syrup
Prometh VC Plain Liquid A

Generic Ingredients: Promethazine + Codeine Phosphate + Phenylephrine Hydrochloride G
Phenergan VC with Codeine Syrup
Pherazine VC with Codeine Syrup
Prometh VC with Codeine Liquid A
Promethist with Codeine Syrup A

Type of Drug

Antihistamine.

Prescribed for

Allergy, motion sickness, nausea, vomiting, nighttime sedation, and pain relief.

General Information

Promethazine hydrochloride, one of the older members of

the phenothiazine antihistamine group, is used alone and in combination with cough suppressants and decongestants.

Cautions and Warnings

Promethazine should be used with caution if you are **allergic** to it or if you cannot tolerate any other phenothiazine drug such as chlorpromazine and prochlorperazine.

Promethazine should be used with care if you have very **low blood pressure; Parkinson's disease;** or **heart, blood, liver, or kidney disease**. This drug should be used under your doctor's strict supervision if you have an **ulcer, epilepsy, glaucoma,** or **urinary difficulties**.

Children with a history of **sleep apnea** (condition characterized by intermittent cessation of breathing during sleep), a family history of **sudden infant death syndrome, liver disease,** or **Reye's syndrome** should not take promethazine.

Possible Side Effects

The suppositories can cause rectal burning or stinging.

▼ Most common: drowsiness, thick mucus, and sedation.

▼ Less common: sore throat and fever; unusual bleeding or bruising; tiredness; weakness; dizziness; feeling faint; clumsiness; unsteadiness; dry mouth, nose, or throat; facial redness; breathing difficulties; hallucinations; confusion; seizure; muscle spasm, especially in the back and neck; restlessness; a shuffling walk; jerky movements of the head and face; shaking and trembling of the hands; blurred vision or other changes in vision; urinary difficulties; rapid heartbeat; sensitivity to the sun; increased sweating; and appetite loss. Children and older adults are more likely to develop difficulty sleeping, excitability, nervousness, restlessness, or irritability.

Drug Interactions

• The sedating effects of promethazine are increased by nervous-system depressants including tranquilizers, alcohol, hypnotics, sedatives, antianxiety drugs, and narcotics. These combinations should be used with extreme caution.

• Use of a monoamine oxidase inhibitor (MAOI) antide-pressant together with promethazine may cause low blood pressure and unusual or uncoordinated movements.

• Promethazine will antagonize the effects of ampheta-mines and other appetite suppressants such as diet pills.

• The combination of promethazine and an oral antithyroid drug may increase the risk of agranulocytosis (condition char-acterized by a reduction in the number of white blood cells).

• The combination of quinidine and promethazine may increase the cardiac effects of both drugs.

• Increasing the dosage of anticonvulsant medication, bromocriptine, guanadrel, guanethidine, or levodopa may be necessary when any of these drugs are taken with prometh-azine.

• Riboflavin requirements are increased in people taking promethazine.

• Promethazine may interfere with blood-sugar tests and home pregnancy tests.

Food Interactions

Take promethazine with food if it upsets your stomach.

Usual Dose

Allergy
    Adult: 12.5 mg before meals and 12.5–25 mg at bedtime.
    Child: 5–12.5 mg 3 times a day and 25 mg at bedtime.

Motion Sickness
    Adult: 25 mg half an hour before travel; repeat in 8–12 hours if needed. Then take 1 dose upon arising and another before dinner.
    Child: 10–25 mg given by mouth or as a suppository.

Nausea and Vomiting
    Adult: 25 mg when needed; repeat up to 6 times a day if necessary.
    Child: 10–25 mg twice a day as needed.

Nighttime Sedation
    Adult: 25–50 mg at bedtime.
    Child: about half the adult dose.

Overdosage

Symptoms include drowsiness; confusion; clumsiness; dry mouth, nose, or throat; hallucinations; seizure; and other promethazine side effects. Overdose victims should be taken to a hospital emergency room for treatment. ALWAYS bring the prescription bottle or container.

Special Information

Be careful when performing tasks requiring concentration and coordination, such as driving, because the drug may cause tiredness, dizziness, or light-headedness; avoid alcohol.

Call your doctor if you develop sore throat; dry mouth, nose, or throat; fever; chills; unusual bleeding or bruising; tiredness; weakness; clumsiness; unsteadiness; hallucinations; seizure; sleeping problems; feeling faint; flushing; breathing difficulties; or any bothersome or persistent side effect.

Maintain good dental hygiene while taking promethazine because dry mouth may cause you to be more susceptible to oral infections. If the dry mouth caused by promethazine is not eased by gum or hard candy or lasts more than 2 weeks, call your doctor or dentist. Any dental work should be completed prior to starting on this drug.

If you forget a dose of promethazine, take it as soon as you remember. If you take it twice a day and it is almost time for your next dose, take 1 dose right away and another in 5 or 6 hours, then continue with your regular schedule. If you take promethazine 3 or more times a day and forget a dose, take it as soon as you remember. If it is almost time for your next dose, take 1 dose right away and another in 3 or 4 hours, then continue with your regular schedule. Never take a double dose.

Special Populations

Pregnancy/Breast-feeding
Babies born to women who took phenothiazines have suffered side effects at birth such as yellowing of the skin and whites of the eyes, nervous-system effects, and blood-clotting problems. Do not take any antihistamine without your doctor's knowledge if you are or might be pregnant—especially during the last 3 months of pregnancy—because newborns may have severe reactions to antihistamines.

Nursing mothers who must take promethazine should bottle-feed.

Seniors
Seniors are more sensitive to side effects.

Generic Name

Propoxyphene Hydrochloride

(proe-POK-sih-fene hye-droe-KLOR-ide) [G]

Brand Name

Darvon

Combination Products

Generic Ingredients: Propoxyphene Hydrochloride +
Aspirin + Caffeine [G]
Darvon Compound-65

Generic Ingredients: Propoxyphene Hydrochloride +
Acetaminophen [G]
Wygesic

The information in this profile also applies to the following
drugs:

Generic Ingredient: Propoxyphene Napsylate
Darvon-N

Generic Ingredients: Propoxyphene Napsylate +
Acetaminophen [G]
Darvocet-N 50   Propacet 100
Darvocet-N 100

Type of Drug

Analgesic.

Prescribed for

Mild to moderate pain.

General Information

A chemical derivative of methadone (a narcotic pain reliever),
propoxyphene hydrochloride is widely used for mild pain. It
is estimated that propoxyphene hydrochloride is about ½ to
⅔ as strong a pain reliever as codeine and about as equally
effective as aspirin. Propoxyphene hydrochloride is more
effective when combined with aspirin or acetaminophen than
when used alone. Propoxyphene hydrochloride is about 30%
more potent than propoxyphene napsylate.

Cautions and Warnings

Do not take propoxyphene hydrochloride if you are **allergic** to it or to similar drugs. Psychological or physical **drug dependence (addiction)** may result when propoxyphene hydrochloride is taken in doses larger than those needed for pain relief for long periods of time. The major sign of psychological dependence is anxiety when the drug is suddenly stopped. People may also become physically addicted to propoxyphene hydrochloride; it can be abused to the same degree as codeine.

Never take more of this medication than is prescribed by your doctor.

Propoxyphene hydrochloride should be considered a **potentially dangerous drug,** especially in the hands of anyone who is severely depressed or addiction-prone. Excessive doses of propoxyphene hydrochloride, either by itself or together with alcohol or other nervous-system depressants, are a major cause of **drug-related deaths**. Many of these deaths have occurred in people with a history of emotional disturbances, suicidal ideas or suicide attempts, and misuse of tranquilizers, alcohol, and other nervous-system depressants.

Possible Side Effects

▼ Common: dizziness, sedation, nausea, and vomiting. These effects usually disappear if you lie down and relax for a few moments.

▼ Less common: constipation, stomach pain, rash, light-headedness, headache, weakness, euphoria, and minor visual disturbances. Taking propoxyphene hydrochloride over long periods of time and in very high doses has caused psychotic reactions and convulsions.

Drug Interactions

• Propoxyphene hydrochloride may cause drowsiness when taken with other drugs that cause drowsiness, such as tranquilizers, sedatives, hypnotics, narcotics, alcohol, and possibly antihistamines.

• Carbamazepine levels may be increased by propoxyphene hydrochloride, resulting in dizziness, nausea, and poor coordination.

• Charcoal tablets decrease the absorption of propoxyphene hydrochloride into the bloodstream.

• Cigarette smoking increases the rate at which this drug is broken down in the liver. Heavy smokers may need more propoxyphene hydrochloride to obtain pain relief but will have to take less of the drug if they stop smoking.

• Cimetidine may interfere with the breakdown of this drug in the liver, causing confusion, disorientation, breathing difficulties, and seizures.

• Propoxyphene hydrochloride may increase the anticoagulant (blood-thinning) effect of warfarin.

Food Interactions

Take propoxyphene hydrochloride with a full glass of water or with food if it upsets your stomach.

Usual Dose

Propoxyphene Hydrochloride: 65 mg every 4 hours as needed.

Propoxyphene Napsylate: 100 mg every 4 hours as needed. Seniors and people with poor liver or kidney function may need to take the medication less often.

Overdosage

Symptoms include a decrease in respiratory rate, changes in breathing pattern, pinpointed pupils, convulsions, extreme sleepiness leading to stupor or coma, and abnormal heart rhythms. The overdose victim should be taken to a hospital emergency room immediately. ALWAYS bring the prescription bottle or container.

Special Information

Use caution while driving or performing any tasks that require you to be awake and alert. Avoid alcohol and other nervous-system depressants.

Call your doctor if you develop nausea or vomiting while taking this drug, or if you develop breathing difficulties.

If you forget a dose, take it as soon as you remember. If it is almost time for your next dose, skip the one you forgot and continue with your regular schedule. Do not take a double dose.

Special Populations

Pregnancy/Breast-feeding

No clinical studies of this medication have been conducted in pregnant women, but a survey of almost 3,000 pregnant women who took propoxyphene hydrochloride found that 46—1.6%—had infants with birth defects. Animal studies show that high doses of the drug can cause problems in a fetus. Pregnant women who must take propoxyphene hydrochloride should talk to their doctor about the risks of this drug.

Small amounts of propoxyphene hydrochloride pass into breast milk. Nursing mothers who must take this drug should consider bottle-feeding.

Seniors

Seniors, especially those with reduced kidney or liver function, are more likely to be sensitive to the effects of this drug and should be treated with smaller dosages.

Generic Name

Propranolol (proe-PRAN-oe-lol) Ⓖ

Brand Name

Inderal

Combination Products

Generic Ingredients: Propranolol + Hydrochlorothiazide Ⓖ
Inderide

Type of Drug

Beta-adrenergic blocking agent.

Prescribed for

High blood pressure, angina pectoris, abnormal heart rhythm, prevention of second heart attack or migraine, tremors, aggressive behavior, side effects of antipsychotic drugs, acute panic, stage fright and other anxieties, and schizophrenia; also used to treat bleeding from the stomach or esophagus, and symptoms of hyperthyroidism (overactive thyroid gland).

General Information

Propranolol hydrochloride is one of 15 beta-adrenergic block-ing drugs, or beta blockers, that interfere with the action of a specific part of the nervous system. Beta receptors are found all over the body and affect many body functions. Each beta blocker has particular characteristics that make it more suit-able for certain conditions or people.

Cautions and Warnings

You should be cautious about taking propranolol if you have **asthma, severe heart failure,** a very **slow heart rate,** or **heart block** (disruption of the electrical impulses that control heart rate) because the drug may aggravate these conditions.

People with **angina** who take propranolol for high blood pressure risk aggravating their angina if they suddenly stop taking the drug. These people should have their drug dosage reduced gradually over 1 to 2 weeks.

Propranolol should be used with caution if you have **liver or kidney disease** because your ability to eliminate this drug from your body may be impaired.

Propranolol reduces the amount of blood pumped by the heart with each beat. This reduction in blood flow may aggra-vate the condition of people with **poor circulation** or **circula-tory disease**.

If you are undergoing **major surgery,** your doctor may want you to stop taking propranolol at least 2 days before surgery.

Possible Side Effects

Side effects are relatively uncommon and usually mild.

▼ Most common: impotence.

▼ Less common: tiredness or weakness, slow heart-beat, heart failure, dizziness, breathing difficulties, bron-chospasm, depression, confusion, anxiety, nervousness, sleeplessness, disorientation, short-term memory loss, emotional instability, cold hands and feet, constipation, diarrhea, nausea, vomiting, upset stomach, increased sweating, urinary difficulties, cramps, blurred vision, rash, hair loss, stuffy nose, facial swelling, aggravation of lupus erythematosus, itching, chest pain, back or joint pain, colitis, drug allergy (symptoms include fever and sore throat), and liver toxicity.

Drug Interactions

• Propranolol may interact with surgical anesthetics to increase the risk of heart problems during surgery. Some anesthesiologists recommend gradually stopping the drug by 2 days before surgery.

• Propranolol may interfere with the normal signs of low blood sugar and with the action of oral antidiabetes medications.

• Propranolol increases the blood-pressure-lowering effect of other blood-pressure-reducing agents including clonidine, guanabenz, and reserpine, as well as calcium channel blockers such as nifedipine.

• Aspirin-containing drugs, indomethacin, sulfinpyrazone, and estrogen drugs may interfere with the blood-pressure-lowering effect of propranolol.

• Cocaine may reduce the effectiveness of all beta blockers.

• Propranolol may worsen the problem of cold hands and feet associated with ergot alkaloids, used to treat migraine. Gangrene is a possibility in people taking both ergot and propranolol.

• The effect of benzodiazepine antianxiety drugs may be increased by propranolol.

• Propranolol will counteract thyroid hormone replacements.

• Calcium channel blockers, flecainide, hydralazine, oral contraceptives, propafenone, haloperidol, phenothiazine tranquilizers—molindone and others—quinolone antibacterials, and quinidine may increase the amount of propranolol in the bloodstream and lead to increased propranolol effects.

• Propranolol should not be taken within 2 weeks of taking a monoamine oxidase inhibitor (MAOI) antidepressant.

• Cimetidine increases the amount of propranolol absorbed into the bloodstream from oral tablets.

• Propranolol may interfere with the effectiveness of some antiasthma medications including theophylline and aminophylline, and especially ephedrine and isoproterenol.

• Combining propranolol and phenytoin or digitalis drugs may result in excessive slowing of the heart, possibly causing heart block.

• Your propranolol dose may have to be reduced if you stop smoking because your liver will break down the drug more slowly after you stop.

Food Interactions

Although it is best to take propranolol without food or on an empty stomach, it is more important to be consistent about taking it with or without food in order to maintain consistent effects.

Usual Dose

30–700 mg a day.

Overdosage

Symptoms include changes in heartbeat—unusually slow, fast, or irregular; severe dizziness or fainting; breathing difficulties; bluish-colored fingernails or palms; and seizures. The victim should be taken to a hospital emergency room. ALWAYS bring the prescription bottle or container.

Special Information

Propranolol is for continuous use. Do not stop taking this drug unless directed to do so by your doctor: Abrupt withdrawal may cause chest pain, breathing difficulties, increased sweating, and unusually fast or irregular heartbeat. When ending propranolol treatment, dosage should be reduced gradually over a period of about 2 weeks.

Call your doctor at once if you develop back or joint pain, breathing difficulties, cold hands or feet, depression, rash, or changes in heartbeat. Propranolol may produce an undesirable lowering of blood pressure, leading to dizziness or fainting; call your doctor if this happens to you. Call your doctor if you experience persistent or bothersome anxiety, diarrhea, constipation, impotence, headache, itching, nausea or vomiting, nightmares or vivid dreams, upset stomach, trouble sleeping, stuffy nose, frequent urination, unusual tiredness, or weakness.

Propranolol may cause drowsiness, light-headedness, dizziness, or blurred vision. Be careful when driving or performing complex tasks.

It is best to take propranolol at the same time each day. If you forget a dose, take it as soon as you remember. If you take propranolol once a day and it is within 8 hours of your next dose, skip the dose you forgot and continue with your regular schedule. If you take it twice a day and it is within 4 hours of your next dose, skip the dose you forgot and continue with your regular schedule. Never take a double dose.

Special Populations

Pregnancy/Breast-feeding

In studies, infants born to women who took a beta blocker while pregnant had lower birth weights, low blood pressure, and reduced heart rates. Propranolol should be avoided by pregnant women.

Propranolol passes into breast milk in concentrations too small to have any effect.

Seniors

Seniors may require less of the drug to achieve results. Seniors taking propranolol may be more likely to suffer from cold hands and feet, reduced body temperature, chest pain, general feelings of ill health, sudden breathing difficulties, increased sweating, or changes in heartbeat.

Propulsid   *see Cisapride, page 210*

Prozac   *see Fluoxetine, page 447*

Generic Name

Quetiapine   (keh-TYE-uh-pene)

Brand Name

Seroquel

Type of Drug

Antipsychotic.

Prescribed for

Psychotic disorders.

General Information

Quetiapine fumarate is effective against a wide variety of symptoms. It may work by antagonizing a number of different types of brain receptors. This means that the drug increases levels of certain neurotransmitters including serotonin, dopamine, and histamine, by preventing them from binding to cell receptors. Quetiapine is broken down by the liver.

Cautions and Warnings

People who are **sensitive** or **allergic** to quetiapine should avoid it.

A potentially fatal condition called **neuroleptic malignant syndrome** (symptoms include convulsions, breathing difficulties, and back, neck, or leg pain) may occur with some antipsychotic drugs. People who have experienced this syndrome with another antipsychotic drug should be cautious when taking quetiapine.

Antipsychotic drugs are often associated with **involuntary, uncoordinated, and uncontrolled movements**. This reaction is most common among older adults, especially women. Call your doctor if you develop any unusual movements while taking quetiapine.

Quetiapine may make you **dizzy** or cause you to **faint** if you rise suddenly from a sitting or lying position. It should be used with caution if you have a history of **heart disease** including heart attack, angina pains, and abnormal heart rhythms. Take this drug with caution if you have a condition or take any drug that can cause **low blood pressure**.

People taking this drug for a long period have developed cataracts, but they have not been directly related to the drug. People taking quetiapine should have an eye exam when they start the drug and every 6 months thereafter to detect any cataract formation.

Quetiapine should be used with caution if you have had a **seizure,** or have a seizure disorder or other condition that may make you more susceptible to seizures, such as Alzheimer's disease.

Quetiapine treatment has been associated with low levels of **thyroid hormone** in the blood. This is usually not a problem, although a small percentage of people taking this drug may need a thyroid supplement.

Quetiapine may cause increases in **blood cholesterol** and **triglyceride** levels.

Quetiapine has caused **liver inflammation** without any symptoms, as measured by increases in enzymes produced by the liver. These enzymes generally return to normal with continued treatment.

The possibility of **suicide** exists in any person with schizophrenia. People at risk of suicide should keep only small amounts of medication at any time.

Possible Side Effects

▼ Most common: dizziness, headache, upset stomach, tiredness, dizziness or fainting when rising from a sitting or lying position, abdominal pain, weight gain, and dry mouth.

▼ Common: swelling in the arms or legs, heart palpitations, spastic movements, difficulty talking, sore throat, runny nose, increased coughing, breathing difficulties, flu symptoms, appetite loss, sweating, and low white-blood-cell counts.

▼ Less common: weight loss, increased blood fats, intolerance to alcohol, dehydration, blood-sugar changes, loss of kidney function, flushing and warmth, electrocardiogram changes, migraine, slow heartbeat, poor blood flow to the brain, stroke, blood clots, irregular pulse, changes in the electrical impulses in the heart, pneumonia, nosebleed, asthma, abnormal dreaming, uncoordinated or abnormal movement, fainting, uncontrollable or excessive movement, confusion, memory loss, psychosis, hallucination, increased sex drive, urinary difficulties, poor coordination, paranoid feelings, unusual walking, muscle spasm, delusion, manic reactions, apathy, depersonalization, stupor, teeth grinding, catatonic reactions, loss of movement on one side of the body, neck or pelvic pain, suicide attempt, feeling unwell, sun sensitivity, chills, facial swelling, fungal infection, salivation, increased appetite, gum irritation or bleeding, difficulty swallowing, gas, stomach irritation, hemorrhoids, mouth sores, thirst, tooth decay, loss of bowel control, stomach contents coming back up into the throat or mouth, rectal bleeding, tongue swelling, itching, acne, eczema, contact dermatitis, raised rash, seborrhea, skin sores, painful menstruation or menstruation accompanied by unusual pain, vaginal irritation, loss of urinary control, painful urination, impotence, abnormal ejaculation, vaginal infection, vaginal discharge, vaginal bleeding, irritation of the external vagina, testicle inflammation, cystitis, frequent urination, loss of periodic bleeding,

Possible Side Effects *(continued)*

oozing of breast milk, eye redness, abnormal vision, dry eyes, ringing or buzzing in the ears, changes in the sense of taste, eyelid inflammation, eye pain, broken bones, muscle weakness, twitching, joint pain, arthritis, leg cramps, bone pain, increased white-blood-cell count, anemia, black-and-blue marks, swollen lymph glands, bluish skin, diabetes, and underactive thyroid gland.

▼ Rare: Rare side effects can occur in almost any part of the body. Contact your doctor if you experience any side effect not listed above.

Drug Interactions

• Drinking alcohol while taking quetiapine can cause drowsiness.

• Quetiapine may antagonize the effects of levodopa and other drugs used to treat Parkinson's disease.

• Combining quetiapine with phenytoin increases the rate at which quetiapine is released from the body by 5 times. You may require an increase in quetiapine dosage to achieve the same effect. Once dosage has been adjusted, special caution should be taken if phenytoin is replaced by another anti-seizure drug that does not stimulate the body's breakdown of quetiapine. Other drugs that have a similar effect on quetiapine are thioridazine, carbamazepine, barbiturates, rifampin, and oral corticosteroids.

• Ketoconazole, itraconazole, fluconazole, and erythromycin may affect quetiapine. Caution should be exercised when combining these drugs with quetiapine.

• Quetiapine may reduce the rate at which the body clears lorazepam.

Food Interactions

Taking quetiapine with food increases the amount of drug absorbed by a small amount. This is not likely to change its effect on your body.

Usual Dose

Adult: 150–750 mg a day.

Overdosage

Overdose victims should be taken to a hospital emergency room at once. ALWAYS bring the prescription bottle or container.

Special Information

Quetiapine may make you drowsy. Take care while driving or performing any task that requires concentration.

Antipsychotic drugs may increase your sensitivity to hot weather and your susceptibility to dehydration by interfering with temperature-control mechanisms. This problem has not been reported with quetiapine, but be sure to call your doctor if anything unusual develops.

Special Populations

Pregnancy/Breast-feeding

Quetiapine should only be taken during pregnancy if the possible benefits outweigh the risks. Talk to your doctor if you become pregnant or are trying to become pregnant while taking this drug.

Quetiapine passes into breast milk. Nursing mothers who must take quetiapine should bottle-feed.

Seniors

Seniors may be more sensitive to side effects, especially dizziness, fainting, and tiredness.

Generic Name

Quinapril (QUIN-uh-pril)

Brand Name

Accupril

Combination Products

Generic Ingredients: Quinapril + Hydrochlorothiazide
Accuretic 10/12.5   Accuretic 20/12.5

The information in this profile also applies to the following drugs:

Generic Ingredient: Perindopril
Aceon

Generic Ingredient: Ramipril
Altace

Type of Drug

Angiotensin-converting enzyme (ACE) inhibitor.

Prescribed for

High blood pressure and congestive heart failure.

General Information

Quinapril and other ACE inhibitors work by preventing the conversion of a hormone called angiotensin I to another hormone called angiotensin II, a potent blood-vessel constrictor. Preventing this conversion relaxes blood vessels, thus reducing blood pressure and relieving the symptoms of heart failure. Quinapril also affects the production of other hormones and enzymes that participate in the regulation of blood-vessel dilation. Quinapril begins working about 1 hour after you take it and lasts for 24 hours.

Some people who start taking an ACE inhibitor after they are already on a diuretic (an agent that increases urination) experience a rapid blood-pressure drop after their first doses or when the dosage is increased. To prevent this from happening, you may be told to stop taking the diuretic 2 or 3 days before starting the ACE inhibitor or to increase your salt intake during that time. The diuretic may then be restarted gradually.

Cautions and Warnings

Do not take quinapril if you have had an **allergic reaction** to it.

Quinapril occasionally causes **very low blood pressure**. Quinapril can affect your **kidneys,** especially if you have congestive **heart failure**. It is advisable for your doctor to check your urine for changes during the first few months of treatment. Dosage adjustment is necessary if you have reduced kidney function.

Rarely, quinapril affects white-blood-cell count, possibly increasing your susceptibility to **infection**. Blood counts should be monitored periodically.

Possible Side Effects

▼ Most common: dizziness, tiredness, headache, and chronic cough. The cough usually goes away a few days after you stop taking the medication.

▼ Less common: nausea, vomiting, and abdominal pain.

▼ Rare: Rare side effects can occur in almost any part of the body. Contact your doctor if you experience any side effect not listed above.

Drug Interactions

• The blood-pressure-lowering effect of quinapril is additive with diuretic drugs and beta blockers. Any other drug that causes a rapid drop in blood pressure should be used with caution if you are taking an ACE inhibitor.

• Quinapril may increase potassium levels in your blood, especially when taken with dyazide or other potassium-sparing diuretics.

• Quinapril may increase the effects of lithium; this combination should be used with caution.

• Antacids and quinapril should be taken at least 2 hours apart.

• Quinapril decreases the absorption of tetracycline by about ⅓, possibly because of the high magnesium content of quinapril tablets.

• Quinapril may increase blood levels of digoxin, possibly increasing the chance of digoxin-related side effects.

• Capsaicin may trigger or aggravate the cough associated with quinapril therapy.

• Indomethacin may reduce the blood-pressure-lowering effect of quinapril.

• Phenothiazine tranquilizers and antiemetics may increase the effects of quinapril.

• Combining allopurinol and quinapril increases the risk of side effects.

Food Interactions

Quinapril is affected by high-fat food and should be taken on an empty stomach, at least 1 hour before or 2 hours after a meal.

Usual Dose

Perindopril: Adult dosage is 4–8 mg a day. Seniors and people with kidney disease may require a lower dosage.

Quinapril: Adult dosage is 10–80 mg once a day. Seniors and people with kidney disease may require a lower dosage.

Accuretic: 1 tablet a day.

Ramipril: Adult dosage is 2.5–20 mg a day. Seniors and people with moderate to severe kidney disease should begin with 1.25 mg a day; dosage may then be increased up to 5 mg a day.

Overdosage

The principal effect of quinapril overdose is a rapid drop in blood pressure, as evidenced by dizziness and fainting. Take the overdose victim to a hospital emergency room at once. ALWAYS bring the prescription bottle or container.

Special Information

ACE inhibitors may cause unexplained swelling of the face, lips, hands, and feet. This swelling can also affect the larynx (throat) and tongue and interfere with breathing. If this happens, go to a hospital emergency room for treatment immediately. Call your doctor if you develop a sore throat, mouth sores, abnormal heartbeat, chest pain, a persistent rash, or loss of taste perception.

You may get dizzy if you rise too quickly from a sitting or lying position.

Avoid strenuous exercise and very hot weather because heavy sweating or dehydration can cause a rapid drop in blood pressure.

Avoid over-the-counter diet pills, decongestants, and other stimulants that can raise blood pressure.

If you forget a dose, take it as soon as you remember. If it is within 8 hours of your next dose, skip the one you forgot and continue with your regular schedule. Do not take a double dose.

Special Populations

Pregnancy/Breast-feeding
ACE inhibitors can cause fetal injury or death. They are not considered safe for use during pregnancy.

Small amounts of quinapril pass into breast milk. Nursing mothers who must take this drug should consider bottle-feeding.

Seniors

Seniors may be more sensitive to the effects of quinapril due to age-related kidney impairment; the starting dosage for seniors is 10 mg daily.

Generic Name

Quinidine (QUIN-ih-dene) Ⓖ

Brand Names

Cardioquin	Quinidex Extentabs
Quinaglute Dura-Tabs	Quinora
Quinalan	

Type of Drug

Antiarrhythmic.

Prescribed for

Abnormal heart rhythms.

General Information

Derived from the bark of the cinchona tree, which also gives us quinine, quinidine works by affecting the flow of potassium into and out of heart muscle cells. This helps quinidine slow the flow of nerve impulses throughout the heart muscle, which allows control mechanisms in the heart to take over and keep the heart beating at a normal, even rate. The 3 kinds of quinidine—gluconate, polygalacturonate, and sulfate—provide different amounts of active drug and cannot be interchanged without dosage adjustments.

Cautions and Warnings

Do not take quinidine if you are **allergic** to it, to quinine, or to a related drug. Quinidine sensitivity may be masked if you have **asthma, muscle weakness,** or an **infection** when you start taking the drug.

Liver toxicity related to quinidine sensitivity occurs rarely. Unexplained fever or liver inflammation may indicate this effect. People with **kidney or liver disease** may require lower dosages.

Quinidine can also cause **abnormal heart rhythms**.

People taking quinidine for long periods may experience sudden fainting or an abnormal heart rhythm. Occasionally, these episodes may be fatal.

Possible Side Effects

▼ Most common: nausea, vomiting, abdominal pain, diarrhea, and appetite loss. These may be accompanied by fever.

▼ Less common: unusual heart rhythms, altering of blood components; irritation of the esophagus, headache, dizziness, feelings of apprehension or excitement, confusion, delirium, muscle ache or joint pain, ringing or buzzing in the ears, mild hearing loss, blurred vision, changes in color perception, sensitivity to bright light, double vision, difficulty seeing at night, flushing of the skin, itching, sensitivity to the sun, cramps, an unusual urge to defecate or urinate, and cold sweat.

▼ Rare: asthma; swelling of the face, hands, and feet; respiratory collapse; and liver problems.

High dosages of quinidine may cause rash, hearing loss, dizziness, ringing in the ears, headache, nausea, or disturbed vision. This group of symptoms, called cinchonism, is usually related to taking a large amount of quinidine but may appear after a single dose of the medication. Cinchonism is not necessarily a toxic reaction, but you should immediately report any sign of it to your doctor. Do not stop taking this drug unless instructed to do so by your doctor.

Drug Interactions

• Quinidine increases the effect of warfarin and other oral anticoagulants (blood thinners).

• Quinidine may increase the effects of metoprolol, procainamide, propafenone, propranolol, and other beta blockers; benztropine, oxybutynin, atropine, trihexyphenidyl, and other anticholinergic drugs; and tricyclic antidepressants.

• The effect of quinidine may be decreased by the following medicines: phenobarbital and other barbiturates, phenytoin and other hydantoins, nifedipine, rifampin, sucralfate, and cholinergic drugs such as bethanechol.

• The effectiveness and side effects of quinidine may be increased by taking amiodarone, some antacids, cimetidine, anything that decreases urine acid levels, and verapamil.

• Quinidine may dramatically increase the amount of digoxin in the blood, causing possible digoxin toxicity. This combination should be monitored closely by your doctor.

• The combination of disopyramide and quinidine may result in increased disopyramide levels and possible side effects; reduced quinidine activity may also result.

• Avoid over-the-counter cough, cold, allergy, and diet preparations. These medications may contain drugs that stimulate the heart and may be dangerous in combination with quinidine

Food Interactions

You may take quinidine with food if it upsets your stomach. Some forms of quinidine are less irritating to the stomach.

Usual Dose

Immediate-Release: extremely variable; generally, 600–1200 mg a day.

Sustained-Release: generally, 600–1800 mg a day.

Overdosage

Overdose produces depressed mental function, including lethargy, decreased breathing, seizures, and coma. Other symptoms are abdominal pain and diarrhea, abnormal heart rhythms, and symptoms of cinchonism (see "Possible Side Effects"). The victim should be taken to a hospital emergency room. ALWAYS bring the prescription bottle or container.

Special Information

Call your doctor if you develop ringing or buzzing in the ears, hearing or visual disturbances, dizziness, headache, nausea, rash, breathing difficulties, or any intolerable side effect.

Do not crush or chew the sustained-release products.

Some side effects of quinidine may lead to oral discomfort including dry mouth, cavities, periodontal disease, and oral

Candida infections. See your dentist regularly while taking this drug.

If you forget to take a dose of quinidine and you remember within 2 hours of your regular time, take it right away. If you do not remember until later, skip the dose you forgot and continue your regular schedule. Do not take a double dose.

Special Populations

Pregnancy/Breast-feeding
Quinidine may cause birth defects. When this drug is considered crucial by your doctor, its potential benefits must be carefully weighed against its risks.

Quinidine passes into breast milk but is considered acceptable for use while breast-feeding. Consult your doctor.

Seniors
Seniors may be more sensitive to the effects of this medication due to decreased kidney function.

Generic Name
Raloxifene (rah-LOX-ih-feen)

Brand Name
Evista

Type of Drug
Selective Estrogen Receptor Modulator (SERM).

Prescribed for
Osteoporosis.

General Information
The female hormone estrogen plays an important role in maintaining bone strength in women by regulating the body's use of calcium. When the ovaries stop producing estrogen after menopause, a woman's risk of developing osteoporosis increases significantly. Raloxifene hydrochloride, which belongs to the SERM class of drugs, is used to increase bone density in postmenopausal women by mimicking the protective effect that estrogen has on bone. This drug

also lowers cholesterol levels by acting like estrogen therapy in the cardiovascular system. Raloxifene has a potential advantage over estrogen therapy in the treatment of osteoporosis because it does not appear to have an estrogen-like effect in the breast or uterus, where the hormone may increase cancer risk. Raloxifene, which is being studied for the treatment and prevention of breast cancer, is broken down in the liver.

Cautions and Warnings

Do not take raloxifene if you are **sensitive** or **allergic** to it, are **pregnant,** or have had **blood-clotting problems** or clots in the lung, leg, eye, or another part of the body.

Only postmenopausal women should use raloxifene.

People with **liver disease** should use this drug with caution.

Possible Side Effects

▼ Most common: infections, flu-like symptoms, hot flashes, joint pain, and sinus irritation.

▼ Common: depression, sleeplessness, rash, nausea, upset stomach, weight gain, muscle aches, leg cramps, sore throat, and cough.

▼ Less common: chest pain, fever, migraine, sweating, vomiting, gas, stomach and intestinal problems, vaginal irritation, vaginal discharge, urinary infection, cystitis, endometrial problems, swelling in the arms or legs, arthritis, pneumonia, and laryngitis.

▼ Rare: coughing up of blood; loss of or changes in speech, coordination, or vision; pain or numbness in the chest, arm, or leg; and shortness of breath. Rare side effects can occur in almost any part of the body. Contact your doctor if you experience any side effect not listed above.

Raloxifene is more likely to cause hot flashes, infection, and chest pain than estrogen therapy but is much less likely to cause abdominal pain, vaginal bleeding, breast pain, and gas.

Drug Interactions

• Taking raloxifene and estrogen therapy is not recommended because the effects of this combination are unknown.

• Raloxifene can increase blood levels of clofibrate, indomethacin, naproxen, ibuprofen, diazepam, and diazoxide.

• Ampicillin can reduce the absorption of raloxifene, but this interaction is not considered important.

• Cholestyramine can significantly reduce the absorption of raloxifene. Separate doses of these drugs by 2 hours or more.

• Raloxifene can reduce the effect of warfarin (a blood thinner). Your warfarin dosage may need an adjustment.

Food Interactions

Raloxifene can be taken with or without food.

Usual Dose

Adult: 60 mg once a day.
Child: not recommended

Overdosage

Little is known about the effects of raloxifene overdose. Call your local poison control center or a hospital emergency room for information. If you seek treatment, ALWAYS bring the prescription bottle or container.

Special Information

Raloxifene can increase your risk of developing a blood clot in the lung, leg, or another part of the body during any extended period of inactivity. Stop taking raloxifene 3 days before surgery, a long period of bed rest, or lengthy plane or car trips.

It is very important for all postmenopausal women age 51 and over to get 1200 mg of calcium and 10 mcg (400 IU) of vitamin D every day, either from food or a dietary supplement. Women age 70 and over require 1200 mg of calcium and 15 mcg (600 IU) of vitamin D daily.

Regular exercise is recommended for all postmenopausal women because it helps build strong bones.

Raloxifene does not reduce the hot flashes or flushes associated with menopause. Call your doctor if you experience hot flashes or flushes while taking raloxifene.

If you forget a dose, take it as soon as you remember. If a whole day has passed without taking your medication, skip the forgotten dose and continue with your regular schedule. Do not take a double dose.

Special Populations

Pregnancy/Breast-feeding

Raloxifene can harm the fetus. It is not considered safe for use during pregnancy.

It is not known if raloxifene passes into breast milk. Nursing mothers who must take it should bottle-feed.

Seniors

Seniors can use raloxifene without special precaution.

Generic Name

Ranitidine (rah-NIT-ih-deen) Ⓖ

Brand Names

Zantac   Zantac 75 Ⓢ

Type of Drug

Antiulcer and histamine H_2 antagonist.

Prescribed for

Duodenal (intestinal) and gastric (stomach) ulcers; also prescribed for gastroesophageal reflux disease (GERD), other conditions characterized by the secretion of large amounts of gastric fluids, and to prevent bleeding in the stomach and upper intestines, stress ulcers, stomach damage caused by nonsteroidal anti-inflammatory drugs (NSAIDs), and the production of stomach acid during surgery.

General Information

Ranitidine hydrochloride and other H_2 antagonists work by turning off the system that produces stomach acid and other secretions. Ranitidine starts working within 1 hour and reaches its peak effect in 1 to 3 hours. Its effect lasts for up to 15 hours. Ranitidine is effective in treating ulcer symptoms and preventing complications of the disease. It is prescribed for short-term and maintenance therapy. Since all H_2 antagonists work in the same way, ulcers that do not respond to one will probably not respond to another. The only difference among H_2 antagonists is their potency. Cimetidine is the least potent, with 1000 mg roughly equal to 300 mg of ranitidine and nizatidine or 40 mg of famotidine. The ulcer-healing rates of all of these drugs are roughly equivalent, as is the risk of side effects.

Cautions and Warnings

Do not take ranitidine if you have had an **allergic reaction** to it or another H$_2$ antagonist. Caution must be exercised by people with **kidney or liver disease** who take ranitidine because the drug is partly broken down in the liver and passes out of the body through the kidneys. Occasionally, reversible **hepatitis or other liver abnormality** may occur, with or without jaundice (symptoms include yellowing of the skin or whites of the eyes). Reducing stomach acid levels in a person with **compromised immune function** may increase the risk of intestinal worm infection.

Possible Side Effects

Side effects with ranitidine are rare.

▼ Most common: dizziness, confusion, hallucinations, depression, sleeplessness, hair loss, inflammation of the pancreas, joint pain, and drug reactions.

▼ Less common: headache, blurred vision, agitation or anxiety, nausea, vomiting, constipation, diarrhea, abdominal discomfort, painful breast swelling, impotence, loss of sex drive, and rash.

▼ Rare: reversible reduction in white-blood-cell or blood-platelet count and hepatitis.

Drug Interactions

• Antacids slightly reduce the effects of ranitidine. To avoid this interaction, separate doses of these drugs by about 2 to 3 hours.

• Ranitidine may interfere with the absorption of diazepam tablets. This interaction is considered minor and is unlikely to affect most people.

• Ranitidine may increase blood concentrations of glipizide, glyburide, theophylline drugs, and procainamide, increasing the risk of side effects. Interactions between ranitidine and glyburide or a theophylline drug are rare.

• Ranitidine may interact with warfarin, an anticoagulant (blood thinner). Your warfarin dosage may need an adjustment.

Food Interactions

You may take ranitidine with or without food.

Usual Dose

150–300 mg a day. People with severe conditions may require up to 600 mg a day. People with severe kidney disease need less medication.

Overdosage

Little is known about the effects of ranitidine overdose, though symptoms are likely to include severe side effects. Induce vomiting with ipecac syrup—available at any pharmacy. Call your doctor or a local poison control center before doing this. If you seek treatment, ALWAYS bring the prescription bottle or container.

Special Information

It may take several days for ranitidine to begin to relieve stomach pain. You must take this drug exactly as directed and follow your doctor's instructions for diet and other treatments to get the maximum benefit from it.

Call your doctor at once if any unusual side effects develop. Especially important are unusual bleeding or bruising, unusual tiredness, diarrhea, dizziness, rash, or hallucinations. Black, tarry stools or vomiting "coffee-ground"-like material may indicate that your ulcer is bleeding.

If you forget a dose, take it as soon as you remember. If it is almost time for your next dose, skip the one you forgot and continue with your regular schedule. Do not take a double dose.

Special Populations

Pregnancy/Breast-feeding

While animal studies of ranitidine reveal no damage to the fetus, this drug should only be used during pregnancy after carefully weighing its potential benefits against its risks.

Large amounts of ranitidine pass into breast milk. Nursing mothers who must take this drug should consider bottle-feeding.

Seniors

Seniors may obtain maximum benefit with smaller dosages. They also may be more susceptible to side effects, especially confusion.

Generic Name

Ranitidine Bismuth Citrate

(rah-NIT-ih-deen BIZ-muth SIH-trate)

Brand Name

Tritec

Type of Drug

Antibacterial and antiulcer combination.

Prescribed for

Duodenal (upper intestinal) ulcer.

General Information

Revolutionary research into the causes of ulcer disease has shown that the microorganism *Heliobacter pylori* is almost always present. This has led to a major change in the treatment of the disease. Drugs that combine an acid blocker with an antibiotic are now used to treat the ulcer and the infection that may be causing it. Ranitidine bismuth citrate, which is prescribed in conjunction with the antibiotic clarithromycin, is a combination of ranitidine and bismuth. Ranitidine turns off the system that produces stomach acid, providing relief from ulcer symptoms. Bismuth works against *H. pylori* by disrupting the bacterial cell wall. It may also prevent bacteria from sticking to cells in the stomach lining and from becoming resistant to antibiotics.

Cautions and Warnings

Ranitidine bismuth citrate should **not be used alone** for active duodenal ulcers. Active ulcer treatment also requires the use of clarithromycin.

If you have taken clarithromycin for *H. pylori* and your **ulcer symptoms persist,** it is likely that you have a resistant form of the bacterium. A different antibiotic may be needed.

Do not take this drug if you are **sensitive** or **allergic** to it.

People with **porphyria** should not take ranitidine bismuth citrate and clarithromycin.

People with **kidney disease** should take ranitidine bismuth citrate and clarithromycin with caution. Some people with kidney disease may require lower dosages.

Ranitidine may interfere with the **Multistix urine test**.

Possible Side Effects

Ranitidine Bismuth Citrate
Side effects can be expected to be minimal. In studies, they are approximately equal to those reported with a placebo (sugar pill). For more information, see "Ranitidine."

Ranitidine Bismuth Citrate in Conjunction with Clarithromycin
   ▼ Most common: diarrhea and changes in sense of taste.
   ▼ Less common: headache, nausea, vomiting, and gynecological problems.
   ▼ Rare: tremors, abdominal discomfort, stomach pain, rash, and drug reactions.

Drug Interactions

• Combining clarithromycin, ranitidine, and bismuth increases blood levels of all 3 drugs. This interaction is beneficial to people taking the combination.
• High-dose antacids may reduce ranitidine and bismuth blood levels.

Food Interactions

This drug may be taken with food if it upsets your stomach.

Usual Dose

Adult: 400 mg 2 times a day for 4 weeks; 500 mg of clarithromycin is taken 3 times a day for the first 2 weeks.
Child: not recommended.

Overdosage

Bismuth overdose may lead to kidney and nervous system toxicity, but this has not been seen with ranitidine bismuth citrate, only with other bismuth products. Ranitidine overdose may cause dizziness, confusion, hallucinations, depression, sleeplessness, hair loss, inflammation of the pancreas, and joint pain; these effects usually are not permanent. Take the victim to a hospital emergency room. ALWAYS bring the prescription bottle or container.

Special Information

Bismuth may cause a temporary darkening of your tongue or stool. This is a harmless effect. Darkening of the stool should not be confused with blood in the stool, which turns it black.

If you forget a dose, take it as soon as you remember. If it is almost time for your next dose, skip the dose you forgot and continue with your regular schedule. Do not take a double dose.

Special Populations

Pregnancy/Breast-feeding

While animal studies of ranitidine bismuth citrate reveal no damage to the fetus, this drug should only be used during pregnancy after carefully weighing its potential benefits against its risks. Information in humans is limited. Of the 4 known cases in which ranitidine bismuth citrate was used in the course of a full-term pregnancy, 1 child was born with birth defects, which doctors considered unrelated to the medication.

It is not known if ranitidine bismuth citrate passes into breast milk, though both ingredients pass into rat breast milk. Nursing mothers who must take this drug should consider bottle-feeding.

Seniors

Seniors may take this drug without special restriction.

Brand Name
Rebetron

Generic Ingredients

Interferon Alfa-2b + Ribavirin

Type of Drug

Antiviral combination.

Prescribed for

Hepatitis C.

General Information

This combination should be used only when interferon alpha, the only other approved treatment for hepatitis C, has failed. Ribavirin is not effective against hepatitis C by itself. The way that this combination works against hepatitis C is not known.

Cautions and Warnings

All people taking this combination must be closely **monitored by their doctors,** including periodic **blood and liver and thyroid function** tests.

People with **kidney disease** or **heart disease** should use this medication with caution. If heart disease worsens during treatment, the drug should be discontinued.

Rebetron can affect both sperm and egg. Men and women taking Rebetron must **use effective contraception** during treatment and for 6 months after treatment is completed. Call your doctor if pregnancy occurs.

People who develop **severe side effects** or become **depressed** while taking this medication should have their interferon dosage temporarily lowered. The medication should be stopped if severe depression develops.

Children as young as age 1 have been treated with interferon alpha, but the combination product has not been studied in **children** of any age.

Possible Side Effects

Some people experience no side effects while taking Rebetron, and most feel well enough to work and travel during treatment.

▼ Most common: depression, fever, tiredness, headache, muscle aches, chills, flu-like symptoms, irritability, nausea, diarrhea, appetite loss, abdominal pain, weakness, joint pain, muscle pain, and feeling unwell.

▼ Common: dry mouth, thirst, dizziness, tingling in the hands or feet, sleep disturbances, vomiting, upset stomach, weight loss, and hemolytic anemia (red-blood-cell destruction).

Possible Side Effects *(continued)*

▼ Less common: loss of concentration, nervousness, constipation, loose stools, changes in sense of taste, sore throat, breathing difficulties, sinus irritation, inflamed injection site (interferon only), chest pain, and sweating,

▼ Rare: confusion, loss of sex drive, stuffy nose, coughing, facial swelling, and cold sores. Other rare side effects can occur in almost any part of the body. Contact your doctor if you experience any side effect not listed above.

Drug Interactions

• Antacids may reduce the amount of ribavirin absorbed.

Food Interactions

High-fat meals can increase the amount of ribavirin absorbed, though the importance of this is not known. These drugs may be taken with or without food.

Usual Dose

Adult (under 166 lbs.): Ribavirin—400 mg in the morning and 600 mg at night. Interferon Alfa—3 million units 3 times a week by injection under the skin.

Adult (166 lbs. and over): Ribavirin—600 mg morning and night. Interferon Alfa—3 million units 3 times a week by injection under the skin.

Child: not recommended.

Overdosage

Little is known about the effects of Rebetron overdose. Take the victim to a hospital emergency room. ALWAYS bring the prescription bottle or container.

Special Information

This medication can make you drowsy. Be careful when driving or performing any task that requires concentration.

Drink lots of water while using Rebetron to make sure you are well hydrated.

Call your doctor at once if hives, itching, chest tightness, coughing, breathing difficulties, visual difficulties, wheezing, low blood pressure, or light-headedness develop. These can be signs of drug allergy.

Rebetron can make you more sensitive to the sun. Avoid spending a lot of time in the sun while taking it.

If you forget to take a dose of interferon, take it as soon as you remember. If it is almost time for your next dose, space your remaining weekly doses throughout the rest of the week. If you forget a dose of ribavirin, take it as soon as you remember. If it is almost time for your next dose, skip the dose you forgot and continue with your regular schedule. Do not take a double dose. Call your doctor if you forget 2 or more doses in a row.

Do not change brands of interferon without your doctor's knowledge—they may not be equivalent.

Special Populations

Pregnancy/Breast-feeding
Rebetron should not be taken by pregnant women or their male partners because of its effect on the sperm, egg, and fetus. Women must be tested monthly to be sure they are not pregnant.

It is not known if the ingredients in Rebetron pass into breast milk. Nursing mothers who must take this medication should bottle-feed.

Seniors
Seniors may use Rebetron without special restriction.

Relafen see Nabumetone, page 699

Generic Name

Repaglanide (reh-PAG-luh-nide)

Brand Name
Prandin

Type of Drug
Antidiabetic.

Prescribed for

Type II diabetes.

General Information

In people with type II diabetes, the pancreas does not make enough insulin or the hormone fails to work. Because insulin regulates the amount of sugar in the blood, lack of this hormone causes blood sugar to rise to unhealthy levels. Repaglanide is the first in a new group of drugs designed to control diabetes by increasing insulin production. When taken with meals, this drug temporarily stimulates the pancreas to release more insulin when it is needed to help process dietary sugar. This helps to stabilize blood sugar. Repaglanide may be used alone or combined with metformin. Repaglanide only works if beta cells in the pancreas are functioning properly.

Cautions and Warnings

Because repaglanide is broken down in the liver, people with **liver problems** may require reduced dosage or more time between doses.

Any antidiabetes drug can **excessively lower blood sugar.** Low blood sugar can develop when you do not consume enough calories, overexert yourself physically, drink alcohol, or combine blood-sugar-lowering drugs.

You may need to temporarily switch to insulin therapy if you have **surgery** or experience **fever, infection,** or **trauma.**

Possible Side Effects

▼ Most common: high or low blood sugar, headache, and respiratory infection.

▼ Common: sinus irritation, runny nose, bronchitis, nausea, diarrhea, and back or joint pain.

▼ Less common: constipation, vomiting, upset stomach, tingling in the hands or feet, chest pain, urinary infection, and tooth problems.

▼ Rare: allergy.

Drug Interactions

• Combining repaglanide and ketoconazole, miconazole, or erythromycin may result in low blood sugar.

• Combining repaglanide and troglitazone, rifampin, barbiturates, or carbamazepine may result in high blood sugar.

• The blood-sugar-lowering effect of all antidiabetes drugs may be increased by sulfa drugs: aspirin, ibuprofen, and other nonsteroidal anti-inflammatory drugs (NSAIDs); chloramphenicol; coumadin-type anticoagulants (blood thinners); probenecid; monoamine oxidase inhibitor (MAOI) drugs; and beta blockers.

• Thiazides and other diuretics, corticosteroid anti-inflammatory drugs, phenothiazines, thyroid drugs, estrogens, oral contraceptives ("the pill"), phenytoin, nicotinic acid, stimulants, calcium channel blockers, and isoniazid may increase blood sugar levels. Your dosage of repaglanide may need to be increased if you combine it with any of these drugs.

Food Interactions

Repaglanide should be taken before meals.

Usual Dose

Adult: 0.5–4 mg 15–30 minutes before each meal, up to 4 times a day.

Child: not recommended.

Overdosage

Little is known about the effects of repaglanide overdose, but symptoms may include very low blood sugar. Take the victim to a hospital emergency room. ALWAYS bring the prescription bottle or container.

Special Information

Measurements of blood sugar and glycosylated hemoglobin (hemoglobin A1$_c$) are essential to your doctor's evaluation of your progress. See your doctor regularly.

Repaglanide must be taken before you eat. If you skip a meal, do not take this drug. If you have an extra meal, take an extra dose of repaglanide before that meal.

The timing of each repaglanide dose is key to its effectiveness. If you forget to take repaglanide before a meal, take it during the meal. If you have already eaten and forgotten your medication, skip the forgotten dose. If you cannot remember to take repaglanide before each meal, talk to your doctor about changing drugs.

Special Populations

Pregnancy/Breast-feeding
Repaglanide should not be taken during pregnancy. Animal studies indicate that it may affect the skeletal development of the fetus. Most experts recommend that diabetes be controlled with insulin during pregnancy.

Repaglanide passes into breast milk. Nursing mothers who must take it should bottle-feed.

Seniors
Some seniors may be more sensitive to the effects of this drug.

Rezulin   *see Troglitazone, page 1064*

Generic Name

Rifampin   (rih-FAM-pin) [G]

Brand Names

Rifadin   Rimactane

Combination Products

Generic Ingredients: Rifampin + Isoniazid
Rifamate

Generic Ingredients: Rifampin + Isoniazid + Pyrazinamide
Rifater

Type of Drug

Antitubercular.

Prescribed for

Tuberculosis, meningitis, and other infections.

General Information

Rifampin, an important agent in the treatment of tuberculosis, is always used with at least one other tuberculosis drug. It is also prescribed to eradicate the organism that causes

meningitis in carriers—people who are not infected themselves but carry the organism and can spread it to others.
Rifampin can be used to treat staphylococcal infections of the
skin, bones, or prostate; legionnaires' disease; and leprosy;
and to prevent meningitis caused by *Haemophilus influenzae,* common among children in day care.

Cautions and Warnings

Do not take this drug if you are **allergic** to it or rifabutin, prescribed for *Mycobacterium avium* complex (an infection
associated with advanced cases of AIDS).

Liver damage and death have been reported in people
taking rifabutin, a drug that is very similar to rifampin. People taking other drugs that may cause liver damage should
avoid rifampin. People with liver disease should be carefully monitored by their doctors and receive reduced
dosage.

Bacterial resistance develops very quickly if rifampin is
used for meningococcus infection. It should not be used for
this purpose.

A few cases of accelerated **lung cancer growth** have been
reported, but a link to rifampin use is not established.
Rifampin has the potential to **suppress the immune system**.

Possible Side Effects

▼ Most common: flu-like symptoms, heartburn, upset
stomach, appetite loss, nausea, vomiting, gas, cramps,
diarrhea, headache, drowsiness, tiredness, menstrual
disturbances, dizziness, fever, pain in the arms and legs,
confusion, visual disturbances, numbness, and hypersensitivity to the drug.

▼ Less common: effects on the blood, kidneys, or
liver.

Drug Interactions

• Severe liver damage may develop when rifampin is combined with other drugs that cause liver toxicity.

• Rifampin may increase your need for oral anticoagulant
(blood-thinning) drugs and may also affect angiotensin-converting enzyme (ACE) inhibitors, especially enalapril; acetaminophen; oral antidiabetes drugs; barbiturates; benzodi-

azepine tranquilizers; beta blockers; chloramphenicol; clofibrate; corticosteroids; cyclosporine; digitalis drugs; disopyramide; estrogens; phenytoin; methadone; mexiletine; quinidine; sulfa drugs; theophylline drugs; tocainide; and verapamil.

• Women taking birth control pills should use another contraceptive method while taking rifampin.

Food Interactions

Take rifampin 1 hour before or 2 hours after a meal, at the same time every day.

Usual Dose

Adult: 600 mg once a day.
Child: 4.5–9 mg per lb. of body weight, up to 600 mg a day.

Overdosage

Symptoms include nausea, vomiting, and tiredness. Unconsciousness is possible in cases of severe liver damage. Brown-red or orange skin discoloration may also develop. Take the victim to a hospital emergency room at once. ALWAYS bring the prescription bottle or container.

Special Information

Rifampin may cause a red-brown or orange discoloration of the urine, stool, saliva, sweat, and tears; this is not harmful. Soft contact lenses may become permanently stained.

Call your doctor if you develop flu-like symptoms, fever, chills, muscle pain, headache, tiredness or weakness, appetite loss, nausea, vomiting, sore throat, unusual bleeding or bruising, yellowing of the skin or whites of the eyes, rash, or itching.

If you take rifampin once a day and miss a dose, take it as soon as you remember. If it is almost time for your next dose, skip the dose you forgot and continue with your regular schedule. Do not take a double dose. Regularly missing doses of rifampin increases the risk of side effects.

Special Populations

Pregnancy/Breast-feeding

Animal studies indicate that rifampin may cause cleft palate and spina bifida (birth defect in which bones of the lower spinal column do not form properly, leaving the spinal canal partially exposed) in the fetus. Pregnant women should use this drug only if absolutely necessary.

This drug may pass into breast milk. Nursing mothers who must take it should bottle-feed.

Seniors

Seniors with liver disease may be more sensitive to the effects of this drug.

Generic Name

Riluzole (RIL-ue-zole)

Brand Name

Rilutek

Type of Drug

Glutamate-release blocker.

Prescribed for

Amyotrophic lateral sclerosis (ALS), also known as Lou Gehrig's disease.

General Information

ALS is a chronic disease of the nervous system. Riluzole, the only drug proven to affect ALS, has a number of different actions, though nobody knows exactly how it works. The drug slows the release of glutamate, which is thought to damage important nerve centers in the brains of people with ALS, and protects other aspects of nerve function. Riluzole extended survival in people with ALS during 18 months of treatment, though muscle strength and nerve function did not improve. Overall, death rates at the end of the studies were the same whether people took riluzole or not. In one study, the average life extension for people taking riluzole was 60 days. Riluzole is broken down in the liver.

Cautions and Warnings

Do not take riluzole if you are **allergic** to it.

Riluzole causes **liver inflammation;** people with severe liver disease should use this drug with caution. Liver function should be evaluated regularly. People with **kidney disease** should also use riluzole with caution.

People of Japanese descent may eliminate riluzole from their bodies twice as slowly as do Caucasians. The drug may be eliminated more slowly due to genetic factors or because of differences in diet such as decreased use of alcohol, nicotine, and caffeine.

Cigarette smoking is likely to increase the rate at which riluzole is broken down by the liver. The drug may break down more quickly in women than in men. There is no indication that either of these factors is important in determining riluzole dosage.

Taking more than 100 mg a day of riluzole increases side effects and is not more effective.

Possible Side Effects

About 14% of people stop taking riluzole because of side effects.

▼ Most common: weakness, nausea, dizziness (twice as common in women), diarrhea, a tingling sensation around the mouth, appetite loss, fainting, and tiredness. These effects increase with dosage.

▼ Common: poor lung function, abdominal pain, pneumonia, and vomiting.

▼ Less common: back pain, headache, upset stomach at high dosages, gas, stuffy nose, runny nose, cough, high blood pressure, joint aches, and swelling in the arms and legs. At high dosages—urinary infection and painful urination, and dizziness when rising from a lying or sitting position.

▼ Rare: aggravation, feeling unwell, mouth infection, eczema, rapid heartbeat, and vein irritation. Other rare side effects can occur in almost any part of the body. Contact your doctor if you experience any side effects not listed above.

Drug Interactions

• Allopurinol, methyldopa, sulfasalazine, and other drugs that are toxic to the liver may interact with riluzole. Combinations of liver-toxic drugs should be taken with caution.

• Caffeine, theophylline, phenacetin, amitriptyline, and quinolone antibacterials may slow the elimination of riluzole, increasing the risk of drug side effects.

• Rifampin and omeprazole may quicken the elimination of riluzole.

• Riluzole can accelerate the breakdown of caffeine, theophylline, and tacrine, but these effects have not actually been seen in people.

Food Interactions

Take riluzole on an empty stomach, at least 1 hour before or 2 hours after meals. Avoid charcoal-broiled foods, which may speed the elimination of riluzole.

Usual Dose

Adult: 50 mg every 12 hours.
Child: not recommended.

Overdosage

Little is known about the effects of riluzole overdose. Take the victim to a hospital emergency room at once. ALWAYS bring the prescription bottle or container.

Special Information

Taking more than 50 mg twice a day will not improve your condition and may increase drug side effects.

Call your doctor at once if you become feverish or ill. This could be a sign of a very low white-blood-cell count.

Riluzole should be taken at the same time each day—morning and evening—to achieve maximum benefit.

Riluzole can make you dizzy, tired, or faint. Be careful when driving or doing any task that requires concentration.

People taking riluzole should not drink to excess.

Store riluzole tablets between 68°F and 77°F and protect them from bright light.

If you forget a dose, take it as soon as you remember. If it is almost time for your next dose, skip the dose you forgot and continue with your regular schedule.

Special Populations

Pregnancy/Breast-feeding

Riluzole is toxic to pregnant lab animals at high dosages. When this drug is considered crucial by your doctor, its potential benefits must be carefully weighed against its risks.

It is not known if riluzole passes into breast milk. Nursing mothers who must take it should bottle-feed.

Seniors

Seniors with kidney or liver disease should use riluzole with caution.

Generic Name

Rimantadine (rih-MAN-tuh-dene)

Brand Name

Flumadine

Type of Drug

Antiviral.

Prescribed for

Influenza A viral infection (type A flu).

General Information

Rimantadine hydrochloride is a synthetic antiviral agent that appears to interfere with the reproduction of various strains of the influenza A virus, a common cause of viral infection. Rimantadine is used both to treat and to prevent type A flu. Annual vaccination against the virus is the best way of preventing the flu, but immunity takes 2 to 4 weeks to develop. In the meantime, rimantadine may be taken to prevent viral infection in high-risk people or people who may experience greater exposure to the virus.

Cautions and Warnings

People with severe **liver or kidney disease** clear this drug from their bodies only half as fast as those with normal organ function; they will need to have their dosage adjusted appropriately.

People with a history of **seizures** are likely to suffer another one while taking rimantadine. Call your doctor if this happens to you.

The influenza virus may become **resistant** to rimantadine in up to 30% of people taking the drug. When this happens, the resistant virus can infect people who are not protected by the vaccine.

Possible Side Effects

▼ Most common: sleeplessness, nervousness, loss of concentration, headache, fatigue, weakness, nausea, vomiting, appetite loss, dry mouth, and abdominal pains.

▼ Less common: diarrhea, upset stomach, dizziness, depression, euphoria (feeling "high"), changes in gait or walk, tremors, hallucinations, convulsions, fainting, ringing or buzzing in the ears, changes in or loss of the senses of taste or smell, breathing difficulties, pallor, rash, heart palpitations, rapid heartbeat, high blood pressure, heart failure, swelling of the ankles or feet, and heart block.

▼ Rare: constipation, swallowing difficulties, mouth sores, agitation, sweating, diminished sense of touch, eye pain or tearing, cough, bronchospasm, increased urination, fever, and fluid oozing from the nipples in women.

Drug Interactions

The importance of rimantadine's drug interactions is not known because there is no established relationship between the amount of drug in the blood and its antiviral effect.

• Aspirin and acetaminophen may reduce the amount of rimantadine in the blood by about 10%.

• Cimetidine increases the rate at which rimantadine is broken down by the liver.

Food Interactions

Rimantadine is best taken on an empty stomach, or at least 1 hour before or 2 hours after meals. You may take it with food if it upsets your stomach.

Usual Dose

Adult and Child (age 10 and over): 100 mg twice a day. People with severe liver or kidney disease—no more than 100 mg a day.

Child (under age 10): 2.25 mg per lb. of body weight, up to 150 mg, taken once a day.

Overdosage

Symptoms include agitation, hallucination, and abnormal heart rhythm. Overdose victims should be made to vomit with ipecac syrup—available at any pharmacy—as soon as possible. Call your local poison control center or a hospital emergency room before giving ipecac. Take overdose victims to a hospital emergency room. ALWAYS bring the prescription bottle or container.

Special Information

Rimantadine may be given to children to prevent influenza infection, but it is not recommended for treatment of their flu symptoms.

Call your doctor if you develop seizures, convulsions, or any other serious or unusual side effects.

If you forget a dose, take it as soon as you remember. If it is almost time for your next dose, skip the dose you forgot and continue with your regular schedule. Do not take a double dose.

Special Populations

Pregnancy/Breast-feeding

In animal studies, rimantadine is toxic to fetuses. When this drug is considered crucial by your doctor, its potential benefits must be carefully weighed against its risks.

Rimantadine passes into breast milk. Nursing mothers who must take it should bottle-feed.

Seniors

Seniors are more likely to suffer from rimantadine side effects of the nervous system, stomach, and intestine and may require reduced dosage due to liver or kidney dysfunction.

Risperdal   *see Risperidone, page 894*

Generic Name

Risperidone (ris-PER-ih-done)

Brand Name

Risperdal

Type of Drug

Antipsychotic.

Prescribed for

Psychotic disorders and schizophrenia.

General Information

Risperidone affects brain receptors for serotonin and dopamine, two important neurohormones. It is broken down in the liver. Between 6% and 8% of Caucasians and a very small number of Asians have little of the liver enzyme that breaks down risperidone and are considered to be "poor metabolizers" of the drug. Because these people break risperidone down very slowly, the drug takes about 5 days to reach a steady level in their blood. People with normal amounts of the enzyme reach a steady level in about 1 day. People with kidney or liver disease require reduced dosage.

Cautions and Warnings

Do not take this drug if you are **sensitive** or **allergic** to it. People taking it for longer than 6 to 8 weeks must be reevaluated at least every 2 months.

A serious set of side effects known as **neuroleptic malignant syndrome (NMS)** has been associated with some antipsychotic drugs. The symptoms that constitute NMS include high fever, muscle rigidity, mental changes, irregular pulse or blood pressure, sweating, and abnormal heart rhythm. NMS is potentially fatal and requires **immediate medical attention**.

Risperidone can produce **uncontrolled movements,** including spasm of the neck muscles, rolling back of the eyes, convulsions, difficulty swallowing, and symptoms associated with Parkinson's disease. These effects usually disappear after the drug has been discontinued. Face, tongue, and jaw symptoms may persist, especially in older women. Contact your doctor immediately if you experience any of these symptoms.

Risperidone can cause a life-threatening abnormal heart rhythm called **torsade de pointes**. The drug should therefore be used with caution in people with **heart disease**. Slow heart rate, electrolyte imbalance, and taking other drugs that carry a risk of torsade de pointes may increase the chances of developing this abnormality.

Risperidone raises levels of a hormone called prolactin. Increased prolactin has been associated with **tumors of the pituitary gland, breast, and pancreas,** but no problems have been noted with risperidone specifically.

Possible Side Effects

▼ Most common: sleepiness, sleeplessness, agitation, anxiety, uncontrolled movements, headache, and nasal stuffiness and irritation.

▼ Less common: dizziness, constipation, nausea, vomiting, upset stomach, abdominal pain, increased saliva, toothache, coughing, upper respiratory infection, sinus infection, sore throat, breathing difficulties, rapid heartbeat, joint or back pain, chest pain, fever, abnormal vision, rash, dry skin, and dandruff.

Other side effects can occur in almost any part of the body. Contact your doctor if you experience any side effect not listed above.

Drug Interactions

• Risperidone may decrease the effects of levodopa.
• Carbamazepine and clozapine may reduce the effect of this drug.

Food Interactions

None known.

Usual Dose

Adult: starting dosage—1 mg 2 times a day. Maintenance dosage—increase gradually up to 6 mg a day if needed.

Senior: starting dosage—0.5 mg 2 times a day. Increase gradually if needed.

Child: not recommended.

Overdosage

Symptoms include drowsiness, rapid heartbeat, low blood pressure, and abnormal and uncontrolled muscle movements. Overdose victims should be taken to a hospital emergency room. ALWAYS bring the prescription bottle or container.

Special Information

Risperidone can make you tired and affect your judgment, an effect that increases with dosage. Be careful when driving or performing any task that requires concentration. Avoid alcohol.

Some antipsychotic drugs can interfere with the body's temperature-regulating mechanism. Avoid extreme heat while you are taking risperidone.

Some people develop a rapid heartbeat and become dizzy or faint when first taking risperidone. This risk can be minimized by starting at a low dose, such as 2 mg a day in adults, or 1 mg in seniors or those with kidney or liver disease.

Risperidone can make you unusually sensitive to the sun. Wear protective clothes and use sunscreen.

If you forget a dose, take it as soon as you remember. If it is almost time for your next dose, skip the dose you forgot and continue with your regular schedule. Call your doctor if you forget 2 doses in a row.

Special Populations

Pregnancy/Breast-feeding

Studies of risperidone in animals show an increase in birth defects and stillbirth. There is also a report of an infant who was born with an abnormally developed brain after the mother took risperidone. Risperidone should not be taken by pregnant women unless the potential benefits are carefully weighed against the risks.

It is not known if risperidone passes into breast milk. Nursing mothers who must take this medication should bottle-feed.

Seniors

Seniors with reduced kidney function require lower dosage. Seniors may also be more sensitive to side effects.

Generic Name

Ritonavir (rih-TON-uh-vere)

Brand Name

Norvir

Type of Drug

Protease inhibitor.

Prescribed for

Human immunodeficiency virus (HIV) infection.

General Information

Part of the multidrug cocktail responsible for the most important gains in the fight against acquired immunodeficiency syndrome (AIDS), ritonavir belongs to a group of anti-HIV drugs called protease inhibitors. Triple-drug cocktails are considered responsible for the first overall reduction in the AIDS death rate, recorded in 1996. Protease inhibitors work in a unique way but are not a cure for HIV infection or AIDS. When the HIV virus attacks a cell, it must be converted into viral DNA. Older drugs, known as reverse transcriptase inhibitors, interfere with this step, but they need help in fighting HIV. Protease inhibitors work at the end of the HIV reproduction process, when proteins are "cut" into strands of exactly the right size to duplicate HIV. The protein is cut by a protease enzyme. Protease inhibitors prevent the mature HIV virus from being formed by interfering with this cutting process. Proteins that are cut to the wrong length or that remain uncut are inactive.

Protease inhibitors are always taken with 1 or 2 nucleoside antiviral drugs such as AZT, ddI, ddC, or 3TC. Protease inhibitors revolutionized HIV treatment because when taken in combination, they reduce the amount of HIV virus in the bloodstream to levels that are often undetectable by current methods—CD_4 cell counts (immune system cells) and viral load (amount of virus in the blood) measurements. Multiple-drug therapy has changed the current view of HIV from a fatal disease to a manageable chronic illness.

People taking a protease inhibitor may still develop infections or other conditions associated with HIV disease.

Because of this, it is very important for you to remain under the care of a doctor or other health care provider. The long-term effects of ritonavir are not known at this time. You may be able to pass the HIV virus to others even if you are on triple-drug therapy.

Cautions and Warnings

Do not take ritonavir if you are **allergic** to it. People with mild or moderate **liver disease** and **cirrhosis** break down ritonavir more slowly than those with normal liver function and may be more likely to develop side effects. People with cirrhosis should receive a reduced dose of ritonavir.

Ritonavir may raise your blood sugar, worsen your **diabetes,** or bring out latent diabetes. Diabetics who take ritonavir may have to have the dosage of their antidiabetes medication adjusted.

Some of ritonavir's drug interactions may be dangerous (see "Drug Interactions").

Ritonavir can affect a wide variety of **blood tests,** including those for triglycerides, liver function, and blood sugar.

Possible Side Effects

▼ Most common: weakness, tiredness, nausea, diarrhea, vomiting, appetite loss, abdominal pains, taste changes, and tingling around the mouth and in the hands or feet.

▼ Rare: Rare side effects can occur in almost any part of the body, including muscles and joints, blood components, and the mouth, stomach and intestines, nervous system, skin, kidneys, and urinary and respiratory tracts. Changes in mental state and sexual function may also occur.

Drug Interactions

• The following drugs should not be combined with ritonavir: amiodarone, astemizole, bepridil, bupropion, cisapride, clozapine, encainide, flecainide, meperidine, piroxicam, propafenone, propoxyphene, quinidine, rifabutin, and terfenadine. Ritonavir can be expected to substantially raise the blood levels of all these drugs, which may cause serious abnormal heart rhythms, blood problems, seizures, and other serious side effects.

• Combining ritonavir with any of the following drugs may cause excessive sedation and breathing difficulties: alprazolam, clorazepate, diazepam, estazolam, flurazepam, midazolam, triazolam, and zolpidem. The effectiveness of other sedative-hypnotics is likely to be reduced by ritonavir. Ritonavir may interact with narcotic pain relievers, but the exact interaction is not predictable.

• Combining rifampin with ritonavir decreases the amount of ritonavir absorbed by about 35%.

• Combining ritonavir with clarithromycin or zidovudine (AZT) raises the amount of both drugs in the blood. Mixing ritonavir with isoniazid increases the amount of isoniazid in the blood.

• Combining ritonavir with didanosine (ddI) may reduce the amount of ddI in the blood by about 15%.

• Combining fluconazole or fluoxetine with ritonavir increases the amount of ritonavir in the blood.

• Combining ritonavir with desipramine substantially increases the amount of desipramine in the blood.

• Do not combine ritonavir oral solution and disulfiram or metronidazole.

• Combining ritonavir with oral contraceptives containing ethinyl estradiol can lower blood hormone levels, possibly reducing their effectiveness. Your doctor may lower the dose of your contraceptive.

• Combining ritonavir with saquinavir, another protease inhibitor, slows the breakdown of saquinavir and increases its blood levels.

• Ritonavir lowers the amount of sulfamethoxazole absorbed into the blood by about 20% and raises trimethoprim by about 20%.

• Combining ritonavir with theophylline reduces the amount of theophylline absorbed by about 40%.

• Taking ritonavir with AZT reduces the amount of AZT in the blood by about 10%.

• Ritonavir is likely to increase the absorption of these drugs into the blood: alpha blockers, antiarrhythmics, anticancer drugs, antidepressants, antiemetics, antifungals, antimalarials, beta blockers, blood-fat reducers, calcium entry blockers, cimetidine, corticosteroids, erythromycin, immunosuppressants, methylphenidate, pentoxifylline, phenothiazines, and warfarin.

• Ritonavir is likely to reduce the amount of these drugs

absorbed into the blood: atovaquone, clofibrate, daunoru-
bicin, diphenoxylate, and metoclopramide.

Food Interactions

To increase the effectiveness of ritonavir capsules, take them
with meals. Ritonavir oral solution should be taken on an
empty stomach, 1 hour before or 2 hours after meals. The
taste of the oral liquid may be improved by mixing it with
chocolate milk, Ensure, or Advera. Do not mix earlier than 1
hour before you take your dose.

Usual Dose

Adult: 600 mg 2 times a day. You may start with a lower
dosage and increase gradually to avoid upset stomach.
Child: not recommended.

Overdosage

Little is known about the effects of ritonavir overdose. Take
the victim to a hospital emergency room at once. ALWAYS
bring the prescription bottle or container.

Special Information

It is imperative to take your HIV medication exactly as prescribed. Missing doses of ritonavir makes you more likely to
become resistant to the drug and to lose the benefits of therapy.

Ritonavir does not cure AIDS. It will not prevent you from
transmitting the HIV virus to another person; you must still
practice safe sex.

Stay in close touch with your doctor while taking ritonavir
and report unusual symptoms.

Ritonavir capsules should be stored in the refrigerator. The
liquid may be kept at room temperature, but only for 30 days;
refrigeration is recommended.

If you forget a dose of ritonavir, take it as soon as you
remember. If it is almost time for your next dose, skip the
dose you forgot and continue with your regular schedule. Do
not take a double dose.

Special Populations

Pregnancy/Breast-feeding
Animal studies indicate that ritonavir may affect the fetus.
When this drug is considered crucial by your doctor, its

potential benefits must be carefully weighed against its risks.

It is not known if ritonavir passes into breast milk. Nursing mothers who must take ritonavir should bottle-feed.

Seniors

Seniors may take ritonavir without special restriction.

Generic Name

Rofecoxib (roe-feh-SOX-ib)

Brand Name

Vioxx

Type of Drug

Cyclooxygenase-2 (COX-2) inhibitor and nonsteroidal anti-inflammatory drug (NSAID).

Prescribed for

Osteoarthritis, painful menstruation, and acute pain.

General Information

Traditional NSAIDs works primarily by blocking the effects of COX-2, a body enzyme that plays an important role in regulating pain and inflammation. But these NSAIDs also have an unwanted effect: They interfere with cyclooxygenase-1 (COX-1), a related enzyme that helps to maintain the stomach's protective lining. NSAIDs that block the effects of this enzyme may produce side effects such as stomach irritation, gas, and stomach ulcers.

COX-2 inhibitors such as rofecoxib are a new class of NSAIDs that interfere only with COX-2, leaving the stomach-protecting COX-1 unaffected. This means that COX-2 inhibitor NSAIDs can relieve pain and inflammation just like traditional NSAIDs but are less likely to cause gastrointestinal (GI) side effects. Another potential advantage of rofecoxib is that it does not cause thinning of the blood or affect blood platelets like older NSAIDs do. Rofecoxib is broken down in the liver.

Cautions and Warnings

Do not take rofecoxib if you are **sensitive** or **allergic** to it or to sulfa drugs. NSAIDs should not be taken by people with **asthma** or **itchy sores** or by those who have had an **allergic reaction to aspirin or another NSAID**.

NSAIDs can cause **GI bleeding and ulcers** and **stomach perforation**. This can occur at any time, with or without warning, in people who take NSAIDs regularly. Minor upper GI problems, such as upset stomach, are common and may occur at any time during NSAID therapy. People who develop bleeding or ulcers and continue NSAID treatment should be aware of the risk of developing more serious side effects.

Rofecoxib should be used with caution by people who have had **ulcers** or **stomach or intestinal bleeding**.

Rofecoxib should not be used by people with severe **kidney disease**.

Rofecoxib can cause **liver irritation** and should be used with caution by people with **hepatitis** or **cirrhosis**. People with moderate liver disease require reduced dosages. The effect of rofecoxib in people with severe liver failure is not known.

African Americans and Hispanics absorb 10% to 15% more rofecoxib than Caucasians. The importance of this fact is unclear.

Possible Side Effects

Side effects are similar to those of traditional NSAIDs. Stomach and intestinal effects are about half as common.

▼ Common: respiratory infection, diarrhea, and nausea.

▼ Less common: abdominal pain, weakness, fatigue, dizziness, flu-like symptoms, swollen legs, high blood pressure, upset stomach, heartburn, sinus irritation, back pain, headache, and urinary infection.

▼ Rare: Rare side effects can occur in almost any part of the body. Contact your doctor if you experience any side effect not listed above.

Drug Interactions

• Combining rofecoxib and an aluminum and magnesium

antacid slightly reduces the amount of drug absorbed. Separate doses of these antacids and rofecoxib by 1 to 2 hours.

• Rofecoxib may raise lithium blood levels and increase the risk of side effects.

• While rofecoxib may be combined with low dosages of aspirin, taking these two drugs together can increase the risk of stomach or intestinal ulcers or other complications.

• Rofecoxib can reduce the blood-pressure-lowering effect of angiotensin-converting enzyme (ACE) inhibitor and diuretic drugs. This combination can also increase the risk of kidney damage after chronic rofecoxib use.

• High dosages of cimetidine (800 mg twice a day) can increase the amount of rofecoxib in the blood, but no dosage adjustment is necessary.

• NSAIDs can reduce the effect of furosemide and thiazide-type diuretics in some people.

• Rofecoxib can elevate methotrexate blood levels by about 25% and increase the risk of methotrexate side effects.

• Rifampin reduces the amount of rofecoxib in the blood by 50%. People taking rifampin should begin with a higher dosage of rofecoxib.

• Rofecoxib may increase the blood-thinning effect of warfarin. Your doctor should check your blood if you are combining these drugs.

Food Interactions

Rofecoxib may be taken without regard to food or meals. For optimal effectiveness, avoid taking this drug with high-fat meals.

Usual Dose

Adult (age 18 and over): 12.5–50 mg once a day.
Child (under age 18): not recommended.

Overdosage

Overdose symptoms are usually limited to lethargy, drowsiness, nausea, vomiting, and stomach pain. Stomach or intestinal bleeding occur. High blood pressure, kidney failure, breathing difficulty, and coma can occur but are rare. Severe allergic reactions may occur following an overdose. In case of overdose, call your local poison control center or a hospital emergency room. You may be told to induce vomiting with ipecac syrup—available at any pharmacy—before taking the victim to an emergency room. If you seek treatment, ALWAYS bring the prescription bottle or container.

Special Information

People taking any NSAID can develop a group of symptoms known as the aspirin triad. This typically occurs in people with asthma. Symptoms include runny nose with or without nasal polyps and severe, potentially fatal bronchial spasm. People who have these symptoms must seek emergency treatment.

Call your doctor if you develop rash, itching, unexplained weight gain, nausea, fatigue, yellowing of the skin or whites of the eyes, flu-like symptoms, lethargy, swelling, black stools, severe stomach pain, persistent headache, or any bothersome or persistent side effect.

If you forget a dose, take it as soon as you remember. If it is almost time for your next dose, skip the forgotten dose and continue with your regular schedule.

Special Populations

Pregnancy/Breast-feeding

Any NSAID may affect fetal heart development during the second half of pregnancy. Pregnant women should not take rofecoxib without their doctor's approval. When this drug is considered crucial by your doctor, its potential benefits must be carefully weighed against its risks.

NSAIDs may pass into breast milk. There is a possibility that a nursing mother taking rofecoxib could affect her baby's heart or cardiovascular system. Nursing mothers who take this drug should bottle-feed.

Seniors

Generally, seniors can take this drug without special precaution. They should use the lowest effective dosage.

Generic Name

Ropinirole (roe-PIN-ih-role)

Brand Name

Requip

Type of Drug

Antiparkinsonian.

Prescribed for

Parkinson's disease.

General Information

Ropinirole relieves symptoms of Parkinson's disease by stimulating dopamine receptors in the brain. A study of people with early Parkinson's disease showed improvement in about 70% of people taking the drug for 10 to 12 weeks, compared to 40% of people taking a placebo (sugar pill). In another study, 28% of people with advanced Parkinson's disease who received ropinirole for 6 months showed improvement compared to 11% of people in the placebo group. Ropinirole is broken down in the liver.

Cautions and Warnings

Do not take ropinirole if you are **sensitive** or **allergic** to it. Ropinirole may cause **low blood pressure** and make you **dizzy or faint** when rising from a sitting or lying position, especially during the early stages of treatment. About 1 in 10 to 15 people who take ropinirole experience **hallucinations** that may be serious enough to require stopping drug therapy.

People stopping other treatments for Parkinson's disease have developed **high fever** and **confusion**. **Breathing difficulties** caused by lung changes have occurred with the use of other antiparkinsonians. These problems have not been associated with ropinirole but there is a risk that you may experience similar problems if you stop taking ropinirole.

Possible Side Effects

Early Parkinson's Disease

▼ Most common: sleepiness or tiredness, nausea, dizziness, upset stomach, vomiting, and virus infection.

▼ Common: general pain, sweating, weakness, fainting, abdominal pain, sore throat, and changes in vision.

▼ Less common: dry mouth, flushing, chest pain, feeling unwell, blood-pressure changes, heart palpitations, rapid heartbeat, hallucinations, confusion, memory loss, very sensitive reflexes, yawning, unusual movements,

Possible Side Effects *(continued)*

difficulty concentrating, appetite loss, gas, swollen arms
or legs, runny nose, sinus irritation, bronchitis, breathing
difficulties, eye problems, urinary infection, impotence,
and poor blood supply to the hands, legs, and feet.

Advanced Parkinson's Disease
  ▼ Most common: abnormal movements, tremor, muscle rigidity, hallucinations, and urinary infection.
  ▼ Common: confusion, constipation, pneumonia,
sweating, abdominal pain, and twitching.
  ▼ Less common: dizziness or fainting when rising
from a sitting or lying position, unusual dreaming,
changes in the way you walk, poor muscle coordination,
memory loss, nervousness, tingling in the hands or feet,
temporary paralysis, diarrhea, difficulty swallowing, gas,
increased salivation, poor urinary control, pus in the
urine, arthritis, breathing difficulties, dry mouth, anemia,
and weight loss.

Drug Interactions

• Ropinirole increases levodopa blood levels and may
worsen uncontrolled muscle spasm that occurs with levodopa. Your doctor may reduce your levodopa dosage.
• Ciprofloxacin, diltiazem, enoxacin, erythromycin, estrogen, fluvoxamine, mexilitene, norfloxacin, tacrine, and cigarette smoking increase ropinirole's effects.
• Phenothiazine tranquilizers, haloperidol and similar tranquilizers, thioxanthene tranquilizers, and metoclopramide
and other drugs that antagonize the effects of dopamine may
reduce the effect of ropinirole.
• Ropinirole increases the sedative effect of tranquilizers,
sleeping pills, and other nervous system depressants.

Food Interactions

You may take this drug with food to prevent nausea.

Usual Dose

Adult: 0.25 mg 3 times a day to start, gradually increasing
to a maximum of 3 mg a day. Dosage is reduced for people
with kidney disease.

Overdosage

Little is known about the effects of ropinirole overdose. Symptoms are likely to include the most common side effects. Take the victim to a hospital emergency room. ALWAYS bring the prescription bottle or container.

Special Information

Take this drug exactly as prescribed.

Ropinirole causes sedation. Be careful when driving or performing any task that requires concentration. Avoid alcohol and other nervous system depressants.

Hallucinations may occur with this drug, especially among seniors. Call your doctor if you develop hallucinations or bothersome or persistent side effects.

If you forget a dose, take it as soon as you remember. Space the remaining daily dosage evenly throughout the day. Go back to your regular schedule the next day. Do not take a double dose.

Special Populations

Pregnancy/Breast-feeding

In animal studies, ropinirole causes birth defects and damages the fetus. When this drug is considered crucial by your doctor, its potential benefits must be carefully weighed against its risks.

Animal studies show that ropinirole passes into breast milk, but it is not known if this occurs in humans. Ropinirole may interfere with milk production. Nursing mothers who must take this drug should bottle-feed.

Seniors

Hallucinations are more likely in seniors.

Generic Name

Rosiglitazone (roe-sih-GLIT-uh-zone)

Brand Name

Avandia

Type of Drug

Antidiabetic.

Prescribed for

Type II diabetes.

General Information

Rosiglitazone reduces the amount of sugar produced by the liver and increases the amount used by muscle, liver, and fat cells. It may also help to control blood-fat levels, which are often elevated in diabetes. Rosiglitazone does not increase the amount of insulin made in the pancreas. It apparently works by affecting genes responsible for the control of sugar and fat use in the body, making cells more sensitive to insulin. This drug is effective for people with type II diabetes, who generally have enough insulin but whose cells do not respond to it. Rosiglitazone can be used alone or combined with metformin. Rosiglitazone is closely related to troglitazone but is considered less harmful to the liver.

Cautions and Warnings

Do not take this drug if you are **sensitive** or **allergic** to it or related drugs. Rosiglitazone is broken down in the liver; people with **liver disease** should not take it. Liver enzyme monitoring is recommended for all people taking rosiglitazone.

Rosiglitazone can raise blood levels of **cholesterol** and other blood fats. It may worsen **heart failure**.

Premenopausal women who are not ovulating may be at risk of becoming pregnant because this drug can trigger **ovulation**.

Weight gain (up to 7½ lbs. over 6 months) was experienced by some people taking rosiglitazone in studies.

Women may achieve maximum benefit with smaller dosages.

Possible Side Effects

▼ Common: respiratory infections, accidental injuries, and headache.

▼ Less common: swelling, back pain, high blood sugar, fatigue, sinus irritation, and diarrhea.

▼ Rare: anemia and low blood sugar.

Drug Interactions

None known.

Food Interactions

This drug may be taken with or without food.

Usual Dose

Adult (age 18 and over): 4–8 mg once a day or in divided doses.

Child: not recommended.

Overdosage

Little is known about the effects of rosiglitazone overdose. Take the victim to a hospital emergency room. ALWAYS bring the prescription bottle or container.

Special Information

Diet, calorie control, exercise, and weight loss are essential to controlling type II diabetes. Do not depend solely on this drug to manage your condition.

Alcohol, smoking, age, and race do not affect the way that rosiglitazone is processed in the body.

Call your doctor if you develop symptoms of liver disease, such as nausea, vomiting, abdominal pain, fatigue, appetite loss, or dark-colored urine.

See your doctor for regular monitoring of blood sugar, gly-cosylated hemoglobin (a more sensitive indicator of long-term diabetes control), and liver function.

If you forget a dose, take it as soon as you remember. If it is almost time for your next dose, skip the dose you forgot and continue with your regular schedule.

Special Populations

Pregnancy/Breast-feeding

The safety of using rosiglitazone during pregnancy is not known. Most experts recommend that diabetes be controlled with insulin during pregnancy.

It is not known if rosiglitazone passes into breast milk. Nursing mothers who must take it should consider bottle-feeding.

Seniors

Seniors may take this drug without special precaution.

Roxicet   *see Percocet, page 792*

see Percocet, page 792

Generic Name

Sacrosidase (sah-KROE-sih-dase)

Brand Name

Sucraid

Type of Drug

Nutritional therapy.

Prescribed for

Sucrase deficiency.

General Information

People with congenital sucrase-isomaltase deficiency (CSID) cannot break down or absorb sugar or starches because they lack the enzyme sucrase. Children with this disorder cannot eat a well-balanced diet because sugar gives them gas, bloating, cramps, and nausea and vomiting. Up to 10% of children with chronic diarrhea of unknown causes have CSID. Undiagnosed CSID can lead to malnutrition and impede proper growth and development. Sacrosidase is an enzyme that mimics the action of sucrase, allowing the body to process sugar normally. It has been safely used in children age 5 months and over.

Cautions and Warnings

Sacrosidase **allergy can be severe and fatal**. The first few doses of sacrosidase should be taken in a doctor's office or medical facility in case an allergic reaction develops.

　　People who are **allergic to yeast, yeast products, or glycerine** should not use this drug.

Possible Side Effects

A very small number of people were included in sacrosidase studies, so the overall number of reported side effects is also small.

　　▼ Common: abdominal pain and vomiting.

　　▼ Less common: nausea, diarrhea, constipation, sleeplessness, headache, nervousness, and dehydration.

　　▼ Rare: severe allergic reactions.

Drug Interactions

None known.

Food Interactions

Sacrosidase should not be mixed or taken with fruit juice. The acidity of juice can reduce the activity of the enzyme.

Usual Dose

Adult and Child (34 lbs. and over): 2 scoops or 44 drops with each meal or snack.

Child (under 34 lbs.): 1 scoop or 22 drops with each meal or snack.

Take half of the dose at the beginning of each meal and the second half at the end of the meal.

Overdosage

Little is known about the effects of sacrosidase overdose. Call your local poison control center or a hospital emergency room for information. If you seek treatment, ALWAYS bring the prescription bottle or container.

Special Information

Bottles of sacrosidase should be thrown away 4 weeks after they have been opened because of the risk of bacterial growth.

Sacrosidase can be mixed with milk, water, or infant formula but it is sensitive to heat and should be served cold. Mixing sacrosidase with warm milk, water, or formula is likely to reduce its effectiveness. Do not mix it with fruit juice.

Special Populations

Pregnancy/Breast-feeding

Sacrosidase is considered safe for use during pregnancy and breast-feeding. Always consult your doctor before using any drug if you are pregnant or nursing.

Seniors

Seniors may use this drug without special precaution.

Generic Name

Salmeterol (sal-METE-er-ol)

Brand Name

Serevent

Type of Drug

Bronchodilator.

Prescribed for

Asthma and bronchospasm.

General Information

Salmeterol xinafoate differs from other bronchodilators in that it does not provide immediate symptom relief but is instead prescribed for long-term prevention. When you start salmeterol treatment, you may need to continue your other asthma inhalers for symptom relief. After a while, however, you should have less need for the other drugs. Salmeterol works like other bronchodilator drugs, such as albuterol, terbutaline, and metaproterenol, but it has a weaker effect on nerve receptors in the heart and blood vessels; for this reason, it is somewhat safer for people with heart conditions. Still, very large doses of salmeterol may lead to abnormal heart rhythms. Salmeterol begins working within 20 minutes after a dose and continues for 12 hours.

Cautions and Warnings

Salmeterol should be used with caution by people with a history of **angina pectoris** (condition characterized by brief attacks of chest pain), **heart disease, high blood pressure, stroke** or **seizure, thyroid disease, prostate disease,** or **glaucoma**.

Used in excess, salmeterol can actually lead to more **breathing difficulties,** rather than breathing relief. In the most extreme cases, people have had **heart attacks** after using excessive amounts of inhalant bronchodilators.

Long-term use of salmeterol, and related drugs, can lead to increases in certain **ovarian tumors**.

Possible Side Effects

▼ Most common: heart palpitations, rapid heartbeat, tremors, dizziness and fainting, shakiness, nervousness, tension, headache, diarrhea, heartburn or upset stomach, dry or sore and irritated throat, respiratory infections, and nasal or sinus conditions.

▼ Less common: nausea and vomiting, joint or back pain, muscle cramps, muscle soreness, muscle ache or pain, giddiness, viral stomach infections, itching, dental pain, not feeling well, rash, and menstrual irregularity.

Drug Interactions

• Monoamine oxidase inhibitors (MAOIs), tricyclic antidepressants, thyroid drugs, other bronchodilator drugs, and some antihistamines may increase the effects of salmeterol.

• The risk of cardiotoxicity may be increased in people taking both salmeterol and theophylline.

• Salmeterol may antagonize the effects of blood-pressure-lowering drugs, especially reserpine, methyldopa, and guanethidine.

Food Interactions

None known.

Usual Dose

Adult and Child (age 12 and over): 2 puffs every 12 hours.
Child (under age 12): not recommended.

Overdosage

Overdose of salmeterol inhalation usually results in exaggerated side effects, including chest pain and high blood pressure, although blood pressure may drop to a low level after a short period of elevation. People who inhale too much salmeterol should see a doctor. ALWAYS bring the prescription bottle or container.

Special Information

Be sure to follow the inhalation instructions that come with the product. Salmeterol should be inhaled during the second half of your inward breath, since this will allow it to reach deeper into your lungs. Wait at least 1 minute between puffs. Do not inhale salmeterol if you have food or anything else in your mouth.

Call your doctor immediately if you develop chest pain, palpitations, rapid heartbeat, muscle tremors, dizziness, headache, facial flushing, or urinary difficulty, or if you continue to experience difficulty in breathing after using salmeterol.

If you forget a dose of salmeterol, take it as soon as you remember. If it is almost time for your next dose, skip the one you forgot and go back to your regular schedule. Do not take a double dose.

Special Populations

Pregnancy/Breast-feeding

When used during childbirth, salmeterol may slow or delay natural labor. It can cause rapid heartbeat and high blood sugar in the mother and rapid heartbeat and low blood sugar in the baby. It is not known whether salmeterol causes birth defects in humans, but it has caused defects in animals. When your doctor considers this drug crucial, its potential benefits must be carefully weighed against its risks.

Salmeterol may pass into breast milk. Nursing mothers who must take this drug should consider bottle-feeding.

Seniors

Seniors should use the same dosage of salmeterol as younger adults.

Generic Name

Saquinavir Mesylate

(suh-QUIN-uh-vere MES-uh-late)

Brand Names

Invirase   Fortovase

Type of Drug

Protease inhibitor.

Prescribed for

Advanced human immunodeficiency virus (HIV) infection.

General Information

Part of the multidrug cocktail responsible for important gains in the fight against acquired immunodeficiency syndrome (AIDS), saquinavir is a member of a group of anti-HIV drugs called protease inhibitors. These drugs work at the end of the HIV reproduction process, when proteins are "cut" into strands of exactly the correct size to duplicate HIV. The protein is cut by an enzyme known as protease. Protease inhibitors prevent the mature HIV virus from being formed by inhibiting this cutting process. Proteins that are cut to the wrong length or that remain uncut are inactive.

Protease inhibitors are always taken with 1 or 2 nucleoside antiviral drugs such as AZT, ddI, ddC, or 3TC. They revolutionized HIV treatment because, when taken in combination, they reduce the amount of HIV virus in the bloodstream to levels that are often undetectable by current methods—CD_4 cell (immune system cell) counts and viral load (amount of virus in the blood) measurements. Multiple-drug therapy has changed the current view of HIV from a fatal disease to a manageable chronic illness.

Cautions and Warnings

Do not take this drug if you are **sensitive** or **allergic** to it.

If a serious **toxic reaction** occurs while taking saquinavir, you should stop the drug until your doctor can determine the cause or until the reaction resolves itself. Then treatment can be resumed.

Use caution if you have moderate to severe **liver disease**.

Saquinavir may raise your **blood sugar,** worsen your **diabetes,** or bring out latent diabetes. People with diabetes who take saquinavir may need the dosage of their antidiabetes medication adjusted.

HIV virus may become **resistant** to saquinavir or other protease inhibitors. For this reason it is essential that you take saquinavir exactly according to your doctor's directions.

Possible Side Effects

Most side effects are mild. Other side effects become more prominent when saquinavir is taken together with antiretroviral drugs; these include weakness, muscle pain, and mouth ulcers.

Possible Side Effects *(continued)*

▼ Most common: diarrhea, nausea, and abdominal discomfort.

▼ Less common: upset stomach, abdominal pain, headache, tingling or numbness in the hands or feet, dizziness, nerve damage, changes in appetite, and rash.

▼ Rare: Rare side effects can occur in almost any part of the body. Contact your doctor if you experience any side effect not listed above.

Drug Interactions

• Rifampin and rifabutin reduce saquinavir blood levels by 80% and 40%, respectively. Do not combine these drugs with saquinavir. Other drugs that can reduce saquinavir blood levels are phenobarbital, phenytoin, carbamazepine, and dexamethasone.

• Blood levels of saquinavir may be elevated by terfenidine, astemizole, ketoconazole, and itraconazole. Other drugs that may elevate saquinavir levels and lead to side effects are calcium channel blockers, clindamycin, dapsone, quinidine, and triazolam.

• Protease inhibitors may drastically increase sildenafil blood levels, increasing the risk of sildenafil side effects including low blood pressure, visual changes, and persistent, painful erection.

Food Interactions

Take saquinavir within 2 hours after a full meal. The amount of saquinavir absorbed into the blood is vastly reduced when it is taken on an empty stomach, thus negating its antiviral effects.

Usual Dose

Invirase
    Adult (age 16 and over): 600 mg 3 times a day, within 2 hours after a full meal.

Fortovase
    Adult (age 16 and over): 1200 mg 3 times a day, within 2 hours after a meal.
    Child (under age 16): dosage varies.

Overdosage

Little is known about the effects of saquinavir overdose. Take the victim to a hospital emergency room. ALWAYS bring the prescription bottle or container.

Special Information

Saquinavir does not cure HIV infection or AIDS. It will not prevent you from transmitting the HIV virus to another person; you must still practice safe sex. You may still develop opportunistic infections or other illnesses associated with advanced HIV disease. The long-term effects of this drug are not known.

It is imperative for you to take this medication exactly according to your doctor's instructions. Missing doses of saquinavir increases the risk that you will become resistant to the drug. It should be taken after meals with your nucleoside antiviral drug. If you forget a dose of saquinavir, take it as soon as you remember. Do not take a double dose.

Special Populations

Pregnancy/Breast-feeding

While animal studies of saquinavir reveal no damage to the fetus, this drug should only be used during pregnancy after carefully weighing its potential benefits against its risks.

It is not known if saquinavir passes into breast milk. Nursing mothers with HIV should always bottle-feed, regardless of whether they take this drug, to avoid transmitting the virus.

Seniors

Seniors can take this drug without special precaution.

Generic Name

Selegiline (seh-LEG-uh-leen) Ⓖ

Brand Names

Atapryl   Eldepryl
Carbex

Type of Drug

Antiparkinsonian and selective monoamine oxidase inhibitor (MAOI).

Prescribed for

Parkinson's disease.

General Information

Selegiline hydrochloride is often combined with levodopa or carbidopa to control Parkinson's disease. Selegiline blocks the effects of the enzyme monoamine oxidase (MAO); it interferes with a form of it found almost exclusively in the brain. Selegiline also stimulates dopamine receptors. In order for any drug to work in Parkinson's disease, it must increase the activity of dopamine in the brain.

Cautions and Warnings

Be cautious about using selegiline if you have had a **reaction** to it.

If you take **Sinemet**—which contains levodopa and carbidopa—and start taking selegiline, you may experience an increase in levodopa side effects. Your Sinemet dosage may need to be reduced.

Taking more than 10 mg of selegiline a day may cause **severe reactions,** including possibly fatal high blood pressure.

Selegiline should not be used with **meperidine or other narcotic drugs** because of the risk of severe, possibly fatal reactions.

Possible Side Effects

Some of selegiline's side effects may be caused by methamphetamine and amphetamine; these potent stimulants are products of the body's breakdown of selegiline. When selegiline dosage is less than 10 mg per day, most side effects are not caused by the drug itself; rather, selegiline increases the side effects of levodopa. It is important for your doctor to reduce your levodopa dosage as much as possible.

▼ Most common: nausea, vomiting, dizziness, light-headedness or fainting, and abdominal pain.

▼ Less common: tremors or uncontrolled muscle movements, loss of balance, inability to move, increasingly slow movements associated with Parkinson's disease, facial grimacing, falling due to loss of balance, stiff

---

Possible Side Effects *(continued)*

neck, muscle cramps, hallucinations, overstimulation, confusion, anxiety, depression, drowsiness, changes in mood or behavior, nightmares or unusual dreams, tiredness, delusions, disorientation, feeling unwell, apathy, sleep disturbances, restlessness, weakness, irritability, generalized aches and pains, migraine or other headaches, muscle pains in the back or legs, ringing or buzzing in the ears, eye pain, finger or toe numbness, changes in sense of taste, dizziness when rising from a sitting or lying position, blood-pressure changes, abnormal heart rhythm, heart palpitations, chest pain, rapid heartbeat, swelling in the arms or legs, constipation, appetite loss, weight loss, difficulty swallowing, diarrhea, heartburn, rectal bleeding, urinary difficulties, impotence, swelling of the prostate, increased sweating, increased facial hair, hair loss, rash, increased sensitivity to the sun, bruising or black-and-blue marks, asthma, blurred or double vision, shortness of breath, speech problems, and dry mouth.

At dosages above 10 mg a day, selegiline may cause muscle twitching or spasms, memory loss, increased energy, transient euphoria (feeling "high"), grinding of the teeth, decreased sensation in the penis, and inability to achieve orgasm in men.

Drug Interactions

• Selegiline should not be used with meperidine or other narcotics because of the risk of severe, possibly fatal reactions (see "Cautions and Warnings").

• Combining fluoxetine with MAOIs other than selegiline has been deadly. This effect has not been seen with selegiline, but the combination should be avoided. Allow 5 weeks between stopping fluoxetine and starting on any MAOI. If you are already taking an MAOI, allow at least 2 weeks between stopping that drug and starting on selegiline.

Food Interactions

Take selegiline with food to avoid nausea or stomach upset, but avoid the following: Chianti and red wine, vermouth, unpasteurized or imported beer, beef or chicken liver, fermented sausages, tenderized or prepared meats, caviar, dried fish, pickled herring, cheese (American, Brie, cheddar, Camembert, Emmentaler, Boursault, Stilton, and others), avocados, yeast extracts, bananas, figs, raisins, soy sauce, miso soup, bean curd, fava beans, caffeine, and chocolate. These foods may cause severe, sudden high blood pressure in people taking selegiline.

Usual Dose

5 mg with breakfast and lunch.

Overdosage

Symptoms may include excitement, irritability, anxiety, low blood pressure, sleeplessness, restlessness, dizziness, weakness, drowsiness, flushing, sweating, heart palpitations, and unusual movements, including grimacing and muscle twitching. Serious overdoses may lead to convulsions, incoherence or confusion, severe headache, high fever, heart attack, shock, and coma. Take the victim to a hospital emergency room. ALWAYS bring the prescription bottle or container.

Special Information

After you have taken selegiline for 2 or 3 days, your doctor will probably reduce your carbidopa or levodopa dosage by 10% to 30%. If the disease is still under control, your dosage may be reduced further.

Contact your doctor if you develop headache, unusual body movements or muscle spasms, mood changes, or any bothersome or persistent side effects. Do not stop taking selegiline or change your dosage without your doctor's knowledge.

Selegiline reduces saliva flow in the mouth and may increase the risk of cavities, gum disease, and oral infections. Use candy, ice, sugarless gum, or a saliva substitute to avoid dry mouth.

If you forget a dose, take it as soon as you remember. If it is almost time for your next dose, take 1 dose right away and another in 5 or 6 hours, then go back to your regular schedule. Do not take a double dose.

Special Populations

Pregnancy/Breast-feeding

The safety of using selegiline during pregnancy is not known. When this drug is considered crucial by your doctor, its potential benefits must be carefully weighed against its risks.

It is not known if selegiline passes into breast milk. Nursing mothers who must take it should consider bottle-feeding.

Seniors

Seniors should receive the lowest effective dosage to minimize side effects.

Brand Name

Septra

Generic Ingredients

Sulfamethoxazole + Trimethoprim [G]

Other Brand Names

Bactrim	Cotrim Pediatric
Bactrim DS	Septra
Bactrim Pediatric	Septra DS
Cotrim	Sulfatrim
Cotrim DS	TMP-SMZ

Type of Drug

Anti-infective.

Prescribed for

A wide variety of infections, including urinary tract infection, bronchitis, and ear infection in children; also prescribed for traveler's diarrhea, pneumocystis carinii pneumonia (PCP), prostate infection, cholera, nocardiosis (lung infection), and *Salmonella* infection.

General Information

Septra is effective in many situations where other drugs are not. It is unique because it interferes with the infecting microorganism's normal use of folic acid in two ways, making it more efficient than other antibacterial drugs.

Cautions and Warnings

Do not take Septra if you have a **folic acid deficiency** or are **allergic** to either ingredient or to any sulfa drug, antidiabetes drug, or thiazide-type diuretic. Septra should be used with caution by people with **liver or kidney disease. Infants**

under 2 months of age should not be given this combination product.

Symptoms such as unusual bleeding or bruising, extreme tiredness, rash, sore throat, fever, pallor, or yellowing of the skin or eyes may be early indications of a serious **blood disorder**. If any of these effects occur, contact your doctor immediately and stop taking the drug. **People taking Septra for PCP** also have compromised immune function. They may not respond to Septra and are more likely to develop the less common side effects.

Septra should not be used for **strep throat** because of a greater chance of treatment failure than with penicillin.

Possible Side Effects

▼ Most common: nausea, vomiting, upset stomach, loss of appetite, and rash or itching.

▼ Less common: reduced levels of red and white blood cells and platelets, allergic reaction (symptoms include rash, itching, hives, and breathing difficulties), drug fever, swelling around the eyes, arthritis-like pain, diarrhea, coating of the tongue, headache, tingling in the arms or legs, depression, convulsions, hallucinations, ringing in the ears, dizziness, difficulty sleeping, apathy, tiredness, weakness, and nervousness. Septra may also affect your kidneys and cause you to produce less urine.

Drug Interactions

• Septra may prolong the effects of anticoagulant (blood-thinning) agents—such as warfarin—and oral antidiabetes drugs.

• The trimethoprim in Septra may reduce the effectiveness of cyclosporine and increase its toxic effect on the kidney.

• The sulfamethoxazole in Septra can increase the amount of phenytoin and methotrexate in the bloodstream, increasing the chance of side effects. Dosage reduction of phenytoin or methotrexate may be needed to adjust for the presence of Septra.

• Older adults taking a thiazide diuretic with Septra are more likely to develop reduced levels of blood platelets and an increased chance of bleeding under the skin.

• Taking Septra together with dapsone can result in increased blood levels of both drugs. Septra can interfere with the elimination of zidovudine (AZT) through the kidneys, increasing the amount of AZT in the blood.

Food Interactions

Take each dose with a full glass of water. Continue to drink plenty of fluids throughout the day to decrease the risk of kidney-stone formation.

Usual Dose

Adult: 2 regular tablets or 1 Septra DS tablet every 12 hours for 5–14 days, depending on the condition being treated.
Child (67–88 lbs.): 4 tsp. (or 2 tablets) every 12 hours.
Child (45–66 lbs.): 3 tsp. (or 1½ tablets) every 12 hours.
Child (23–44 lbs.): 2 tsp. (or 1 tablet) every 12 hours.
Child (under 22 lbs.): 1 tsp. every 12 hours.
Child (under age 2 months): not recommended.

Overdosage

Large overdoses can cause exaggerated side effects. Call your local poison control center or emergency room for more information. If you go to the hospital for treatment, ALWAYS bring the prescription bottle or container.

Special Information

Take Septra exactly as prescribed for the full length of the prescription. Do not stop taking it just because you are beginning to feel better. Take each dose with a full glass of water and drink plenty of fluids all day to lower the risk of kidney-stone formation.

Call your doctor if you develop sore throat, rash, unusual bleeding or bruising, or any other persistent or intolerable side effect.

You may develop unusual sensitivity to bright light, particularly sunlight. If you have a history of light sensitivity or if you have sensitive skin, avoid prolonged exposure to sunlight while using Septra.

If you miss a dose of Septra, take it as soon as possible. If you take it twice a day and it is almost time for your next dose, take 1 dose as soon as you remember and another in 5 to 6 hours, then go back to your regular schedule. If you take Septra 3 or more times a day and it is almost time for your next dose, take 1 dose as soon as you remember and another in 2 to 4 hours, then continue with your regular schedule. Never take a double dose.

Special Populations

Pregnancy/Breast-feeding
Septra may affect folic acid in the fetus throughout pregnancy and should be used with caution. It should never be taken near term because of the effects of sulfamethoxazole on the newborn, including yellowing of the skin or eyes. Talk to your doctor about Septra's risks versus its benefits if the drug is to be used during pregnancy.

Septra is not recommended for use if you are nursing because of possible effects on the newborn infant.

Seniors
Seniors are more likely to be sensitive to the effects of this drug, especially if they have liver or kidney problems; dosage adjustments may be required.

Serevent   *see Salmeterol, page 912*

see Salmeterol, page 912

Generic Name

Sertraline (SER-truh-lene)

Brand Name
Zoloft

Type of Drug
Selective serotonin reuptake inhibitor (SSRI).

Prescribed for
Depression; also prescribed for obsessive-compulsive disorder.

General Information
Sertraline and other SSRIs, which are chemically unrelated to the older tricyclic and tetracyclic antidepressant drugs, work by preventing the movement of the neurohormone

serotonin into nerve endings. This forces serotonin to remain in the spaces surrounding nerve endings, where it works. Sertraline is effective in treating common symptoms of depression. It can help improve mood and mental alertness, increase physical activity, and improve sleep patterns. Sertraline takes about 4 weeks to work and stays in the body for several weeks after you stop taking it. This fact may be important as your doctor considers when to start or stop treatment. Significant weight loss is uncommon with sertraline, although the drug may cause a weight loss of 1 to 2 lbs.

Cautions and Warnings

Do not take sertraline if you are **allergic** to it.

Serious, **potentially fatal reactions** may occur if sertraline and a **monoamine oxidase inhibitor (MAOI)** antidepressant are taken together (see "Drug Interactions").

Sertraline is broken down in the liver; people with severe **liver disease** should use caution with this drug and be treated with lower doses. People with **reduced kidney function** should take sertraline with caution.

A small number of **manic** or **hypomanic** patients may experience an activation of their condition while taking sertraline.

Sertraline should be used with caution by people who suffer from **seizure** disorders.

SSRIs may affect **blood platelets,** though their exact effect is not known. Some people have had abnormal bleeding while taking these drugs.

Sertraline causes low blood levels of **uric acid,** but has not caused kidney failure.

The possibility of **suicide** exists in people with severe depression and may be present until the condition has significantly improved. Depressed patients should only be allowed to carry small quantities of sertraline with them to limit the possibility of overdose.

Possible Side Effects

▼ Most common: dry mouth; headache; dizziness; tremors; nausea; diarrhea or loose stools; sleeplessness; tiredness; male sexual dysfunction or abnormal ejaculation, in 15% of men; female sexual dysfunction, in 1.7% of women; and feeling unwell.

Possible Side Effects *(continued)*

▼ Common: excessive sweating, constipation, upset stomach, and agitation.

▼ Less common: heart palpitations, chest pain, nervousness, anxiety, tingling or numbness in the hands or feet, twitching, muscle spasm, confusion, rash, muscle and joint ache, gas, appetite increase or decrease, menstrual disorders, sore throat, runny nose, yawning, changes in vision, ringing or buzzing in the ears, frequent urination, fever, back pain, chills, confusion, reduced skin sensation, rash, nightmares, depersonalization, weight gain, vomiting, and changes in sense of taste.

▼ Rare: Rare side effects can occur in almost any part of the body and can affect your skin, urinary function, gastrointestinal tract, and dreaming. Contact your doctor if you experience any side effect not listed above.

Drug Interactions

• At least 5 weeks should elapse between stopping sertraline and starting an MAOI antidepressant. Two weeks should elapse between stopping an MAOI and starting sertraline. Taking these 2 drugs too close together or at the same time may cause serious, life-threatening reactions.

• Sertraline may prolong the effects of diazepam and other benzodiazepine drugs.

• Cimetidine increases blood levels of sertraline by about 50%.

• People taking warfarin may experience an increase in its effect if they start taking sertraline. Your doctor should reevaluate your warfarin dosage.

• Sertraline may affect lithium blood levels.

• Sertraline may slow the rate at which tolbutamide (prescribed for diabetes) is released from the body. The clinical importance of this interaction is not known.

• Combining alcohol with sertraline is not recommended.

Food Interactions

To maintain consistent blood levels, sertraline should be taken on an empty stomach at least 1 hour before or 2 hours after meals.

Usual Dose

50–200 mg once a day, morning or night. Seniors, people with kidney or liver disease, and people taking several different drugs should take the lowest effective dose.

Overdosage

Symptoms are tiredness, nausea, vomiting, rapid heartbeat, anxiety, dilated pupils, and changes in heartbeat. Overdose victims should be taken to a hospital emergency room at once. ALWAYS bring the prescription bottle or container.

Special Information

Sertraline may make you dizzy or drowsy. Take care when driving or performing tasks that require alertness and concentration.

Do not drink alcohol while taking sertraline.

Be sure your doctor knows if you are pregnant, breast-feeding, or taking other drugs, including over-the-counter drugs, while taking sertraline. Notify your doctor if you experience any unusual side effect.

If you forget a dose, take it as soon as you remember. If it is almost time for your next dose, skip the one you forgot and continue with your regular schedule. Do not take a double dose.

Special Populations

Pregnancy/Breast-feeding

Animal studies with up to 4 times the human dose show that sertraline can affect the fetus. Do not take sertraline if you are or might be pregnant without first weighing its potential benefits against its risks with your doctor.

It is not known if sertraline passes into breast milk. Nursing mothers who must take this drug should consider bottle-feeding.

Seniors

Seniors with liver or kidney disease should take a lower dose.

Serzone   *see Nefazodone, page 707*

Generic Name

Sevelamer (seh-VEL-ah-mer)

Brand Name

Renagel

Type of Drug

Phosphate binder.

Prescribed for

High blood-phosphate levels in people with end-stage renal disease (ESRD).

General Information

People with ESRD, a form of kidney disease, tend to retain phosphorous. High phosphate levels, in turn, can effect calcium balance in the body and cause deposits of this mineral to build up in the wrong places. Sevelamer hydrochloride helps to reduce phosphate levels by limiting the amount of phosphorous absorbed from food. Sevelamer also lowers levels of total and low-density lipoprotein (LDL) cholesterol.

Cautions and Warnings

Do not take sevelamer if you are **sensitive** or **allergic** to it or have a **low phosphate level** or a **bowel obstruction**.

Use this drug with caution if you have had **gastrointestinal (GI) surgery** or have **difficulty swallowing** or severe **stomach or intestinal problems**.

Possible Side Effects

▼ Most common: headache, infection, pain, blood pressure changes, blood clotting problems, diarrhea, upset stomach, and vomiting.

▼ Common: nausea.

▼ Less common: cough, gas, and constipation.

▼ Rare: Rare side effects can occur in almost any part of the body. Contact your doctor if you experience any side effect not listed above.

Drug Interactions

• Sevelamer may interfere with other drugs taken at the same time. Take sevelamer either 1 hour before or 3 hours after other medications.

Food Interactions

Sevelamer should be taken with meals.

Usual Dose

Adult: 2–4 capsules with each meal; maximum dosage is 30 capsules a day.

Child: There is no information on the use of this drug in children. Those receiving it must be closely monitored by their doctors.

Overdosage

Symptoms include drug side effects. Call your local poison control center or a hospital emergency room for more information. If you seek treatment, ALWAYS bring the prescription bottle or container.

Special Information

Sevelamer can interfere with the absorption of vitamins from food. Take a supplemental multivitamin while using this drug.

It is important to take sevelamer with each meal. If you forget a dose, skip it and continue to take the drug with subsequent meals.

Do not chew or dismantle the capsules before swallowing them.

Special Populations

Pregnancy/Breast-feeding

In animal studies, sevelamer interfered with fetal bone development. It also interferes with the absorption of vitamins and nutrients, which are essential for a healthy pregnancy. When this drug is considered crucial by your doctor, its potential benefits must be carefully weighed against its risks.

It is not known if sevelamer passes into breast milk. Nursing mothers who must take it should consider bottle-feeding.

Seniors

Seniors may take this drug without special precaution.

Generic Name

Sibutramine (sih-BYUE-trah-meen)

Brand Name

Meridia

Type of Drug

Appetite suppressant.

Prescribed for

Weight loss.

General Information

Sibutramine works by increasing levels of norepinephrine, serotonin, and dopamine in the brain. By preventing the re-uptake of these chemicals into nerve endings, sibutramine stimulates areas of the brain associated with appetite control. About 6 in 10 people who take sibutramine in conjunction with a diet and exercise program lose 4 lbs. or more during the first 4 weeks of treatment and are likely to lose about 5% of their total body weight in 6 to 12 months.

Cautions and Warnings

Do not take sibutramine if you are **allergic** to it.

People taking sibutramine may develop **drug dependency**.

People taking sibutramine may eventually become resistant to the drug, requiring increased dosage to achieve the same effect.

People who have had a **stroke** or who have **heart disease** should not take sibutramine.

People with **narrow-angle glaucoma** should take this drug with caution because it can dilate pupils.

Sibutramine should not be taken by people with severe **liver or kidney disease**.

Sibutramine can **raise blood pressure and pulse rate,** especially if you already have high blood pressure. Check your blood pressure and pulse regularly.

Rarely, people taking sibutramine develop a group of symptoms called **serotonin syndrome,** consisting of one or more of the following symptoms: excitement, a mild manic reaction, restlessness, loss of consciousness, confusion, disorientation, anxiety, agitation, muscle weakness, muscle spasms, tremors, involuntary muscle movements on one side of the body, shivering and dilated pupils, sweating, vomiting, and rapid heartbeat. Serotonin syndrome requires immediate medical treatment.

Other weight loss drugs that act on the nervous system like sibutramine does can cause a rare condition called pulmonary hypertension. This has not been reported with sibutramine.

Rapid weight loss can cause or worsen **gallstones**.

Possible Side Effects

▼ Most common: headache, dry mouth, sleeplessness, appetite loss, constipation, runny nose, and sore throat.

▼ Common: back pain, flu-like symptoms, injuries, weakness, dizziness, nervousness, increased appetite, nausea, joint pain, and sinus irritation.

▼ Less common: abdominal pain, chest pain, neck pain, allergy, rapid heartbeat, flushing, migraine, high blood pressure, heart palpitations, anxiety, depression, tingling in the hands or feet, tiredness, stimulation, emotional instability, rash, sweating, herpes infections, acne, upset stomach, stomach irritation, vomiting, rectal problems, painful menstruation, urinary or vaginal infections, excessive menstrual flow, thirst, swelling, muscle aches, tendon inflammation, joint problems, increased cough, laryngitis, changes in sense of taste, and ear problems.

▼ Rare: seizures, agitation, leg cramps, gas, tooth problems, abnormal thinking, bronchitis, breathing difficulties, bleeding problems, and kidney problems.

Drug Interactions

• Cimetidine, erythromycin, and ketoconazole can mildly increase sibutramine blood levels, but this effect is not considered important.

• Do not drink alcohol to excess while taking sibutramine.

• Do not combine monoamine oxidase inhibitor (MAOI) drugs and sibutramine. This combination could lead to serotonin syndrome (see "Cautions and Warnings").

• Do not combine sibutramine and other weight loss pills that act on the nervous system (usually these are prescription-only diet pills), triptan-type migraine drugs, dihydroer-gotamine, antidepressants, decongestants, cough medications, lithium, or L-tryptophan.

• Stimulants found in some over-the-counter medications—such as decongestants, weight loss pills, or cough, cold, or allergy drugs—can raise blood pressure or heart rate when combined with sibutramine.

Food Interactions

Sibutramine can be taken with or without food.

Usual Dose

Adult and Child (age 16 and over): 10–15 mg once a day.
Child (under age 16): not recommended

Overdosage

Little is known about the effects of sibutramine overdose, though symptoms may include rapid heartbeat. Take the victim to a hospital emergency room. ALWAYS bring the prescription bottle or container.

Special Information

Call your doctor if you develop an allergic reaction such as rash or hives or experience any bothersome or persistent side effect.

This drug can cause an inability to concentrate. Be careful when driving or performing any task that requires concentration or good judgment.

If you forget a dose, take it as soon as you remember. If it is almost time for your next dose, skip the forgotten dose and continue with your regular schedule. Do not take a double dose.

Special Populations

Pregnancy/Breast-feeding

Pregnant women should not take sibutramine under any circumstances. Women of childbearing age should be sure to use effective contraception while taking this medication.

It is not known if sibutramine passes into breast milk. Nursing mothers who must take it should consider bottle-feeding.

Seniors
Seniors with reduced kidney or liver function should receive the lowest effective dosage.

Generic Name

Sildenafil Citrate (sil-DEN-a-fil SIH-trate)

Brand Name

Viagra

Type of Drug

Anti-impotence agent.

Prescribed for

Erectile disfunction (ED).

General Information

The chemical nitric oxide is released in the penis during sexual stimulation. Nitric oxide results in the release of the enzyme cyclic guanosine monophosphate (cGMP), which causes more blood to flow into the penis, producing an erection. cGMP is broken down by the enzyme phosphodiesterase type 5 (PDE5). In men with low levels of cGMP, sildenafil helps achieve and maintain an erection by inhibiting PDE5, thus causing higher levels of cGMP. ED can be the result of nerve, blood vessel, or psychological problems. This drug, which is effective in about 70% of men, only helps when poor blood flow is the cause of the dysfunction. Women have reported some benefit from sildenafil, though it has been widely studied only in men. It starts working in 30 to 60 minutes and its effects last 2 to 4 hours, though some have noted an effect as long as 24 hours or more.

Cautions and Warnings

Sildenafil **lowers blood pressure** and should be avoided if you have high (greater than 170/100) or low (less than 90/50) blood pressure. Several people have died from a sudden blood pressure drop after combining sildenafil with other medications that can reduce blood pressure.

People with **heart disease** may experience heart problems with sildenafil, including a heart attack. These reactions can occur during or shortly after sexual activity.

Avoid sildenafil if you have had a **heart attack, stroke,** or life-threatening **abnormal heart rhythm** in the past 6 months, or if you have **heart failure,** unstable **angina pectoris, damage to the penis,** or a progressive eye disease called **retinitis pigmentosa.**

People taking sildenafil have experienced difficulties seeing blue or green colors. This happens because sildenafil affects an enzyme in the eye. The effect clears up after the drug passes out of your body.

People with **kidney or liver damage** retain sildenafil in their bodies longer than people whose kidneys and liver function normally. People with kidney or liver problems should always begin with the lowest possible dosage.

People with **priapism** (painful erection lasting more than 6 hours) or a condition that predisposes them to priapism—such as **leukemia** or **multiple myeloma**—should be cautious about taking sildenafil.

Possible Side Effects

▼ Most common: headache and flushing.

▼ Less common: upset stomach, stuffy nose, urinary infection, diarrhea, rash, dizziness, seizure, anxiety, prolonged and possibly painful erection, double vision, visual changes, blood-shot eyes, burning eyes, swelling in the eye, and blood vessel diseases in the retina.

▼ Rare: Rare side effects can occur in almost any part of the body. Contact you doctor if you experience any side effect not listed above.

Drug Interactions

• Combining cimetidine with sildenafil leads to a substantial (more than 50%) increase in the amount of sildenafil in the blood. Erythromycin, ketoconazole, itraconazole, and protease inhibitors—used to combat HIV—drugs can cause sildenafil blood levels to almost double.

• Rifampin can be expected to reduce the effect of sildenafil by reducing the amount of drug in the blood.

• Do not combine sildenafil with nitrates and other drugs that lower blood pressure. The combination can cause a sudden, rapid drop in blood pressure.

Food Interactions

Taking sildenafil with a high-fat meal reduces the amount of drug absorbed.

Usual Dose

Adult: 50 mg taken about 1 hour before sexual activity. Individual doses can range from 25–100 mg.

Senior: Begin with 25 mg and gradually increase dosage as needed.

Overdosage

Sildenafil overdose is likely to produce exaggerated drug side effects. Call your local poison control center for more information.

Special Information

Call your doctor and do not engage in sexual activity if the erection produced by sildenafil is painful or lasts 4 or more hours, or if you experience dizziness, nausea, or chest pain after taking sildenafil.

People who use organic nitrates for gardening or other purposes can experience a severe and dangerous blood pressure drop if they take sildenafil. It is not known how long you have to wait after taking sildenafil to resume nitrate use.

Sildenafil does not protect against sexually transmitted diseases.

Special Populations

Pregnancy/Breast-feeding

There is no evidence that sildenafil harms the fetus. This drug is not intended for use by pregnant women or nursing mothers.

Seniors

Men age 65 and over eliminate sildenafil more slowly than younger men and should begin with the 25 mg dosage.

Brand Name

Sinemet

Generic Ingredients

Carbidopa + Levodopa [G]

Other Brand Names

Sinemet CR

The information in this profile also applies to the following drug:

Generic Ingredient: Carbidopa
Lodosyn

Type of Drug

Antiparkinsonian.

Prescribed for

Parkinson's disease.

General Information

In Sinemet, levodopa is the active ingredient that affects Parkinson's disease; carbidopa slows the breakdown of levodopa, making more available to the brain. This combination is so effective that your dosage of levodopa may be reduced by about 75%, which results in fewer side effects. Unfortunately, people eventually develop a resistance to levodopa in any form. Carbidopa is sold under the brand name Lodosyn for people who need individual doses of both carbidopa and levodopa.

Cautions and Warnings

Do not take Sinemet if you are **allergic** to either of its ingredients. If you are switching from levodopa to Sinemet, you should stop taking levodopa 8 hours before your first dose of Sinemet. The sustained-release form of Sinemet has a lesser incidence of **nervous-system side effects**; the immediate-release version may produce such effects even at lower dosages.

Possible Side Effects

▼ Common: uncontrolled muscle movements, appetite loss, nausea, vomiting, stomach pain, dry mouth, difficulty swallowing, drooling, shaky hands, headache, dizziness, numbness, weakness, feeling faint, grinding of the teeth, confusion, sleeplessness, nightmares, hallucinations, anxiety, agitation, tiredness, feeling unwell, and euphoria (feeling "high").

▼ Less common: heart palpitations; dizziness when rising quickly from a sitting or lying position; sudden extreme slowness of movement ("on-off" phenomenon); changes in mental state, including paranoia, psychosis, depression, and a slowdown of mental functioning; difficulty urinating; muscle twitching; eyelid spasms; lockjaw; burning sensation on the tongue; bitter taste; diarrhea; constipation; gas; flushing; rash; sweating; unusual breathing; blurred or double vision; pupil dilation; hot flashes; weight changes; and darkening of urine or sweat.

▼ Rare: Rare side effects can occur in almost any part of the body. Contact your doctor if you experience any side effect not listed above.

The drug may affect blood tests for kidney and liver function.

Drug Interactions

• Sinemet's effectiveness may be increased by anticholinergic drugs such as trihexyphenidyl.

• Methyldopa (an antihypertensive drug) may increase the amount of levodopa available in the central nervous system and may have a slight effect on Sinemet as well.

• People taking guanethidine or a diuretic to treat high blood pressure may need less of either if they start taking Sinemet.

• Reserpine, benzodiazepine tranquilizers, antipsychotic drugs, phenytoin, and papaverine may interfere with Sinemet. Vitamin B_6 interferes with levodopa but not with Sinemet.

• Combining Sinemet and a monoamine oxidase inhibitor (MAOI) may cause a rapid increase in blood pressure. MAOIs should be stopped 2 weeks before starting on Sinemet.

• Sinemet may increase the effects of ephedrine, amphetamines, epinephrine, and isoproterenol. This interaction, which may also occur with antidepressant drugs, can result in adverse effects on the heart.

Food Interactions

Immediate-release Sinemet may be taken with food to reduce upset stomach. Sinemet CR, the sustained-release form, should be taken on an empty stomach.

Usual Dose

Three Sinemet strengths are available: 10/100, 25/100, and 25/250. The first number represents carbidopa content, the second the levodopa content, in mg. Dosage must be individualized based on previous drug treatment. Dosage adjustments are made by adding or omitting ½–1 tablet a day. Maximum daily dosage is eight 25/250-tablets. Sinemet CR is started at dosages roughly equal to 10% more levodopa a day than was being taken previously.

If extra carbidopa is needed, your doctor may prescribe Lodosyn to be taken together with Sinemet. Lodosyn is added in steps of no more than 25 mg a day until the desired effect is achieved.

Overdosage

Symptoms include exaggerated side effects. Take the victim to a hospital emergency room. ALWAYS bring the prescription bottle or container.

Special Information

Sinemet can cause tiredness or an inability to concentrate: Be careful when driving or doing any task that requires concentration.

Call your doctor if you experience dizziness; light-headedness or fainting spells; changes in mood or mental state; abnormal heart rhythm or heart palpitations; difficulty urinating; persistent nausea, vomiting, or other stomach complaints; or uncontrollable movements of the face, eyelids, mouth, tongue, neck, arms, hands, or legs.

This drug may cause darkening of urine or sweat. This effect is not harmful, but may interfere with urine tests for diabetes. Make sure all your doctors know you are taking this medication.

Take Sinemet exactly as prescribed.

If you forget a dose, take it as soon as you remember. If it is within 2 hours of your next dose, skip the one you forgot and continue with your regular schedule. Do not take a double dose.

Special Populations

Pregnancy/Breast-feeding

Both of the ingredients in Sinemet cause birth defects in animals. When this drug is considered crucial by your doctor, its potential benefits must be carefully weighed against its risks.

The ingredients in Sinemet may pass into breast milk and are considered unsafe for infants. Nursing mothers who must take this drug should bottle-feed.

Seniors

Seniors may require reduced dosage. They are also more likely to develop abnormal heart rhythms or other cardiac side effects, especially if they have heart disease.

Singulair see Leukotriene Antagonist/Inhibitor, page 570

Generic Name

Spironolactone (spih-ROE-noe-lak-tone) Ⓖ

Brand Name

Aldactone

Type of Drug

Diuretic (agent that increases urination) and aldosterone antagonist.

Prescribed for

High blood pressure, cirrhosis, and congestive heart failure (CHF), and for people with low blood potassium who require a diuretic.

General Information

Spironolactone interferes with aldosterone, a hormone that helps to regulate fluid levels in the body. Too much aldosterone results in high sodium levels (which leads to water retention) and loss of potassium. A mild diuretic that blocks the effects of aldosterone and is generally combined with hydrochlorothiazide or another diuretic, spironolactone is very useful in removing excess body fluids in conditions associated with high aldosterone levels. In people with CHF, whose aldosterone levels can be 20 times higher than normal, it is important to reduce water retention because it can worsen their condition. Spironolactone helps the body to release sodium and remove excess body fluids while retaining potassium.

Cautions and Warnings

Do not use this drug if you have **kidney failure** or **high blood potassium**.

People taking spironolactone should have their potassium levels checked periodically.

Possible Side Effects

▼ Less common: drowsiness, lethargy, headache, gastrointestinal upset, cramps and diarrhea, rash, mental confusion, fever, feeling unwell, painful enlargement of the breasts, impotence, and irregular menstrual cycles or deepening of the voice in women.

Drug Interactions

• Spironolactone increases the action of other antihypertensive drugs and is frequently used for this effect, though dosages of those drugs may need to be reduced by up to 50%.

• Spironolactone may interfere with anticoagulant (blood-thinning) drugs and mitotane (an anticancer drug).

• Combining a potassium supplement and spironolactone can lead to dangerously high blood levels of potassium. Do not take any extra potassium unless prescribed by your doctor.

• Combining spironolactone and angiotensin-converting enzyme (ACE) inhibitor drugs may significantly increase

blood potassium. Be sure your doctor monitors your potassium levels if you combines these drugs.
* Aspirin can interfere with the diuretic effect of spironolactone but does not alter its effect on high blood pressure or CHF.
* Combining spironolactone with alcohol, barbiturates, or narcotics can lead to dizziness or fainting when rising suddenly from a lying position.
* Combining spironolactone and a corticosteroid can lead to very low blood potassium.
* Spironolactone may alter your response to drugs used during general anesthesia.
* Lithium generally should not be combined with any diuretic.
* Combining nonsteroidal anti-inflammatory drugs (NSAIDs) such as indomethacin and potassium-sparing diuretics has led to severe elevations of blood potassium.
* Spironolactone may increase digoxin blood levels and the risk of severe digoxin side effects. Your doctor may have to adjust your digoxin dosage.

Food Interactions

Food appears to increase the amount of spironolactone absorbed. Take this drug at the same time every day with food.

Usual Dose

Adult: Starting dosage is 50–100 mg a day in divided doses for high blood pressure, 100–200 mg a day in divided doses for high fluid levels related to other diseases, and 25 mg a day for CHF.
Child: 1–2 mg per lb. of body weight a day.

Overdosage

Symptoms may include drowsiness, confusion, rash, nausea, vomiting, dizziness, and diarrhea. Rarely, coma may occur in people with severe liver disease. High blood potassium may also occur, especially in people with kidney disease. Call your local poison control center or a hospital emergency room for more information. If you seek treatment, ALWAYS bring the prescription bottle or container.

Special Information

Take the drug exactly as prescribed.

High blood levels of potassium associated with use of spironolactone may cause weakness, lethargy, drowsiness, muscle pain or cramps, and muscular fatigue. Be careful when driving or performing any task that requires concentration.

People who have high blood pressure should not self-medicate with over-the-counter cough, cold, or allergy remedies containing stimulants because these drugs may counteract spironolactone's effectiveness and have an adverse effect on the heart.

If you forget a dose, take it as soon as you remember. If it is almost time for your next dose, skip the one you forgot and continue with your regular schedule. Do not take a double dose.

Special Populations

Pregnancy/Breast-feeding
Spironolactone crosses into the fetal circulation. When this drug is considered crucial by your doctor, its potential benefits must be carefully weighed against its risks.

This drug passes into breast milk. Nursing mothers who must take it should consider bottle-feeding.

Seniors
Seniors are more sensitive to the effects of this drug, especially high blood-potassium levels.

Type of Drug
Statin Cholesterol-Lowering Agents

Brand Names

Generic Ingredient: Atorvastatin
Lipitor

Generic Ingredient: Cerivastatin
Baycol

Generic Ingredient: Fluvastatin
Lescol

Generic Ingredient: Lovastatin
Mevacor

Generic Ingredient: Pravastatin
Pravachol

Generic Ingredient: Simvastatin
Zocor

Prescribed for

High blood levels of cholesterol, low-density lipoprotein (LDL) cholesterol, and triglyceride; also prescribed for atherosclerosis (hardening of the arteries), diabetes-related blood-fat problems, preventing heart attacks and strokes, and reducing the risk of cardiac bypass surgery. Some of these drugs may also be used for blood-fat disorders related to kidney disease and inherited blood-fat problems.

General Information

High blood-fat levels are believed to play a role in the development of cardiovascular disease. Statin drugs help to lower blood-fat levels by blocking the effects of the enzyme HMG-CoA reductase, which in turn interferes with the production of cholesterol in the body. They also increase levels of high-density lipoprotein (HDL) cholesterol, the "good" cholesterol considered to have a beneficial effect on heart health. Statin drugs are proven to slow the progression of atherosclerosis, help prevent heart attacks, and reduce the risk of dying from heart disease.

These drugs begin working quickly. Blood-fat levels are significantly improved after 1 to 2 weeks of treatment. Maximum effect occurs in 4 to 6 weeks, persists for the remainder of drug therapy, and continues for 4 to 6 weeks after you stop taking these drugs. These drugs are generally not recommended for people under age 30, though they may be prescribed for teenagers under certain circumstances. With the exception of cerivastatin, only a small amount of these drugs enters the bloodstream. They are largely broken down in the liver.

Cautions and Warnings

Do not take any of these drugs if you are **allergic** to them. It is possible to be allergic to one of these drugs and tolerate another.

People with a history of **liver disease** and those who drink **large amounts of alcohol** should avoid these drugs because they may aggravate or cause liver disease. About 1 in 100 people who take these drugs develops high liver-enzyme counts; the risk of this effect is highest with lovastatin and lowest with atorvastatin and cerivastatin. Your doctor should take a blood sample to test your liver function every month or so during the first year of treatment.

Rarely, people taking these drugs develop **muscle aches or weakness,** which can be a sign of a more serious condition.

People with **kidney failure** who take pravastatin or simvastatin must be closely monitored by their doctors.

People in early studies of lovastatin developed **cloudy vision,** due to an effect on the lens of the eye, but this effect has not been seen in further studies. Report any changes in vision to your doctor.

Possible Side Effects

Side effects are usually mild and temporary. Rare side effects associated with these drugs can occur in almost any part of the body. Contact your doctor if you experience any side effect not listed below.

Atorvastatin
▼ Most common: headache.
▼ Common: muscle aches.
▼ Less common: gas, upset stomach, itching, rash, allergy, and infection.

Cerivastatin
▼ Most common: headache, runny nose, and sore throat.
▼ Common: upset stomach, joint pain, sinus irritation, urinary problems, and accidents.
▼ Less common: dizziness, weakness, sleeplessness, nausea, vomiting, diarrhea, cramps, gas, constipation, heartburn, leg pain, muscle aches, cough, itching, rash, chest pain, and swelling in the arms or legs.

Fluvastatin
▼ Most common: respiratory infection.
▼ Common: headache, muscle aches, diarrhea, abdominal pain or cramps, changes in sense of taste, flu-like symptoms, and allergy.
▼ Less common: dizziness, sleeplessness, nausea, vomiting, constipation, gas, tooth problems, arthritis, joint pain, runny nose, cough, sore throat, sinus irritation, itching, rash, and fatigue.

Possible Side Effects *(continued)*

Lovastatin

▼ Common: stomach pain, cramps, gas, and constipation.

▼ Less common: headache, dizziness, heartburn, upset stomach, itching, rash, allergy, infection, nausea, vomiting, diarrhea, muscle aches or pain, joint pain, blurred vision, and eye irritation.

Pravastatin

▼ Most common: generalized pain.

▼ Common: headache, nausea, vomiting, diarrhea, abdominal pain or cramps, and common cold symptoms.

▼ Less common: dizziness, constipation, heartburn, upset stomach, muscle aches, cough, runny nose, chest pain, itching, rash, flu-like symptoms, fatigue, and urinary difficulties.

Simvastatin

▼ Less common: headache, weakness, nausea, vomiting, diarrhea, abdominal pain or cramps, constipation, gas, upset stomach, and respiratory infection.

Drug Interactions

• Drinking alcohol regularly increases the amount of fluvastatin in the blood by 30%.

• Antacids reduce atorvastatin blood levels, though cholesterol lowering may not be affected. Separate doses of these drugs by at least 1 hour.

• The cholesterol-lowering effects of these drugs and cholestyramine are additive. Take a statin drug 1 hour before or 4 hours after cholestyramine. Colestipol reduces atorvastatin blood levels, but this combination more effectively lowers blood-fat levels than either drug used alone.

• Combining these drugs and cyclosporine, erythromycin, gemfibrozil, or niacin can lead to severe muscle aches or degeneration or other muscle problems. These combinations should be avoided.

• Digoxin can reduce fluvastatin blood levels. Statin drugs can increase the amount of digoxin in the blood by about 20%.

• Isradipine may increase the clearance of lovastatin from the body.

• Itraconazole can increase statin blood levels by 20 times. Avoid this combination by temporarily stopping your cholesterol medication if you take itraconazole.

• Rifampin may reduce fluvastatin blood levels.

• Atorvastatin increases blood levels of oral contraceptives ("the pill"), which can lead to side effects. If you must take both drugs, talk to your doctor about lowering your contraceptive dosage.

• These drugs may increase the effects of warfarin. People taking these drugs together should be periodically examined by their doctors. Warfarin dosage adjustment may be necessary.

• Propranolol can reduce the effectiveness of these drugs.

Food Interactions

Lovastatin must be taken with meals. Other statin drugs may be taken with or without food.

Usual Dose

Atorvastatin
    Adult: 10–80 mg a day.
    Senior: 10–20 mg a day. Dosage should be adjusted monthly based on how well the drug is working.

Cerivastatin
    Adult: 0.3 mg a day, taken in the evening; 0.2 mg may be used when moderate to severe kidney damage is present.

Fluvastatin
    Adult: 20–40 mg a day, taken in the evening. Dosage may be adjusted up to 80 mg based on how well the drug is working.

Lovastatin
    Adult: 20–80 mg a day, usually taken with your evening meal. Dosage should be adjusted monthly based on how well the drug is working.

Pravastatin
    Adult: 10–40 mg, taken at bedtime.
    Senior: 10–20 mg, taken at bedtime. Dosage should be adjusted monthly based on how well the drug is working.

Simvastatin
 Adults: 5–40 mg, taken in the evening.
 Senior: 5–20 mg, taken in the evening. Dosage may be adjusted monthly based on how well the drug is working.

Overdosage

People taking overdoses of these drugs have experienced no specific symptoms and have recovered without a problem after the drug was removed from their stomachs by making them vomit. Overdose victims should be taken to a hospital emergency room for evaluation and treatment. ALWAYS bring the prescription bottle or container.

Special Information

Call your doctor if you develop blurred vision or muscle aches, pain, tenderness, or weakness, especially if you are also feverish or don't feel well.

Statin drugs are prescribed in combination with a low-fat diet. Following your doctor's dietary instructions will help reduce your blood fats and keep them low. Do not take more cholesterol-lowering medication than your doctor has prescribed. Do not stop taking it without your doctor's knowledge.

These drugs may cause increased sensitivity to the sun. Use sunscreen and wear protective clothing.

If you forget a dose, take it as soon as you remember. If it is almost time for your next dose, skip the one you forgot and continue with your regular schedule. Do not take a double dose.

Special Populations

Pregnancy/Breast-feeding
Pregnant women and those who might become pregnant must not take any of these drugs.

These drugs may pass into breast milk. Nursing mothers who must take them should bottle-feed.

Seniors
Seniors are more sensitive to the effects of some statin drugs and may require reduced dosage.

Generic Name

Stavudine (STAV-ue-dene)

Brand Name

Zerit

Type of Drug

Antiviral.

Prescribed for

Advanced human immunodeficiency virus (HIV) infection.

General Information

Stavudine is a synthetic nucleoside antiviral drug that inhibits the reproduction of the HIV virus by interfering with viral DNA duplication. Stavudine can also interfere with DNA in human cells and may affect the duplication of some body cells. The drug is eliminated primarily through the kidneys.

Cautions and Warnings

Stavudine should be taken only by adults with **advanced HIV infection** who cannot take or tolerate other AIDS treatments, or whose disease has progressed despite treatment with other antiviral drugs. There is no proof that stavudine prolongs the lives of people with AIDS.

People taking stavudine or any other anti-HIV drug may continue to develop **opportunistic infections** and other complications of the disease, and should remain under the direct care of a doctor.

Peripheral neuropathy is the most common side effect of stavudine (see "Special Information"). People who have had these symptoms before are more likely to have this problem while taking stavudine.

Pancreatic inflammation occurs in 1% of people taking stavudine and has been associated with 14 deaths in people taking this drug.

Stavudine is approved only for adults with AIDS, although in children who were studied for as long as 3 years, stavudine acted similarly to the way it acts in adults.

Possible Side Effects

▼ Most common: peripheral neuropathy, which can produce tingling, burning, numbness, or pain in the hands, arms, feet, or legs; diarrhea; nausea; vomiting; headache; fever; chills; weakness; abdominal pain; back pain; muscle or joint ache; generalized pain; not feeling well; sleeplessness; anxiety; depression; nervousness; breathing difficulties; appetite and weight loss; rash; itching; and sweating.

▼ Common: allergic reactions; flu-like symptoms; swollen lymph glands, usually felt under the arms or in the neck; chest pain; constipation; upset stomach; and dizziness.

▼ Less common: pelvic pain, tumors, hypertension (high blood pressure), swelling, flushing, stomach ulcers, confusion, migraine headache, sleepiness, tremors, nerve pain, asthma, pneumonia, skin tumors, conjunctivitis, visual disturbances, painful urination, genital pain, painful menstruation, and vaginitis.

▼ Rare: frequent urination, blood in the urine, impotence, fainting, inflammation of the pancreas, nerve pain, and peeling skin.

Food and Drug Interactions

None known.

Usual Dose

Adult: 30–40 mg every 12 hours. Dosage reduction may be needed in seniors.

Child: not recommended.

Overdosage

Chronic overdose can produce peripheral neuropathy (see "Special Information") and liver toxicity. Call your local poison control center for more information. Overdose victims should be taken to a hospital emergency room for treatment. ALWAYS bring the prescription bottle or container.

Special Information

Peripheral neuropathy (symptoms include tingling, pain, or numbness in the hands, arms, legs, or feet) occurs in 15% to

20% of people who take stavudine. If the drug is stopped, symptoms may disappear, although they can actually worsen for a time after you stop taking stavudine. If the symptoms do go away, your doctor may restart stavudine treatment at a lower daily dosage.

Your stavudine dosage will be reduced if you develop symptoms of neuropathy or if you have reduced kidney function.

Stavudine does not cure AIDS. It will not prevent you from transmitting the virus to another person; you must still practice safe sex. Stavudine may not prevent some illnesses associated with AIDS from developing. The long-term effects of stavudine are not known.

It is very important to take stavudine according to your doctor's directions. If you forget a dose, take it as soon as you remember. If it is almost time for your next dose, take the dose you forgot, take the next 2 doses 8 hours apart, and then go back to your regular schedule. Do not take a double dose. Call your doctor if you skip more than 2 consecutive doses.

Special Populations

Pregnancy/Breast-feeding
Animal studies show that stavudine passes to the fetus and causes birth defects, but there is no direct information on what happens in humans. Stavudine should be taken during pregnancy only if it is absolutely necessary.

Animal studies show that stavudine passes into breast milk, but it is not known if this occurs in humans. In any case, mothers who are HIV positive should bottle-feed their babies to avoid transmitting the virus through their milk.

Seniors
Older adults are likely to have reduced kidney function and may need to have their daily dose adjusted accordingly.

Generic Name

Sucralfate (sue-KRAL-fate) Ⓖ

Brand Name

Carafate

Type of Drug

Antiulcer.

Prescribed for

Short-term (less than 8-week) treatment of duodenal (intestinal) ulcer; also used for stomach ulcer, irritation, and bleeding; gastroesophageal reflux disease (GERD); irritation of the esophagus and mouth; throat ulcer; and prevention of stress ulcer and stomach bleeding.

General Information

Sucralfate works within the gastrointestinal (GI) tract by exerting a soothing local effect on ulcer tissue; very little of the drug is absorbed into the bloodstream. After the drug binds to proteins in the damaged mucous tissue within the ulcer, it forms a barrier to the normal acids and enzymes of the GI tract. This barrier protects ulcer tissue from further damage, allowing it to heal naturally. Sucralfate is not an antacid and works differently than cimetidine, omeprazole, and other antiulcer drugs, but it is as effective in treating duodenal ulcer disease as these drugs.

Cautions and Warnings

Duodenal ulcer is a chronic disease. Short-term treatments like sucralfate can completely heal an ulcer, but this does not reduce the risk of having another ulcer.

Small amounts of aluminum are absorbed while you take sucralfate. This can be a problem for people with chronic **kidney failure** and for those on **dialysis**.

Possible Side Effects

Side effects are usually minimal.
  ▼ Most common: constipation.
  ▼ Less common: diarrhea, nausea, upset stomach, indigestion, dry mouth, rash, itching, back pain, dizziness, and sleepiness.

Drug Interactions

• Sucralfate may decrease the effects of digoxin, ketoconazole, phenytoin, quinidine, tetracycline, warfarin, and ciprofloxacin, norfloxacin, and other quinolone antibacterials. Separate these drugs and sucralfate by 2 hours to avoid this effect.

• Do not take antacids 30 minutes before or after taking sucralfate.

• Do not take aluminum-containing antacids at all while you are taking sucralfate. This combination increases aluminum absorption into the bloodstream and may lead to aluminum toxicity.

Food Interactions

Take each dose on an empty stomach, at least 1 hour before or 2 hours after meals.

Usual Dose

Adult: starting dosage—1 tablet 4 times a day for active ulcers. Maintenance dosage—1 tablet 2 times a day.

Child: not recommended.

Overdosage

Little is known about the effects of sucralfate overdose, though the risk associated with it is thought to be minimal. Call your local poison control center or a hospital emergency room for more information. If you seek treatment, ALWAYS bring the prescription bottle or container.

Special Information

Complete the full course of drug therapy.

Notify your doctor if you develop constipation, diarrhea, or other GI side effects.

If you forget a dose, take it as soon as you remember. If it is almost time for your next dose, skip the one you forgot and continue with your regular schedule. Do not take a double dose.

Special Populations

Pregnancy/Breast-feeding

While animal studies of sucralfate reveal no damage to the fetus, this drug should only be used during pregnancy after carefully weighing its potential benefits against its risks.

It is not known if sucralfate passes into breast milk. Nursing mothers who must take it should consider bottle-feeding.

Seniors

Seniors may take sucralfate without special restriction.

Type of Drug

Sulfa Drugs

Brand Names

Generic Ingredient: Sulfadiazine G
Only available in generic form.

Generic Ingredient: Sulfamethizole
Thiosulfil Forte

Generic Ingredient: Sulfamethoxazole G
Gantanol

Generic Ingredient: Sulfasalazine G
Azulfidine   Azulfidine EN-Tabs

Generic Ingredient: Sulfisoxazole G
Gantrisin

*Generic Ingredients: Triple Sulfa (Sulfathiazole +
Sulfacetamide + Sulfabenzamide)* G
Dayto Sulf   Trysul
Gyne-Sulf   V.V.S.
Sultrin

Prescribed for

Urinary and other infections; may also be prescribed for
rheumatoid, juvenile, and psoriatic arthritis; ulcerative and
other forms of colitis; Crohn's disease; ankylosing spondylitis; and psoriasis. Sulfisoxazole has also been used to prevent middle ear infection. Triple sulfa is used only to treat
vaginal infection.

General Information

In use for many years, sulfa drugs are prescribed for infections in various parts of the body but are particularly helpful
for urinary tract infections. They kill bacteria and some fungi
by interfering with the metabolic processes of these organisms. Some organisms may become resistant to the effects of
sulfa drugs.

Sulfasalazine is different from the other sulfa drugs in that
only about 1/3 of it is absorbed into the bloodstream; the rest
remains in the intestines. Because of its specific anti-inflam-

matory and immune system effects, sulfasalazine is effective against colitis, intestinal irritation, and arthritis and other inflammatory conditions.

Cautions and Warnings

Do not take sulfa drugs if you are **allergic** to them or any drug chemically related to the sulfa drugs including thiazide and loop diuretics, carbonic anhydrase inhibitors, and sulfonylurea-type oral antidiabetes drugs—which do not include metformin. Do not use any sulfa drug if you are allergic to PABA-containing sunscreens or local anesthetics, or if you have **porphyria**. Sulfasalazine should not be used by people with aspirin allergy or by **children under age 2**.

Sulfa drugs can cause **increased sensitivity to the sun or bright light**. Use sunscreen and wear protective clothing.

Men taking sulfasalazine may have **low sperm count** or become **infertile**. This effect reverses when the drug is stopped.

Sulfa drugs should be taken by people with severe **kidney or liver disease** only after a doctor has evaluated their condition and need for the drug.

Deaths in people taking sulfasalazine have been related to a variety of effects on the blood, liver damage, and nervous system changes. Call your doctor if anything unusual develops while taking a sulfa drug.

Possible Side Effects

▼ Most common: headache, itching, rash, skin sensitivity to strong sunlight, nausea, vomiting, abdominal or stomach cramps or pain, feeling unwell, hallucination, dizziness, ringing or buzzing in the ears, and chills.

▼ Less common: blood diseases or changes in blood composition, arthritic pain, diarrhea, appetite loss, drowsiness, hearing loss, itchy eyes, fever, hair loss, and yellowing of the skin or whites of the eyes. Sulfasalazine may reduce sperm count.

Drug Interactions

• Sulfa drugs may increase the effects of sulfonylurea-type oral antidiabetes drugs, methotrexate, warfarin, and phenytoin and other hydantoin antiseizure drugs. Dosages of these drugs may have to be reduced by your doctor.

• Cyclosporine blood levels may be reduced by sulfa drugs, possibly increasing kidney toxicity.

• Sulfa drugs may increase blood levels of indomethacin, probenecid, and aspirin and other salicylates, increasing the risks of side effects.

• When methenamine and a sulfa drug are taken together, an insoluble substance may form in acid urine. Avoid this combination.

• Erythromycin increases the effect of sulfa drugs against infections caused by *Haemophilus influenzae,* a common cause of middle-ear infections.

• The effects of folic acid and digoxin may be antagonized by sulfasalazine; dosage increases may be needed.

Food Interactions

Sulfa drugs should be taken on an empty stomach with a full glass of water. Sulfasalazine may be taken with food if it upsets your stomach.

Usual Dose

Sulfadiazine
  Adult: 2–4 g a day.
  Child (age 2 months and over): 34–68 mg per lb. of body weight a day.
  Child (under age 2 months): not recommended, except to treat certain infections present at birth. In these cases, dosage is 11.3 mg per lb. of body weight, 4 times a day.

Sulfamethizole
  Adult: 1.5–4 g a day.
  Child (age 2 months and over): 13–20 mg per lb. of body weight a day, in divided doses.

Sulfamethoxazole
  Adult: 2–3 g a day.
  Child (age 2 months and over): 23–27 mg per lb. of body weight a day.

Sulfasalazine
  Adult: 1–4 g a day in evenly divided doses.
  Child (age 2 and over): 18–27 mg per lb. of body weight a day, in evenly divided doses.
  Child (under age 2): not recommended.

Sulfisoxazole
   Adult: 2–8 g a day, in 4–6 divided doses.
   Child (age 2 months and over): 34–68 mg per lb. of body weight a day, in 4–6 divided doses.

Triple Sulfa
   Adult: 1 applicator's worth twice a day for 4–6 days, then ¼–½ applicator's worth twice a day; or 1 intravaginal tablet morning and evening for 10 days.

Overdosage

Symptoms include appetite loss, nausea, vomiting and colic, dizziness, headache, drowsiness, unconsciousness, and high fever. Take the victim to a hospital emergency room at once. ALWAYS take the prescription bottle or container.

Special Information

Sulfa drugs often cause increased sensitivity to the sun. Use sunscreen or wear protective clothing.

Sore throat, fever, chills, unusual bleeding or bruising, rash, and drowsiness are signs of serious blood disorders and should be reported to your doctor at once. Contact your doctor if you experience ringing in the ears, blood in the urine, or breathing difficulties.

Be sure to take the full course of medication as prescribed, even if you notice an improvement in your symptoms.

Sulfasalazine may turn your urine orange-yellow. This is a harmless reaction. Skin discoloration has also occurred. This drug may permanently stain soft contact lenses.

Sulfa drugs may interfere with some tests for sugar in the urine.

If you forget a dose, take it as soon as you remember. If you take the drug twice a day and it is almost time for your next dose, take 1 dose right away, another after 5 to 6 hours, and then go back to your regular schedule. If you take the drug 3 or more times a day and it is almost time for your next dose, take 1 dose right away, another after 2 to 4 hours, and then go back to your regular schedule. Never take a double dose.

Special Populations

Pregnancy/Breast-feeding
Sulfa drugs pass into the fetal circulation and may affect the fetus. Malformations have been seen in animal studies. Sulfa drugs are not recommended during pregnancy. When a sulfa

drug is considered crucial by your doctor, its potential benefits must be carefully weighed against its risks.

Small amounts of sulfa drugs pass into breast milk. Nursing mothers who must take them should consider bottle-
feeding, especially if their babies are premature, deficient in
the enzyme G-6-PD, or have hyperbilirubinemia (condition in
which there is too much bilirubin in the blood).

Seniors
Seniors with kidney or liver problems should take sulfa drugs
with caution.

Type of Drug
Sulfonylurea Antidiabetes Drugs

Brand Names

Generic Ingredient: Acetohexamide 🅖
Dymelor

Generic Ingredient: Chlorpropamide 🅖
Diabinese

Generic Ingredient: Glimepiride
Amaryl

Generic Ingredient: Glipizide 🅖
Glucotrol   Glucotrol XL

Generic Ingredient: Glyburide 🅖
DiaBeta   Micronase
Glynase PresTab

Generic Ingredient: Tolazamide 🅖
Tolinase

Generic Ingredient: Tolbutamide 🅖
Orinase

Prescribed for

Diabetes mellitus. Chlorpropamide may also be used to treat
diabetes insipidus (a hormonal condition unrelated to blood
sugar).

General Information

These medicines work by stimulating the production and release of insulin from the pancreas. They differ from each other in how long they take to start working, the duration of their effectiveness, and the amount of each required to produce a roughly equivalent antidiabetic effect (see table). These drugs do not lower blood sugar directly; they require some working pancreas cells. The "second-generation" antidiabetes drugs (glimepiride, glipizide, and glyburide) belong to the same chemical class as the older "first generation" ones, but lower doses of the second-generation agents are required to accomplish the same effect.

Drug	Equivalent dose (mg)	Hours to start working	Hours of Effectiveness
Acetohexamide	500	1	12 to 24
Chlorpropamide	250	1	up to 60
Glimepiride	4	1	24
Glipizide	10	1 to 1½	10 to 16
Glyburide (DiaBeta, Micronase)	5	2 to 4	24
Glyburide (Glynase PresTab)	3	1	12 to 24
Tolazamide	250	4 to 6	12 to 24
Tolbutamide	1000	1	6 to 12

Cautions and Warnings

Mild stress, such as **infection, minor surgery,** or **emotional upset,** reduces the effectiveness of these drugs. You must be under your doctor's continuous care while taking any of these drugs.

These drugs are **not a form of oral insulin** or a substitute for insulin. They do not lower blood sugar by themselves.

Studies conducted in the 1960s and confirmed in 1999 found that people taking oral sulfonylurea antidiabetes drugs are more likely to have **fatal heart trouble** than those who can control their diabetes with diet alone or diet plus insulin.

These drugs can cause **low blood sugar** (see "Overdosage") that may require medical attention.

These drugs should be used with caution if you have serious **liver, kidney, or endocrine disease;** monitor your blood sugar very closely.

Possible Side Effects

▼ Most common: loss of appetite, nausea, vomiting, and stomach upset. At times you may experience weakness or tingling in the hands and feet.

▼ Less common: Oral sulfonylurea antidiabetes drugs may produce abnormally low blood sugar levels when too much is taken for your immediate requirements.

▼ Rare: yellowing of the skin or whites of the eyes, itching, and rash. Usually these reactions will disappear in time. If they persist, contact your doctor.

Drug Interactions

• The following drugs may increase your need for oral sulfonylurea antidiabetes drugs: beta blockers, calcium channel blockers, cholestyramine, corticosteroids, diazoxide, estrogens, isoniazid, nicotinic acid, oral contraceptives, phenothiazines, phenytoin and other hydantoin drugs, rifampin, stimulants, thiazide diuretics, thyroid replacement drugs, charcoal tablets, and anything that makes your urine less acidic.

• The following drugs may decrease your need for oral sulfonylurea antidiabetes drugs: androgens (male hormones), sulfa drugs, aspirin and other salicylates, bishydroxycoumarin, chloramphenicol, cimetidine, clofibrate, dicumarol, famotidine, fenfluramine, fluconazole, gemfibrozil, itraconazole, ketoconazole, ranitidine, magnesium-containing products, methyldopa, miconazole, monoamine oxidase inhibitor (MAOI) drugs, nizatidine, oxyphenbutazone, phenylbutazone, probenecid, warfarin, phenyramidol, sulfinpyrazone, tricyclic antidepressants, large doses of vitamin C, and citrus fruits and other foods that make your urine more acidic.

• Mixing insulin with one of these medicines may lead to severely low blood sugar. This combination must be used only under a doctor's supervision.

• Mixing these drugs with alcohol can cause flushing and breathlessness. Other possible effects are throbbing pain in the head and neck, breathing difficulties, nausea, vomiting, increased sweating, excessive thirst, chest pains, palpitations, lowered blood pressure, weakness, dizziness, blurred vision, and confusion. If you experience any of these reactions, contact your doctor immediately.

• Combining ciprofloxacin with glyburide can increase its blood-sugar-lowering effect.

• Chlorpropamide may increase the effects of barbiturates.

• Glyburide may alter the effectiveness of oral anticoagulant (blood-thinning) drugs. Dosage may have to be adjusted by your doctor.

• These drugs may increase the effects of digitalis drugs.

• The stimulants in many over-the-counter cough, cold, and allergy remedies may affect your blood sugar; avoid them unless your doctor advises otherwise.

Food Interactions

All these drugs except glipizide may be taken with food. Glipizide should be taken 30 minutes before a meal for best results.

Usual Dose

Acetohexamide: 250–1500 mg a day.

Chlorpropamide: starting dose—1–2 g a day. Your doctor will then raise or lower your dose according to your response. Maintenance dose—0.25–2 g a day; rarely, 3 g a day may be prescribed.

Glimepiride: 4–8 mg once a day.

Glipizide: 5 mg once a day. Seniors may be started on 2.5 mg a day. Doses up to 40 mg a day divided into 2 doses may be needed to control more severe diabetes. Single daily doses should not exceed 15 mg.

Glyburide: DiaBeta/Micronase—2.5–20 mg once a day, usually with breakfast or the first main meal. Seniors may start with 1.25 mg a day. Glynase PresTab—1.5–12 mg a day, usually with breakfast or the first main meal. Seniors may start with 0.75 mg a day. Glynase PresTab is not equivalent to DiaBeta or Micronase and may not be substituted for either of them. DiaBeta and Micronase are interchangeable.

Tolazamide: moderate diabetes—100–250 mg a day. Severe diabetes—500–1000 mg a day.

Tolbutamide: starting dose—1–2 g a day. Your doctor will then raise or lower your dosage based on your response. Maintenance dose—0.25–2 g a day; rarely, 3 g a day may be prescribed.

Overdosage

A mild overdose causes low blood sugar (symptoms include tingling of the lips and tongue, nausea, lethargy, yawning, confusion, agitation, nervousness, rapid heartbeat, increased sweating, tremors, and hunger). This can be treated by consuming sugar in such forms as candy, orange juice, or glucose tablets. Ultimately, low blood sugar may lead to convulsions, stupor, and coma. Call your doctor, local poison control center, or hospital emergency room to find out if the overdose victim should be taken to a hospital emergency room. ALWAYS bring the prescription bottle or container.

Special Information

Treating diabetes is your responsibility. Follow your doctor's instructions about diet, body weight, exercise, personal hygiene, and all measures to avoid infection.

Call your doctor if you develop low blood sugar (see "Overdosage") or high blood sugar (symptoms include excessive thirst or urination and sugar or ketones in the urine), if you are not feeling well, or if you have symptoms such as itching, rash, yellowing of the whites of the eyes, abnormally light-colored stools, a low-grade fever, sore throat, diarrhea, or unusual bruising or bleeding.

Do not stop taking these drugs, except under your doctor's supervision. If you forget a dose, take it as soon as you remember. If it is almost time for your next dose, skip the one you forgot and continue with your regular schedule. Do not take a double dose.

Special Populations

Pregnancy/Breast-feeding

Animal studies have shown that all these drugs except glyburide cause birth defects or interfere with fetal development. Check with your doctor before taking an oral sulfonylurea antidiabetes drug if you are or might be pregnant. Pregnant women are best treated with insulin because oral sulfonylurea antidiabetes drugs generally will not control their blood sugar, and high blood sugar increases the risk of birth defects.

These drugs pass into breast milk. They may lower blood-sugar levels in an infant. Nursing mothers taking one of these medications should bottle-feed.

Seniors

Seniors, especially those with reduced kidney function, are very sensitive to the blood-sugar-lowering effects and side effects of these drugs. Low blood sugar, the major sign of drug overdose, may be more difficult to identify in seniors and is more likely to cause nervous-system side effects. Seniors taking these drugs must keep in close contact with their doctors and follow their directions.

Synthroid   *see Thyroid Hormone Replacements, page* 1005

Generic Name

Tacrine   (TAK-reen)

Brand Name

Cognex

Type of Drug

Cholinesterase inhibitor.

Prescribed for

Alzheimer's disease.

General Information

Tacrine was the first pill proven to raise levels of acetylcholine in the brain. People with Alzheimer's disease (degenerative condition of the nervous system) develop a shortage of this important neurohormone early in the course of the disease. Low levels of acetylcholine may account for the gradual memory loss and decline in reasoning ability associated with Alzheimer's, though this theory is under question. Tacrine is not effective in treating problems that develop later as a result of Alzheimer's effect on other brain systems.

Studies show that 10% to 25% of people with Alzheimer's benefit from taking tacrine though 12% stop taking it because of side effects. Larger dosages are most effective. In a 30-week Alzheimer's study, people who took 120 or 160 mg of tacrine a day continued to get better for the first 24 weeks. After that, their condition slowly worsened. People taking 80 mg improved for the first 18 weeks, then declined.

Cautions and Warnings

People who are **sensitive** or **allergic** to tacrine or similar drugs and those who have had **liver disease** or **jaundice** (yellow discoloration of the skin or whites of the eyes) should not take this drug.

Tacrine may **slow heart rate,** adversely affecting some people with heart disease.

Tacrine increases the production of stomach acid. People with a history of ulcers and those taking nonsteroidal anti-inflammatory drugs (NSAIDs) should be aware that tacrine may increase the risk of **stomach or intestinal bleeding**.

People with **asthma, bladder obstruction or other disease,** or **seizure disorders** should take this drug with caution.

Women may be more likely to develop side effects, especially liver inflammation.

Possible Side Effects

▼ Most common: liver inflammation, headache, nausea or vomiting, diarrhea, and dizziness.

▼ Common: upset stomach, appetite loss, abdominal pain, confusion, poor muscle coordination, sleeplessness, agitation, runny nose, rash, and muscle aches.

▼ Less common: fatigue, chest pain, weight loss, back pain, weakness, constipation, gas, tiredness, tremors, depression, abnormal thinking, anxiety, hallucinations, hostility, coughing, respiratory infections, flushing, urinary infection, frequent urination, poor urinary control, and bleeding under the skin.

▼ Rare: Rare side effects can occur in almost any part of the body. Contact your doctor if you experience any side effect not listed above.

Drug Interactions

• Tacrine is likely to increase the effects of some curare-type muscle relaxants used during surgery. Be sure your surgeon knows you are taking it.

• Tacrine increases theophylline concentrations twofold, requiring theophylline dosage reduction to avoid side effects.

• Cimetidine increases the absorption of tacrine by 50%. Do not combine these drugs without your doctor's knowledge.

• Tacrine interferes with all anticholinergic drugs.

• Cigarette smoking speeds the rate at which tacrine is broken down by the liver.

Food Interactions

This drug is best taken on an empty stomach, though it may be taken with food if it upsets your stomach.

Usual Dose

40–160 mg a day, divided into 4 doses.

Overdosage

Symptoms are salivation, severe nausea or vomiting, increased sweating, slow heartbeat, low blood pressure, collapse, and convulsions. Muscles may become increasingly weak; this can lead to death if the respiratory muscles are involved. Take the victim to a hospital emergency room. ALWAYS bring the prescription bottle or container.

Special Information

Call your doctor if you develop very light-colored or black and tarry stools, or if you vomit material that resembles coffee grounds. Report yellowing of the skin or whites of the eyes, rash, or other side effects that are bothersome or persistent. Your doctor may have to stop treatment if you develop liver inflammation; your doctor will need to take blood samples for at least the first 18 weeks of treatment to watch for signs of this problem.

Abruptly stopping tacrine or reducing dosage by 80 mg or more at a time is likely to cause behavioral changes and a noticeable worsening of Alzheimer's symptoms. Do not alter dosage or stop using tacrine without your doctor's knowledge.

For best results, take tacrine at the same time each day. If you forget a dose, take it as soon as possible. If it is almost time for the next dose, space the remaining daily dosage evenly throughout the day. Go back to your regular schedule the next day. Call your doctor if you miss more than 1 dose.

Special Populations

Pregnancy/Breast-feeding

The safety of using tacrine during pregnancy is not known. When this drug is considered crucial by your doctor, its potential benefits must be carefully weighed against its risks.

It is not known if tacrine passes into breast milk. Nursing mothers who must take it should bottle-feed.

Seniors

Seniors with liver disease are more likely to experience severe side effects.

Generic Name

Tacrolimus (tak-ROE-lim-us)

Brand Name

Prograf

Type of Drug

Immunosuppressant.

Prescribed for

Organ transplantation.

General Information

Formerly known as FK506, tacrolimus is derived from a bacterium and is used to prevent the rejection of transplanted organs. The drug is used in liver transplants and has been studied in kidney, bone marrow, heart, pancreas, and small bowel transplants, among others. Tacrolimus works by blocking the activity of T-cells, which protect the body against invading microorganisms or foreign substances, producing immune-system suppression.

Cautions and Warnings

Transplant patients who are **sensitive** or **allergic** to tacrolimus should be given another drug. Some people may also be allergic to chemically modified castor oil, which is used in tacrolimus injection.

Tacrolimus may cause **kidney damage,** especially when taken in high dosages. This effect has been seen in 33% to 40% of liver transplant patients. To avoid excess kidney damage, this drug should not be taken with cyclosporine (an organ transplant drug). Administration of these drugs should be separated by at least 24 hours.

About 10% to 44% of liver transplant patients who take tacrolimus develop mild elevations of blood potassium.

Tremors, headaches, muscle function changes, changes in mental state and sense perception, or other nervous system problems occur in about half of the people receiving liver transplants. **Seizure** has also occurred. In some cases, these side effects may be associated with large amounts of tacrolimus in the blood.

As with other immune suppressants, people taking tacrolimus have an increased risk of developing a **lymphoma or other malignancy**. The risk increases with the degree of immune suppression and the length of time that the drug is taken. A disorder related to **Epstein-Barr virus** (EBV) infection has also been reported.

People with **kidney disease** should receive lower dosages. People who experience post-transplant reduction in liver function may develop kidney damage. Mild to moderate **high blood pressure** is a common side effect of tacrolimus and may be a sign of kidney damage. People taking this drug should measure their blood pressure regularly.

Possible Side Effects

▼ Most common: headache, tremors, sleeplessness, tingling in the hands or feet, diarrhea, nausea, constipation, appetite loss, vomiting, liver or kidney abnormalities, high blood pressure, urinary infection, infrequent urination, anemia, increased white-blood-cell counts, reduced blood-platelet counts, changes in blood-potassium level, reduced blood magnesium, high blood sugar, fluid in the lungs and other lung problems, breathing difficulties, itching, rash, abdominal pain, pain, fever, weakness, back pain, abdominal-fluid buildup, and retention of fluid.

▼ Less common: abnormal dreaming, anxiety, confusion, depression, dizziness, instability, hallucination, poor coordination, muscle spasms, psychosis, tiredness, unusual thoughts, double vision or other visual

Possible Side Effects *(continued)*

disturbances, ringing or buzzing in the ears, upset stomach, yellowing of the skin or whites of the eyes, difficulty swallowing, gas, stomach bleeding, fungal infection of the mouth, blood in the urine, chest pain, rapid heartbeat, low blood pressure, diabetes, black-and-blue marks, muscle and joint aches, leg cramps, muscle weakness, asthma, bronchitis, coughing, sore throat, pneumonia, stuffy and runny nose, sinus irritation, voice changes, sweating, and herpes infection.

Drug Interactions

• Tacrolimus should not be taken at the same time as other immune suppressants so as to avoid excessive suppression of the immune system.

• Tacrolimus may cause more kidney damage when combined with other drugs that also cause kidney problems including aminoglycoside antibiotics, amphotericin B, cisplatin, and cyclosporine.

• Antifungal drugs, bromocriptine, calcium channel blockers, cimetidine, clarithromycin, danazol, diltiazem, erythromycin, methylprednisolone, and metoclopramide may increase tacrolimus blood levels and side effects.

• Carbamazepine, phenobarbital, phenytoin, rifampin, and rifampicin may reduce tacrolimus blood levels.

• Vaccination may be less effective during tacrolimus use. Live vaccines such as those for measles, mumps, rubella, oral polio, and BCG should be avoided.

Food Interactions

Take this drug at least 1 hour before or 2 hours after meals.

Usual Dose

Adult and Child: 0.075–0.15 mg per lb. of body weight a day divided into 2 doses. Children may require more than adults. Dosing is usually started at higher dosage and then reduced to the lowest effective level.

Overdosage

Overdose is likely to produce severe side effects. Take the victim to a hospital emergency room. ALWAYS bring the prescription bottle or container.

Special Information

It is extremely important to take this drug exactly as prescribed. If you forget a dose, take it as soon as you remember. If it is almost time for your next dose, skip the forgotten
dose and continue with your regular schedule. Do not take a
double dose. Call your doctor if you forget 2 or more doses
in a row.

People taking tacrolimus require regular testing to monitor
their progress.

Call your doctor at the first sign of fever; sore throat; tiredness; weakness; nervousness; unusual bleeding or bruising;
tender or swollen gums; convulsions; irregular heartbeat;
confusion; numbness or tingling of your hands, feet, or lips;
breathing difficulties; severe stomach pain with nausea; or
blood in the urine. Other side effects should be brought to
your doctor's attention.

Maintain good dental hygiene while taking tacrolimus
and use extra care when brushing and flossing because the
drug increases your risk of oral infection. See your dentist
regularly.

Tacrolimus should be continued as long as prescribed by
your doctor. Do not stop taking it because of side effects or
other problems. If you cannot tolerate the oral form, this drug
may be given by injection, though the oral capsules are
preferable.

Special Populations

Pregnancy/Breast-feeding

Tacrolimus passes into the fetal circulation, and in animals
causes miscarriage, birth defects, and reduced fertility. In
humans, babies born to mothers taking this drug have had
high blood potassium and poor kidney function. When this
drug is considered crucial by your doctor, its potential benefits must be carefully weighed against its risks.

Tacrolimus passes into breast milk. Nursing mothers who
must take tacrolimus should bottle-feed.

Seniors

Seniors may require reduced dosage due to loss of kidney
function.

Generic Name

Tamoxifen Citrate (tuh-MOX-ih-fen SYE-trate) Ⓖ

Brand Name

Nolvadex

The information in this profile also applies to the following drug:

Generic Ingredient: Toremifene Citrate
Fareston

Type of Drug

Anti-estrogen.

Prescribed for

Breast cancer. Tamoxifen is also used for painful breasts in women; swollen or painful breasts and breast cancer in men; and pancreatic, endometrial, and liver cell cancer.

General Information

Tamoxifen is effective in treating estrogen-positive breast cancer in women. It works by blocking the effects of estrogen in breast tissue. When used together with chemotherapy after mastectomy, tamoxifen can prevent or delay the recurrence of breast cancer. It is used to treat metastatic breast cancer (that which has spread) and to prevent breast cancer in women at high risk. Up to 60% of women whose breast cancer has metastasized may benefit from taking tamoxifen. Toremifene is used only to treat breast cancer, not to prevent it.

Cautions and Warnings

Visual difficulties have occurred in people taking tamoxifen for 1 year or more in dosages at least 4 times above the maximum recommended dosage. A few cases of decreased visual clarity and other vision problems have been reported at normal dosages.

People taking tamoxifen have experienced **liver inflammation** and, rarely, more serious liver abnormalities. Very high dosages of this drug (15 mg per lb. of body weight) may cause **liver cancer**.

Possible Side Effects

Side effects are generally mild. Lowering drug dosage can sometimes control severe reactions.

▼ Most common: hot flashes, weight changes, fluid retention, vaginal discharge, menstrual changes, and nausea. Increased bone and tumor pain sometimes occur shortly after starting tamoxifen. These may be a sign of a good response to the drug and usually decline rapidly.

▼ Less common: vomiting, vaginal bleeding, skin changes, and kidney problems.

▼ Rare: high blood-calcium levels, swelling of the arms or legs, changes in sense of taste, vaginal itching, depression, dizziness, light-headedness, headache, visual difficulties, and reduced white-blood-cell or platelet count. Ovarian cysts have occurred in premenopausal women with advanced breast cancer who took tamoxifen.

Drug Interactions

• The effects of warfarin and other anticoagulant (blood-thinning) drugs may be increased by tamoxifen. Tamoxifen may increase blood-calcium levels.

• Bromocriptine may increase tamoxifen blood levels.

Food Interactions

Tamoxifen may be taken with food or milk if it upsets your stomach.

Usual Dose

Tamoxifen: 10–20 mg in the morning and evening.

Toremifene: 60 mg once a day.

Overdosage

Symptoms may include breathing difficulties, convulsions, tremors, overactive reflexes, dizziness, and unsteadiness. Take the victim to a hospital emergency room. ALWAYS bring the prescription bottle or container.

Special Information

Take this medication according to your doctor's directions. Inform your doctor if you become very weak or sleepy or if you experience confusion, pain, swelling of the legs, breathing difficulties, blurred vision, bone pain, hot flashes, nausea or vomiting, weight gain, irregular periods, dizziness, headache, or appetite loss. Call your doctor if you vomit shortly after taking a dose of tamoxifen. Your doctor may tell you to take another dose immediately or wait until the next dose.

Women taking tamoxifen should use a condom, diaphragm, or other non-hormonal contraceptive during sexual intercourse until treatment is complete.

If you forget a dose, call your doctor. If you cannot reach your doctor, skip the forgotten dose and continue your regular schedule. Do not take a double dose.

Special Populations

Pregnancy/Breast-feeding
Tamoxifen can harm the fetus and cause vaginal bleeding and spontaneous abortion. It should not be taken by any pregnant women. Women of childbearing age taking tamoxifen must use barrier contraception to prevent pregnancy. Contact your doctor at once if you think you may be pregnant.

It is not known if tamoxifen passes into breast milk. Nursing mothers who must take it should bottle-feed.

Seniors
Seniors may take tamoxifen without special restriction.

Generic Name

Tamsulosin (tam-SUE-loe-sin)

Brand Name

Flomax

Type of Drug

Alpha blocker.

Prescribed for

Benign prostatic hyperplasia (BPH).

General Information

Tamsulosin hydrochloride and similar drugs block nerve endings known as alpha$_1$ receptors. In BPH, tamsulosin works by relaxing smooth muscles in the prostate and neck of the bladder. This effect is produced by blocking alpha$_1$ receptors in the affected muscles. Despite the fact that tamsulosin alleviates the urinary symptoms of BPH, the drug's long-term effect on complications of BPH or the need for urinary surgery is not known. Alpha blockers are broken down in the liver.

Cautions and Warnings

Tamsulosin may cause **dizziness and fainting,** especially after the first few doses. This is known as the first-dose effect and may be minimized by limiting the first dose to 1 mg at bedtime. The first-dose effect occurs in about 1% of people and may recur if the drug is stopped for a few days and then restarted.

Do not take this drug if you are **allergic** or **sensitive** to any alpha blocker.

Tamsulosin may slightly reduce **cholesterol levels** and improve the high-density lipoprotein (HDL)/low-density lipoprotein (LDL) ratio, a positive step for people with blood-cholesterol problems.

Red- and white-blood-cell counts may be slightly reduced by other alpha blockers. This effect should be monitored in people taking tamsulosin.

Possible Side Effects

▼ Most common: dizziness, weakness, and headache.

▼ Less common: low blood pressure; rapid heartbeat; abnormal heart rhythms; chest pain; flushing in the face, arms, or legs; fainting; vomiting; dry mouth; diarrhea; constipation; abdominal pain or discomfort; gas; breathing difficulties; stuffy nose; sinus inflammation; cold or flu-like symptoms; cough; bronchitis; worsening of asthma; nosebleed; sore throat; runny nose; shoulder, neck, or back pain; pain in the arms or legs; joint pain; arthritis; muscle pain; blurred vision or other visual disturbances; conjunctivitis (pinkeye); eye pain; nervousness; tingling in the hands or feet; tiredness; anxiety; difficulty sleeping; frequent urination; urinary infection; itching; rash; sweating; swelling of the face, arms, or legs; and fever.

▼ Rare: depression, reduced sex drive or abnormal sexual function, fluid retention, and weight gain.

Drug Interactions

• Tamsulosin may interact with beta-blocking drugs to produce a higher rate of dizziness or fainting after taking the first dose of tamsulosin.

• The blood-pressure-lowering effect of tamsulosin may be reduced by indomethacin.

• When taken with blood-pressure-lowering drugs, tamsulosin produces severe reduction of blood pressure.

• The blood-pressure-lowering effect of clonidine may be reduced by tamsulosin.

Food Interactions

None known.

Usual Dose

Starting dosage—0.4 mg a half hour after the same meal each day. Dosage may be increased by 0.8 mg a day if there has been no response after 2 weeks.

Overdosage

Symptoms may include severe side effects. Take the victim to a hospital emergency room at once. ALWAYS bring the prescription bottle or container.

Special Information

Take tamsulosin exactly as prescribed and do not stop taking it unless directed to do so by your doctor. Avoid over-the-counter drugs that contain stimulants because they may increase your blood pressure.

Tamsulosin may cause dizziness, headache, and drowsiness, especially 2 to 6 hours after you take your first dose, though these effects may persist after the first few doses. Wait 12 to 24 hours after taking the first dose before driving or doing any task that requires concentration. You should take it at bedtime to minimize this problem.

Call your doctor if you develop severe dizziness, heart palpitations, or any bothersome or persistent side effect.

If you forget a dose, take it as soon as you remember. If it is almost time for your next dose, skip the forgotten dose and continue with your regular schedule. If you forget your medication for several days in a row, you will have to begin again at the lower dosage of 0.4 mg a day regardless of the dosage you were taking before.

Special Populations

Pregnancy/Breast-feeding
Tamsulosin is intended only for men. The safety of using tamsulosin during pregnancy and breast-feeding is not known.

Seniors
Seniors may be more sensitive to the action and side effects of tamsulosin.

Generic Name

Tazarotene (tuh-ZAR-oe-tene)

Brand Name

Tazorac

Type of Drug

Anti-acne.

Prescribed for

Mild to moderate acne, and psoriasis. Also, prescribed for actinic keratosis.

General Information

Tazarotene is converted to its active form after it is applied to the skin. A retinoid related to vitamin A, tazarotene is in the same family as retinoic acid—the active ingredient in Retin-A anti-acne products.

Cautions and Warnings

Women who are or might be **pregnant** should not use this drug.

Tazarotene may cause a temporary **burning** or **stinging** sensation. It may cause severe burning if applied to eczema. Other skin medications and makeup can make the skin very dry and should be avoided while you are using tazarotene. It may also be advisable to "rest" your skin between using other drugs or makeup and starting tazarotene.

Tazarotene can cause **rash, allergy,** or a severe **toxic reaction,** especially if used together with another drug that sensi-

tizes the skin such as a tetracycline antibiotic, a fluoroquinolone, or a phenothiazine tranquilizer.

Possible Side Effects

▼ Most common: peeling skin, a burning or stinging
sensation, dry skin, redness, and itching.

▼ Common: irritation, skin pain, cracking, swelling,
and skin discoloration.

Drug Interactions

None known.

Usual Dose

Adult: Gently clean your face and apply a thin layer of
tazarotene to the affected area every evening.

Overdosage

Accidental ingestion of tazarotene may cause symptoms similar to vitamin A overdose. Call your local poison control center for information about what to do in the case of tazarotene
ingestion.

Special Information

If skin irritation, redness, itching, or peeling is excessive, stop
using tazarotene until your skin is completely healed.
Extreme wind or cold may worsen skin irritation.

Applying excessive amounts of tazarotene to your skin can
cause redness, peeling skin, or other discomfort.

Special Populations

Pregnancy/Breast-feeding

Tazarotene caused birth defects in lab animals. Women who
are or might be pregnant should not use this drug.

It is not known if tazarotene passes into breast milk. Nursing mothers should be aware when using this drug that some
may be passed on to their babies.

Seniors

Seniors may use this drug without special restriction.

Generic Name

Terazosin (ter-AY-zoe-sin) Ⓖ

Brand Name

Hytrin

Type of Drug

Alpha blocker.

Prescribed for

High blood pressure and benign prostatic hyperplasia (BPH).

General Information

Terazosin and similar drugs block nerve endings known as alpha$_1$ receptors. Terazosin lowers blood pressure by dilating (widening) blood vessels and reducing pressure within them. The maximum blood-pressure-lowering effect of terazosin is seen between 2 and 6 hours after taking a single dose. Terazosin's effect lasts for 24 hours.

In BPH, terazosin works by relaxing smooth muscles in the prostate and neck of the bladder. This effect is produced by blockage of alpha$_1$ receptors in the affected muscles. Despite the fact that terazosin alleviates the urinary symptoms of BPH, the drug's long-term effect on complications of BPH or the need for urinary surgery is not known. Alpha blockers are broken down in the liver.

Cautions and Warnings

Terazosin may cause **dizziness and fainting,** especially after the first few doses. This is known as the first-dose effect and may be minimized by limiting the first dose to 1 mg at bedtime. The first-dose effect occurs in about 1% of people and may recur if the drug is stopped for a few days and then restarted.

Do not take this drug if you are **allergic** or **sensitive** to any alpha blocker.

Terazosin may slightly reduce **cholesterol levels** and improve the high-density lipoprotein (HDL)/low-density lipoprotein (LDL) ratio, a positive step for people with blood-cholesterol problems.

Red- and white-blood-cell counts may be slightly reduced by terazosin.

People taking terazosin may experience a weight gain of about 2 lbs.

Possible Side Effects

▼ Most common: dizziness, weakness, and headache.

▼ Less common: low blood pressure; rapid heartbeat; abnormal heart rhythms; chest pain; flushing in the face, arms, or legs; fainting; vomiting; dry mouth; diarrhea; constipation; abdominal pain or discomfort; gas; breathing difficulties; stuffy nose; sinus inflammation; cold or flu-like symptoms; cough; bronchitis; worsening of asthma; nosebleed; sore throat; runny nose; shoulder, neck, or back pain; pain in the arms or legs; joint pain; arthritis; muscle pain; blurred vision or other visual disturbances; conjunctivitis (pinkeye); eye pain; nervousness; tingling in the hands or feet; tiredness; anxiety; difficulty sleeping; frequent urination; urinary infection; itching; rash; sweating; swelling of the face, arms, or legs; and fever.

▼ Rare: depression, reduced sex drive or abnormal sexual function, fluid retention, and weight gain.

Drug Interactions

• Terazosin may interact with beta-blocking drugs to produce a higher rate of dizziness or fainting after taking the first dose of terazosin.

• The blood-pressure-lowering effect of terazosin may be reduced by indomethacin.

• When taken with other blood-pressure-lowering drugs, terazosin produces severe reduction of blood pressure.

• The blood-pressure-lowering effect of clonidine may be reduced by terazosin.

Food Interactions

None known.

Usual Dose

Starting dosage—1 mg at bedtime. Dosage may be increased in increments of 1–5 mg to a total of 20–40 mg a day. Terazosin may be taken once or twice a day. Dosages of 10 mg a day are generally needed to control the symptoms of BPH.

Overdosage

Symptoms may include drowsiness, poor reflexes, and very low blood pressure. Take the victim to a hospital emergency room at once. ALWAYS bring the prescription bottle or container.

Special Information

Take terazosin exactly as prescribed and do not stop taking it unless directed to do so by your doctor. Avoid over-the-counter drugs that contain stimulants because they may increase your blood pressure.

Terazosin may cause dizziness, headache, and drowsiness, especially 2 to 6 hours after you take your first dose, though these effects may persist after the first few doses. Wait 12 to 24 hours after taking the first dose before driving or doing any task that requires concentration. You should take it at bedtime to minimize this problem.

Call your doctor if you develop severe dizziness, heart palpitations, or any bothersome or persistent side effect.

If you forget a dose, take it as soon as you remember. If it is almost time for your next dose, skip the forgotten dose and continue with your regular schedule. Never take a double dose.

Special Populations

Pregnancy/Breast-feeding

Large dosages of terazosin damage the fetus in animal studies. When this drug is considered crucial by your doctor, its potential benefits must be carefully weighed against its risks.

It is not known if terazosin passes into breast milk. Nursing mothers who must take it should consider bottle-feeding.

Seniors

Seniors may be more sensitive to the action and side effects of terazosin.

Generic Name

Terbinafine (ter-BIN-uh-feen)

Brand Name

Lamisil

Type of Drug

Antifungal.

Prescribed for

Fungus infections of the skin, fingernails, or toenails.

General Information

Terbinafine hydrochloride is a general-purpose antifungal. It can cure common athlete's foot, jock itch, and ringworm faster than other drugs of this type. It is also effective against *Candida* and other fungal infections of the skin. Terbinafine is unique because it accumulates in the skin and continues to kill fungus organisms even after you stop using it. Most other antifungals do not kill the fungus; they only stop it from growing.

Cautions and Warnings

Do not take this product if you are **allergic** to terbinafine or any other ingredient in the product. **Kidney or liver disease** can increase the amount of terbinafine in your blood by 50%.

Terbinafine cream is only meant to be applied to the skin. Do not put it into your eyes or use it for a vaginal infection. **Do not swallow** terbinafine cream. Only the capsules are meant for oral use.

Terbinafine should be used only for specific fungal infections and only as prescribed. Rarely, people taking terbinafine have experienced severe eyesight changes or a severe drop in **white-blood-cell count,** leading to serious **infection** and fever. Call your doctor if anything unusual develops.

Possible Side Effects

Cream

▼ Most common: itching and irritation of the skin immediately after application.

▼ Less common: burning, irritation, and dryness of the skin.

Possible Side Effects (continued)

Tablets
  ▼ Most common: headache.
  ▼ Common: diarrhea and rash.
  ▼ Less common: upset stomach, abdominal pain, nausea, gas, itching, liver irritation, taste changes, and temporary eyesight changes.
  ▼ Rare: severe reactions of the liver or skin, low white-blood-cell count, and allergic reactions.

Drug Interactions

• Cimetidine and terfenadine increase the amount of terbinafine in the blood.
• Do not combine terbinafine and rifampin.
• Terbinafine may reduce the effect of cyclosporine.
• Terbinafine may increase the effect of caffeine.

Food Interactions

Take terbinafine tablets 1 hour before or 2 hours after eating.

Usual Dose

Cream: Apply to affected areas morning and night for 1–4 weeks.

Tablets: 250 mg a day for 6 or 12 weeks, depending on condition being treated.

Overdosage

Terbinafine overdose may lead to tiredness, poor muscle coordination, breathing difficulties, and bulging of the eyes. Overdose victims should be taken to a hospital emergency room. ALWAYS bring the prescription bottle or container.

Special Information

Do not put terbinafine cream in contact with your eyes, nose, mouth, or any other mucous membrane tissues.
  Do not stop using terbinafine before your prescription is complete, even if your rash clears up. The full prescription may be necessary to eliminate the offending fungus.

Do not cover the cream with plastic wrap or anything else that restricts ventilation unless so instructed by your doctor.

Call your doctor if your skin becomes red, burns, itches, blisters, swells, or if oozing develops.

If you forget to administer a dose, do so as soon as you remember. If it is almost time for your next dose, skip the one you forgot and continue with your regular schedule.

Special Populations

Pregnancy/Breast-feeding

The effect of terbinafine during pregnancy is not known. Women who are pregnant should not use terbinafine because the treatment of toenail or fingernail fungus infections can be postponed until after pregnancy.

Terbinafine passes into breast milk. Nursing mothers who must use this drug should bottle-feed.

Seniors

Seniors may use terbinafine without special restriction.

Generic Name

Terbutaline (ter-BUE-tuh-leen)

Brand Names

Brethaire

Brethine

Bricanyl

Type of Drug

Bronchodilator.

Prescribed for

Asthma, bronchospasm, and premature labor.

General Information

Terbutaline sulfate is similar to other bronchodilator drugs, such as metaproterenol and isoetharine, but it has a weaker effect on nerve receptors in the heart and blood vessels. For this reason, it is somewhat safer for people with heart conditions.

Terbutaline tablets begin to work within 30 minutes and continue working for 4 to 8 hours. Terbutaline inhalation begins working in 5 to 30 minutes and continues for 3 to 6 hours. Terbutaline injection starts working in 5 to 15 minutes and lasts for 1½ to 4 hours.

Cautions and Warnings

Terbutaline should be used with caution by people with a history of **angina pectoris** (condition characterized by brief attacks of chest pain), **heart disease, high blood pressure, stroke, seizure, thyroid disease, prostate disease,** or **glaucoma**.

Using excessive amounts of terbutaline can lead to **increased difficulty breathing** rather than relief. In the most extreme cases, people have had heart attacks after using excessive amounts of inhalant.

Possible Side Effects

▼ Most common: heart palpitations, abnormal heart rhythm, tremors, dizziness and fainting, shakiness, nervousness, tension, drowsiness, headache, nausea and vomiting, and heartburn or upset stomach.

▼ Less common: rapid heartbeat, chest pain and discomfort, angina, weakness, sleeplessness, wheezing, bronchial spasms and difficulty breathing, dry throat, sore or irritated throat, flushing, sweating, and changes in sense of smell and taste.

Drug Interactions

• Terbutaline's effects may be increased by monoamine oxidase inhibitors (MAOIs), tricyclic antidepressants, thyroid drugs, other bronchodilator drugs, and some antihistamines.

• The risk of cardiac toxicity may be increased in people taking both terbutaline and theophylline.

• Terbutaline is antagonized by beta-blocking drugs such as propranolol.

• Terbutaline may antagonize the effects of blood-pressure-lowering drugs, especially reserpine, methyldopa, and guanethidine.

Food Interactions

Terbutaline tablets are more effective when taken on an empty stomach—1 hour before or 2 hours after meals—but can be taken with food if they upset your stomach.

Usual Dose

Inhaler
   Adult and Child (age 12 and over): 1 or 2 puffs every 4–6 hours.

Tablets
   Adult and Child (age 15 and over): 2.5–5 mg every 6 hours, 3 times a day. Do not take more than 15 mg a day.
   Child (age 12–14): 2.5 mg 3 times a day. Do not take more than 7.5 mg a day.
   Child (under age 12): not recommended.

Overdosage

Overdose of terbutaline inhalation usually results in exaggerated side effects, including chest pain and high blood pressure, although blood pressure may drop to a low level after a short period of elevation. People who inhale too much terbutaline should see a doctor.

Overdose of terbutaline tablets is more likely to trigger changes in heart rate, palpitations, unusual heart rhythms, chest pain, high blood pressure, fever, chills, cold sweats, nausea, vomiting, and dilation of the pupils. Convulsions, sleeplessness, anxiety, and tremors may also develop, and the victim may collapse.

If the overdose was taken within the past 30 minutes, give the victim ipecac syrup—available at any pharmacy—to induce vomiting and to remove any remaining medication from the stomach. DO NOT GIVE IPECAC SYRUP IF THE VICTIM IS UNCONSCIOUS OR CONVULSING. If symptoms have already begun to develop, the victim should be taken to a hospital emergency room. ALWAYS bring the prescription bottle or container.

Special Information

If you are inhaling terbutaline, be sure to follow the inhalation instructions that come with the product. The drug should be inhaled during the second half of your inward breath, since this will allow it to reach deeper into your lungs. Wait at least 1 minute between puffs if you use more than 1 puff per dose. Do not inhale terbutaline if you have food or anything else in your mouth.

Do not take more terbutaline than your doctor prescribes. Taking more than you need could actually worsen your symptoms. If your condition worsens rather than improves after taking terbutaline, stop taking it and call your doctor.

Call your doctor immediately if you develop chest pain, palpitations, rapid heartbeat, muscle tremors, dizziness, headache, facial flushing, or urinary difficulty, or if you continue to experience difficulty in breathing after using the medication.

If you forget a dose of terbutaline, take it as soon as you remember. If it is almost time for your next dose, skip the one you forgot and return to your regular schedule. Do not take a double dose.

Special Populations

Pregnancy/Breast-feeding
When used during childbirth, terbutaline can slow or delay labor. Terbutaline should not be taken after the first 3 months of pregnancy: It can cause rapid heartbeat and high blood sugar in the mother, and rapid heartbeat and low blood sugar in the fetus. It is not known if terbutaline causes birth defects in humans, but it has caused defects in pregnant animals. When your doctor considers this drug crucial, its potential benefits must be carefully weighed against its risks.

Terbutaline passes into breast milk. Nursing mothers who must take this drug should consider bottle-feeding.

Seniors
Seniors are more sensitive to the effects of terbutaline. Follow your doctor's directions closely and report any side effects at once.

Generic Name

Terconazole (ter-KON-uh-zole)

Brand Names

| Terazol 3 | Terazol 7 |

Type of Drug

Antifungal.

Prescribed for

Fungal infections of the vagina.

General Information

Terconazole is available as a vaginal cream or suppository. It may also be applied to the skin to treat common fungal infections. Exactly how it works is unknown.

Cautions and Warnings

Do not use terconazole if you are **allergic** to it. Proper diagnosis is essential for effective treatment. Do not use this product without first consulting your doctor.

Possible Side Effects

▼ Most common: headache, which affects 1 in 4 women who use it.

▼ Rare: painful menstruation, genital pain, body pain, abdominal pain, fever, chills, vaginal burning or irritation, and itching. Application of terconazole cream to the skin can cause unusual sensitivity to the sun.

Food and Drug Interactions

None known.

Usual Dose

Vaginal Suppositories or Cream: 1 applicator's worth or 1 suppository into the vagina at bedtime for 3 or 7 days, depending on formulation.

Topical: Apply to affected areas of skin twice a day for up to 1 month.

Overdosage

Terconazole overdose may cause irritation and accidental ingestion may cause upset stomach. Call your local poison control center or hospital emergency room for more information.

Special Information

When using the vaginal cream, insert the whole applicatorful of cream high into the vagina. Be sure to complete the full course of treatment prescribed. Call your doctor if you develop burning or itching.

Refrain from sexual intercourse or use a condom to avoid reinfection while using this product. Using sanitary napkins may keep terconazole from staining your clothing.

If you forget a dose, administer it as soon as you remember. If it is almost time for your next dose, skip the dose you forgot and continue with your regular schedule. Do not administer a double dose.

Special Populations

Pregnancy/Breast-feeding

Pregnant women should avoid using the vaginal cream during the first 3 months of pregnancy; during the last 6 months, it should be used only if absolutely necessary.

Terconazole may cause problems in breast-fed infants. Nursing mothers who must use this drug should bottle-feed.

Seniors

Seniors may take this medication without special restriction.

Generic Name

Testosterone (tes-TOS-ter-one)

Brand Names

Androderm Transdermal System
Testoderm Transdermal System

The information in this profile also applies to the following drug:

Generic Ingredient: Methyltestosterone G
Android-10   Testred
Android-25   Virilon
Oreton Methyl

Type of Drug

Hormone replacement.

Prescribed for

Impotence due to hormone deficiency and testosterone replacement in men who have lost their testicle function or have low blood levels of testosterone. Androgen may be prescribed for boys before they reach puberty to maintain secondary sex characteristics if testosterone is lacking or if puberty is delayed. In women, testosterone may be used to treat metastatic cancer (cancer that has spread from one part of the body to another) and breast enlargement or pain in women who have just given birth.

General Information

Testosterone is the principal androgen (male hormone). In men, testosterone is produced in the testicles. Women make small amounts of testosterone in their ovaries and in the adrenal gland. Testosterone is responsible for the growth and development of male sex organs as well as secondary sex characteristics such as beard, pubic, chest, and underarm hair; vocal cord thickening, which lowers the voice; and muscle and fat distribution. Androgens are also responsible for the adolescent growth spurt.

Weekly testosterone injection of 200 mg, for up to 1 year, has been studied as a reversible male contraceptive.

Cautions and Warnings

The following people should avoid testosterone: **pregnant women, men with breast or prostate cancer,** those who are **allergic** to it, and people with **heart or kidney disease,** who may respond to the drug by retaining fluid.

Some athletes have taken testosterone in order to improve performance, but this is unsafe and ineffective. Male hormones may cause very **high blood calcium levels** in women with breast cancer and in people who are immobilized; these groups should avoid taking testosterone. Continuous use of high dosages of male hormones may cause life-threatening **liver problems**. Taking male hormones for an extended period of time causes **reduced sperm count and semen volume**.

Men taking testosterone as hormone replacement may develop **enlarged breasts**.

Sometimes, people taking male hormones develop a condition called **acute intermittent porphyria** (symptoms include abdominal pain, nausea and vomiting, constipation, neurotic or psychotic behavior, and nerve irritation).

Blood **cholesterol** may rise while you are taking testosterone. People with heart disease; those who have had a stroke or transient ischemic attack (TIA)—"mini-stroke;" and those who have blood vessel disease, such as claudication, should be cautious about taking a male hormone.

A man using a **scrotal testosterone patch** may transfer some hormone to his sexual partner, which may result in unwanted changes in the partner's secondary sex characteristics.

Testosterone must be used with caution in **children**. They should be treated only by specialists who are experienced with testosterone and understand its effects on children's bone development.

Possible Side Effects

▼ Most common: women—menstrual irregularities, a deepening voice, hairiness, acne, and enlargement of the clitoris. Men—breast soreness or enlargement and excessive erections.

▼ Common: men and women—swelling of the feet or lower legs, rapid weight gain, dizziness, headache, tiredness, flushing or redness, bleeding, nausea, vomiting, yellowing of the skin or whites of the eyes, confusion, depression, thirst, increased urination, and constipation. Men—chills, pain in the scrotum or groin, prostate cancer, and difficult urination.

▼ Less common: men and women—mild acne, diarrhea, increased pubic hair, and difficulty sleeping. Men—impotence, irritation or infection of the skin of the scrotum, and decreased testicle size.

▼ Rare: men and women—male pattern baldness, oily skin, jaundice, and changes in liver function tests.

Drug Interactions

• Testosterone may increase the effects of anticoagulants (blood thinners) such as warfarin.

• Combining testosterone and imipramine (an antidepressant) may lead to a paranoid reaction.

• Testosterone may interfere with laboratory tests of thyroid function; it does not affect the thyroid gland or normal thyroid function.

Food Interactions

You may take this drug with food if it upsets your stomach. Food does not interfere with testosterone skin patches.

Usual Dose

Oral Tablets
  Men: 10–30 mg a day.
  Women: 50–200 mg a day.

Skin Patches
Apply nightly. Testoderm patches should be placed on clean dry skin of the scrotum. Androderm is applied to clean dry skin on your back, abdomen, upper arm, or thigh. Androderm dosage starts at 2 patches a night. Dosage may be adjusted to 1 or 3 patches nightly.

Overdosage

Symptoms resemble drug side effects. Call your local poison control center or a hospital emergency room for more information. If you seek treatment, ALWAYS bring the prescription package or container.

Special Information

If you are using a testosterone skin patch, apply it as directed by your doctor.

Take this drug exactly as prescribed. If you forget a dose, take it as soon as possible. If it is almost time for your next dose, skip the dose you forgot and continue with your regular schedule. Do not take a double dose.

Special Populations

Pregnancy/Breast-feeding

Testosterone is not safe for use during pregnancy. Taking this drug during pregnancy, especially during the first 3 months, results in excessive masculinization of the fetus.

It is not known if testosterone passes into breast milk. Nursing mothers who must take it should bottle-feed.

Seniors

Seniors who take testosterone may have an increased risk of developing prostate disease, including cancer. A marked increase in sex drive may also develop.

Type of Drug

Tetracycline Antibiotics (TEH-tra-SIKE-lene)

Brand Names

Generic Ingredient: Demeclocycline
Declomycin

Generic Ingredient: Doxycycline [G]

Bio-Tab	Monodox
Doryx	Periostat
Doxy Caps	Vibramycin
Doxychel Hyclate	Vibra-Tabs

Generic Ingredient: Meclocycline Sulfosalicylate
Meclan

Generic Ingredient: Minocycline Hydrochloride [G]

Dynacin	Vectrin
Minocin	

Generic Ingredient: Oxytetracycline [G]

Terramycin	Uri-Tet

Generic Ingredient: Tetracycline Hydrochloride [G]

Ala-Tet	Tetracap
Nor-Tet	Tetracyn
Panmycin	Tetralan
Sumycin	Topicycline

Prescribed for

Infection including gonorrhea; infection of the mouth, gums, and teeth; Rocky Mountain spotted fever and other types of fever caused by ticks and lice including Lyme disease; urinary tract infection; and respiratory infection such as pneumonia or bronchitis. Doxycycline has been prescribed to treat and prevent traveler's diarrhea. Tetracycline hydrochloride has been used to treat amebic dysentery.

General Information

Tetracycline antibiotics are effective against a variety of bacterial infection. They work by interfering with the normal growth cycle of the invading bacteria, preventing reproduction. This allows the body's normal defenses to fight off the infection. This process is described as bacteriostatic (inhibiting bacterial growth). Tetracycline may be substituted for penicillin in people who are allergic to it.

They have been successfully used to treat skin infection but are not considered the first-choice antibiotic. Tetracycline hydrochloride and meclocycline have been used successfully in the treatment of adolescent acne, in low dosages over a long period of time.

Cautions and Warnings

Tetracycline should not be given to people with **liver disease** or **kidney or urinary problems**.

If the antibiotic that your doctor has prescribed does not work, a number of things may have happened. You may not have taken the drug long enough. You may be the victim of a superinfection, in which another organism—usually a fungus—unaffected by the tetracycline antibiotic begins to grow in the same area as the bacteria being treated. If this happens, it may seem like a relapse or new infection. Only your doctor can determine which drug to take for it.

Avoid prolonged **exposure to the sun** if you are taking high dosages of tetracycline, especially demeclocycline, because these antibiotics may interfere with your body's normal sunscreening mechanism, making you more prone to severe sunburn.

If you are **allergic** to any tetracycline antibiotic, you are probably allergic to them all. Do not use tetracycline if you are allergic to it.

Tetracycline should not be used by **children under age 8** because they have been shown to interfere with the development of the long bones and may retard growth. Permanent tooth discoloration may also result.

People taking demeclocycline may experience **diabetes insipidus syndrome** (symptoms include excessive thirst, urination, and weakness). The severity of this condition depends on the amount of drug taken and is reversible when the drug is withdrawn.

Minocycline may cause **light-headedness, dizziness,** or **fainting**.

Tetracycline has been associated with **pseudotumor cerebri** (condition characterized by increased pressure in the brain—symptoms include headache and blurred vision).

Possible Side Effects

▼ Most common: upset stomach, nausea, vomiting, diarrhea, and rash.

▼ Less common: hairy tongue and itching and irritation of the anal or vaginal region. If these symptoms appear, call your doctor immediately. Periodic physical examinations and laboratory tests should be given to those who are on long-term tetracycline therapy.

▼ Rare: appetite loss, peeling skin, sensitivity to the sun, fever, chills, anemia, brown spotting of the skin, reduced kidney function, and liver damage.

Drug Interactions

• Tetracycline may interfere with bactericidal (bacteria-killing) agents such as penicillin. You should not take both kinds of antibiotics for the same infection.

• Antacids, mineral supplements, and multivitamins containing bismuth, calcium, zinc, magnesium, or iron may reduce the effectiveness of tetracycline—with the exception of doxycycline and minocycline. Sodium bicarbonate powder may also be a problem if used as an antacid. Separate doses of an antacid, mineral supplement, vitamin with minerals, or sodium bicarbonate and a tetracycline antibiotic by at least 2 hours.

• Tetracycline may increase the effect of anticoagulant (blood-thinning) drugs such as warfarin. Your anticoagulant dosage may need an adjustment.

• Barbiturates, carbamazepine, and hydantoin antiseizure drugs may reduce doxycycline's effectiveness. More doxycycline or a different antibiotic may be required.

• Cimetidine, ranitidine, and other H_2-antagonists may reduce the effectiveness of tetracycline.

• Tetracycline may increase digoxin side effects in a small number of people. This effect may last for months after the tetracycline has been withdrawn. If you are taking this combination, be vigilant for the appearance of digoxin side effects; call your doctor if they develop.

• Tetracycline may reduce insulin requirements for diabetics. If you are using this combination, be sure to carefully monitor your blood-sugar level.

• Tetracycline may increase or decrease blood-lithium levels.

• These drugs may reduce the effectiveness of oral contraceptives ("the pill"). Breakthrough bleeding or pregnancy is possible; you should use another method of contraception in addition to an oral contraceptive while taking one of these antibiotics.

Food Interactions

Take all tetracycline antibiotics, except for doxycycline and minocycline, on an empty stomach, 1 hour before or 2 hours after meals and with 8 oz. of water. The antibacterial effect of these antibiotics may be neutralized when they are taken with food, dairy products such as milk or cheese, or antacids. Doxycycline and minocycline may be taken with food or milk.

Usual Dose

Demeclocycline
 Adult: 600 mg a day.
 Child (age 9 and over): 3–6 mg per lb. of body weight a day.
 Child (under age 9): not recommended.

Doxycycline Hydrochloride
 Adult and Child (age 9 and over, and over 100 lbs.): starting dosage—200 mg in 2 doses of 100 mg given 12 hours apart. Maintenance dosage—100 mg a day in 1 or 2 doses. For gonorrhea, take 300 mg in 1 dose and then a second 300-mg dose in 1 hour; for syphilis, 300 mg a day for not less than 10 days.
 Child (age 9 and over, but under 100 lbs.): starting dosage—2 mg per lb. of body weight divided into 2 doses. Maintenance dosage—1 mg per lb. of body weight as a single daily dose.

Your doctor may double the maintenance dosage for severe infection. An increased incidence of side effects is observed with dosages over 200 mg a day.

Meclocycline Sulfosalicylate
Apply to affected area morning and night.

Minocycline Hydrochloride
 Adult: starting dosage—200 mg. Maintenance dosage—100 mg every 12 hours. Alternate dosage: starting dosage—100-200 mg. Maintenance dosage—50 mg 4 times a day.
 Child (age 9 and over): starting dosage—2 mg per lb. of body weight. Maintenance dosage—1 mg per lb. every 12 hours.
 Child (under age 9): not recommended.

Oxytetracycline and Oral Tetracycline Hydrochloride
   Adult: 250–500 mg 4 times a day.
   Child (age 9 and over): 10–20 mg per lb. of body weight a day in 4 equal doses.
   Child (under age 9): not recommended.

Tetracycline Hydrochloride Ointment and Solution
Apply to affected area morning and night.

Overdosage

Overdose is most likely to affect the stomach and digestive system. Call your local poison control center or a hospital emergency room for more information. ALWAYS bring the prescription bottle or container if you go for treatment.

Special Information

Do not take any antibiotic after the expiration date on the label. Decomposed tetracycline may cause serious kidney damage.

   Since the action of tetracycline depends on its concentration within the invading bacteria, it is imperative that you completely follow the doctor's directions and complete the full course of treatment prescribed.

   Call your doctor if you develop excessive thirst, urination, and weakness; blue-gray discoloration of the skin or mucous membranes (with minocycline); appetite loss; headache; vomiting; changes in vision; abdominal pain with nausea and vomiting; yellowing of the skin or whites of the eyes; or any persistent or intolerable side effect including dizziness, light-headedness, or unsteadiness; burning or cramps in the stomach; diarrhea with nausea and vomiting; or itching of the mouth, rectal, or vaginal areas (may indicate the presence of a superinfection). Call your doctor if your child develops tooth discoloration.

   Avoid excessive exposure to the sun while taking tetracycline, especially demeclocycline, because these drugs may cause susceptibility to sunburn.

   Tetracycline may cause dizziness, light-headedness, or fainting. Be careful when driving or performing any task that requires concentration.

   If you are using tetracycline hydrochloride topical solution or meclocycline sulfosalicylate for acne, apply the product generously to your skin until the area to be treated is completely wet. Stinging or burning may occur but this lasts only a few minutes. Tetracycline hydrochloride solution may stain your skin yellow but the stain usually washes away. Do not apply the solution or cream inside your eyes, nose, or mouth.

If you miss a dose of oral tetracycline, take it as soon as possible. If you take the drug once a day and it is almost time for your next dose, space the missed dose and your next dose 10 to 12 hours apart, then go back to your regular schedule. If you take tetracycline twice a day and it is almost time for your next dose, space the missed dose and your next dose by 5 to 6 hours, then go back to your regular schedule. If you take the drug 3 or more times a day and it is almost time for your next dose, space the missed dose and your next dose by 2 to 4 hours, then go back to your regular schedule. Never take a double dose.

Special Populations

Pregnancy/Breast-feeding

Tetracycline should not be taken if you are pregnant, especially during the last 5 months of pregnancy. It interferes with the formation of skull and bone structures in the fetus.

Tetracycline passes into breast milk. It interferes with the development of a child's skull, bones, and teeth. Nursing mothers who must take tetracycline should bottle-feed.

Seniors

Seniors, especially those with poor kidney function, are more likely to suffer from less common side effects.

Generic Name

Thalidomide (thal-IH-doe-mide)

Brand Name

Thalomid

Type of Drug

Immune-system modulator.

Prescribed for

Erythema nodosum leprosum (ENL)—a painful skin condition associated with leprosy.

General Information

Thalidomide was first introduced in the early 1960s as a mild sedative. It was found to cause birth defects and was quickly removed from the market. Thalidomide was never released for prescription in the United States as a sedative but it was finally approved by the Food and Drug Administration (FDA) in 1998 for ENL under a very strict distribution system called S.T.E.P.S. (System for Thalidomide Education Prescription Safety). Only doctors who are registered with the S.T.E.P.S. program can prescribe thalidomide. The exact way that thalidomide works is not known, but it appears to suppress excessive amounts of tumor necrosis factor (TFN) and also affects the movement of white blood cells. Thalidomide is also being studied for leprosy, scleroderma and other skin conditions, and prostate and other cancers. It has been used for severe weight loss, especially in people with acquired immunodeficiency syndrome (AIDS), but does not appear to be effective.

Cautions and Warnings

As little as 1 dose of thalidomide can cause **birth defects**. It should not be taken by pregnant women under any circumstances. Women who might become pregnant should consider taking thalidomide only if other treatments have failed. Men taking thalidomide can also transmit the drug to the fetus. To protect the health of the fetus, these men should use a condom during intercourse with a pregnant partner; using 2 methods of barrier contraception is preferred.

A **drug sensitivity or allergic reaction** to thalidomide (symptoms include rash, fever, rapid heartbeat, and low blood pressure) may be cause to temporarily stop your treatment.

Thalidomide should not be used as the sole treatment for ENL by people with **neuritis** (nerve irritation).

Thalidomide frequently causes **nerve damage** (symptoms include numbness, tingling, or pain in the hands or feet) that may be permanent. It generally occurs after a few months of regular treatment but can also develop after taking thalidomide for a short time.

Thalidomide can cause a rapid drop in white-blood-cell count, increasing the risk of **infection**.

Thalidomide can increase the level of HIV RNA in people with AIDS, but the importance of this finding is unclear.

Thalidomide is generally not recommended for *children under age 18,* though a small number of children have been safely treated with the drug.

Possible Side Effects

▼ Most common: tiredness, fainting, headache, and stomach pain.

▼ Common: muscle weakness; tingling, burning, numbness, or pain in the hands, arms, feet, or legs; rash; dizziness; tremors; constipation; diarrhea; nausea; mouth infections; sinus irritation; back pain; fever, alone or with chills and sore throat; infections; and feeling unwell.

▼ Less common: dry mouth, liver inflammation, gas, dry skin, mood change, leg swelling, acne, fungal skin infections, nail problems, itching, sweating, loss of appetite, tooth pain, impotence, anemia, low white-blood-cell count, swollen lymph glands, runny nose, abdominal pain, accidental injuries, and a rigid or painful neck.

▼ Rare: blood in the urine, decreased urination, irregular heartbeat, low blood pressure, and agitation. Other rare side effects can occur in almost any part of the body. Contact your doctor if you experience any side effect not listed above.

Drug Interactions

• Combining thalidomide with alcohol, barbiturates, chlorpromazine, reserpine, sedatives, tricyclic antidepressants, tranquilizers, or other nervous system depressants can cause extreme tiredness. Avoid this combination.

• Combining thalidomide and chloramphenicol, cisplatin, dapsone, didanosine, ethambutol, ethionamide, hydralazine, isoniazid, lithium, metronidazole, nitrofurantoin, nitrous oxide, phenytoin, stavudine, vincristine, or zalcitabine may worsen peripheral neuropathy (symptoms include tingling, burning, numbness, or pain in the hands or feet) or increase your risk of developing it.

Food Interactions

For optimal effectiveness, do not take thalidomide with a high-fat meal.

Usual Dose

Adult: 100–400 mg a day.

Overdosage

Symptoms are likely to be common side effects. Take the victim to a hospital emergency room. ALWAYS bring the prescription bottle or container.

Special Information

Women of childbearing age who take thalidomide should have weekly pregnancy tests. Women with irregular periods may have to be tested every 2 weeks. Stop taking the drug at once if you are or think you may be pregnant.

Medications that interfere with oral contraceptives ("the pill") must be avoided if you are taking thalidomide because they increase the risk of an unwanted pregnancy. These drugs include protease inhibitor—used in the treatment of human immunodeficiency virus (HIV) infection; griseofulvin; rifampin; rifabutin; phenytoin; and carbamazepine.

Drowsiness is common with thalidomide. Be careful when driving or performing any task that requires concentration.

Thalidomide can make you dizzy or faint if you rise suddenly from a lying position. Sitting up for a few minutes before attempting to stand may help prevent this problem.

Thalidomide can increase your sensitivity to the sun. Use sunscreen and wear protective clothing while taking this drug.

Take this drug exactly as prescribed. Do not stop taking it without your doctor's knowledge.

If you forget a dose, take it as soon as you remember. If it is almost time for your next dose, skip the one you forgot and continue with your regular schedule. Do not take a double dose.

Special Populations

Pregnancy/Breast-feeding

Women who are or might be pregnant should never take thalidomide, especially during the first 2 months of pregnancy. Women of childbearing age who take thalidomide should use 2 reliable methods of contraception (for example, an oral contraceptive and a condom). Contraception must be used for at least 1 month before treatment is begun, during treatment, and for 1 month after treatment has been completed.

It is not known if thalidomide passes into breast milk but it could cause serious reactions in a nursing infant. Nursing mothers who must take thalidomide should bottle-feed.

Seniors
Seniors may take this drug without special restrictions.

Type of Drug
Thiazide Diuretics (THYE-uh-zide dye-ur-RET-iks)

Brand Names

Generic Ingredient: Bendroflumethiazide
Naturetin

Generic Ingredient: Benzthiazide
Exna

Generic Ingredient: Chlorothiazide G
Diurigen   Diuril

Generic Ingredient: Chlorthalidone G
Hygroton   Thalitone

Generic Ingredient: Hydrochlorothiazide G
Esidrix   Hydro-Par
Ezide   Oretic
HydroDIURIL

Generic Ingredient: Hydroflumethiazide G
Diucardin   Saluron

Generic Ingredient: Indapamide G
Lozol

Generic Ingredient: Methyclothiazide G
Aquatensen   Enduron

Generic Ingredient: Metolazone
Mykrox   Zaroxolyn

Generic Ingredient: Polythiazide
Renese

Generic Ingredient: Quinethazone
Hydromox

Generic Ingredient: Trichlormethiazide ☐G
Diurese   Naqua
Metahydrin

Prescribed for

Congestive heart failure (CHF), cirrhosis of the liver, kidney malfunction, hypertension (high blood pressure), and other conditions where it is necessary to rid the body of excess water.

General Information

Thiazide diuretics increase urine production by affecting the movement of sodium and chloride in the kidney. Thiazide diuretics reduce sodium, magnesium, bicarbonate, chloride, and potassium-ion levels. Calcium elimination is moderated and uric acid is retained as a result of thiazide treatment. Thiazide diuretics may also raise blood sugar. These drugs are used in the treatment of any disease where it is desirable to eliminate large quantities of water. Thiazide diuretics are often taken with other drugs to treat high blood pressure and other conditions. The exact way in which they reduce blood pressure is not known; sodium elimination is of primary importance. These diuretics begin to work within 2 hours and produce their effect in 2 to 6 hours. The differences between thiazide diuretic drugs lie in duration of effect—6 to 12 hours for some and as long as 48 to 72 hours for others—and quantity of drug absorbed.

Cautions and Warnings

Do not take a thiazide diuretic if you are **allergic** or **sensitive** to any drugs in this group or to sulfa drugs. If you have a history of allergy or bronchial asthma, you may also have a sensitivity or allergy to thiazide diuretics. Thiazide diuretics may aggravate **lupus erythematosus** (chronic condition affecting the body's connective tissue).

Thiazides may raise total **cholesterol**, low-density lipoprotein (LDL) cholesterol, and total triglyceride levels. They should be used with caution by people with moderate to high blood-cholesterol or triglyceride levels. Thiazides should be used with caution if you have severe **kidney disease** because they may precipitate kidney failure; only metolazone and indapamide may be safely given in this group. People with severe **liver disease** should be treated carefully with diuretics because minor changes in electrolyte (body-fluid) balance may cause hepatic coma.

Switching between brands of metolazone is not recommended. They are not equivalent.

Possible Side Effects

▼ Most common: Thiazide diuretics cause loss of body potassium. Symptoms of low potassium include dry mouth, thirst, weakness, lethargy, drowsiness, restlessness, muscle pain or cramp, muscular tiredness, low blood pressure, decreased frequency of urination and decreased urine production, abnormal heart rate, and upset stomach including nausea and vomiting. Potassium supplements are given to prevent this problem — or you may eat high-potassium foods such as bananas, citrus fruits, melons, and tomatoes.

▼ Less common: appetite loss, abdominal pain, bloating, diarrhea, constipation, dizziness, yellowing of the skin or whites of the eyes, headache, tingling of the toes and fingers, restlessness, changes in blood composition, increased sensitivity to the sun, rash, itching, fever, breathing difficulties, allergic reaction, dizziness when rising quickly from a sitting or lying position, muscle spasm, impotence and reduced sex drive, weakness, and blurred vision.

Drug Interactions

• Thiazide diuretics increase the action of other blood-pressure-lowering drugs. Consequently, people with high blood pressure often take more than 1 drug.

• The risk of developing imbalances in electrolytes is increased if you take medications such as digitalis drugs, amphotericin B, and adrenal corticosteroids while taking a thiazide diuretic.

• If you begin taking a thiazide diuretic, your insulin or antidiabetic dosage may have to be modified.

• Thiazide diuretics may increase the risk of allopurinol side effects.

• Thiazide diuretics may decrease the effects of oral anticoagulant (blood-thinning) drugs.

• Antigout drug dosage may have to be modified since thiazide diuretics raise blood uric-acid levels.

• Thiazide diuretics may prolong the white-blood-cell-reducing effects of chemotherapy drugs.

• Thiazide diuretics may increase the effects of diazoxide, leading to symptoms of diabetes.

• Combining thiazide diuretics and loop diuretics may lead to an extreme diuretic effect and extreme effect on blood-electrolyte levels.

• Thiazide diuretics may increase the action of vitamin D, possibly leading to high blood-calcium levels.

• Propantheline and other anticholinergics may increase the effects of thiazide diuretics.

• Thiazide diuretics increase the risk of lithium side effects.

• Cholestyramine and colestipol block the absorption of thiazide diuretics. Thiazide diuretics should be taken more than 2 hours before cholestyramine or colestipol.

• Methenamine and other urinary agents may reduce the effect of thiazide diuretics.

• Certain nonsteroidal anti-inflammatory drugs (NSAIDs), particularly indomethacin, may reduce the effectiveness of thiazide diuretics. Sulindac, another NSAID, may increase the effect of thiazide diuretics.

Food Interactions

Thiazide diuretics may be taken with food if they upset your stomach. Your doctor may recommend high-potassium foods like bananas and orange juice to offset the potassium-lowering effect of these drugs.

Usual Dose

Bendroflumethiazide
Starting dosage—not more than 20 mg 1–2 times a day. Maintenance dosage—2.5–5 mg a day.

Benzthiazide
Starting dosage—50–200 mg a day. Daily dosages over 100 mg should be divided into 2 doses. Maintenance dosage—50–150 mg a day.

Chlorothiazide
Adult: 0.5–1 g 1–2 times a day. Often people respond to intermittent therapy, that is, taking the drug on alternate days or 3–5 days a week. This reduces side effects.

Child (age 6 months and over): 10 mg per lb. of body weight a day in 2 equal doses.

Child (under age 6 months): not more than 15 mg per lb. of body weight a day in 2 equal doses.

Chlorthalidone

50–100 mg a day or 100 mg on alternate days or 3 days a week. 150 or 200 mg a day is sometimes required; dosages of more than 200 mg a day generally do not produce greater response.

Hydrochlorothiazide

Adult: 25–200 mg a day depending on the condition being treated. Maintenance dosage—25–100 mg a day. 200 mg a day is sometimes required.

Child (age 6 months and over): 1 mg per lb. of body weight a day in 2 doses.

Child (under age 6 months): 1.5 mg per lb. of body weight a day in 2 doses.

Hydroflumethiazide

Starting dosage—50 mg 1–2 times a day. Maintenance dosage—25–200 mg a day. Daily dosages of more than 100 mg should be divided into separate doses.

Indapamide

1.25–2.5 mg every morning. Dosage may be increased to 5 mg a day.

Methyclothiazide

2.5–10 mg a day.

Metolazone

Dosage is individualized. Zaroxolyn—2.5–20 mg once a day. Mykrox—0.5 mg once a day, in the morning. Dosage may be increased to 1 mg a day.

Polythiazide

1–4 mg a day.

Quinethazone

50–100 mg a day. Occasionally, dosages of 100 mg are divided into 2 doses. 150–200 mg a day is sometimes required.

Trichlormethiazide

2–4 mg a day.

Overdosage

Symptoms include tingling in the arms or legs, weakness, fatigue, fainting, dizziness, changes in heartbeat, feeling unwell, dry mouth, restlessness, muscle pain or cramp, urinary difficulties, nausea, and vomiting. Take the victim to a hospital emergency room at once. ALWAYS bring the prescription bottle or container.

Special Information

Ordinarily, diuretics are prescribed early in the day to prevent excessive nighttime urination from interfering with sleep.

Thiazide diuretics cause excess urination at first but it subsides after several weeks.

Contact your doctor if you develop muscle pain, sudden joint pain, weakness, cramps, nausea, vomiting, restlessness, excessive thirst, tiredness, drowsiness, increased heart or pulse rate, diarrhea, or dizziness. People with diabetes may experience increased blood-sugar levels and need dosage adjustments of their antidiabetic medication.

Avoid alcohol and other medications while taking a thiazide diuretic, unless directed by your doctor.

Avoid over-the-counter medications for the treatment of coughs, colds, and allergy if you have hypertension or CHF because such medication may contain stimulants.

If you forget a dose, take it as soon as you remember. If it is almost time for your next dose, skip the one you forgot and continue with your regular schedule. Do not take a double dose.

Special Populations

Pregnancy/Breast-feeding

Thiazide diuretics enter the fetal circulation and may cause side effects in the newborn such as jaundice, blood problems, and low potassium levels. Diuretics are used to treat specific medical conditions during pregnancy but their routine use during a normal pregnancy is improper. When any of these drugs is considered crucial by your doctor, its potential benefits must be carefully weighed against its risks.

Thiazide diuretics pass into breast milk. Nursing mothers who must take diuretics should bottle-feed.

Seniors

Seniors are more sensitive to side effects, especially dizziness.

Type of Drug

Thyroid Hormone Replacements

Brand Names

Generic Ingredient: Levothyroxine Sodium Ⓖ
Eltroxin   Levoxine
Levo-T   Levoxyl
Levothroid   Synthroid

Generic Ingredient: Liothyronine Sodium Ⓖ
Cytomel

Generic Ingredient: Liotrix Ⓖ
Thyrolar

Generic Ingredient: Thyroglobulin
Only available in generic form.

Generic Ingredient: Thyroid Hormone Ⓖ
Armour Thyroid   Thyroid Strong
S-P-T   Thyrar

Prescribed for

Hypothyroidism (underactive thyroid gland).

General Information

The major differences between these drugs are their sources and hormone content. Thyroid hormone is made from beef and pork thyroid. It is effective but lacks standardization, making it difficult for doctors to control dosage. Synthetic drugs are more desirable because their content is easily standardized, ensuring that you receive the correct amount of hormone.

Basically, there are 2 important thyroid hormones: levothyroxine and liothyronine. Levothyroxine is converted to liothyronine in the body. This process slows the absorption of levothyroxine and lowers the risk of side effects. Liothyronine's potency and its potential for side effects make it less desirable for older adults. Thyroglobulin and liotrix contain both levothyroxine and liothyronine; since levothyroxine is converted naturally to liothyronine, there is no advantage in taking both hormones. These considerations make levothyroxine the treatment of choice for thyroid hormone replacement.

Generic versions of these drugs may not be equivalent to their brand-name counterparts—do not switch brands without your doctor's knowledge.

Cautions and Warnings

If you have **hyperthyroid disease** (symptoms include headache, nervousness, sweating, rapid heartbeat, chest pain, and other signs of central nervous system [CNS] stimulation) or **high output of thyroid hormone**, you should not use these drugs.

If you have **heart disease** or **hypertension** (high blood pressure), thyroid hormone replacement therapy should not be used unless it is clearly indicated and supervised by your doctor. If you develop chest pain or other signs of heart disease while taking this drug, call your doctor immediately.

These drugs should not be used to treat **infertility** unless the person also has hypothyroidism.

Thyroid hormone replacements have been prescribed for **weight loss**. Thyroid treatments do not work in people with a normal thyroid status unless large dosages are used—these dosages may produce serious or fatal side effects, especially when taken with appetite-suppressing drugs.

Thyroid hormone replacement therapy increases metabolism and may worsen the symptoms of other endocrine system—hormone-related—diseases including **diabetes** and **Addison's disease**. Adjustments in the levels of treatment for these diseases may be needed when you begin using these drugs.

Possible Side Effects

Side effects are rare except during the start of therapy or when dosage is adjusted.

▼ Most common: heart palpitations, rapid heartbeat, abnormal heart rhythms, weight loss, chest pain, hand tremor, headache, diarrhea, nervousness, menstrual irregularity, inability to sleep, sweating, and intolerance to heat. These symptoms may be controlled by adjusting dosage.

Drug Interactions

• Colestipol and cholestyramine may reduce the effect of these drugs. Take your thyroid hormone replacement and either colestipol or cholestryamine 4 to 5 hours apart.

• The combination of maprotiline and a thyroid hormone replacement may increase the risk of abnormal heart rhythms. Your doctor may have to adjust the dosage of your thyroid hormone replacement.

• Aspirin and other salicylate drugs may increase the effectiveness of thyroid hormone replacements.

• Estrogen drugs may increase your need for thyroid hormone replacement therapy.

• Avoid taking over-the-counter drugs that contain stimulants—such as many of the products used to treat cough, cold, or allergy—which affect the heart and may cause symptoms of overdose.

• These drugs may increase the effect of anticoagulants (blood thinners) like warfarin. Your anticoagulant dosage must be reduced.

• People with diabetes may need to have their doctors increase their insulin or oral antidiabetic drug dosages when they start taking a thyroid hormone replacement.

• These drugs may reduce the effectiveness of beta blockers. Beta-blocker dosage may need to be increased.

• Dosage adjustment of theophylline may be required if you take a thyroid hormone replacement.

Food Interactions

Thyroid hormone replacements should be taken as a single dose, preferably before breakfast.

Usual Dose

Levothyroxine
Starting dosage—as little as 25 mcg a day, which is then increased in steps of 25 mcg once every 3–4 weeks depending upon response. Maintenance dosage—100–400 mcg a day. It is essential to take levothyroxine at the same time each day.

Liothyronine
Adult: 5–100 mcg a day.
Senior and Child: begin at the low end of the dosage range and increase slowly until the desired effect has been achieved.

Liotrix

Adult: a single "½"–"2" tablet a day, depending on the condition being treated and your response to therapy. Liotrix tablets are rated according to their approximate equivalent to thyroid hormone. A "½" tablet is roughly equal to 30 mg of thyroid hormone, a "1" tablet to 60 mg, a "2" tablet to 120 mg, and so on.

Senior and Child: Begin at the low end of the dosage range and increase slowly until the desired effect has been achieved.

Thyroglobulin and Thyroid Hormone

Starting dosage—15–30 mg, or ¼–½ grain a day, which is then increased in 15-mg steps every 1–2 weeks until response is satisfactory. Maintenance dosage—30–180 mg a day.

Overdosage

Symptoms include headache; irritability; nervousness; sweating; rapid heartbeat with unusual stomach rumbling—with or without cramps; chest pain; heart failure; and shock. Take the victim to a hospital emergency room immediately. ALWAYS bring the prescription bottle or container.

Special Information

Thyroid hormone replacement therapy is usually a lifelong treatment. Take the drug as prescribed and do not stop taking it unless instructed by your doctor.

Do not switch brands, especially in the case of levothyroxine, without your doctor's or pharmacist's knowledge. Different brands of the same thyroid hormone replacement are not always equivalent.

Call your doctor if you develop nervousness, diarrhea, excessive sweating, chest pain, increased pulse rate, heart palpitations, intolerance to heat, or any bothersome or persistent side effect.

Children beginning thyroid hormone replacement therapy may lose some hair during the first few months but this is only temporary and the hair generally grows back.

If you forget a dose, take it as soon as you remember. If it is almost time for your next dose, skip the one you forgot and continue with your regular schedule. Do not take a double dose. Call your doctor if you miss 2 or more consecutive doses.

Special Populations

Pregnancy/Breast-feeding

Small amounts of these drugs enter the fetal bloodstream. These medications have not been associated with any problems when used to maintain normal thyroid function in the mother. Pregnant women who have been taking a thyroid hormone replacement should continue their treatment under medical supervision.

Small amounts of these drugs pass into breast milk. Nursing mothers who must take them should consider bottle-feeding.

Seniors

Seniors, who may be more sensitive to the effects of these drugs, generally require reduced dosage.

Generic Name

Tiagabine (tee-UH-gah-bene)

Brand Name

Gabitril

The information in this profile also applies to the following drug:

Generic Ingredient: Gabapentin
Neurontin

Type of Drug

Anticonvulsant.

Prescribed for

Partial seizure.

General Information

The exact way in which tiagabine hydrochloride works is not known but may be related to its ability to improve the activity of GABA, the major inhibitor of nerve transmission in the brain and central nervous system (CNS). This means that tiagabine probably slows GABA-related nerve impulses that lead to a seizure. The medication achieves maximum blood levels in 45 minutes. It is broken down in the liver.

Cautions and Warnings

Do not take this drug if you are **sensitive** or **allergic** to it. Several people taking tiagabine have developed a **severe rash**.

People with **liver disease** should take this drug with caution and receive reduced dosages. People with **kidney disease** require reduced dosages of gabapentin.

Suddenly stopping any antiepileptic drug can increase the frequency of seizures. Dosage should be reduced gradually.

In studies, a small number of people **died suddenly** while taking gabapentin. It is not known if these deaths were caused by the drug.

A feeling of **severe weakness** has developed in a small number of people taking tiagabine. The weakness goes away when the medication is reduced or stopped.

Tiagabine may bind to parts of the eye. There is no evidence that this produces long-term effects. Tell your doctor if you experience any changes in vision.

Possible Side Effects

Tiagabine

▼ Most common: dizziness, weakness, nervousness, and nausea.

▼ Common: poor concentration, speech or language problems, abdominal or other pain, tremor, sleeplessness, confusion, tiredness, diarrhea, vomiting, sore throat, and rash.

▼ Less common: forgetfulness, tingling in the hands or feet, depression, emotional upset, walking unusually, hostility, rolling of the eyeballs, agitation, hunger, mouth sores, cough, itching, and flushing.

Gabapentin

▼ Most common: tiredness, dizziness, weakness, and abnormal eyeball movement.

▼ Common: fatigue, double vision, blurred vision, and tremors.

▼ Less common: weight gain, back pain, upset stomach, dry mouth or throat, constipation, dental problems, muscle aches, runny nose, sore throat, speech problems, memory loss, depression, abnormal thinking, twitching, itching, abrasions, and impotence.

Possible Side Effects *(continued)*

▼ Rare: leg swelling, increased appetite, broken bones, poor coordination, low red- and white-blood-cell counts, and flushing.

Drug Interactions

• Taking tiagabine with other medications for seizure control, including carbamazepine, phenytoin, phenobarbital, and valproate may affect the amount of each in the blood. Dosage adjustments may be necessary.

Food Interactions

Take tiagabine with food but avoid high-fat meals, which slow its absorption. Gabapentin may be taken with or without food.

Usual Dose

Tiagabine
    Adult (age 19 and over): starting dosage—4 mg once a day. Dosage may be increased in steps of 4 or 8 mg to 56 mg a day. Higher amounts should be divided into 2 or 4 doses a day.
    Child (age 12–18): starting dosage—4 mg once a day. Dosage may be increased in steps of 4 or 8 mg to 32 mg a day. Higher amounts should be divided into 2 doses a day.

Gabapentin
    Adult and Child (age 12 and over): 300–600 mg 3 times a day.
    Child (under age 12): not recommended.

Overdosage

Tiagabine: Symptoms include tiredness, loss of consciousness, agitation, confusion, difficulty talking, hostility, depression, weakness, and muscle spasm.

Gabapentin: Symptoms include double vision, slurred speech, drowsiness, diarrhea, lethargy, weakness, breathing difficulties, sedation, droopy eyelids, and excitation.

Take the victim to a hospital emergency room. ALWAYS bring the prescription bottle or container.

Special Information

This drug may make you dizzy or tired, or interfere with your concentration. Be extremely careful when driving or performing any task that requires concentration. Avoid alcohol or other nervous system depressants.

Tell your doctor if you experience changes in vision, rash, or any bothersome or persistent side effect.

If you forget a dose, take it as soon as you remember. If it is almost time for your next dose, take the dose you forgot and space the remaining daily dosage evenly throughout the day. Do not take a double dose.

Special Populations

Pregnancy/Breast-feeding

This medication causes birth defects in lab animals. Seizure disorder itself has been associated with an increased risk of birth defects. Discuss with your doctor the need to control seizure and the potential benefits and risks of taking this medication during pregnancy.

Tiagabine may pass into breast milk. It is not known if gabapentin does so. Nursing mothers who must take either drug should consider bottle-feeding.

Seniors

Seniors may take tiagabine without special precaution but may require reduced dosage of gabapentin.

Generic Name

Ticlopidine (tih-KLOE-pih-dene) [G]

Brand Name

Ticlid

Type of Drug

Anticoagulant (blood thinner).

Prescribed for

Reducing risk of stroke; also used to treat intermittent claudication and chronic circulatory occlusion, and to reduce the damage caused by stroke. It is used before open heart surgery to reduce the expected drop in platelet count, during coronary artery bypass surgery or stent placement to improve the chance of success, in some forms of kidney disease to help improve kidney function, and in sickle cell disease to reduce the number and severity of sickle cell attacks.

General Information

Ticlopidine hydrochloride makes blood platelets less "sticky," reducing the risk of blood clotting and the possible consequences of clot formation. It interferes with the functioning of the platelet cell membrane, changing platelet cells irreversibly until they are replaced by new ones. Maximum effect (60% to 70% reduction in platelet function) is seen 8 to 11 days after administration of 250 mg of ticlopidine twice a day. In studies, people taking ticlopidine regularly for 2 to 5 years experienced a 24% reduction in incidence of stroke.

Cautions and Warnings

Ticlopidine can cause severe **reductions in white-blood-cell counts,** greatly increasing the risk of infection. Some cases have been fatal. Your doctor should take white-blood-cell counts 2 weeks after you begin taking ticlopidine and continue testing every 2 weeks for the first 3 months of treatment. Only people showing signs of infection need to be tested after that period. Blood counts usually return to normal 1 to 3 weeks after you stop taking the drug.

Blood-platelet counts can also be depressed, leading to spontaneous bruising or bleeding. **Gastrointestinal bleeding** can also worsen during use of ticlopidine.

Do not take this medication if you are **allergic** to it or have an **active bleeding site such as an ulcer, reduced blood-cell counts,** or severe **liver disease**.

Ticlopidine causes an 8% to 10% increase in blood **cholesterol** within a month after you start taking the drug.

People being switched from an anticoagulant or thrombolytic to ticlopidine should stop the former drug and allow it to clear the system before starting ticlopidine.

People with severe **kidney disease** may need less ticlopidine.

Possible Side Effects

Side effects occur in 60% of all people. About 13% of ticlopidine patients stop taking the drug because of stomach side effects.

▼ Most common: diarrhea, nausea, upset stomach, rash, and stomach pain.

▼ Less common: reduced white-blood-cell counts, vomiting, bruising, gas, itching, dizziness, appetite loss, and liver function changes.

Drug Interactions

• Antacids reduce the absorption of ticlopidine. Separate doses by at least 1 hour.

• Taking cimetidine on a regular basis can reduce the clearance of ticlopidine from the body by 50%, increasing the risk of drug toxicity and side effects.

• Combining aspirin and ticlopidine may increase the risk of bleeding. Do not combine these drugs.

• Ticlopidine may slightly reduce blood levels of digoxin. This is not a problem for most people, but dosage adjustment may be needed.

• Ticlopidine reduces the body's clearance of theophylline; your doctor may need to reduce your theophylline dosage.

Food Interactions

Ticlopidine should be taken with meals to reduce stomach upset and maximize absorption of the drug. Take it at the same time each day to gain maximum benefit.

Usual Dose

250 mg taken twice a day with food.

Overdosage

Overdose may lead to increased bleeding and liver inflammation. Other possible effects include stomach bleeding, convulsions, breathing difficulties, and low body temperature. Take the victim to a hospital emergency room. ALWAYS bring the prescription bottle or container.

Special Information

Call your doctor if you have fever, chills, sore throat, or other indication of infection; severe or persistent diarrhea; rash; bleeding under the skin; yellowing of the skin or whites of the eyes; dark urine; light-colored stools; or any bothersome or persistent side effect.

Bleeding may be more difficult to stop if you are taking ticlopidine. Be sure your doctor, dentist, and other health care professionals know that you are taking this medication.

If you miss a dose, take it as soon as you can. If it is 4 hours or less until your next dose, skip the missed dose and continue with your regular schedule. Do not take a double dose.

Special Populations

Pregnancy/Breast-feeding
The safety of using ticlopidine during pregnancy is not known. When this drug is considered crucial by your doctor, its potential benefits must be carefully weighed against its risks.

Ticlopidine may pass into breast milk. Nursing mothers who must take it should bottle-feed.

Seniors
Seniors may be more sensitive to the effects of ticlopidine.

Generic Name

Timolol (TIM-oe-lol) G

Brand Names

Betimol	Timoptic
Blocadren	Timoptic-XE

The information in this profile also applies to the following drugs:

Generic Ingredient: Nadolol G
Corgard

Generic Ingredient: Sotalol
Betapace

Type of Drug

Beta-adrenergic blocking agent.

Prescribed for

High blood pressure, abnormal heart rhythms, prevention of second heart attack or migraine, tremors, stage fright and other anxieties, and glaucoma.

General Information

Timolol is one of many beta-adrenergic blocking drugs, or beta blockers, that interfere with the action of a specific part of the nervous system. Beta receptors are found all over the body and affect many body functions. Each beta blocker has particular characteristics that make it more suitable for certain conditions or people. When applied as eyedrops, timolol reduces ocular pressure (pressure inside the eye) by reducing the production of eye fluids and by slightly increasing the rate at which these fluids flow through and leave the eye.

Cautions and Warnings

You should be cautious about taking timolol if you have **asthma, severe heart failure,** a **very slow heart rate,** or **heart block** (disruption of the electrical impulses that control heart rate) because the drug may aggravate these conditions.

People with **angina** who take timolol for high blood pressure risk aggravating their angina if they suddenly stop taking the drug. These people should have their drug dosage reduced gradually over 1 to 2 weeks.

Timolol should be used with caution if you have **liver or kidney disease** because your ability to eliminate the drug from your body may be impaired.

Timolol reduces the amount of blood pumped by the heart with each beat. This reduction in blood flow may aggravate the condition of people with **poor circulation** or **circulatory disease**.

If you are undergoing **major surgery,** your doctor may want you to stop taking timolol at least 2 days before surgery.

Timolol eyedrops should not be used by people who cannot tolerate oral beta-blocking drugs, such as propranolol.

Possible Side Effects

Side effects are relatively uncommon and usually mild.
  ▼ Most common: impotence.

Possible Side Effects *(continued)*

▼ Less common: unusual tiredness or weakness, slow heartbeat, heart failure, dizziness, breathing difficulties, bronchospasm, depression, confusion, anxiety, nervousness, sleeplessness, disorientation, short-term memory loss, emotional instability, cold hands and feet, constipation, diarrhea, nausea, vomiting, upset stomach, increased sweating, urinary difficulties, cramps, blurred vision, rash, hair loss, stuffy nose, facial swelling, aggravation of lupus erythematosus, itching, chest pain, back or joint pain, colitis, drug allergy (symptoms include fever and sore throat), and liver toxicity.

Drug Interactions

• Timolol may interact with surgical anesthetics to increase the risk of heart problems during surgery. Some anesthesiologists recommend gradually stopping the drug by 2 days before surgery.

• Timolol may interfere with the signs of low blood sugar and with the action of oral antidiabetes drugs.

• Timolol increases the blood-pressure-lowering effects of other blood-pressure-reducing agents, including clonidine, guanabenz, and reserpine; and calcium channel blockers such as nifedipine.

• Aspirin-containing drugs, indomethacin, sulfinpyrazone, and estrogen drugs may interfere with the blood-pressure-lowering effect of timolol.

• Cocaine may reduce the effectiveness of all beta blockers.

• Timolol may worsen the problem of cold hands and feet associated with ergot alkaloids, used to treat migraine. Gangrene is a possibility in people taking both an ergot and timolol.

• Timolol will counteract thyroid hormone replacements.

• Calcium channel blockers, flecainide, hydralazine, oral contraceptives, propafenone, haloperidol, phenothiazine tranquilizers (molindone and others) quinolone antibacterials, and quinidine may increase the amount of timolol in the bloodstream and lead to increased timolol effects.

• Timolol should not be taken within 2 weeks of taking a monoamine oxidase inhibitor (MAOI) antidepressant.

• Cimetidine increases the amount of timolol absorbed into the bloodstream from oral tablets.

• Timolol may interfere with the effectiveness of some anti-asthma drugs including theophylline and aminophylline, and especially ephedrine and isoproterenol.

• Combining timolol and phenytoin or digitalis drugs may result in excessive slowing of the heart, possibly causing heart block.

• If you stop smoking while taking timolol, your dose may have to be reduced because your liver will break down the drug more slowly afterward.

• If you use other glaucoma eye medications, separate them to avoid physically mixing them.

• Small amounts of timolol eyedrops are absorbed into the bloodstream and may interact with other drugs in the same way as oral beta blockers, although this is unlikely.

Food Interactions

None known.

Usual Dose

Tablets: 10–60 mg a day divided into 2 doses.

Eyedrops: 1 drop twice a day.

Overdosage

Symptoms include changes in heartbeat—unusually slow, unusually fast, or irregular—severe dizziness or fainting, breathing difficulties, bluish-colored fingernails or palms, and seizures. The victim should be taken to a hospital emergency room. ALWAYS bring the prescription bottle or container.

Special Information

Timolol is taken continuously. Do not stop taking this drug unless directed to do so by your doctor: Abrupt withdrawal may cause chest pain, breathing difficulties, increased sweating, and unusually fast or irregular heartbeat. When ending timolol treatment, dosage should be reduced gradually over a period of about 2 weeks.

Call your doctor at once if you develop back or joint pain, breathing difficulties, cold hands or feet, depression, rash, or changes in heartbeat. Timolol may produce an undesirable lowering of blood pressure, leading to dizziness or fainting; call your doctor if this happens to you. Call your doctor if you experience persistent or bothersome anxiety, diarrhea, constipation, impotence, headache, itching, nausea or vomiting, nightmares or vivid dreams, upset stomach, trouble sleeping, stuffy nose, frequent urination, unusual tiredness, or weakness.

Timolol can cause drowsiness, dizziness, light-headedness, or blurred vision. Be careful when driving or performing complex tasks.

It is best to take timolol at the same time each day. If you forget a dose, take it as soon as you remember. If you take timolol twice a day and it is within 4 hours of your next dose, skip the dose you forgot and continue with your regular schedule. Do not take a double dose.

To avoid infection, do not touch the eyedropper tip to your finger, eyelid, or any other surface. Wait at least 5 minutes before using another eyedrop or eye ointment.

If you forget a dose of timolol eyedrops, administer it as soon as you remember. If it is almost time for your next dose, skip the dose you forgot and continue with your regular schedule. Do not take a double dose.

Special Populations

Pregnancy/Breast-feeding

Infants born to women who took a beta blocker while pregnant had lower birth weights, low blood pressure, and reduced heart rates. Timolol should be avoided by pregnant women.

Timolol passes into breast milk. Nursing mothers who must use it should bottle-feed.

Seniors

Seniors may require less of the drug to achieve results. Seniors taking timolol may be more likely to suffer from cold hands and feet, reduced body temperature, chest pain, general feelings of ill health, sudden breathing difficulties, sweating, or changes in heartbeat.

Generic Name

Tizanidine (tih-ZAN-ih-dene)

Brand Name

Zanaflex

Type of Drug

Skeletal muscle relaxant.

Prescribed for

Spastic muscle movements.

General Information

Tizanidine hydrochloride is prescribed for people who suffer from uncontrolled muscle spasms usually associated with a nervous system condition. It is presumed to work on the central nervous system by affecting nerves that control major muscle systems; it has no direct effect on skeletal muscles. Tizanidine begins working between 1 to 2 hours after it is taken and lasts for 3 to 6 hours.

Cautions and Warnings

Do not take tizanidine if you are sensitive or **allergic** to it.

Tizanidine can cause **low blood pressure**. This effect usually begins within 1 hour after taking the drug and reaches its height after 2 to 3 hours. Low blood pressure triggered by tizanidine is associated with **slow heart rate, light-headedness,** and **dizziness** when rising from a sitting or lying position.

About 50% of people taking tizanidine experience some **sedation**. Sedation usually begins 30 minutes after taking the drug and continues to get worse for about 1 hour. Sedative effects usually start during the first week of treatment or do not occur at all.

Tizanidine may cause **liver injury**. About 1 of 20 people who take this drug experience some liver inflammation, although most cases resolve once the drug is stopped. Several people have died from liver failure after taking tizanidine; it should be avoided by people with liver disease.

People taking tizanidine have experienced **hallucinations, delusion,** and **psychotic symptoms**.

Tizanidine should be used with caution by people who have **reduced kidney function**. These people need smaller-than-usual doses.

Possible Side Effects

▼ Most common: dry mouth, sleepiness, tiredness, and weakness.

Possible Side Effects *(continued)*

▼ Common: dizziness.

▼ Less common: uncontrolled muscle movement, nervousness, constipation, sore throat, vomiting, frequent urination, urinary infection, liver inflammation, double vision, flu symptoms, runny nose, speech disorders, fever, depression, anxiety, tingling in the hands or feet, rash, sweating, skin sores, diarrhea, abdominal pain, and upset stomach.

▼ Rare: Rare side effects can occur in almost any part of the body Contact your doctor if you experience any side effect not listed above.

Drug Interactions

• Avoid combining alcohol and tizanidine or increased sedation may result.

• Women who combine oral contraceptives and tizanidine should receive reduced dosages of the latter to avoid increased side effects.

• Tizanidine may increase the effects of blood-pressure-lowering drugs.

• Tizanidine may delay the effects of acetaminophen.

Food Interactions

Tizanidine may be taken without regard to food or meals, though it may work faster with food.

Usual Dose

Adult: 8 mg every 6–8 hours as needed, up to 3 doses a day. Do not exceed 36 mg a day.

Child: not recommended.

Overdosage

Little is known about the effects of tizanidine overdose, but it may lead to very slow breathing. Overdose victims should be taken to a hospital emergency room. ALWAYS bring the prescription bottle or container.

Special Information

People taking tizanidine should be careful not to exceed the prescribed dosage since little is known about using higher dosages over an extended period.

Be careful when driving or performing any task that requires concentration.

If you take tizanidine on a regular basis and forget a dose, take it as soon as you remember. If it is almost time for your next dose, skip the one you forgot and continue with your regular schedule. Do not take a double dose.

Special Populations

Pregnancy/Breast-feeding

Tizanidine should only be taken during pregnancy if absolutely necessary and after its potential benefits have been carefully weighed against its risks.

Tizanidine may pass into breast milk. Nursing mothers who must take this drug should consider bottle-feeding.

Seniors

Seniors should use tizanidine with caution.

Generic Name

Tocainide (toe-KAY-nide)

Brand Name

Tonocard

Type of Drug

Antiarrhythmic.

Prescribed for

Abnormal heart rhythms; also prescribed for muscular dystrophy and trigeminal neuralgia (tic douloureux).

General Information

Tocainide hydrochloride works in the same way as lidocaine, one of the most widely used injectable antiarrhythmic drugs. Tocainide slows the speed at which nerve impulses are carried through the heart's ventricle, helping the heart to maintain a stable rhythm by making heart muscle cells less easily excited. Tocainide affects different areas of the heart than do other widely used oral antiarrhythmic drugs. Tocainide is usually prescribed as a follow-up to intravenous lidocaine for people with life-threatening arrhythmias.

Cautions and Warnings

People taking tocainide may develop **bone-marrow depression,** a drastic **drop in white-blood-cell count, low platelet count,** or other **abnormalities of blood components**. Because these abnormalities happen most often during the first 3 months on tocainide, you should have weekly blood counts throughout that period.

This drug should not be used by people who are **allergic** to it, to lidocaine, or to local anesthetics.

Some people using tocainide may develop **respiratory difficulties,** including fluid buildup in the lungs, pneumonia, and irritation of the lungs. Immediately report any cough, wheezing, shortness of breath, or breathing difficulties to your doctor. Tocainide should not be used by people with **heart failure** because the drug can actually worsen that condition.

Like other antiarrhythmic drugs, tocainide may occasionally **worsen heart rhythm problems**. It has not actually been proven to help people live longer.

Possible Side Effects

▼ Most common: nausea, dizziness, fainting, tingling in the hands or feet, and tremors. These reactions are generally mild and short-lived, and usually go away when dosage is reduced or when you take tocainide with food.

▼ Less common: vomiting, reduced appetite, lightheadedness, confusion, disorientation, hallucinations, nervousness, mood or self-awareness changes, poor muscle coordination, blurred or double vision, increased sweating, giddiness, restlessness, anxiety, low blood pressure, slowing of the heart rate, heart palpitations, chest pains, cold sweats, headache, drowsiness, lethargy, ringing or buzzing in the ears, visual disturbances, rolling of the eyes, diarrhea, unusual feelings of heat or cold, joint inflammation and pain, and muscle aches.

▼ Rare: Rare side effects can affect your mental state, breathing, taste, smell, memory, speech, stomach and intestines, blood, urinary tract, sexual function, blood flow to the arms and legs, and muscles and joints. Contact your doctor if you experience any side effect not listed above.

Drug Interactions

• Tocainide taken with metoprolol or other beta-blocking drugs may cause too rapid a drop in blood pressure and slow the heart.

• Tocainide may produce additive cardiac side effects if taken with other antiarrhythmic drugs.

• Tocainide may increase the effects of other drugs that depress bone-marrow function, leading to low levels of white blood cells and blood platelets.

• Cimetidine and rifampin reduce the amount of tocainide absorbed into the bloodstream. Ranitidine, which can be used instead of cimetidine, does not have this effect.

Food Interactions

None known.

Usual Dose

Adult: 1200–1800 mg a day in 2–3 doses. Seniors and people with kidney or liver disease usually require lower doses.

Overdosage

The first symptoms of tocainide overdose are usually tremors or other nervous system effects. Other, more serious, side effects may follow. Victims should be taken to an emergency room for treatment at once. ALWAYS bring the prescription bottle or container.

Special Information

Be sure to report any side effects to your doctor, particularly breathing difficulties after exertion, cough, wheezing, tremors, palpitations, rash, easy bruising or bleeding, fever, chills, sore throat or mouth, or mouth sores.

Tocainide can make you dizzy or drowsy. Be careful while driving or performing other complex tasks.

Do not take more or less of this drug than prescribed. If you forget a dose and remember within 4 hours of your regular time, take it right away. If you do not remember until later, skip the dose you forgot and go back to your regular schedule. Do not take a double dose.

Special Populations

Pregnancy/Breast-feeding

In animal studies, tocainide caused spontaneous abortions

and stillbirths. When this drug is considered crucial by your doctor, its potential benefits must be carefully weighed against its risks.

Tocainide passes into breast milk. Nursing mothers who must take this drug should bottle-feed.

Seniors

Seniors are more sensitive to the side effects of this drug, especially dizziness and low blood pressure.

Generic Name

Tolcapone (TOL-kap-one)

Brand Name

Tasmar

Type of Drug

COMT inhibitor.

Prescribed for

Parkinson's disease.

General Information

Tolcapone is believed to block the effects of an enzyme known as COMT, which is found throughout the body. COMT is an essential part of the process by which natural stimulants or catecholamines, including L-DOPA, are eliminated. This extends levodopa's beneficial effect on Parkinson's disease.

Cautions and Warnings

Do not take this drug if you are **sensitive** or **allergic** to it. Tolcapone can cause **liver irritation and injury,** which may be fatal. Liver function should be evaluated monthly during the first 3 months of drug therapy, then every 6 weeks for the next 3 months. People with **cirrhosis of the liver** should receive about half the usual dose. Other forms of liver disease do not affect tolcapone dosage.

Tolcapone increases levodopa side effects, including **low blood pressure, dizziness, or fainting,** and **uncontrolled muscle movements.**

Possible Side Effects

▼ Most common: abnormal muscle movements, sleep disturbances, stiffness, vivid dreams, tiredness, confusion, nausea, appetite loss, diarrhea, vomiting, muscle cramps, dizziness, and fainting.

▼ Common: hallucinations, constipation, dry mouth, abdominal pain, respiratory infections, sweating, falling, and fatigue.

▼ Less common: loss of balance, changes in muscular activity, tingling in the hands or feet, upset stomach, gas, arthritis, neck pain, chest pain, low blood pressure, chest discomfort, breathing difficulties, sinus congestion, flu-like symptoms, urine discoloration, and difficulty urinating.

▼ Rare: agitation, irritability, hyperactivity, minor skin bleeding, hair loss, a burning sensation, feeling unwell, fever, cataracts, and eye inflammation.

Drug Interactions

• Do not combine tolcapone and any monoamine oxidase inhibitor (MAOI) drug except selegiline.

• Tolcapone may increase the blood-thinning effects of warfarin; do not combine these drugs.

• Tolcapone increases levodopa side effects.

Food Interactions

Take this drug at least 1 hour before or 2 hours after meals.

Usual Dose

Adult: 100–200 mg 3 times a day.
Child: not recommended.

Overdosage

Common symptoms include nausea, vomiting, and dizziness. Take the victim to a hospital emergency room. ALWAYS bring the prescription bottle or container.

Special Information

Nausea, dizziness or fainting, hallucinations, and other side effects are more likely when you first start taking this drug.

Call your doctor if you experience any bothersome or persistent side effect.

Tolcapone can make you tired and dizzy. Be careful when driving or performing any task that requires concentration.

Your doctor may reduce your dosage of levodopa or carbidopa when you begin taking tolcapone.

If you forget a dose, take it as soon as you remember. If it is almost time for your next dose, skip the forgotten dose and continue with your regular schedule.

Special Populations

Pregnancy/Breast-feeding

The safety of using tolcapone during pregnancy is not known, though there is a risk that it may be toxic to a pregnant woman. It is always prescribed with levodopa, which is known to cause birth defects. When tolcapone is considered crucial by your doctor, its potential benefits must be carefully weighed against its risks.

Tolcapone may pass into breast milk. Nursing mothers who must take it should consider bottle-feeding.

Seniors

Seniors may be more sensitive to side effects, especially hallucinations.

Generic Name

Tolterodine (tole-TER-oe-deen)

Brand Name

Detrol

Type of Drug

Anticholinergic.

Prescribed for

Overactive bladder.

General Information

Tolterodine improves bladder control by interfering with nerve receptors that control bladder muscles. By dulling the response of these receptors to nervous system stimulation, tolterodine can prevent bladder muscle contractions and the resulting urgent need to urinate. Tolterodine does not work the same for everyone. Because most of this drug is broken down in the liver, drug response as well as dosage may depend on your degree of liver function. People with liver disease should not take more than 1 mg twice a day.

Cautions and Warnings

Do not take this drug if you are **sensitive** or **allergic** to it, are **retaining urine,** or have a **stomach obstruction** or **uncontrolled narrow-angle glaucoma**. People being treated for narrow-angle glaucoma should use tolterodine with caution.

Possible Side Effects

▼ Most common: dry mouth and headache.

▼ Common: dizziness, fainting, abdominal pain, constipation, diarrhea, upset stomach, nausea, and tiredness.

▼ Less common: sleepiness, visual problems, very dry eyes, bronchitis, coughing, sore throat, runny nose, sinus irritation, respiratory infection, painful urination, frequent urination, urinary retention, joint pain, back pain, chest pain, high blood pressure, fungus infections, flu-like symptoms, and weight gain.

▼ Rare: tingling in the hands or feet, nervousness, itching, rash, dry skin, gas, and vomiting.

Drug Interactions

• Fluoxetine may increase tolterodine blood levels and side effects.

• Erythromycin, clarithromycin, ketoconazole, itraconazole, and miconazole can interfere with the breakdown of tolterodine in the liver. People taking any of these drugs should take no more than 1 mg a day of tolterodine.

Food Interactions

Tolterodine can be taken with or without food.

Usual Dose

Adult: 1–2 mg 2 times a day.
Child: not recommended.

Overdosage

Symptoms may include dry mouth and other side effects. Take the victim to a hospital emergency room. ALWAYS bring the prescription bottle or container.

Special Information

This drug can blur your vision.

If you forget a dose, take it as soon as you remember. If it is almost time for your next dose, skip the forgotten dose and continue with your regular schedule. Do not take a double dose.

Special Populations

Pregnancy/Breast-feeding

Large dosages of tolterodine caused fetal harm and birth defects in animal studies. When this drug is considered crucial by your doctor, its potential benefits must be carefully weighed against its risks.

Tolterodine may pass into breast milk. Nursing mothers who must take it should bottle-feed.

Seniors

Seniors may take tolterodine without special precaution.

Generic Name

Topiramate (toe-PYE-ruh-mate)

Brand Name

Topamax

Type of Drug

Anticonvulsant.

Prescribed for

Partial onset seizure.

General Information

Topiramate has a broad spectrum of antiepileptic activity, but the exact way in which it affects seizures is not known. Topiramate reaches peak blood levels within 2 hours. It passes out of the body through urine.

Cautions and Warnings

Do not take topiramate if you are **sensitive** or **allergic** to it. People who **suddenly stop taking topiramate** may worsen their seizures. Anticonvulsant drugs should be reduced gradually.

People with moderate to severe **kidney disease** should receive half the usual dose; other dosage adjustments may be needed. People with **liver disease** may clear topiramate from their bodies more slowly than others do, but the reasons for this are not well understood. About 1.5% of people taking topiramate develop **kidney stones**. This effect may be avoided by drinking several glasses of water a day during treatment.

Possible Side Effects

Side effects usually affect the central nervous system.

▼ Most common: slow reflexes; slow thought processes; difficulty concentrating; speech or language problems, especially word-finding; tiredness; dizziness; weakness; poor muscle coordination; tingling in the hands or feet; tremors; depression; nausea; respiratory infections; and visual disturbances, including double vision.

▼ Less common: back or chest pain, leg pain, hot flushes, body odor, swelling, abnormal coordination, agitation, mood changes, aggressive reactions, reduced touch sensation, apathy, emotional instability, depersonalization, itching, rash, upset stomach, appetite loss, abdominal pain, constipation, dry mouth, breast pain, menstrual disorders, painful menstruation, sore throat, sinus inflammation, breathing difficulties, eye pain, weight loss, loss of white blood cells, muscle ache, and hearing loss.

▼ Rare: chills, sweating, gum irritation, blood in the urine, and nosebleeds. Other rare side effects can occur in almost any part of the body. Contact your doctor if you experience any side effect not listed above.

Drug Interactions

• Certain other anticonvulsant drugs—phenytoin, carba-mazepine, and valproic acid—reduce topiramate levels.

• Topiramate increases the depressive effect of alcohol and other nervous system depressants. Avoid these combinations.

• Combining topiramate with a carbonic anhydrase inhibitor drug may increase your risk of kidney stones.

• Topiramate reduces the effect of oral contraceptive pills and digoxin.

Food Interactions

None known.

Usual Dose

Adult: starting dosage—50 mg a day. Increase gradually to 200 mg twice a day. People with moderate to severe kidney failure should begin with ½ the usual dose.

Child: not recommended.

Overdosage

Overdose is likely to cause nervous system depression. Overdose victims must be taken to a hospital emergency room immediately. ALWAYS bring the prescription bottle or container.

Special Information

Drink several glasses of water or other fluids every day to avoid developing kidney stones.

Be careful when driving or performing any task that requires concentration.

If you forget a dose, take it as soon as you remember. If it is almost time for your next dose, skip the dose you forgot and continue with your regular schedule. Do not take a double dose.

Special Populations

Pregnancy/Breast-feeding

Animal studies indicate that topiramate may cause birth defects. When this drug is considered crucial by your doctor, its potential benefits must be carefully weighed against its risks.

Animal studies show that topiramate passes into breast milk. Nursing mothers who must take it should consider bottle-feeding.

Seniors
Lower dosage may be needed because of age-related kidney impairment.

Toprol XL *see Metoprolol, page 657*

Generic Name

Tramadol (TRAM-uh-dol)

Brand Name

Ultram

Type of Drug

Non-narcotic pain reliever.

Prescribed for

Mild to moderate pain.

General Information

Tramadol hydrochloride is a synthetic compound that works in the central nervous system (CNS) to relieve pain. The exact way in which this drug works is unknown, but it binds to opioid receptors and reduces the uptake of two important neurohormones, serotonin and norepinephrine, into nerves. Pain relief begins about an hour after you take a dose and reaches its maximum effect in 2 to 3 hours. Like the narcotic pain relievers, tramadol can cause dizziness, tiredness, nausea, constipation, sweating, and itching. Unlike the narcotics, this drug causes little interference with breathing and does not cause histamine reactions. It has no effect on heart function.

Cautions and Warnings

Do not take this drug if you are **sensitive** or **allergic** to it or are **intoxicated** with drugs, alcohol, or narcotics. People who must take tranquilizers, sedatives, or other nervous system depressants should take reduced doses of tramadol.

Large dosages of tramadol may **interfere with breathing**, especially when combined with alcohol.

Tramadol use should be avoided in people who have had **abdominal conditions** or a **head injury** because the drug may interfere with diagnosing the injury or understanding its severity.

Seizure has occurred in people taking oral doses of 700 mg or intravenous doses of 300 mg.

People who are dependent on narcotics and take tramadol may experience **withdrawal symptoms**.

People with **reduced kidney function** or **liver disease** should receive reduced dosage.

Possible Side Effects

▼ Most common: dizziness or fainting, nausea, constipation, headache, tiredness, vomiting, itching, weakness, sweating, upset stomach, dry mouth, and diarrhea.

▼ Less common: feeling unwell, warmth and flushing, nervousness, anxiety, agitation, euphoria (feeling "high"), emotional instability, trouble sleeping, abdominal pain, appetite loss, gas, rash, visual disturbances, urinary difficulties, and symptoms of menopause.

▼ Rare: Rare side effects can affect your senses, mental state, heart, stomach and intestines, liver, blood, and urinary tract. Headaches, fainting, and allergies can also occur. Contact your doctor if you experience any side effect not listed above.

Drug Interactions

• Carbamazepine reduces tramadol's effectiveness. People taking this combination may need twice the usual dosage of tramadol.

• The combination of tramadol and monoamine oxidase inhibitor (MAOI) antidepressant may cause severe reactions and should be used with caution.

• Quinidine may slow the breakdown of tramadol. The full impact of this interaction is not known.

Food Interactions

None known.

Usual Dose

Adult and Child (age 16 and over): 50–100 mg every 4–6 hours; do not exceed 400 mg a day. People with cirrhosis should receive 50 mg every 12 hours. People with severe kidney disease should receive no more than 100 mg every 12 hours.

Senior: do not exceed 300 mg a day.

Child (under age 16): not recommended.

Overdosage

Overdose can be deadly. Symptoms include breathing difficulties and seizure. Take the victim to a hospital emergency room at once. ALWAYS bring the prescription bottle or container.

Special Information

Drowsiness may occur: Be careful when driving or performing any task that requires concentration.

Do not drink alcohol while taking tramadol. Hypnotics, opioids, and psychotropic drugs interact adversely with tramadol.

If you forget a dose, take it as soon as you remember. If it is almost time for your next dose, skip the one you forgot and continue with your regular schedule. Do not take a double dose.

Special Populations

Pregnancy/Breast-feeding

Tramadol is toxic to animal fetuses and passes into the fetal circulation in humans. When this drug is considered crucial by your doctor, its potential benefits must be carefully weighed against its risks.

This drug passes into breast milk. Nursing mothers who must take it should bottle-feed.

Seniors

Seniors may be more sensitive to side effects and should not take more than 300 mg a day.

Generic Name

Trandolapril (tran-DOE-luh-pril)

Brand Name

Mavik

Combination Products

Generic Ingredients: Trandolapril + Verapamil
Tarka

Type of Drug

Angiotensin-converting enzyme (ACE) inhibitor.

Prescribed for

High blood pressure.

General Information

Trandolapril and other ACE inhibitors work by preventing the conversion of a hormone called angiotensin I to another hormone called angiotensin II, a potent blood vessel constrictor. Preventing this conversion relaxes blood vessels, thus reducing blood pressure and relieving symptoms of heart failure. Trandolapril also affects the production of other hormones and enzymes that participate in the regulation of blood-vessel dilation.

Some people who start taking trandolapril after they are already on a diuretic (agent that increases urination) experience a rapid drop in blood pressure after their first doses or when their dosage is increased. To prevent this from happening, your doctor may tell you to stop taking your diuretic 2 or 3 days before starting trandolapril or to increase your salt intake during that time. The diuretic may then be restarted gradually.

Trandolapril is prescribed for high blood pressure alone or with hydrochlorthiazide or another blood-pressure-lowering drug. The brand-name product, Tarka, contains trandolapril and verapamil, a calcium channel blocker.

Cautions and Warnings

Do not take trandolapril if you are **allergic** to it. Trandolapril causes very **low blood pressure**.

Trandolapril may affect **kidney function,** especially if you have congestive **heart failure.** Your doctor should check your urine for protein content during the first few months of treatment. Dosage adjustment of trandolapril is necessary if you have reduced kidney function or liver cirrhosis.

Trandolapril may affect white-blood-cell count, possibly increasing your susceptibility to **infection.** Your doctor should periodically monitor your blood counts.

Possible Side Effects

▼ Most common: dizziness, fatigue, headache, nausea, and chronic cough. The cough usually goes away a few days after you stop taking the medication.

▼ Less common: chest tightness or pain, dizziness when rising from a sitting or lying position, fainting, abdominal pain, nausea, vomiting, diarrhea, bronchitis, urinary tract infection, breathing difficulties, weakness, and rash.

▼ Rare: Rare side effects can occur in almost any part of the body. Contact your doctor if you experience any side effect not listed above.

Drug Interactions

• The blood-pressure-lowering effect of trandolapril is additive with diuretic drugs and beta blockers. Any other drug that causes a rapid drop in blood pressure should be used with caution if you are taking trandolapril.

• Trandolapril may increase blood-potassium levels, especially when taken with Dyazide or other potassium-sparing diuretics.

• Trandolapril may increase the effects of lithium; this combination should be used with caution.

• Antacids and trandolapril should be taken at least 2 hours apart.

• Capsaicin may trigger or aggravate the cough associated with trandolapril therapy.

• Indomethacin may reduce the blood-pressure-lowering effects of trandolapril.

• Phenothiazine tranquilizers and antiemetics may increase the effects of trandolapril.

• The combination of allopurinol and trandolapril increases the chance of side effects.

• Trandolapril increases blood levels of digoxin, which may increase the chance of digoxin-related side effects.

Food Interactions

You may take trandolapril with food if it upsets your stomach.

Usual Dose

Trandolapril: 1 mg a day; 2 mg a day in African Americans. Daily dosage may be adjusted up to 6 mg a day. Daily dosages greater than 4 mg may be taken in 2 doses.

Trandolapril-Verapamil Combination: Dosage for adults age 18 and over is 1 tablet a day. This sustained-release combination is available in a variety of strengths.

Overdosage

The principal effect of trandolapril overdose is a rapid drop in blood pressure, as evidenced by dizziness or fainting. Take the overdose victim to a hospital emergency room immediately. ALWAYS bring the prescription bottle or container.

Special Information

Trandolapril may cause swelling of the face, lips, hands, or feet. This swelling may also affect the larynx (throat) or tongue and interfere with breathing. If this happens, go to a hospital emergency room at once. Call your doctor if you develop sore throat, mouth sores, abnormal heartbeat, chest pain, persistent rash, or loss of taste perception.

You may get dizzy if you rise too quickly from a sitting or lying position. Avoid strenuous exercise or very hot weather because heavy sweating or dehydration can cause a rapid drop in blood pressure.

While taking trandolapril, avoid over-the-counter diet pills, decongestants, and other stimulants that can raise blood pressure.

If you take trandolapril once a day and forget a dose, take it as soon as you remember. If it is within 8 hours of your next dose, skip the one you forgot and continue with your regular schedule. If you take trandolapril twice a day and miss a dose, take it right away. If it is within 4 hours of your next dose, take 1 dose immediately and another in 5 or 6 hours, then go back to your regular schedule. Never take a double dose.

Special Populations

Pregnancy/Breast-feeding
ACE inhibitors can cause fetal injury or death. Women who are or might be pregnant should not take ACE inhibitors. If you become pregnant, stop taking this drug and call your doctor immediately.

Relatively small amounts of trandolapril pass into breast milk, and the effect on a nursing infant is likely to be minimal. However, nursing mothers who must take this drug should consider bottle-feeding.

Seniors
Seniors may be more sensitive to the effects of this drug due to age-related losses in kidney or liver function.

Generic Name

Trastuzumab (tras-TUE-zue-mab)

Brand Name

Herceptin

Type of Drug

Antineoplastic.

Prescribed for

Breast cancer.

General Information

Trastuzumab, which works differently than chemotherapy or hormonal anticancer drugs, is used to treat breast cancer in women whose tumor cells produce excessive amounts of a protein called HER2, which stands for human epidermal growth factor receptor 2. This overproduction of the HER2 protein is believed to fuel the cancer's growth. Trastuzumab works by binding to particles of the HER2 protein on the surface of cancerous cells and blocking the protein's effect.

This action can slow the growth of tumors or reduce their size. Trastuzumab can be used alone or, for women who have not received chemotherapy, combined with paclitaxel. Trastuzumab is prescribed for breast cancer that has metastasized (spread) to other parts of the body.

Cautions and Warnings

Do not use trastuzumab if you are **allergic** to it or benzyl alcohol.

Cardiac health must be periodically evaluated while you are taking this drug. Using trastuzumab can lead to **congestive heart failure** and serious **heart ventricle disorders**. People who develop these conditions while taking trastuzumab may have to stop taking it.

Trastuzumab can cause **anemia** and a **low white-blood-cell count**. Periodic blood tests are necessary.

Possible Side Effects

▼ Most common: chills or fever during the first infusion of trastuzumab, nausea, vomiting, rash, diarrhea, dizziness, sleeplessness, appetite loss, cough, breathing difficulties, sore throat, runny nose, abdominal pain, weakness, back pain, headache, infection, and pain.

▼ Common: heart failure, rapid heartbeat, depression, tingling in the hands or feet, swelling in the arms or legs, fluid retention, sinus irritation, and flu-like symptoms.

▼ Less common: nerve pain or inflammation, anemia, low white-blood-cell count, acne, cold sores, bone pain, joint pain, and urinary infection.

▼ Rare: Rare side effects can occur in almost any part of the body. Contact your doctor if you experience any side effect not listed above.

Drug Interactions

• Trastuzumab should not be combined with any other drugs during intravenous infusion.

Food Interactions

None known.

Usual Dose

Adult: 0.9–3.6 mg per lb. of body weight given weekly by

IV infusion in a hospital or medical clinic or your doctor's office.

Child: not recommended.

Overdosage

Symptoms may include chills, shaking, fever, nausea, vomiting, pain, dizziness, fainting, difficulty breathing, headache, rash, and weakness. Medical attention is necessary.

Special Populations

Pregnancy/Breast-feeding

The safety of using trastuzumab during pregnancy is not known, though it is likely to affect the fetus. When this drug is considered crucial by your doctor, its potential benefits must be carefully weighed against its risks.

Trastuzumab passes into breast milk. Nursing mothers should not breast-feed during drug treatment or for 6 months after treatment is finished.

Seniors

Seniors are more likely to develop cardiac side effects.

Generic Name

Trazodone (TRAY-zoe-done) Ⓖ

Brand Names

Desyrel   Desyrel Dividose

Type of Drug

Antidepressant.

Prescribed for

Depression with or without anxiety, cocaine withdrawal, panic disorder, agoraphobia (fear of open spaces), and aggressive behaviors.

General Information

Trazodone hydrochloride is chemically different from other antidepressants. It is just as effective as other drugs in treating the symptoms of depression but may be less likely to cause side effects. Symptoms can often be relieved as early as 2 weeks after starting trazodone, but 4 or more weeks may be required to achieve maximum benefit.

Cautions and Warnings

Do not use trazodone if you are **allergic** to it. Do not use trazodone if you are recovering from a **heart attack**. People with a previous history of **heart disease** should not use trazodone because it may cause abnormal heart rhythms.

Though rare, painful and sustained erections have occurred with trazodone. If this happens, stop taking the drug and call your doctor. One-third of these cases may require surgery or may lead to a permanent inability to achieve erection.

Possible Side Effects

▼ Most common: upset stomach; constipation; abdominal pains; a bad taste in the mouth; nausea; vomiting; diarrhea; palpitations; rapid heartbeat; rash; swelling of the arms or legs; blood pressure changes; breathing difficulties; dizziness; anger; hostility; nightmares; vivid dreams; confusion; disorientation; loss of memory or concentration; drowsiness; fatigue; lightheadedness; difficulty sleeping; nervousness; excitement; headache; loss of coordination; tingling in the hands or feet; tremor of the hands or arms; ringing or buzzing in the ears; blurred vision; red, tired, and itchy eyes; stuffy nose or sinuses; loss of sex drive; muscle ache and pain; appetite loss; weight gain or loss; increased sweating; clamminess; and feeling unwell.

▼ Less common: drug allergy, chest pain, heart attack, delusions, hallucinations, agitation, difficulty speaking, restlessness, numbness, weakness, seizures, increased sex drive, reverse ejaculation, impotence, missed or early menstrual periods, gas, increased salivation, anemia, reduced levels of certain white blood cells, muscle twitches, blood in the urine, reduced urine flow, increased urinary frequency, and increased appetite. Trazodone may cause elevations in levels of body enzymes, which are used to measure liver function.

Drug Interactions

• Trazodone may increase digoxin or phenytoin blood levels and the risk of side effects.

• Trazodone may increase the effects of sedatives, tranquilizers, alcohol, and other drugs that depress the nervous system.

• Trazodone may cause a small reduction in blood pressure. Your dosage of high blood pressure medication may have to be reduced slightly when you start taking trazodone. Clonidine (a drug used to treat high blood pressure) may be inhibited by trazodone. These interactions must be evaluated by your doctor.

• Little is known about the potential interaction between trazodone and monoamine oxidase inhibitor (MAOI) antidepressants. It is usually recommended that one antidepressant be discontinued 2 weeks before taking another. Caution should be used when combining trazodone and an MAOI.

Food Interactions

Take trazodone with food to increase effectiveness and reduce the risk of upset stomach, dizziness, and light-headedness.

Usual Dose

Adult: 150 mg a day with food, to start. This dose may be increased by 50 mg a day every 3–4 days, to a maximum of 400 mg a day. Severely depressed people may be prescribed as much as 600 mg a day.

Overdosage

Drowsiness and vomiting are the most frequent symptoms of trazodone overdose. Others include very severe side effects, especially those affecting mood and heart function. Fever may be present at first, but as time passes body temperature will drop below normal. Victims must be taken to a hospital emergency room immediately. ALWAYS bring the prescription bottle or container.

Special Information

Be careful when driving or performing any task that requires concentration. Avoid alcohol or other depressant drugs while taking trazodone.

Call your doctor if you develop any side effect, especially blood in the urine, dizziness, or light-headedness. Trazodone may cause dry mouth, irregular heartbeat, nausea, vomiting, or breathing difficulties.

If you forget a dose, take it as soon as possible. If it is within 4 hours of your next dose, skip the dose you forgot and go back to your regular schedule. Do not take a double dose.

Special Populations

Pregnancy/Breast-feeding

Trazodone may damage the fetus and generally should not be taken by women who are or might be pregnant. When this drug is considered crucial by your doctor, its potential benefits must be carefully weighed against its risks.

Trazodone passes into breast milk. Nursing mothers who must take it should consider bottle-feeding.

Seniors

Seniors may be more sensitive to trazodone's effects and should start with lower doses.

Generic Name

Tretinoin (TRET-in-oin) G

Brand Names

Avita   Retin-A
Renova

The information in this profile also applies to the following drug:

Generic Ingredients: Mequinol + Tretinoin
Solagé

Type of Drug

Anti-acne; and antiwrinkling agent and skin irritant.

Prescribed for

Acne and other skin conditions, skin cancer, acute promyelo-cytic leukemia (APL), wrinkling, and liver spots caused by chronic sun exposure.

General Information

Tretinoin, also known as retinoic acid or vitamin A acid, works against acne by decreasing the cohesiveness of skin cells, causing the skin to peel. Tretinoin is usually not effective in treating severe acne.

Medical research shows that regular application of tretinoin cream to aging skin prevents wrinkling and may even reverse the wrinkling process for some people. Tretinoin causes a temporary "plumping" of the skin when it is applied, peeling the outer layer. This gives the appearance of improved skin and reduced wrinkling. Some tretinoin— about 5%—is absorbed through the skin. When used to treat APL, a blood cancer, tretinoin causes the leukemia cells to mature and reduces the spread of APL cells; the exact way it works is not known.

Cautions and Warnings

Do not use tretinoin if you are **allergic** to it or any of its components.

This drug may increase the **skin-cancer-causing effects** of ultraviolet light. If you apply this drug to your skin you should allow a "rest period" between uses of tretinoin and other skin irritants or peeling agents. You must also limit sun exposure to treated areas and avoid sunlamps. If you cannot avoid sun exposure, use sunscreen and protective covering.

Do not apply tretinoin close to your eyes, the sides of the nose, or to mucous membrane tissue.

People with APL are at high risk for severe side effects. About 25% of people with APL treated with tretinoin develop a group of symptoms called retinoic acid-APL syndrome. These symptoms include fever, breathing difficulties, weight gain, and fluid in the lungs. Low blood pressure and loss of heart function may also occur.

Forty percent of people who take oral tretinoin develop a rapid **increase in white-blood-cell count,** which is associated with greater risk of life-threatening complications. Sixty percent of people taking tretinoin develop **high blood-cholesterol or triglyceride levels**.

Retinoids such as tretinoin have been associated with **pseudotumor cerebri** (increased pressure in the brain), especially in children. Early signs of this problem include swelling in the eyes, headache, nausea, vomiting, and visual difficulties.

There is limited information on children's use of tretinoin, though children ages 1 to 16 have used this medication.

Possible Side Effects

Skin Products

▼ Most common: burning, stinging, tingling, itching, swelling, or blistering of the skin; formation of crusts on the skin near the application site; and temporary skin discoloration and greater sun sensitivity. All side effects disappear after the drug has been stopped.

▼ Common: skin irritation.

▼ Less common: dry skin, crusting, and rash.

Capsules

▼ Most common: headache, fever, weakness, and fatigue. These generally go away with time.

▼ Common: skin changes, dry skin and membranes, bone pain and inflammation, itching, sweating, visual disturbances and other eye problems, hair loss, earache or a feeling of fullness in the ears, not feeling well, shivering, bleeding, infection, swelling in the arms or legs, pain, chest discomfort, weight gain, breathing difficulties, pneumonia, wheezing, abdominal pain, diarrhea, constipation, upset stomach, abnormal heart rhythms, blood-pressure changes, vein irritation, dizziness, tingling in the hands or feet, sleeplessness, depression, confusion, and bleeding in the brain.

▼ Less common: muscle aches, pain in the side, skin irritation, facial swelling, loss of color, lymph system problems, asthma, swollen larynx, gas, swollen liver, hepatitis, ulcer, heart failure, heart attack, heart inflammation, kidney problems including kidney failure, painful urination, frequent urination, enlarged prostate, agitation, hallucination, an unusual walk, convulsions, coma, depression, paralysis of the face, and a variety of nervous system problems.

▼ Rare: hearing loss.

Drug Interactions

Skin Products

• Other skin irritants will cause excessive sensitivity, irritation, and side effects. Among the substances that cause this interaction are medications that contain sulfur in topical form, resorcinol, benzoyl peroxide, or salicylic acid; abrasive soaps or skin cleansers; cosmetics, creams, or ointments with a severe drying effect; and products with a high alcohol, astringent, spice, or lime content.

• Tretinoin increases the absorption of minoxidil through the skin when they are applied together, leading to lower blood pressure.

Capsules

• Combining ketoconazole, and other drugs that affect systems in the liver that break down tretinoin, with tretinoin causes a substantial increase in tretinoin blood levels.

Food Interactions

Tretinoin capsules are better absorbed when taken with food.

Usual Dose

Skin Products: Wash the affected area thoroughly and apply a small amount of tretinoin at bedtime.

Capsules: Dosage is individualized for each person. Doses are calculated from height and weight.

Overdosage

Ingesting tretinoin is like taking vitamin A and can be extremely dangerous for pregnant women, who should not take more vitamin A than is contained in their prenatal vitamins. Infants who swallow tretinoin should be taken to a hospital emergency room for treatment. Symptoms of accidental ingestion include headache, facial flushing, abdominal pain, dizziness, and weakness. These symptoms have resolved without apparent aftereffects.

Special Information

Your acne may worsen during the first few weeks of treatment because the drug is acting on deeper, hidden lesions. This is beneficial and is not a reason to stop using tretinoin. Results should be seen in 2 to 3 weeks but may not reach maximum effect for 6 weeks; normal cosmetics can be used during this time.

Keep this drug away from your eyes, nose, mouth, and mucous membranes. Avoid skin exposure to sunlight or sunlamps.

Applying too much tretinoin will cause skin irritation and peeling but will not increase its effectiveness. Use your fingertip, a gauze pad, or a cotton swab when applying tretinoin to acne lesions to reduce the chances of applying too much medication.

You may feel warmth and slight stinging when you apply tretinoin. If you develop a burning sensation, peeling, redness, or are uncomfortable, stop using tretinoin for a short time.

Extreme weather or wind may cause severe irritation of skin treated with tretinoin.

If you forget a dose of tretinoin, do not apply the forgotten dose. Skip it and continue with your regular schedule. Do not apply a double dose.

Special Populations

Pregnancy/Breast-feeding
At very high doses, tretinoin causes birth defects in animals. A pregnant woman taking tretinoin capsules is likely to deliver a severely deformed infant. When applied to the skin, tretinoin is rapidly broken down. When this drug is considered crucial by your doctor, its potential benefits must be carefully weighed against its risks. Women who need to take tretinoin capsules should be tested for pregnancy before treatment is started. Use 2 reliable forms of contraception while you are taking tretinoin and for 1 month after treatment has ended.

It is not known if tretinoin passes into breast milk. Nursing mothers who must take tretinoin should bottle-feed.

Seniors
Seniors may use this product without special restriction.

Generic Name

Triazolam (trye-AY-zuh-lam) Ⓖ

Brand Name

Halcion

The information in this profile also applies to the following drugs:

Generic Ingredient: Quazepam
Doral

Generic Ingredient: Temazepam Ⓖ
Restoril

Type of Drug

Benzodiazepine sedative.

Prescribed for

Insomnia and sleep disturbances.

General Information

Triazolam is a member of the group of drugs known as benzodiazepines. Benzodiazepines work by a direct effect on the
brain. They make it easier to go to sleep and decrease the
number of times you wake up during the night. Triazolam has
the shortest action of drugs in this class. While this virtually
eliminates "hangover," it may also cause some people to
wake up earlier than they would like because the drug has
stopped working. Temazepam is considered to be an intermediate-acting sedative and generally remains in your body
long enough to give you a good night's sleep with minimal
hangover.

Cautions and Warnings

Triazolam has been associated with **memory loss,** especially when higher doses are taken. This effect, known as
traveler's amnesia, is most common among people who
take this medication to adjust to time zone changes during
travel; it may be linked to the use of alcoholic beverages
and to attempts at starting daily activity too soon after waking up.

If you abruptly stop taking triazolam, you may experience
rebound sleeplessness, where sleeplessness is worse during
the first 1 to 3 nights after you stop the drug than it was
before you started it.

People with respiratory disease may experience **sleep
apnea** (intermittent cessation of breathing during sleep)
while taking triazolam.

People with **kidney or liver disease** should be carefully
monitored while taking triazolam. Take the lowest possible
dose to help you sleep.

Clinical **depression** may be increased by triazolam, which can depress the nervous system. Intentional overdose is more common among depressed people who take sleeping pills than among those who do not.

All benzodiazepines can be **addictive** if taken for long periods of time and can cause drug withdrawal symptoms if suddenly discontinued. Withdrawal symptoms include tremors, muscle cramps, insomnia, agitation, diarrhea, vomiting, sweating, and convulsions.

Possible Side Effects

▼ Common: drowsiness, headache, dizziness, talkativeness, nervousness, apprehension, poor muscle coordination, light-headedness, daytime tiredness, muscle weakness, slowness of movement, hangover, and euphoria (feeling "high").

▼ Rare: Rare side effects can affect your heart, stomach and intestines, urinary tract, blood, muscles, and joints. Contact your doctor if you experience any side effect not listed above.

Drug Interactions

• As with all benzodiazepines, the effects of triazolam are enhanced if it is taken with alcohol, antihistamines, tranquilizers, barbiturates, anticonvulsants, tricyclic antidepressants, or monoamine oxidase inhibitors (MAOIs).

• Oral contraceptives, cimetidine, disulfiram, itraconazole, ketoconazole, nefazadone, and isoniazid may increase the effect of triazolam by interfering with the drug's breakdown in the liver. Probenecid may also increase triazolam's effect.

• Cigarette smoking, rifampin, and theophylline may reduce the effect of triazolam.

• Triazolam decreases the effectiveness of levodopa.

• Triazolam may increase the amount of zidovudine (an AIDS drug—also known as AZT), phenytoin, or digoxin in your blood, increasing the chances of side effects.

• Mixing clozapine and benzodiazepines has led to respiratory collapse in a few people. Triazolam should be stopped at least 1 week before starting clozapine treatment.

• The effects of triazolam may be increased by the macrolide antibiotics—azithromycin, erythromycin, and clarithromycin.

Food Interactions

Triazolam may be taken with food if it upsets your stomach.

Usual Dose

Quazepam
   Adult (age 18 and over): 7.5–15 mg at bedtime. Dosage must be individualized for maximum benefit. Seniors should take the lowest effective dose.
   Child (under age 18): not recommended.

Temazepam
   Adult: 15–30 mg at bedtime. The dose must be individualized for maximum benefit.
   Senior: starting dose—5 mg at bedtime. Dosage may be increased if needed.
   Child (under age 18): not recommended.

Triazolam
   Adult (age 18 and over): 0.125–0.5 mg about 30 minutes before sleep.
   Senior: starting dose—0.125 mg, then increase in 0.125 mg steps until the desired effect is achieved.
   Child (under age 18): not recommended.

Overdosage

The most common symptoms of overdose are confusion, sleepiness, depression, loss of muscle coordination, and slurred speech. Coma may also occur. Overdose victims must be made to vomit with ipecac syrup—available at any pharmacy—to remove any remaining drug from the stomach. Call your doctor or a poison control center before doing this. If 30 minutes have passed since the overdose was taken or if symptoms have begun to develop, the victim must immediately be taken to a hospital emergency room. ALWAYS bring the prescription bottle or container.

Special Information

Never take more triazolam than your doctor has prescribed.
   Avoid alcohol and other nervous system depressants while taking triazolam.
   Exercise caution while performing tasks that require concentration and coordination. Triazolam may make you tired, dizzy, or light-headed.

If you take triazolam daily for 3 or more weeks, you may experience some withdrawal symptoms when you stop taking it.

Benzodiazepines, including triazolam, can cause a morning-after hangover. Do not take triazolam unless circumstances will allow for a full night's sleep and some time before you need to be alert and active.

If you forget to take a dose of triazolam and remember within 1 hour of your regular time, take it as soon as you remember. If you do not remember until later, skip the dose you forgot and continue your regular schedule. Do not take a double dose.

Special Populations

Pregnancy/Breast-feeding

Triazolam should absolutely not be used by pregnant women.

Triazolam passes into breast milk. Nursing mothers who must take it should bottle-feed.

Seniors

Seniors are more susceptible to the effects of triazolam.

Type of Drug

Tricyclic Antidepressants

Brand Names

Generic Ingredient: Amitriptyline Ⓖ
Elavil

Generic Ingredients: Amitriptyline + Perphenazine Ⓖ

Etrafon	Triavil 2-25
Etrafon A	Triavil 4-10
Etrafon 2-10	Triavil 4-25
Etrafon Forte	Triavil 4-50
Triavil 2-10	

Generic Ingredients: Amitriptyline + Chlordiazepoxide Ⓖ
Limbitrol   Limbitrol DS 10-25

Generic Ingredient: Amoxapine Ⓖ
Asendin

Generic Ingredient: Clomipramine [G]
Anafranil

Generic Ingredient: Desipramine [G]
Norpramin

Generic Ingredient: Doxepin [G]
Sinequan

Generic Ingredient: Imipramine [G]
Tofranil   Tofranil-PM

Generic Ingredient: Nortriptyline [G]
Aventyl   Pamelor
Aventyl Pulvules

Generic Ingredient: Protriptyline [G]
Vivactil

Generic Ingredient: Trimipramine
Surmontil

Prescribed for

Depression, with or without symptoms of anxiety or sleep disturbance; chronic pain due to migraine, tension headache, diabetic disease, tic douloureux, cancer, herpes lesions, and arthritis; pathologic laughing or weeping caused by brain disease; bulimia; sleep apnea; peptic ulcer disease; cocaine withdrawal; panic disorder; eating disorder; premenstrual depression; and skin problems. Clomipramine is prescribed only for obsessive compulsive disorder (OCD).

General Information

Tricyclic antidepressants block the passage of stimulant chemicals—norepinephrine or serotonin—in and out of nerve endings, producing a sedative effect. They also counteract the effects of the neurohormone acetylcholine. Recent theory maintains that antidepressants work by causing long-term changes in the way nerve endings function. Tricyclic antidepressants can elevate mood, increase physical activity and mental alertness, and improve appetite and sleep patterns after 2 to 4 weeks of use.

Tricyclic antidepressants have been used in treating nighttime bed-wetting but do not produce long-lasting results. The combination of amitriptyline and perphenazine, a tranquilizer, is used to treat anxiety, agitation, and depression associated with chronic physical or psychiatric disease. The combination of amitriptyline and chlordiazepoxide, an antianxiety drug, is used to treat anxiety and depression. Tricyclic antidepressants are broken down in the liver.

Cautions and Warnings

Do not take one of these drugs if you are **allergic** or **sensitive** to any tricyclic antidepressant. These drugs should not be used if you are recovering from a **heart attack**; rapid heartbeat and fainting when rising from a sitting or lying position are problems associated with protryptiline.

These drugs should be taken with caution if you have a history of **epilepsy or other convulsive disorders; seizure,** which may be a special problem with clomipramine; **difficulty urinating; glaucoma; heart disease; liver disease;** or **hyperthyroidism.** Antidepressants may aggravate the condition of people who are schizophrenic or paranoid and may cause people with **bipolar (manic-depressive) disorder** to switch phase. These reactions are also possible when changing or stopping antidepressants.

Suicide is always a risk in severely depressed people, who should only be allowed to have minimal quantities of medication in their possession.

Amoxapine may cause very **high fever, muscle rigidity, changes in mental state, irregular pulse or blood pressure, sweating, abnormal heart rhythms,** and **rapid heartbeat.** This group of symptoms is associated with neuroleptic malignant syndrome (NMS), which may be **fatal.** If these symptoms develop, stop taking your medication at once and call your doctor. Clomipramine may also cause very high fever, especially when used with other drugs; this may also be a sign of NMS.

Amoxapine may increase the risk of potentially irreversible involuntary muscle movements associated with tardive dyskinesia (symptoms include lip smacking or puckering, puffing of the cheeks, rapid or worm-like tongue movements, uncontrolled chewing motions, and uncontrolled arm and leg movements). This condition is more common among the elderly, especially women.

Possible Side Effects

▼ Most common: sedation and anticholinergic effects including blurred vision; disorientation; confusion; hallucinations; muscle spasm or tremors; seizures or convulsions; dry mouth; constipation, especially in older adults; difficulty urinating; worsening glaucoma; and sensitivity to bright light.

▼ Less common: blood-pressure changes, abnormal heart rate, heart attack, anxiety, restlessness, excitement, numbness and tingling in the extremities, poor coordination, rash, itching, fluid retention, fever, allergy, changes in blood composition, nausea, vomiting, appetite loss, upset stomach, diarrhea, enlargement of the breasts in men and women, changes in sex drive, and blood-sugar changes.

▼ Rare: Rare side effects can occur in almost any part of the body. Contact your doctor if you experience any side effect not listed above.

Drug Interactions

• Combining a tricyclic antidepressant with a monoamine oxidase inhibitor (MAOI) antidepressant may cause high fever, convulsions, and death. Do not take an MAOI until at least 2 weeks after amitriptyline has been discontinued. People who must take both an MAOI and a tricyclic antidepressant require close medical observation.

• Tricyclics interact with guanethidine and clonidine (drugs used to treat high blood pressure). Tell your doctor if you are taking any drug for high blood pressure.

• Tricyclics increase the effects of barbiturates, tranquilizers, alcohol, and other sedative drugs. Barbiturates may decrease the effectiveness of a tricyclic antidepressant.

• Combining a tricyclic antidepressant and a thyroid drug enhances the effects of both, possibly causing abnormal heart rhythms. The combination of reserpine and a tricyclic antidepressant may cause overstimulation.

• Oral contraceptives ("the pill") may reduce the effect of a tricyclic antidepressant, as may smoking. Charcoal tablets may prevent antidepressant absorption by the blood. Estrogen may increase or decrease the effect of a tricyclic antidepressant.

• Bicarbonate of soda, acetazolamide, quinidine, and procainamide increase the effect of a tricyclic antidepressant.
Combining a tricyclic antidepressant and cimetidine, methylphenidate, or phenothiazine drugs such as thorazine and
compazine may cause severe side effects.

Food Interactions

You may take a tricyclic antidepressant with food if it upsets
your stomach.

Usual Dose

Amitriptyline
   Adult and Child (age 12 and over): 25 mg 3 times a day,
increased to 150 mg a day if necessary.
   Senior: lower dosages are recommended, generally 30–50
mg a day.
   Child (under age 12): not recommended.

Amoxapine
   Adult and Child (age 17 and over): 100–400 mg a day. Hos-
pitalized patients may need up to 600 mg a day.
   Senior: lower dosages are recommended. People over age
60 usually take 50–300 mg a day.
   Child (under age 17): not recommended.

Clomipramine
   Adult: 25–250 mg a day.
   Child: 25–100 mg a day.

   This drug may be taken at bedtime to minimize daytime
sedation.

Desipramine
   Adult and Child (age 12 and over): 75–300 mg a day. People
taking high dosages should have regular heart examinations
to check for side effects.
   Senior: lower dosages are recommended, usually 25–150
mg a day.
   Child (under age 12): not recommended.

Doxepin and Imipramine
   Adult: start with about 75 mg a day in divided doses, then
increase or decrease as needed. The final daily dosage may
be less than 75 or up to 200 mg. Long-term depression may
be treated with sustained-release medication taken daily at
bedtime or several times a day.

Senior: starting dosage—30–40 mg a day. Maintenance dosage—usually less than 100 mg daily.

Child (doxepin: age 12 and over; imipramine: age 6 and over): 25 mg a day, given 1 hour before bedtime for nighttime bed-wetting. If bed-wetting does not cease within a week, daily dosage is typically increased to 50–75 mg depending on age—more than 75 mg a day increases side effects without increasing effectiveness. Doses are often taken in mid-afternoon and at bedtime. The dosage should be gradually reduced to help prevent bed-wetting from recurring. Doxepin concentrate should be diluted with about 4 oz. of milk, water, or juice just before it is taken. Do not mix with soda or grape juice.

Nortriptyline
Adult: 25 mg 3 times a day, increased to 150 mg a day if necessary.
Senior: lower dosages are recommended, generally 30–50 mg a day.
Child (age 6–17): 10–20 mg a day.
Child (under age 6): not recommended.

Protriptyline
Adult: 15–60 mg a day in 3–4 divided doses. Protriptyline must not be taken as a single bedtime dose because of its stimulant effect.
Senior: lower dosages are recommended, usually up to 20 mg a day. Seniors taking more than 20 mg a day should have regular heart examinations.
Child: not recommended.

Trimipramine
Adult: 75 mg a day in divided doses to start, then increased as necessary to 150–200 mg. The entire daily dosage may be taken at bedtime or divided into several doses a day. Hospitalized adults may receive up to 300 mg a day.
Senior: starting dosage—50 mg a day. Maintenance dosage—up to 100 mg daily.
Child: not recommended.

Overdosage

Symptoms include confusion, inability to concentrate, hallucinations, drowsiness, lowered body temperature, abnormal heart rate, heart failure, enlarged pupils, convulsions, severely lowered blood pressure, stupor, and coma. Overdose victims should be taken to a hospital emergency room immediately. ALWAYS bring the prescription bottle or container.

Special Information

Avoid alcohol and other depressants while taking any tricyclic antidepressant. Do not stop taking your medication without your doctor's knowledge. Abruptly stopping a tricyclic antidepressant may cause nausea, headache, and feelings of ill health.

Tricyclic antidepressants may cause drowsiness, dizziness, and blurred vision. Be careful when driving or doing any task that requires concentration. Avoid prolonged exposure to the sun.

Call your doctor immediately if you develop seizure, breathing difficulties or rapid breathing, fever and sweating, blood-pressure changes, muscle stiffness, loss of bladder control, or unusual tiredness or weakness. Dry mouth may lead to an increase in dental cavities and gum bleeding and disease. Maintain good dental hygiene while taking a tricyclic antidepressant.

If your symptoms are unchanged after 6 to 8 weeks of treatment with an antidepressant, contact your doctor.

When used for nighttime bed-wetting, doxepin and imipramine are often ineffective.

If you forget a dose, skip it and go back to your regular schedule. Do not take a double dose.

Special Populations

Pregnancy/Breast-feeding

Tricyclic antidepressants cross into the fetal circulation. Birth defects including heart, breathing, and urinary problems have been reported when women took a tricyclic antidepressant during the first 3 months of pregnancy. When any of these drugs is considered crucial by your doctor, its potential benefits must be carefully weighed against its risks.

Small amounts of these drugs pass into breast milk. Nursing mothers who must take a tricyclic antidepressant should bottle-feed.

Seniors

Seniors are more sensitive to the effects of these drugs, especially abnormal heart rhythms and other cardiac side effects, and often require reduced dosage.

Trimox   *see Penicillin Antibiotics, page 785*

Triphasil   *see Contraceptives, page 254*

Type of Drug

Triptan-Type Antimigraine Drugs
(TRIP-tan)

Brand Names

Generic Ingredient: Naratriptan
Amerge

Generic Ingredient: Rizatriptan
Maxalt

Generic Ingredient: Sumatriptan
Imitrex

Generic Ingredient: Zolmitriptan
Zomig

Prescribed for

Migraine. Sumatriptan injection can be used for cluster headaches.

General Information

Triptan-type drugs are used to alleviate symptoms of migraine, which include severe headaches as well as nausea, vomiting, and increased sensitivity to light and sound. These drugs work by affecting specific serotonin (5HT) receptors in the brain. This action constricts (narrows) blood vessels in the brain, which are usually dilated (widened) during a migraine attack. Triptan-type drugs mainly interfere with one type of serotonin receptor, known as 5-HT$_{1B/1D}$, and do not affect other serotonin receptors. While these drugs can alleviate symptoms of migraine, they do not prevent attacks.

Triptan-type drugs are only recommended after analgesics (pain relievers)—such as aspirin, acetaminophen, and other nonsteroidal anti-inflammatory drugs (NSAIDs)—have failed to relieve symptoms. If you experience serious, incapacitating migraines more often than twice a month, your doctor may recommend taking other medications on a regular basis to reduce the number and severity of attacks including beta blockers, calcium channel blockers, tricyclic antidepressants, MAOIs, methysergide, and cyproheptadine. Triptan-type drugs generally start to relieve migraine symptoms in about 1 hour; rizatriptan works fastest. They are broken down partially in the liver.

Cautions and Warnings

Do not use these drugs if you are **allergic** to them.

These drugs should only be prescribed after you have been diagnosed with migraine (sumatriptan injection may be used for cluster headaches) because they are not effective in treating other types of headache or pain.

Zolmitriptan and naratriptan should not be used if you have uncontrolled **high blood pressure**.

It is strongly recommended that triptan-type drugs not be taken by **people at risk for heart disease,** as indicated by factors including high blood pressure, high blood cholesterol, smoking, obesity, diabetes, and a family history of heart disease. If you have any of these risk factors, your doctor must evaluate you heart disease risk before prescribing one of these drugs. People who take triptan-type drugs regularly or who develop risk factors for heart disease should be reevaluated by their doctors. Rarely, serious cardiac problems have occurred after taking one of these drugs.

People have experienced **chest, neck, or jaw tightness and pain** after taking one of these drugs, but these sensations are rarely associated with heart problems.

Do not take these drugs if your **headache is different** in any way. A change in the characteristics of your headache may signal a much more serious problem. Call your doctor at once.

Strokes and some fatalities have occurred in people taking sumatriptan, though they may have happened because a stroke-related headache was treated with sumatriptan rather than as a symptom of stroke. People with migraine are more likely to have a stroke or bleeding in the brain. Sumatriptan has been associated with **seizures**.

Rizatriptan must be used with caution by people with severe **kidney problems** or moderate to severe **liver disease**. People with severe kidney or liver disease should not take naratriptan.

These drugs can collect in the eye and cause **eye disorders** if taken over a long period. Have your eyes checked regularly.

Possible Side Effects

Side effects are usually mild or moderate and do not last long and are the same in men and women regardless of age. Some reported side effects (nausea, vomiting, dizziness, fainting, a feeling of ill health, drowsiness, and sedation) are also migraine symptoms. Side effects may increase with dosage, especially tingling in the hands or feet; chest, neck, jaw, or throat tightness or heaviness; dizziness; tiredness; weakness; and nausea. Rare side effects can affect the heart and blood vessels, nervous system, skin, stomach and intestines, urinary and reproductive systems, blood, muscles and bones, eyes, ears, nose, throat, and other parts of the body. Contact your doctor if you experience any side effect not listed below.

Naratriptan
▼ Less common: nausea; tingling in the hands or feet; dizziness; fatigue; drowsiness; pain or pressure in the neck, throat, or jaw; and pain.

Rizatriptan
▼ Common: dizziness, tiredness, fatigue, and nausea.
▼ Less common: tingling in the hands or feet; headache; pain or pressure in the neck, throat, chest, or jaw; pain, and dry mouth.

Sumatriptan
▼ Common: tingling and nasal discomfort.
▼ Less common: unusual sensations of warmth or cold, flushing, heart palpitations, heaviness, tightness, pressure, eye problems, and weakness. At high dosages, agitation, eye irritation, and painful urination may occur.

Zolmitriptan
▼ Most common: tightness in the jaw or neck, tingling, a warm or burning sensation, tiredness, dizziness, and fainting.

Possible Side Effects *(continued)*
▼ Less common: diminished sensitivity to stimulation, heart palpitations, chest pain or pressure, sweating, and muscle aches.

Drug Interactions

• Cimetidine doubles the time that zolmitriptan remains in the blood. You may need a lower dosage of zolmitriptan if you are combining these drugs.

• Oral contraceptives ("the pill") increase naratriptan and zolmitriptan blood levels and the risk of side effects.

• Ergotamine and dihydroergotamine may add to the effects of triptan-type drugs. Allow at least 24 hours between taking these drugs.

• Do not combine triptan-type drugs.

• Monoamine oxidase inhibitor (MAOI) drugs can increase blood levels of sumatriptan, zolmitriptan, and rizatriptan, and the risk of their side effects. Do not combine these drugs. Stop taking an MAOI at least 2 weeks before starting on sumatriptan, zolmitriptan, or rizatriptan.

• Propranolol may significantly increase zolmitriptan blood levels.

• Rarely, combining a triptan-type drug with a selective serotonin reuptake inhibitor (SSRI) antidepressant such as fluoxetine, fluvoxamine, or sertraline can cause weakness, overly sensitive reflexes, and poor coordination. This interaction does not occur with paroxetine.

Food Interactions

These drugs may be taken with or without food.

Usual Dose

Naratriptan
    Adult (age 18 and over): 1–2.5 mg as soon as migraine symptoms begin or at any time during the attack. If symptoms do not go away, you may take another tablet in 4 hours. Do not take more than 5 mg a day.
    Child: not recommended.

Rizatriptan Tablets
    Adult (age 18 and over): 5–10 mg as soon as migraine

symptoms begin or at any time during the attack. If symptoms do not go away, you may take another tablet in 2 hours. Do not take more than 30 mg a day. People also taking propranolol should take no more than 5 mg of rizatriptan at a time, up to 15 mg a day.

Child: not recommended.

Rizatriptan Tablets (Disintegrating)
Dosage is the same as for regular rizatriptan tablets, but these tablets can be taken without fluid. Do not take the tablet out of its protective packaging until just before you swallow it. Make sure your hands are dry and place the tablet on your tongue, where it will dissolve and be swallowed with your saliva. For people with phenylketonuria (PKU disease): orally disintegrating tablets have 1.05 mg of phenylalanine per 5 mg.

Sumatriptan Tablets
Adult (age 18 and over): 25–50 mg as soon as migraine symptoms begin or at any time during the attack. If symptoms do not go away, you may take another 25–50 mg every 2 hours. Do not take more than 300 mg a day. People with liver disease should take the lowest effective dosage.

Child: not recommended.

Sumatriptan Nasal Spray
Adult (age 18 and over): 1–2 sprays of the 5 mg nasal spray or 1 spray of the 20 mg spray into 1 nostril only. Higher dosages may increase side effects. The dose may be repeated 2 or more hours later if symptoms return. Do not take more than 40 mg (8 sprays of the 5-mg or 2 sprays of the 20-mg) a day.

Sumatriptan Injection
Adult (age 18 and over): 6 mg as a subcutaneous injection; the dose may be repeated if symptoms return. Do not take more than 12 mg every 1–2 days. Single doses larger than 6 mg are not more effective and are not recommended.

Child: not recommended.

Zolmitriptan
Adult (age 18 and over): 1.25–5 mg as soon as migraine symptoms begin or at any time during the attack. If symptoms do not go away, you may take another tablet in 2 hours; do not take more than 10 mg a day. People with liver disease should take the lowest effective dosage.

Child: not recommended.

Overdosage

Overdose can be expected to cause sedation, convulsions, tremors, swelling, redness in the arms or legs, physical inactivity, slowed breathing, bluish discoloration of the lips or skin under the fingernails, weakness, dilated pupils, paralysis, increased blood pressure, light-headedness, neck tension, or poor coordination. Take the victim to a hospital emergency room. ALWAYS bring the prescription bottle or container.

Special Information

Tell your doctor if you have high blood pressure, high cholesterol, diabetes, obesity, or a history of smoking.

Stop taking the drug and contact your doctor at once if you develop shortness of breath; wheezing; heart palpitations; swelling in the eyelids, face, or lips; rash; lumps; hives; severe tightness in the chest or throat; or sudden abdominal pain.

These drugs may make you tired or dizzy. Be careful when driving or performing any task that requires concentration.

These drugs can increase your sensitivity to the sun. Use sunscreen and wear protective clothing.

These drugs are meant only to treat migraine or cluster headache. They do not work for other types of headache or pain.

Take your medication at the first sign of a migraine—usually pain or aura. You may enhance the effect of the drug if you lie down in a quiet, dark room.

Avoid alcohol because it can worsen your headaches.

Read and follow the product instructions.

Call your doctor if the usual dosage does not relieve 3 consecutive headaches, if your headaches become more frequent or worse, or if you develop chest pain; difficulty swallowing or breathing; high blood pressure; chest pressure, tightness, or heaviness; nausea; vomiting; or any bothersome or persistent side effect.

People taking one of these medicines should have their eyes checked periodically.

Special Populations

Pregnancy/Breast-feeding

Animal studies have shown possible toxic effects on the fetus. When any of these drugs is considered crucial by your doctor, its potential benefits must be carefully weighed against its risks.

Sumatriptan passes into breast milk. Animal studies show that other triptan-type drugs may pass into breast milk. Nursing mothers who must take any of these drugs should consider bottle-feeding.

Seniors

Rizatripan, sumatriptan, and zolmitriptan may be taken without special precaution. Seniors are more likely to develop naratriptan side effects; this drug is not recommended for them.

Generic Name

Troglitazone (troe-GLIT-uh-zone)

Brand Name

Rezulin

Type of Drug

Antidiabetic.

Prescribed for

Type II diabetes and polycystic ovary syndrome.

General Information

Troglitazone reduces the amount of sugar produced by the liver and increases the amount used by muscle, liver, and fat cells. Troglitazone apparently works by affecting genes responsible for the control of sugar and fat use in the body, making cells more sensitive to insulin. This drug is effective for people with type II diabetes, who generally have enough insulin but whose cells do not respond to it. Troglitazone must be combined with a sulfonylurea-type antidiabetes drug or metformin.

Cautions and Warnings

Do not take troglitazone if you are **allergic** or **sensitive** to it. Troglitazone is broken down in the liver; it should be taken with caution by people who have **hepatitis** or **liver disease**; it may be toxic to the liver in some people.

Troglitazone should be used with caution if you have **heart failure**. Animals given 14 times the maximum human dosage of troglitazone developed enlarged hearts, a sign of heart failure. This effect has not been seen in people taking troglitazone, but increased blood volume, another sign of heart failure, occurred in some people taking the drug. Since people with heart failure were not included in studies of troglitazone, caution is advised.

Premenopausal women who are not ovulating may be at risk of becoming pregnant because troglitazone can trigger **ovulation**.

Possible Side Effects

In studies, the side effects of troglitazone were about the same as those for a placebo (sugar pill).

▼ Most common: infections, headache, and pain.

▼ Common: accidental injury, weakness, dizziness, back pain, nausea, runny nose, diarrhea, urinary infection, swelling, and sore throat.

▼ Rare: yellowing of the skin or whites of the eyes, hepatitis, liver failure, and death.

Drug Interactions

• Troglitazone may reduce the effectiveness of oral contraceptives ("the pill") containing norethindrone and ethinyl estradiol. Higher-dose contraceptives or another contraceptive method may be needed.

• Combining troglitazone and insulin may lead to very low blood sugar; insulin dosage may have to be reduced. Combining troglitazone and glyburide (a sulfonylurea-type antidiabetes drug) can also excessively lower blood sugar.

• Troglitazone can stimulate the breakdown of other drugs also metabolized in the liver.

• Cyclosporine, tacrolimus, terfenadine, and blood-fat reducers may be affected by troglitazone; dosage adjustments may be needed.

• Cholestyramine may reduce the amount of troglitazone absorbed into the blood by 70%. Separate doses of these drugs by several hours.

Food Interactions

For optimal effectiveness, take troglitazone with meals.

Usual Dose

Adult: 400–600 mg a day.

Overdosage

Little is known about the effects of troglitazone overdose, though symptoms may resemble side effects. Call your local poison control center or a hospital emergency room for more information. If you seek treatment, ALWAYS bring the prescription bottle or container.

Special Information

If you are also taking insulin, be sure to follow your doctor's directions for dosage reduction. Your blood sugar and insulin requirements can change if you have fever, trauma, infection, or surgery.

If you forget a dose, take it with your next meal. If it is almost time for your next dose, skip the forgotten dose and continue with your regular schedule. Do not take a double dose.

Special Populations

Pregnancy/Breast-feeding
The safety of using troglitazone during pregnancy is not known, though it does not affect pregnant animals or their fetuses. Most experts recommend that diabetes be controlled with insulin during pregnancy.

It is not known if troglitazone passes into breast milk, though it does in animal studies. Nursing mothers who must take this drug should bottle-feed.

Seniors
Seniors may take this drug without special precaution.

Brand Name

Tussionex Pennkinetic Ⓐ

Generic Ingredients

Hydrocodone + Chlorpheniramine

Type of Drug

Cough suppressant and antihistamine.

Prescribed for

Cough and other symptoms of a cold or other respiratory condition.

General Information

Tussionex Pennkinetic is one of many cough suppressant-antihistamine combinations that may be prescribed to treat a cough or congestion that has not responded to other medication. The narcotic cough-suppressant ingredient in this combination, hydrocodone, is more potent than codeine.

Cautions and Warnings

Do not use Tussionex Pennkinetic if you are **allergic** to any of its ingredients. Those allergic to codeine may also be allergic to Tussionex Pennkinetic. Chronic (long-term) use of this drug may lead to drug dependence or **addiction**. Tussionex Pennkinetic may cause **drowsiness, tiredness,** or **loss of concentration**. Use with caution if you have a history of **convulsions, glaucoma,** stomach **ulcer, hypertension** (high blood pressure), **thyroid disease, heart disease,** or **diabetes**.

Possible Side Effects

▼ Most common: light-headedness, dizziness, sleepiness, nausea, vomiting, increased sweating, itching, rash, sensitivity to bright light, chills, and dryness of the mouth, nose, or throat.

▼ Less common: euphoria (feeling "high"), weakness, agitation, uncoordinated muscle movement, disorientation and visual disturbances, minor hallucinations, appetite loss, constipation, facial flushing, rapid heartbeat, palpitations, feeling faint, urinary difficulties, reduced sexual potency, low blood sugar, anemia, yellowing of the skin or whites of the eyes, blurred or double vision, ringing or buzzing in the ears, wheezing, and nasal stuffiness.

Drug Interactions

• Do not use alcohol or other depressant drugs because they increase the depressant effect of Tussionex Pennkinetic.

• This drug should not be combined with monoamine oxidase inhibitor (MAOI) antidepressants.

Food Interactions

Take Tussionex Pennkinetic with food if it upsets your stomach.

Usual Dose

1 tsp. every 12 hours.

Overdosage

Symptoms include depression, slowed breathing, flushing, and upset stomach. Take the victim to a hospital emergency room. ALWAYS bring the prescription bottle or container.

Special Information

This drug causes sedation. Be careful when driving or doing any task that requires concentration.

If you forget a dose, take it as soon as you remember. If it is almost time for your next dose, skip the one you forgot and continue with your regular schedule. Do not take a double dose.

Special Populations

Pregnancy/Breast-feeding

Antihistamines pass into the circulation of the fetus but have not caused birth defects. Taking narcotics during pregnancy may lead to drug dependency in newborns or breathing difficulties if narcotics are used just prior to delivery. When this drug is considered crucial by your doctor, its potential benefits must be carefully weighed against its risks.

The ingredients in this product pass into breast milk and may affect an infant's breathing if abused. Nursing mothers who must take this drug should consider bottle-feeding.

Seniors

Seniors are more likely to be sensitive to both ingredients in Tussionex Pennkinetic and to experience depressant effects; dizziness, light-headedness or fainting when rising suddenly from a sitting or lying position; confusion; difficult or painful urination; feeling faint; dry mouth, nose, or throat; nightmares; excitement; nervousness; restlessness; or irritability.

Brand Name

Tussi-Organidin NR ⑤

Generic Ingredients

Codeine Phosphate + Guaifenesin Ⓖ

Other Brand Names

Cheracol	Halotussin AC ⑤ Ⓐ
Gani-Tuss NR	Mytussin AC
Guiatuss AC	Robafen AC
Guiatussin with Codeine	Robitussin A-C ⑤

Type of Drug

Cough suppressant and expectorant.

Prescribed for

Cough due to a cold or other upper respiratory infection.

General Information

In Tussi-Organidin NR, codeine is the ingredient that suppresses cough. Guaifenesin, an expectorant, increases the production of mucus and other bronchial secretions, making coughs more productive. Many experts question the effectiveness of guaifenesin, especially for removing the mucus that accumulates during serious respiratory conditions such as bronchitis, bronchial asthma, emphysema, cystic fibrosis, or chronic sinusitis. Drinking plenty of fluid works as well as any expectorant for the average cold or upper-respiratory cough. Expectorants do not suppress your cough.

Cautions and Warnings

Do not take Tussi-Organidin NR if you are **allergic** or **sensitive** to any of its ingredients. Chronic (long-term) use of codeine may lead to drug dependence or **addiction**.

Possible Side Effects

▼ Most common: light-headedness, dizziness, sedation or sleepiness, nausea, vomiting, diarrhea, stomach pain, and sweating.

Possible Side Effects *(continued)*

▼ Less common: euphoria (feeling "high"), weakness, headache, agitation, uncoordinated muscle movement, minor hallucinations, disorientation and visual disturbances, dry mouth, appetite loss, constipation, facial flushing, rapid heartbeat, palpitations, feeling faint, urinary difficulties or hesitancy, reduced sex drive or potency, itching, rash, anemia, lowered blood sugar, and yellowing of the skin or whites of the eyes. Narcotic analgesics (pain relievers) such as codeine may aggravate convulsions in those who have had them.

Drug Interactions

• Codeine has a general depressant effect and may affect breathing. Tussi-Organidin NR should be taken with extreme care in combination with alcohol, sedatives, tranquilizers, antihistamines, or other depressant drugs.

Food Interactions

Tussi-Organidin NR should be taken with a full glass of water or other fluid.

Usual Dose

2 tsp. every 4 hours as needed for cough relief.

Overdosage

Symptoms include breathing difficulties, pinpointed pupils, lack of response to pain stimulation, cold or clammy skin, slow heartbeat, low blood pressure, convulsions, heart attack, or extreme tiredness progressing to stupor and then coma. Take the victim to a hospital emergency room immediately. ALWAYS bring the prescription bottle or container.

Special Information

Codeine is a respiratory depressant and affects the central nervous system (CNS), producing sleepiness, tiredness, or an inability to concentrate. Be careful when driving or doing any task that requires concentration. Report persistent or bothersome side effects to your doctor.

If you take Tussi-Organidin NR 3 or more times a day and forget a dose, take it as soon as you remember. If it is almost time for your next dose, take 1 dose right away and another in 3 or 4 hours, then go back to your regular schedule. Do not take a double dose.

Special Populations

Pregnancy/Breast-feeding

Taking narcotics during pregnancy may lead to drug dependency in newborns or breathing difficulties if narcotics are used just prior to delivery. When Tussi-Organidin NR is considered crucial by your doctor, its potential benefits must be carefully weighed against its risks.

Codeine passes into breast milk and may affect an infant's breathing if abused. Nursing mothers who must take Tussi-Organidin NR should consider bottle-feeding.

Seniors

Seniors are more sensitive to the effects of codeine.

Ultram   see Tramadol, page 1032

Generic Name

Valacyclovir (val-ay-SYE-kloe-vere)

Brand Name

Valtrex

Type of Drug

Antiviral.

Prescribed for

Herpes zoster (shingles) and recurrent genital herpes.

General Information

Valacyclovir hydrochloride is rapidly converted to the antiviral acyclovir in the liver and intestine after it is absorbed into the blood. Acyclovir, the form valacyclovir takes in order to work, fights the herpes virus by inhibiting and inactivating an enzyme that is key to viral reproduction and by affecting the growing viral DNA chain.

Cautions and Warnings

Do not take valacyclovir if you are **allergic** to it, acyclovir, or any component of the tablet.

Some people with advanced **HIV disease**, or who have had a **bone marrow transplant** or an **organ transplant**, developed a potentially fatal condition known as TTP (blood-clotting disorder) while taking valacyclovir. This drug should not be taken by anyone with **AIDS** or a **compromised immune system**.

Possible Side Effects

▼ Most common: headache, diarrhea, dizziness, weakness, constipation, abdominal pain, appetite loss, nausea, and vomiting.

▼ Less common: aching joints, tingling in the hands or feet, stomach gas, fatigue, rash, not feeling well, leg pain, sore throat, a bad taste in the mouth, sleeplessness, and fever.

Drug Interactions

• Cimetidine and probenecid slow the rate at which valacyclovir is converted to acyclovir, but this does not change valacyclovir's effectiveness. No adjustments in valacyclovir dosage are necessary.

• Cimetidine and probenecid may decrease acyclovir elimination from your body and increase drug blood levels, raising the risk of side effects.

• Combining acyclovir and zidovudine (an AIDS drug—also known as AZT) may lead to severe drowsiness or lethargy.

Food Interactions

None known.

Usual Dose

Adult: shingles—1000 mg 3 times a day for 7 days. Genital herpes—500 mg twice a day for 5 days. Dosage is reduced in people with kidney disease.

Child (age 12 and under): not recommended.

Overdosage

Little is known about the effects of valacyclovir overdose. It may lead to kidney damage due to deposits of drug crystals in the kidney. Call your local poison control center for more information.

Special Information

Treatment with valacyclovir must be started as soon as possible after shingles is diagnosed. All information on the effectiveness of this drug was gathered from cases in which treatment was begun within 72 hours of diagnosis.

Women with genital herpes have an increased risk of cervical cancer. Check with your doctor about the need for an annual Pap smear.

Herpes may be transmitted even if you do not have symptoms of active disease. To avoid giving the condition to a sexual partner, do not have intercourse while visible herpes lesions are present. A condom should protect against transmission of the herpes virus, but spermicidal products or diaphragms do not. Valacyclovir alone will not prevent herpes transmission.

Call your doctor if valacyclovir does not relieve your symptoms, if side effects become severe, or if you become pregnant or want to begin breast-feeding.

Check with your dentist or doctor about how to take care of your teeth if you notice swelling or tenderness of the gums.

If you forget a dose of valacyclovir, take it as soon as you remember. If it is almost time for your next dose, skip the dose you forgot and continue with your regular schedule. Do not take a double dose.

Special Populations

Pregnancy/Breast-feeding

Acyclovir crosses into the circulation of the fetus. Animal studies have shown that large doses of acyclovir—up to 125 times the human dose—cause damage to both mother and fetus. When this drug is considered crucial by your doctor, its potential benefits must be carefully weighed against its risks.

Acyclovir passes into breast milk. Nursing mothers who must take it should consider bottle-feeding.

Seniors

People age 50 and over with shingles tend to have more severe attacks and respond best to valacyclovir treatment if the drug is started within 48 to 72 hours of the first sign of rash. Seniors with reduced kidney function should receive lower dosages.

Generic Name

Valproic Acid (val-PROE-ik) G

Brand Names

Depakene

Depakote

Depakote Sprinkle

Type of Drug

Anticonvulsant and antimanic.

Prescribed for

Petit mal and absence seizure and bipolar (manic-depressive) disorder; also prescribed for grand mal, myoclonic, and other seizures; prevention of fever convulsions in children; migraine; and anxiety or panic attacks.

General Information

Valproic acid is chemically unrelated to other drugs used in the treatment of seizure disorders. It may work by increasing levels of gamma-aminobutyric acid (GABA) and improving its effects in the brain. Valproic acid also has a stabilizing effect on cell membranes within the brain, which may account for some of the drug's other effects. It is broken down in the liver. The information in this profile applies to both forms of the drug: valproic acid (Depakene) and its related compound, divalproex sodium (Depakote). Divalproex sodium is made up of equal quantities of valproic acid and sodium valproate.

Cautions and Warnings

Do not take valproic acid if you are **allergic** to it.

Use this drug with caution if you have a history of **liver problems**. Liver failure, sometimes resulting in death, has occurred in people taking valproic acid. **Children under age 2** are at increased risk for liver failure associated with valproic acid, especially if they are also taking other anticonvulsants or have congenital disorders of metabolism, severe seizure disorders, mental retardation, or organic brain disease. After age 2, the risk of a fatal liver reaction decreases sharply. Ammonia in the bloodstream, another factor that worsens liver disease, may also occur with valproic acid.

If it is going to occur, serious liver disease usually develops during the first 6 months of valproic acid treatment and is often preceded by feeling unwell, weakness, tiredness, facial swelling, appetite loss, yellowing of the skin or whites of the eyes, vomiting, and loss of seizure control. Your doctor should check your liver function before beginning valproic acid treatment and periodically thereafter.

Valproic acid can affect **platelet function**, leading to bruising, bleeding, or changes in blood-clotting function.

Possible Side Effects

Side effects worsen as dosage increases.

▼ Most common: nausea, vomiting, indigestion, sedation or sleepiness, weakness, rash, emotional upset, depression, psychosis, aggression, hyperactive behavior, and changes in blood components.

▼ Less common: diarrhea, stomach cramps, constipation, increased or decreased appetite, headache, loss of eye-muscle control, drooping eyelids, double vision, spots before the eyes, loss of muscle control or coordination, and tremors.

Drug Interactions

• Valproic acid may increase the depressive effects of alcohol, sleeping pills, tranquilizers, phenobarbital, primidone, and other depressant drugs. It may slightly increase blood levels of clozapine or zidovudine (an AIDS drug—also known as AZT).

• Dosages of carbamazepine, clonazepam, ethosuximide, lamotrigine, and phenytoin may have to be adjusted when you begin taking valproic acid.

• Valproic acid may affect oral anticoagulant (blood-thinning) drugs; your anticoagulant dose may have to be adjusted.

• Aspirin, cimetidine, chlorpromazine, erythromycin, and felbamate may increase the risk of valproic acid side effects.

- Rifampin may reduce the effectiveness of valproic acid.
- Valproic acid may increase the need for levocarnitine.
- Valproic acid may increase the risk of bleeding or bruising if combined with other drugs that affect platelet "stickiness." These include aspirin, which also increases valproic acid side effects, and other nonsteroidal anti-inflammatory drugs (NSAIDs), dipyridamole, sulfinpyrazone, and ticlopidine.
- Valproic acid may cause false-positive reactions in the urine ketone tests used in diabetes.
- Charcoal tablets interfere with the absorption of valproic acid.

Food Interactions

Food slows the absorption of valproic acid slightly, but you may take it with food if it upsets your stomach. The syrup form can be mixed with food to improve its taste.

Do not take divalproex sodium with milk. Depakote Sprinkle can be taken whole or mixed with 1 tsp. of pudding, applesauce, or other soft food. Swallow the mixture promptly—do not chew.

Usual Dose

7–27 mg per lb. a day. Valproic acid is best taken in 1 dose at bedtime to minimize sedative effects. Daily dosages greater than 250 mg should be split into 2 or more doses a day. The dosage of divalproex sodium is measured in terms of the equivalent dosage of valproic acid.

Overdosage

Overdose may result in restlessness, hallucinations, flapping tremors of the hands, coma, and death. Call your local poison control center or take the victim to a hospital emergency room immediately. ALWAYS bring the prescription bottle or container.

Special Information

This medication may cause drowsiness: Be careful while driving or performing any task that requires concentration.

Do not chew or crush the capsules or tablets.

Do not switch brands of valproic acid without your doctor's knowledge. In at least 1 case, seizures resulted when a person was switched to a new product after 3 seizure-free years on another brand of valproic acid.

Valproic acid can cause mouth, gum, and throat irritation or bleeding, and increased risk of mouth infections. Maintain good dental hygiene while taking this drug. Dental work should be delayed if your blood counts are low.

People with a seizure disorder should carry special identification indicating their condition and any drugs being taken.

If you take valproic acid once a day and forget a dose, take it as soon as possible. If you do not remember until the next day, skip the dose you forgot and continue with your regular schedule. If you take valproic acid 2 or more times a day and forget a dose, take it as soon as possible if you remember within 6 hours of your regular time. Take the remaining daily dosage at evenly spaced intervals. Go back to your regular schedule the next day. Never take a double dose.

Special Populations

Pregnancy/Breast-feeding
Taking valproic acid during the first 3 months of pregnancy may increase the risk of birth defects. Pregnant women should take valproic acid only after discussing with their doctors its potential benefits and risks.

Valproic acid passes into breast milk and may affect a nursing infant. Nursing mothers who must take this drug should consider bottle-feeding.

Seniors
Seniors are more likely to experience side effects due to reduced kidney or liver function and may require lower dosage.

Generic Name

Venlafaxine (ven-luh-FAX-ene)

Brand Names

Effexor   Effexor XR

Type of Drug

Antidepressant.

Prescribed for

Depression.

General Information

Chemically different from other antidepressant drugs, venlafaxine may work by inhibiting the ability of nerve endings in
the brain to absorb serotonin, norepinephrine, and dopamine.
Venlafaxine passes out of the body primarily via the urine.

Cautions and Warnings

People with severe **kidney or liver disease** may require
reduced dosages.

Venlafaxine can raise **blood pressure**. If this happens, your
dosage of venlafaxine may have to be reduced. Venlafaxine
has not been fully studied in people with recent **heart attack**
or unstable **heart disease**, although a small study revealed no
unusual changes in their cardiograms.

Possible Side Effects

Side effects increase with dosage.

▼ Most common: blurred vision, tiredness, dry
mouth, dizziness, sleeplessness, nervousness, tremors,
weakness, sweating, nausea, constipation, appetite loss,
vomiting, impotence, and abnormal ejaculation.

▼ Less common: changes in sense of taste, ringing in
the ears, dilated pupils, high blood pressure, rapid heartbeat, anxiety, reduced sex drive, agitation, chills, yawning, and inability to experience orgasm.

▼ Rare: Rare side effects can occur in almost any part
of the body. Contact your doctor if you experience any
side effect not listed above.

Drug Interactions

• Taking venlafaxine within 2 weeks of taking a monoamine
oxidase inhibitor (MAOI) antidepressant may cause severe
reactions including high fever, muscle rigidity or spasm,
mental changes, and fluctuations in pulse, temperature, or
breathing rate. People stopping venlafaxine should wait at
least 1 week before starting an MAOI.

• Cimetidine can increase venlafaxine blood levels,
although the effect on the body may be minimal.

Food Interactions

Take each dose with food.

Usual Dose

Adult: 3.75–225 mg a day, divided into 2–3 doses. Some people may benefit from doses up to 375 mg a day. People with severe kidney or liver disease should receive half the usual daily dosage. Those with moderate kidney disease may need their daily dosage reduced by only 25%.

Child (under age 18): not recommended.

Overdosage

Symptoms may include tiredness, mild convulsions, and cardiac effects. Contact your local poison control center or a hospital emergency room for more information. Overdose victims should be taken to a hospital emergency room. ALWAYS bring the prescription bottle or container.

Special Information

Call your doctor if you develop rash, hives, or any other allergic-type reaction.

Venlafaxine may make you tired; be careful when driving or performing any task that requires concentration. Avoid alcohol.

If you forget a dose, take it as soon as you remember. If it is almost time for your next dose, skip the dose you forgot and continue with your regular schedule. Do not take a double dose.

Do not suddenly stop taking this drug. Venlafaxine dosage should be gradually reduced over a 2-week period.

Special Populations

Pregnancy/Breast-feeding

Animal studies of venlafaxine suggest that it may cause low birth weight and other problems. When this drug is considered crucial by your doctor, its potential benefits must be carefully weighed against its risks.

Venlafaxine passes into breast milk. Nursing mothers who must take this drug should consider bottle-feeding.

Seniors

Seniors may be more sensitive to side effects.

Generic Name

Verapamil (vuh-RAP-uh-mil) Ⓖ

Brand Names

Calan	Isoptin SR
Calan SR	Verelan
Covera HS	Verelan PM
Isoptin	

Type of Drug

Calcium channel blocker.

Prescribed for

Angina pectoris and Prinzmetal's angina, high blood pressure, abnormal heart rhythm, asthma, cardiomyopathy, migraine, nighttime leg cramps, and bipolar (manic-depressive) disorder.

General Information

Verapamil hydrochloride is one of many calcium channel blockers available in the U.S. These drugs block the passage of calcium, an essential factor in muscle contraction, into the heart and smooth muscles. Such blockage of calcium interferes with the contraction of these muscles, which in turn dilates (widens) the veins and vessels that supply blood to them. This dilating effect reduces blood pressure, the amount of oxygen used by the heart muscle, and the risk of blood vessel spasm. Verapamil is therefore useful in treating not only high blood pressure but also angina pectoris (brief attacks of chest pain), a condition related to poor oxygen supply to the heart muscle.

Verapamil affects the movement of calcium only into muscle cells; it has no effect on calcium in the blood.

The sustained-release brands of verapamil should be used only for high blood pressure.

Cautions and Warnings

Verapamil may cause **low blood pressure** in some people.

People taking a beta-blocking drug who begin taking verapamil may develop **heart failure**.

Do not take this drug if you have had an **allergic reaction** to it.

Verapamil may cause **angina** when treatment is first started, when dosage is increased, or if the drug is rapidly withdrawn. This can be avoided by reducing dosage gradually.

Studies have shown that people taking calcium channel blockers—usually those taken several times a day, not those taken only once daily—have a greater risk of having a **heart attack** than do people taking beta blockers or other medication for the same purposes. Discuss this with your doctor to be sure you are receiving the best possible treatment.

In small numbers of people, verapamil can lead to an unusual **slowing of heart rate**.

People with **hypertrophic cardiomyopathy** (progressive weakening and destruction of heart muscle) who are receiving up to 720 mg a day of verapamil are at risk of developing severe cardiac side effects. Most of these effects respond to dosage reduction, and people generally may continue on verapamil at a lower dosage.

People with **kidney disease** or severe **liver disease** should use this drug with caution and may require dosage adjustments.

Verapamil may slow the transmission of nerve impulses to muscle in people with **Duchenne's muscular dystrophy,** possibly causing respiratory muscle failure.

Possible Side Effects

Verapamil generally causes fewer side effects than other calcium channel blockers.

▼ Most common: rash; low blood pressure; slowed heartbeat; heart failure or lung congestion marked by coughing, wheezing, or breathing difficulties; tiredness or weakness; swelling of the ankles, feet, or legs; headache; dizziness; light-headedness; constipation; and nausea.

▼ Rare: chest pain, rapid or irregular heartbeat, unusual production of breast milk, bleeding or tender gums, fainting, flushing, and feeling warm. Other rare side effects can occur in almost any part of the body. Contact your doctor if you experience any side effect not listed above.

Some people taking verapamil have experienced heart attack and abnormal heart rhythm, but the occurrence of these effects has not been directly linked to verapamil.

Drug Interactions

• If you take verapamil for long periods of time, your dosage of digoxin or digitoxin will have to be lowered drastically.

• Disopyramide should not be taken within 48 hours of taking verapamil.

• People taking verapamil together with quinidine may experience very low blood pressure, slow heartbeat, and fluid in the lungs.

• Verapamil's effectiveness and its side effects may be reversed by taking calcium products, including antacids.

• Verapamil may interact with beta-blocking drugs to cause heart failure, very low blood pressure, or increased angina. Low blood pressure can also result from taking verapamil with fentanyl (a narcotic pain reliever).

• Verapamil may cause unexpected blood pressure reduction in patients also taking other medication to control their high blood pressure.

• Cimetidine and ranitidine increase the amount of verapamil in the blood and may account for a slight increase in its effect.

• The combination of dantrolene and verapamil may lead to high blood-calcium levels and heart muscle depression. If you are taking dantrolene, a calcium channel blocker other than verapamil should be prescribed by your doctor.

• Verapamil may increase the effects of carbamazepine, cyclosporine, and theophylline products, increasing the chance of side effects with those drugs.

• Verapamil may decrease the amount of lithium in your body, leading to a possible loss of antimanic control, lithium toxicity, and psychotic symptoms.

• Rifampin, barbiturates, phenytoin and similar antiseizure medicines, vitamin D, and sulfinpyrazone may decrease verapamil's effects.

Food Interactions

Take immediate-release products at least 1 hour before or 2 hours after meals. Take sustained-release products with food if they upset your stomach.

Usual Dose

120–480 mg a day, according to your needs.

Overdosage

Overdose of verapamil can cause low blood pressure. Symptoms are dizziness, weakness, and slowed heartbeat. If you have taken an overdose of verapamil, call your doctor or go to an emergency room. ALWAYS bring the prescription bottle or container.

Special Information

Call your doctor if you develop abnormal heart rhythm, swelling in the arms or legs, breathing difficulties, increased heart pain, dizziness, light-headedness, or low blood pressure. Do not stop taking verapamil abruptly.

If you forget to take a dose of verapamil, take it as soon as you remember. If it is almost time for your next dose, skip the one you forgot and continue with your regular schedule. Do not take a double dose.

Special Populations

Pregnancy/Breast-feeding

Verapamil may cause birth defects or interfere with fetal development. When this drug is considered crucial by your doctor, its potential benefits must be carefully weighed against its risks.

Verapamil passes into breast milk. Nursing mothers who must take this drug should bottle-feed.

Seniors

Seniors are more sensitive to side effects, especially low blood pressure.

Viagra   *see Sildenafil Citrate, page 933*

Vancenase AQ   *see Corticosteroids, Nasal, page 274*

Vasotec   *see Enalapril, page 371*

Veetids *see Penicillin Antibiotics, page 785*

Generic Name

Warfarin (WOR-far-in) Ⓖ

Brand Name

Coumadin

The information in this profile also applies to the following drugs:

Generic Ingredient: Anisindione
Miradon

Generic Ingredient: Dicumarol Ⓖ
Only available in generic form.

Type of Drug

Oral anticoagulant (blood thinner).

Prescribed for

Blood clots or coagulation; also prescribed for reducing the risk of small cell carcinoma of the lung, recurrent heart attack or stroke, and transient ischemic attack (TIA).

General Information

Warfarin prevents the formation of blood clots or coagulation by suppressing the body's production of vitamin-K-dependent factors essential to the coagulation process. If you are taking warfarin, you must take it exactly as prescribed. Notify your doctor at the earliest sign of unusual bleeding or bruising; blood in your urine or stool; or black, tarry stools. Warfarin may be affected by many other drugs, and these interactions may be dangerous (see "Drug Interactions"). Warfarin may also be extremely dangerous if not used properly. Periodic tests to monitor blood clotting are required for proper control of warfarin therapy.

Cautions and Warnings

Do not take warfarin if you are **allergic** to it. Anisindione is usually reserved for people allergic to warfarin.

Warfarin must be taken with care if you have any **blood-clotting disease**. Use of warfarin may be dangerous and should be discussed with your doctor if you have: **cramp-like pains and minor vaginal bleeding** that may or may not be followed by a spontaneous abortion during the first 20 weeks of pregnancy; past or planned eye or nervous system surgery; protein C deficiency—a hereditary condition; **liver inflammation or disease; kidney disease;** any **infection** being treated with an antibiotic; active **tuberculosis;** severe or prolonged **dietary deficiencies; stomach ulcer or bleeding; bleeding from the genital or urinary areas; high blood pressure;** severe **diabetes; vein irritation;** disease of the large bowel, such as **diverticulitis or ulcerative colitis;** and subacute bacterial **endocarditis.**

People with **congestive heart failure** may be more sensitive to dicumarol than to other anticoagulants.

Anisindione can cause **hepatitis** and **agranulocytosis** (condition characterized by a reduction in the number of white blood cells).

Anticoagulant therapy may increase the release of **microplaques** into the bloodstream. These microplaques may block very small blood vessels, leading to purple toe syndrome (condition that occurs when pressure exerted by normal walking leads to bleeding into the skin of your toes). This usually goes away when anticoagulant treatment is stopped but it may be a sign of a more serious problem present in another part of your body.

Women taking anticoagulants may be at risk of **ovarian bleeding** when they ovulate.

People taking warfarin must be extremely careful to **avoid cuts, bruises, or other injuries** that may cause internal or external bleeding.

Possible Side Effects

Warfarin and Dicumarol

▼ Most common: bleeding, which may occur with usual dosages and even when the results of blood tests used to monitor anticoagulant therapy are normal. If you bleed abnormally while you are taking anticoagulants, call your doctor immediately.

Possible Side Effects *(continued)*

▼ Less common: abdominal cramps, nausea, vomiting, diarrhea, fever, anemia, adverse effects on blood components, hepatitis, jaundice (symptoms include yellowing of the skin or whites of the eyes), itching, rash, hair loss, sore throat or mouth, red or orange urine, painful or persistent erection, and purple toe syndrome.

Anisindione
▼ Common: rash.
▼ Less common: headache, sore throat, blurred vision, hepatitis, liver or kidney damage, jaundice (symptoms include yellowing of the skin or whites of the eyes), red or orange urine, and changes in blood components.

Drug Interactions

Anticoagulants may have more drug interactions than any other kind of medication. Your doctor and pharmacist should keep records of all drugs you take in order to anticipate possible interactions. It is essential that your doctor and pharmacist know about every medication you are taking including over-the-counter (OTC) drugs containing aspirin.

• Drugs that may increase the effect of warfarin include the following: acetaminophen; aminoglycoside antibiotics; amiodarone; androgen; aspirin and other salicylate drugs; beta blockers; cephalosporin antibiotics; chloral hydrate; chloramphenicol; chlorpropamide; cimetidine; clofibrate; corticosteroids; cyclophosphamide; dextrothyroxine; diflunisal; disulfiram; erythromycin; fluconazole; gemfibrozil; glucagon; hydantoin antiseizure drugs—blood levels of the hydantoins may also be increased in this interaction; ifosfamide (an influenza virus vaccine); isoniazid; ketoconazole; loop diuretics; lovastatin; metronidazole; miconazole; mineral oil; moricizine; nalidixic acid; nonsteroidal anti-inflammatory drugs (NSAIDs); omeprazole; penicillin; phenylbutazone; propafenone; propoxyphene; quinidine; quinine; quinolone antibacterials; sulfa drugs; sulfinpyrazone; tamoxifen; tetracycline antibiotics; thioamines; thyroid hormones; and vitamin E.

• Some drugs decrease the effect of warfarin and the interaction may be just as dangerous. Some examples are alcohol, aminoglutethimide, ascorbic acid (vitamin C), barbiturates, carbamazepine, cholestyramine, dicloxacillin, glutethimide, ethchlorvynol, etretinate, meprobamate, griseofulvin, estrogen, oral contraceptives ("the pill"), chlorthalidone, nafcillin, rifampin, spironolactone, sucralfate, thiazide-type diuretics, trazodone, and vitamin K.

Food Interactions

Warfarin is best taken on an empty stomach because food slows the rate at which it is absorbed by the blood. Vitamin K counteracts the effects of warfarin. Avoid eating large quantities of vitamin-K-rich foods, such as spinach and other green, leafy vegetables. Any change in dietary habits or alcohol intake may affect warfarin's action.

Usual Dose

Warfarin: 2–15 mg or more a day; dosage must be individualized.

Anisindione: 300 mg the first day, 200 mg the second day, 100 mg the third day, and 25–250 mg daily thereafter.

Dicumarol: 200–300 mg the first day, then 25–200 mg a day.

Overdosage

The primary symptom is bleeding. Bleeding may make itself known by the appearance of blood in the urine or stool, an unusual number of black-and-blue marks, oozing of blood from minor cuts, or bleeding from the gums after brushing the teeth. If bleeding does not stop within 10 to 15 minutes, call your doctor. Your doctor may tell you to skip a dose of warfarin or go to a hospital or doctor's office for blood evaluations, or may give you a prescription for vitamin K, which antagonizes the effect of warfarin. This last approach has some dangers because it may complicate subsequent anticoagulant therapy.

Special Information

Do not change warfarin brands without your doctor's knowledge. Different brands may not be equivalent.

Do not stop taking warfarin unless directed to do so by your doctor.

Do not stop or start ANY other medication without your doctor's or pharmacist's knowledge. Avoid alcohol, aspirin and other salicylates, and drastic changes in your diet, since all of these may affect your response.

Call your doctor if you develop unusual bleeding or bruising, red or black tarry stool, or red or dark-brown urine.

Warfarin may turn your urine a red or orange color. This is different from blood in the urine—which causes urine to appear red or brownish in color—and generally happens only if your urine has less acid in it than normal.

If you forget a dose, take it as soon as you remember, then continue with your regular schedule. If you do not remember until the next day, skip the missed dose and continue with your regular schedule. Do not take a double dose. Call your doctor if you miss a dose.

Special Populations

Pregnancy/Breast-feeding

Warfarin is not considered safe for use during pregnancy. It passes into the fetal circulation and causes bleeding, brain and other abnormalities, and stillbirth in 30% of fetuses. In some pregnant women, the benefits of taking warfarin may outweigh its risks, but the drug should not be used during the first 3 months of pregnancy. Pregnant women who need an anticoagulant are often given heparin because it does not cross into the fetal bloodstream.

Warfarin and dicumarol pass into breast milk in an inactive form. Full-term babies are not affected by warfarin but dicumarol may affect a nursing child. The effect on premature babies is not known. Nursing mothers who must take dicumarol should bottle-feed.

Seniors

Seniors may be more sensitive to the effects of warfarin and obtain maximum benefit with smaller dosages.

Wellbutrin SR   see Bupropion, page 140

Xalatan   see Latanoprost, page 564

Type of Drug

Xanthine Bronchodilators (ZAN-thene)

Brand Names

Generic Ingredient: Aminophylline [G]
Phyllocontin   Truphylline

Generic Ingredient: Dyphylline [G]
Dilor   Lufyllin-400
Dilor-400   Neothylline
Lufyllin

Generic Ingredient: Oxtriphylline [G]
Choledyl SA

Generic Ingredient: Theophylline [G]

Aerolate*	Theo-24
Aquaphyllin [A]	Theo-Dur
Asmalix	Theo-Sav
Bronkodyl	Theo-X
Elixomin	Theobid Duracaps
Elixophyllin	Theochron
Lanophyllin [S]	Theoclear-80 [A]
Quibron-T Dividose	Theoclear L.A.
Quibron-T/SR Dividose	Theocron
Respbid	Theolair [A]
Slo-bid Gyrocaps	Theolair-SR
Slo-Phyllin [A]	Theospan-SR
Slo-Phyllin Gyrocaps	Theostat-80
Sustaire	Theovent
T-Phyl	Uniphyl

Some products in this brand-name group are alcohol- or sugar-free. Consult your pharmacist.

Prescribed for

Asthma and bronchospasm associated with emphysema, bronchitis, and other diseases; also prescribed for essential tremors and chronic obstructive pulmonary disease (COPD).

General Information

Xanthine bronchodilators are a mainstay of therapy for bronchial asthma and similar diseases. Although the dosage of each of these drugs is different, they all work by relaxing bronchial muscles and helping to reverse spasms. The exact way in which they work is not known.

Some xanthine bronchodilators are sustained-release products that act throughout the day. These minimize potential side effects by avoiding the peaks and valleys associated with immediate-release xanthine drugs. They also allow you to reduce the total number of daily doses.

Initial treatment with a xanthine bronchodilator requires your doctor to take blood samples to assess how much of the drug is in your blood. Dosage adjustments may be required based on these blood tests and on your response to the therapy. Because dyphylline is not eliminated by the liver, it is not subject to many of the drug interactions or limitations placed on the other xanthine bronchodilators.

Cautions and Warnings

Do not use a xanthine bronchodilator if you are **allergic** or **sensitive** to any of these medications. If you have a **stomach ulcer,** congestive **heart failure, heart disease, liver disease, low blood-oxygen levels,** or **high blood pressure,** or are an **alcoholic,** you should use this drug with caution. People with **seizure disorders** should not take a xanthine bronchodilator unless they are receiving appropriate anticonvulsant medicines. Theophylline may cause or worsen preexisting **abnormal heart rhythm**. Any change in heart rate or rhythm warrants your doctor's immediate attention.

Status asthmaticus, a medical condition in which the breathing passages are almost completely closed, does not respond to oral bronchodilators. Victims of this condition must be taken to a hospital emergency room at once for treatment.

Serious side effects, including convulsions, serious arrhythmias, and death, may be among the initial signs of drug toxicity. Periodic monitoring by your physician is mandatory if you are taking one of these drugs.

Dosage of dyphylline must be altered in the presence of **kidney failure**.

Possible Side Effects

Side effects are directly related to the amount of drug in your blood. As long as you stay in the proper range—below 20 mcg per ml of blood—you should experience few, if any, problems.

Possible Side Effects *(continued)*

▼ Most common: nausea; vomiting; stomach pain; diarrhea; irritability; restlessness; difficulty sleeping; rectal irritation or bleeding, especially with suppositories; and rapid breathing.

▼ Less common: excitability, high blood sugar, muscle twitching or spasms, heart palpitations, seizures, brain damage, or death. These effects are more likely when drug levels reach 35 mcg per ml or more.

▼ Rare: vomiting blood, regurgitating stomach contents while lying down, fever, headache, rash, hair loss, and dehydration.

Drug Interactions

• Taking two xanthine bronchodilators together may increase side effects.

• Xanthine bronchodilators are often given in combination with a stimulant drug such as ephedrine. Such combinations can cause excessive stimulation and should be used only as your doctor specifically directs.

• Reports have indicated that combining erythromycin, flu vaccine, allopurinol, beta blockers, calcium channel blockers, cimetidine—and, rarely, ranitidine—oral contraceptives, corticosteroids, disulfiram, ephedrine, interferon, mexiletine, quinolone antibacterials, or thiabendazole with a xanthine bronchodilator will increase blood levels of the xanthine bronchodilator. Higher blood levels mean the possibility of more side effects. Tetracycline may also increase the risk for xanthine bronchodilator side effects.

• The following drugs may decrease theophylline levels: aminoglutethimide, barbiturates, charcoal, ketoconazole, rifampin, sulfinpyrazone, sympathomimetic drugs, and phenytoin and other hydantoin anticonvulsants. The hydantoin level may also be reduced.

• Smoking cigarettes or marijuana makes xanthine bronchodilators less effective by increasing the rate at which your liver breaks them down. This does not apply to dyphylline.

• Drugs that may either increase or decrease xanthine bronchodilator levels include carbamazepine, isoniazid, and furosemide and other loop diuretics. Persons combining a xanthine bronchodilator with one of these drugs must be evaluated individually. Again, consult your doctor when combining xanthine bronchodilators with any of these drugs.

• People with an overactive thyroid clear xanthine bronchodilators faster and may require a larger dose. People with an underactive thyroid have the opposite reaction. Correcting thyroid function through medical or surgical treatment will normalize your response to a xanthine bronchodilator.

• A xanthine bronchodilator may counteract the sedative effect of valium and other benzodiazepine tranquilizers.

• Xanthine bronchodilators may interfere with or interact with a number of different drugs used during anesthesia. Your doctor may temporarily alter your bronchodilator dose or change drugs to avoid this problem.

• Blood lithium levels may be lowered by xanthine bronchodilators.

• Probenecid may increase the effects of dyphylline by interfering with its removal from the body through the kidneys.

• Xanthine bronchodilators may counteract the sedative effects of propofol.

Food Interactions

To obtain a consistent effect from your medication, take it at the same time each day on an empty stomach, at least 1 hour before or 2 hours after meals.

Theophylline is eliminated from the body faster if your diet is high in protein and low in carbohydrates. Eating charcoal-broiled beef also aids theophylline elimination. Conversely, the rate at which your body eliminates theophylline is reduced by a high-carbohydrate, low-protein diet. You may take some food with a liquid or immediate-release xanthine bronchodilator if it upsets your stomach. Dyphylline is not affected in this way.

Caffeine—a xanthine derivative—may add to the side effects of the xanthine bronchodilators, except dyphylline. Avoid large amounts of caffeine-containing products, such as coffee, tea, cola, cocoa, and chocolate, while taking one of these drugs.

Usual Dose

Aminophylline
   Adult (age 16 and over): 100–200 mg every 6 hours. Sustained-release—200–500 mg a day in 1–3 doses.

Child (under age 16): 50–100 mg every 6 hours, or 1–2.5 mg per lb. of body weight every 6 hours.

Dyphylline
Adult: up to 7 mg per lb. of body weight 4 times a day. Dosage is reduced when kidney failure is present.

Oxtriphylline
Adult: about 2 mg per lb. of body weight, 3 times a day. Sustained-release—400–600 mg every 12 hours.
Child (age 1–9): 2.8 mg per lb. of body weight 4 times a day.

Theophylline
Adult: up to 6 mg per lb. of body weight a day, to a maximum daily dose of 900 mg. Sustained-release—same dosage, but taken 1–3 times a day.
Child (age 12–16): up to 8.1 mg per lb. of body weight a day.
Child (age 9–11): up to 9 mg per lb. of body weight a day.
Child (age 1–8): up to 10.9 mg per lb. of body weight a day.
Infant (6–52 weeks): Your doctor will calculate total daily dosage in mg by a formula that factors in age and weight. Under 6 months, give ⅓ the total daily dosage every 8 hours; age 26 weeks–1 year, give ¼ the total daily dosage every 6 hours.
Premature Infant (25 days and over): 0.68 mg per lb. of body weight every 12 hours.
Premature Infant (under 24 days): 0.45 mg per lb. of body weight every 12 hours.

Dosage of xanthine bronchodilators is often calculated on the basis of theophylline equivalents, and must be tailored to your specific condition. The best dose is the lowest that will control your symptoms. Children break down xanthine bronchodilators faster than adults and usually require more drug per lb. of body weight.

Overdosage

The first symptoms of overdose are loss of appetite, nausea, vomiting, nervousness, difficulty sleeping, headache, and restlessness. These symptoms are followed by rapid or abnormal heart rhythm, unusual behavior, extreme thirst, delirium, convulsions, very high temperature, and collapse. These serious toxic symptoms are rarely experienced after overdose by mouth, which generally produces loss of appetite, nausea, vomiting, and stimulation. The overdose victim should be taken to a hospital emergency room immediately. ALWAYS bring the prescription bottle or container.

Special Information

Do not chew or crush coated or sustained-release capsules or tablets. Doing so could result in the immediate release of large amounts of the drug, possibly causing serious side effects.

To ensure consistent effectiveness, take your medication at the same time and in the same way, with or without food, every day.

Call your doctor if you develop nausea, vomiting, heartburn, sleeplessness, jitteriness, restlessness, headache, rash, severe stomach pain, convulsions, or a rapid or irregular heartbeat. Acute drug toxicity may descend abruptly, with little or no warning; serious side effects such as convulsions, life-threatening arrhythmias, and death may result. Periodic monitoring by your physician is mandatory if you are taking a xanthine bronchodilator.

Do not change xanthine bronchodilator brands without notifying your doctor or pharmacist. Different brands of the same bronchodilator may not be identical in their effect on your body.

If you forget to take a dose of your xanthine bronchodilator, take it as soon as you remember. If it is almost time for your next dose, skip the one you forgot and continue with your regular schedule. Do not take a double dose.

Special Populations

Pregnancy/Breast-feeding

Xanthine bronchodilators pass into the fetal circulation. They do not cause birth defects, but they may produce dangerous drug levels in a newborn's bloodstream. Babies born to women who take one of these drugs may be nervous, jittery, and irritable, and may gag or vomit when fed. Pregnant women who must use a xanthine bronchodilator to control asthma or other conditions should talk with their doctors about the risks of this medication.

These drugs pass into breast milk and may cause a nursing infant to be nervous and irritable or to have difficulty sleeping. Nursing mothers who must use one of these drugs should bottle-feed.

Seniors, especially men age 55 and over, may take longer to clear the xanthine bronchodilators from their bodies. Seniors with heart failure or other cardiac conditions, chronic lung disease, a viral infection with fever, or reduced liver function may require a lower dosage of this medication to account for the clearance effect.

Generic Name

Zalcitabine (zal-SYE-tuh-bene)

Brand Name

Hivid

Type of Drug

Antiviral.

Prescribed for

Human immunodeficiency virus (HIV) infection, either alone or in combination with zidovudine (AZT).

General Information

Zalcitabine, also known as ddC or dideoxycytidine, was first approved for use in multiple-drug treatment of acquired immunodeficiency syndrome (AIDS), but it can be used alone in people who cannot tolerate AZT or whose disease has progressed while taking AZT. Zalcitabine interferes with the reproduction of the HIV virus by interrupting its internal DNA manufacturing process. DNA carries the essential genetic messages that direct all life processes; by acting on the DNA of HIV, zalcitabine interferes with the life of the HIV virus. Zalcitabine was originally approved because of its ability to increase levels of CD4 cells in the blood. CD4 cells represent the level of immune function and are considered an important indicator of the severity of an HIV infection.

Zalcitabine has been compared with didanosine (ddI) as a single-drug treatment for HIV infection. In these studies, both drugs were equally effective in prolonging the time to the next AIDS-defining event, but survival comparisons favored zalcitabine. When zalcitabine was given with AZT to people who had not previously received AZT, the combination was better than AZT alone. People who had been taking AZT and then added zalcitabine did not benefit more than people who took either drug alone.

Cautions and Warnings

Zalcitabine has caused **severe, potentially fatal side effects**. Although it is rare, people taking zalcitabine, AZT, or didanosine can develop lactic acidosis (a potentially fatal metabolic imbalance).

Between 22% and 35% of people taking zalcitabine experience **nervous system inflammation,** which is generally signaled by numbness and burning pain in the hands and feet. These symptoms may be followed by sharp shooting pains or a severe and continuous burning pain. If the drug is continued, these pains may become permanent. People who already have signs of this kind of nerve damage should not take zalcitabine. Stop taking zalcitabine if the numbness, burning, and pain become moderately uncomfortable. If the symptoms improve on their own after you stop taking the drug, you may, after consultation with your doctor, start taking zalcitabine again in a smaller dosage.

Fatal inflammation of the pancreas has occurred in less than 1% of people taking zalcitabine. People with a history of pancreatic inflammation should take this drug only after careful consideration. Symptoms of inflammation of the pancreas include major changes in blood-sugar levels, rising blood levels of triglycerides, a drop in blood calcium, nausea, vomiting, and abdominal pain. People who develop pancreatic inflammation must stop taking zalcitabine.

Mouth ulcers developed in about 3% of people taking zalcitabine during clinical studies. Infrequently, people taking zalcitabine develop **ulcers of the esophagus**. People taking zalcitabine may develop heart failure. People who already have **heart failure** should take this drug only after careful consideration.

Do not take zalcitabine if you are **allergic** to it or any ingredient in the zalcitabine tablet. Zalcitabine may worsen the condition of people with **liver disease**. Death from liver failure may also occur with zalcitabine. **Alcohol abuse** aggravates the liver problems associated with zalcitabine.

Possible Side Effects

▼ Most common: mouth sores, nausea and vomiting, appetite loss, abdominal pain, itching, rash, headache, muscle ache, joint pain, tiredness, sore throat, fever, chest pain, and weight loss.

▼ Less common: swallowing difficulties, constipation, stomach irritation and ulcers, night sweats, and foot pain.

▼ Rare: Rare side effects can occur in almost any part of the body. Contact your doctor if you experience any side effect not listed above.

Drug Interactions

• Chloramphenicol, cisplatin, dapsone, didanosine, disulfiram, ethionamide, glutethimide, gold, hydralazine, iodoquinol, isoniazid, metronidazole, nitrofurantoin, phenytoin, ribavirin, vincristine, and other drugs that can cause nervous system inflammation should be avoided while taking zalcitabine.

• Drugs such as probenecid, foscarnet, cimetidine, amphotericin, and aminoglycoside-type antibiotics may interfere with the elimination of zalcitabine from the kidneys, increasing the risk of side effects.

• Drugs that may cause inflammation of the pancreas—including intravenous pentamidine—should not be taken with zalcitabine.

• Taking metoclopramide together with zalcitabine moderately reduces the amount of zalcitabine absorbed into the blood.

Food Interactions

Food interferes with the amount of zalcitabine absorbed and the speed at which it is absorbed into the blood. Take zalcitabine on an empty stomach, or 1 hour before or 2 hours after meals.

Usual Dose

Adult and Child (age 13 and over): 0.75 mg every 8 hours. For people with poor kidney function, dosage may be reduced to 0.75 mg once or twice a day.

Overdosage

Zalcitabine overdose victims generally experience side effects of the drug, especially inflammation of the nervous system. Victims should be taken to a hospital emergency room for testing and monitoring. ALWAYS bring the prescription bottle or container.

Special Information

Zalcitabine is not an AIDS cure. It will not prevent you from transmitting the HIV virus to another person; you must still practice safe sex. Patients may still develop AIDS-related opportunistic infections while taking this drug.

Zalcitabine may cause anemia and affect other components of the blood. Your doctor should perform blood tests to check for any changes.

People taking zalcitabine must take care of their teeth and gums to minimize the risk of oral infections.

Call your doctor if you develop any of the following symptoms of zalcitabine toxicity: numbness and burning pain in the hands and feet; sharp, shooting pains or a severe and continuous burning pain; nausea; vomiting; or abdominal pain.

If you forget to take a dose of zalcitabine, take it as soon as you remember. If it is almost time for your next dose, allow 2 to 4 hours to pass between the dose you took late and your next dose, and then continue with your regular schedule. Do not take a double dose. Call your doctor for more specific advice if you forget to take several doses.

Special Populations

Pregnancy/Breast-feeding

In animal studies, zalcitabine causes the development of malformed fetuses. When this drug is considered crucial by your doctor, its potential benefits must be carefully weighed against its risks. Use effective contraception while taking zalcitabine.

It is not known if zalcitabine passes into breast milk. Nursing mothers who are HIV positive should always bottle-feed, regardless of whether they take this drug, to avoid transmitting the virus.

Seniors

People with reduced kidney function, including older adults, should receive smaller doses of zalcitabine than those with normal kidneys.

Generic Name

Zaleplon (zah-LEP-lon)

Brand Name

Sonata

Type of Drug

Hypnotic.

Prescribed for

Insomnia.

General Information

Zaleplon works on the same nerve receptors as the benzodiazepine-type drugs, though it is chemically different from
them. Zaleplon usually works within an hour. It is removed
from the body relatively quickly and causes little or no
"morning-after hangover" effect, which may occur with other
sleeping pills. Zaleplon is broken down in the liver.

Cautions and Warnings

People with moderate **liver disease** should take the lowest
effective dosage.

Take zaleplon just before you go to bed. Taking it during the
day causes **tiredness** and an **inability to concentrate** and may
interfere with normal activities.

People taking zaleplon nightly for an extended period of
time may become **anxious** and have **trouble sleeping** when
they stop the drug.

The effect of zaleplon in people with **respiratory illness** is
not known.

Possible Side Effects

In studies, side effects were similar in people taking zaleplon and those taking a placebo (sugar pill).

▼ Most common: headache.

▼ Common: abdominal pain, weakness, muscle
aches, memory loss, dizziness, and tiredness.

Possible Side Effects *(continued)*

▼ Less common: fever, difficulty swallowing, tingling in the hands or feet, tremors, eye pain, unusually sensitive hearing, changes in sense of smell, and painful menstrual periods.

▼ Rare: anxiety, feeling unwell, fainting, nosebleeds, visual problems, ear pain, loss of a sense of reality or sense of self, hallucinations, reduced sensitivity to stimulation, increased sensitivity to the sun, appetite loss, and colitis. Other rare side effects can occur in almost any part of the body. Contact you doctor if you experience any side effect not listed above.

Drug Interactions

A number of drug interactions are possible, some of which may not appear below.

• Do not combine zaleplon and diphenhydramine (an over-the-counter antihistamine and sleeping pill).

• Zaleplon increases the depressant effects of alcohol and other nervous system depressants, imipramine, and thioridazine.

• Rifampin reduces zaleplon's effect.

• Combining zaleplon and cimetidine can almost double zaleplon blood levels. People taking cimetidine regularly for heartburn, ulcers, or stomach acid reduction should begin with the lowest effective dosage of zaleplon.

Food Interactions

Take this drug on an empty stomach, at least 1 hour before or 2 hours after meals. High-fat meals can reduce its effectiveness.

Usual Dose

Adult: 5–10 mg at bedtime.
Senior: begin with 5 mg nightly and increase if needed.
Child: not recommended.

Overdosage

Symptoms include dizziness, tiredness, and an inability to concentrate or perform complicated tasks. Take the victim to a hospital emergency room. ALWAYS bring the prescription bottle or container.

Special Information

Sleeping pills sometimes cause memory loss of events that occur during the several hours after a dose. Call your doctor if this happens.

If you see no improvement with this drug in 7 to 10 days, call your doctor.

Taking zaleplon during the day will make you drowsy and interfere with your concentration and coordination. Use it just before bedtime.

If you find that you need a larger dose of zaleplon to help you sleep, you may be developing a tolerance to the drug.

Sometimes, people who stop taking zaleplon after using it for 2 weeks or more have difficulty sleeping or become anxious. These are drug withdrawal symptoms and usually go away after 1 or 2 nights. More severe symptoms are rare.

Special Populations

Pregnancy/Breast-feeding

Taking zaleplon in the weeks just before delivery may cause tiredness or listlessness in newborns. Zaleplon should not be taken during pregnancy.

Small amounts of zaleplon pass into breast milk. Nursing mothers who must take it should bottle-feed.

Seniors

Seniors may be more sensitive to side effects.

Generic Name

Zanamivir (zuh-NAM-ih-veer)

Brand Name

Relenza

Type of Drug

Antiviral.

Prescribed for

Influenza A or B viral infection (type A or B flu).

General Information

Zanamivir is the first antiviral agent to be approved for treating flu symptoms. It must be inhaled within 2 days of the beginning of symptoms. It is inhaled directly into the nose and throat, where the influenza virus typically takes hold. Studies of zanamivir in people age 12 and over (average age was 34) suggest that people using this product feel better about 1 day sooner. Zanamivir is used to treat uncomplicated cases of the flu and is not intended for flu prevention.

Cautions and Warnings

Do not use zanamivir if you are **sensitive** or **allergic** to any ingredients in the inhalation.

People with **chronic lung problems** like asthma may not benefit from zanamivir inhalations. Also, zanamivir can cause **bronchospasm** (breathing difficulty) in a small number of people with asthma.

People using this drug are still contagious and should be careful about spreading the virus to others.

Individual virus particles can become **resistant** to zanamivir, but it is not yet known if virus infections will become resistant to zanamivir.

The safety of zanamivir in people with **severe liver disease** and in **children under age 12** is not known.

Possible Side Effects

▼ Less common: headache; diarrhea; nausea; vomiting; stuffy nose; nasal irritation; bronchitis; cough; sinus irritation; ear, nose, and throat infections; and dizziness.

▼ Rare: feeling unwell, tiredness, fever, abdominal pain, muscle aches, joint pain, and itching.

Drug Interactions

None known.

Food Interactions

Do not have any food in your mouth when you use this product.

Usual Dose

Adult and Child (age 12 and over): 2 inhalations 2 times a day for 5 days. Make sure to take 2 doses on your first day of treatment, even if they are only 2 hours apart.

Child (under age 12): not recommended.

Overdosage

Little is known about the effects of zanamivir overdose or accidental ingestion. Call your local poison control center or a hospital emergency room for more information.

Special Information

Make certain to complete the full 5-day course of zanamivir treatment, even if you start to feel better sooner.

Ask your doctor or pharmacist to instruct you on how to use the Diskhaler device that comes with each 5-day package of zanamivir. The drug comes in a small blister pack that is inserted into the Diskhaler. The blister pack is punctured inside the device and the powdered medication inside is drawn into the throat and nasal passages when you inhale through the Diskhaler.

Make certain that you do not have any food in your mouth when you use this product.

Special Populations

Pregnancy/Breast-feeding

Zanamivir may pass into the fetal circulation in extremely small amounts. When this drug is considered crucial by your doctor, its potential benefits must be carefully weighed against its risks.

It is not known if this drug passes into breast milk. Nursing mothers using zanamivir should consider bottle-feeding.

Seniors

Seniors may use this product without special restriction.

Zestril   *see Lisinopril, page 585*

Zestoretic   *see Lisinopril, page 585*

Ziac   *see Bisoprolol, page 127*

Generic Name

Zidovudine   (zih-DOE-vuh-dene) Ⓖ

Brand Name

Retrovir

Type of Drug

Antiviral.

Prescribed for

Human immunodeficiency virus (HIV) infection.

General Information

Zidovudine, also known as azidothymidine, compound S, and AZT—which it is commonly called—was approved for use in the U.S. before being tested completely for safety and effectiveness because of the severity of the specific disease it is designed to treat. AZT inhibits the production of several viruses, including the HIV virus that causes acquired immunodeficiency syndrome (AIDS). It works by interfering with specific enzymes within the virus that are responsible for essential steps in HIV's reproduction process. It has been generally recognized that AZT helps people with AIDS to live longer, although an international study of AIDS patients questions this claim. Treatment recommendations emphasize that AZT should be used to fight the HIV virus only in the later stages of the illness, when symptoms have developed and CD4 cell counts (an indication of the severity of the disease) are below 500. The true safety and effectiveness of AZT after prolonged use, and in people with less-advanced HIV disease, are not known.

Cautions and Warnings

AZT may cause severe reductions in white- and red-blood-cell counts and should be taken with caution by people with **bone-marrow disease** or those whose bone marrow has already been compromised by other treatments. Your doctor should take a blood count every 2 weeks; if problems develop, the dosage should be reduced.

In rare instances, people taking AZT or other nucleoside-type antivirals have developed **lactic acidosis** (a potentially fatal metabolic imbalance). Symptoms of lactic acidosis may include unexplained rapid breathing, breathing difficulties, and reduced blood-bicarbonate levels—which your doctor can detect with a routine blood test.

People with **impaired kidney or liver function** should use this drug with caution.

Prolonged use of AZT may cause **muscle irritation and abnormalities** similar to those caused by HIV infection.

Possible Side Effects

Adults

▼ Most common: anemia, reduced white-blood-cell counts, headache, nausea, sleeplessness, and muscle aches.

▼ Less common: Less common side effects can occur in almost any part of the body. Contact your doctor if you experience any side effect not listed above.

Children

▼ Most common: anemia, reduced white-blood-cell counts, vomiting, abdominal pain, fever, and sleeplessness.

▼ Less common: headache, blood infection, nervousness, and irritability.

▼ Rare: nausea, diarrhea, weight loss, seizures, heart failure and other cardiac abnormalities, blood in the urine, and bladder infections.

Drug Interactions

• Combining AZT with other drugs that can damage your kidneys, including pentamidine, dapsone, amphotericin B, flucytosine, vincristine, vinblastine, adriamycin, and alfa- and beta-interferon, increases the risk of loss of some kidney function.

• Probenecid may reduce the rate at which your body eliminates AZT, increasing the amount of the drug in your blood and the risk for side effects. Other drugs that can reduce the liver's ability to break down AZT are acetaminophen, aspirin, indomethacin, and trimethoprim; combining any of these drugs with AZT may lead to increased side effects.

• Acyclovir is often used in combination with AZT to combat opportunistic infections in AIDS patients; however, this combination may cause lethargy or seizures.

• Other drugs that can cause anemia, including ganciclovir or zalcitabine, should be used carefully in combination with AZT because of the risk of worsening drug-related anemia.

• Taking AZT together with rifampin or rifampicin may reduce the amount of AZT absorbed into the blood.

• Taking phenytoin and AZT together may affect the amounts of both drugs in the blood, usually increasing the amount of AZT. The effect on phenytoin blood levels varies. This combination can result in either too much phenytoin (leading to phenytoin side effects) or too little phenytoin (leading to a possible increase in the number of seizures). Your doctor should check your phenytoin levels if you are also taking AZT.

Food Interactions

AZT is best taken on an empty stomach, but you may take it with food if it upsets your stomach.

Usual Dose

Adult: symptomatic AIDS—100 mg every 4 hours around the clock, even if sleep must be interrupted. Dosage may be reduced if side effects develop. Asymptomatic AIDS—100 mg every 4 hours during waking hours. Combination therapy with zalcitabine—200 mg of AZT with 0.8 mg of zalcitabine every 8 hours.

Pregnancy: AZT is used to prevent transmission of HIV infection to the fetus. After 14 weeks of pregnancy—100 mg 5 times a day, until labor starts. During labor and delivery— intravenously, until the umbilical cord is clamped.

Child (age 3 months–12 years): up to 100 mg every 6 hours.

Infant: about 1 mg per lb. of body weight every 6 hours by mouth, starting within 12 hours of birth and continuing through 6 weeks of age. The drug may be given intravenously if necessary.

Overdosage

The most serious effect of AZT overdose is suppression of

bone marrow and its ability to make red and white blood cells. Take the victim to a hospital emergency room at once. ALWAYS bring the prescription bottle or container.

Special Information

AZT does not cure AIDS. It will not decrease the risk of your transmitting the HIV virus to another person; you must still practice safe sex. AZT may not prevent some illnesses associated with AIDS or AIDS-related complex (ARC) from continuing to develop.

See your doctor if any significant change in your health occurs. Periodic blood counts are very important while taking AZT to detect possibly serious side effects. Avoid acetaminophen, aspirin, and other drugs that may increase AZT toxicity.

Be sure to take this drug exactly as prescribed—around the clock if needed, even though it will interfere with your sleep. Do not take more AZT than your doctor has prescribed.

People taking AZT must take especially good care of their teeth and gums to minimize the risk of developing oral infections.

If you miss a dose of AZT, take it as soon as possible. If it is almost time for your next dose, allow 2 to 4 hours to pass between the dose you took late and your next dose, and then continue with your regular schedule. Do not take a double dose.

Protect AZT capsules and liquid from light.

Special Populations

Pregnancy/Breast-feeding

If you are HIV-positive and pregnant, talk to your doctor about taking or continuing your AZT. AZT treatment in HIV-positive women who are pregnant has been shown to sharply reduce the risk of transmitting the HIV virus to babies. Treatment should begin by the 14th week of pregnancy and continue through delivery. The baby should also be given AZT for the first 6 weeks of life. Studies have shown that the risk of birth defects is not increased by taking AZT during pregnancy.

It is not known if AZT passes into breast milk. Nursing mothers with HIV should always bottle-feed, regardless of whether they take this drug, to avoid transmitting the virus.

Seniors

Seniors may be at a greater risk of side effects due to reduced kidney function.

Zithromax *see Azithromycin, page 101*

Zocor *see Statin Cholesterol-Lowering Agents, page 942*

Zoloft *see Sertaline, page 924*

Generic Name

Zolpidem (ZOLE-pih-dem)

Brand Name

Ambien

Type of Drug

Sedative.

Prescribed for

Insomnia.

General Information

Zolpidem is a nonbenzodiazepine sleeping pill that works in the brain in much the same way as do benzodiazepine sleeping pills and tranquilizers. Unlike the benzodiazepines, however, zolpidem has little muscle-relaxing or antiseizure effects. It is meant for short-term use—7 to 10 days—and should not be taken regularly for longer than that without your doctor's knowledge. Unlike a benzodiazepine, zolpidem causes little or no "hangover," and there are no rebound effects after stopping the drug. Zolpidem is broken down in the liver.

Cautions and Warnings

Sleeping problems often result from a **physical or psychological illness**. Zolpidem does not affect the underlying causes of insomnia. It should be taken only with your doctor's knowledge. If you cannot sleep after 7 to 10 days of taking zolpidem, contact your doctor.

Zolpidem has caused **amnesia** (memory loss), but this happens mostly at dosages larger than 10 mg a night.

Suddenly stopping zolpidem after having taken it for some time may produce **drug withdrawal** (symptoms include fatigue, nausea, flushing, light-headedness, crying, vomiting, stomach cramps, panic, nervousness, and general discomfort). People with a history of substance abuse may be more likely to develop **drug dependence** on zolpidem.

Zolpidem is a nervous system depressant and may cause **loss of coordination and concentration**. It should be taken just before bedtime. Zolpidem may interfere with normal activities the next day, especially if taken with alcohol.

People with **liver disease** require reduced dosage. People with severe **kidney disease** should be monitored for side effects.

Zolpidem should be avoided in the presence of severe **depression**, severe **lung disease, sleep apnea** (condition characterized by intermittent cessation of breathing during sleep), and **drunkenness** or you run the risk of increasing the depressive effects of zolpidem or worsening your overall condition.

Possible Side Effects

Short-Term Use (10 Days or Less)

▼ Most common: drowsiness, dizziness, and diarrhea.

▼ Less common: chest pain, fatigue, unusual dreams, memory loss, anxiety, nervousness, difficulty sleeping, appetite loss, vomiting, and runny nose.

▼ Rare: Rare side effects can occur in almost any part of the body. Contact your doctor if you experience any side effect not listed above.

Long-Term Use

▼ Most common: drowsiness and a feeling of being drugged.

▼ Common: headache, allergy symptoms, back pain, flu-like symptoms, lethargy, sensitivity to light, depression, upset stomach, constipation, abdominal pain, muscle and joint pain, upper respiratory infection, sinus irritation, sore throat, rash, urinary infection, heart palpitations, and dry mouth.

Possible Side Effects *(continued)*

▼ Rare: Rare side effects can occur in almost any part
of the body. Contact your doctor if you experience any
side effect not listed above.

Drug Interactions

• Avoid combining zolpidem with alcohol and other nervous system depressants including tranquilizers, narcotics,
barbiturates, antidepressants, and antihistamines. Taking a
benzodiazepine such as diazepam with zolpidem may result
in excessive depression, tiredness, sleepiness, breathing difficulties, or similar symptoms.

Food Interactions

For the most rapid and complete effect, take zolpidem on an
empty stomach at least 2 hours after a meal.

Usual Dose

Adult (age 18 and over): 10 mg immediately before bed-
time.
Senior: 5 mg immediately before bedtime.
Child: not recommended.

People with severe liver disease should take 5 mg.

Overdosage

Overdose results in excessive nervous system depression,
from unconsciousness to light coma. Combining zolpidem
with alcohol or other nervous system depressants may be
fatal or affect other body organs. Take the victim to a hospital
emergency room at once. ALWAYS bring the prescription
bottle or container.

Special Information

Zolpidem may cause tiredness, drowsiness, and an inability
to concentrate. Be careful when driving or performing any
task that requires concentration on the day following a dose.

People taking zolpidem on a regular basis may develop a
drug withdrawal reaction if the medication is stopped suddenly (see "Cautions and Warnings").

If you forget a dose, take it as soon as you remember. If it is almost time for your next dose, skip the forgotten one and continue with your regular schedule. Do not take a double dose.

Special Populations

Pregnancy/Breast-feeding
Animal studies with large dosages show that zolpidem may affect the fetus. When this drug is considered crucial by your doctor, its potential benefits must be carefully weighed against its risks.

Small amounts of zolpidem pass into breast milk. Nursing mothers who must take this drug should bottle-feed.

Seniors
Seniors, who are likely to be more sensitive to zolpidem and its side effects, should take the lowest effective dosage.

Zyrtec   see *Cetirizine*, page 183

Zyprexa   see *Olanzapine*, page 751

Twenty Questions to Ask Your Doctor and Pharmacist About Your Prescription

1. What is the name of this medication?

2. What results may be expected from taking it?

3. How long should I wait before reporting if this medication does not help me?

4. How does the medication work?

5. What is the exact dosage of the medication?

6. What time of day should I take it?

7. Do alcoholic beverages have an effect on this medication?

8. Do I have to take special precautions with this medication in combination with other prescription medications I am taking?

9. Do I have to take special precautions with this medication in combination with over-the-counter (OTC) medications?

10. Does food have any effect on this medication?

11. Are there any special instructions I should have about how to use this medication?

12. How long should I continue to take this medication?

13. Is my prescription renewable?

14. For how long a period may my prescription be renewed?

15. Which side effects should I report, and which ones may I disregard?

16. May I save any unused part of this medication for future use?

17. How should I store this medication?

18. How long may I keep this medication without it losing its strength?

19. What should I do if I miss a dose of this medication?

20. Does this medication come in a less expensive, generic form?

Other Points to Remember for Safe Drug Use

- Store your medications in a sealed, light-resistant container to maintain maximum potency, and be sure to follow any special storage instructions listed on your prescription bottle or container, such as "refrigerate," "do not freeze," "protect from light," or "keep in a cool place." Protect all medications from excessive humidity.
- Make sure you tell the doctor everything that is wrong. The more information your doctor has, the more effective will be your treatment.
- Make sure each doctor you see knows about all the medications you use regularly, including prescription and over-the-counter (OTC) medications.
- Keep a record of any bad reaction you have had to a medication.
- Fill each prescription you are given. If you do not fill a prescription, make sure your doctor knows you are not taking the medication.
- Do not take extra medication without consulting your doctor or pharmacist.
- Follow the label instructions exactly. If you have any questions, call your doctor or pharmacist.
- Report any unusual symptoms that develop after taking any medication.
- Do not save unused medication for future use unless you have consulted your doctor. Dispose of unused medication by flushing it down the toilet.
- Never keep medications where children may see or reach them.
- Always read the label before taking your medication. Do not trust your memory.

- Consult your pharmacist for guidance on the use of medications.
- Do not share your medication with anyone. Your prescription was written for you and only you.
- Be sure the label stays on the container until the medication is used or destroyed.
- Keep the label facing up when pouring liquid medication from the bottle.
- Do not use a prescription medication unless it has been specifically prescribed for you. Whenever you travel, carry your prescription in its original container.
- If you move to another city, ask your pharmacist to forward your prescription records to your new pharmacy. Carry important medical facts about yourself in your wallet. Such things as drug allergies, chronic diseases (e.g., diabetes), and special requirements may be very useful.
- Do not hesitate to discuss the cost of medical care with your doctor or pharmacist.
- Exercise your right to make decisions about purchasing medications:
  1. If you suffer from a chronic condition, you will probably save money by buying in larger quantities.
  2. Choose your pharmacist as carefully as you choose your doctor.
  3. Remember, the cost of your prescription includes the professional services offered by your pharmacy. If you want more service, you may have to pay for it.

Safe Use of Eyedrops

To administer eyedrops, lie down or tilt your head back. Hold the dropper above your eye, gently squeeze your lower lid to form a small pouch, and release the drop or drops of medication inside your lower lid while looking up. Release the lower lid, keeping your eye open. Do not blink for 40 seconds. Press gently on the bridge of your nose at the inside corner of your eye for 1 minute to help circulate the drug in your eye. To avoid infection, do not touch the dropper tip to your finger, eyelid, or any other surface. Wait at least 5 minutes before using another eyedrop or eye ointment.

THE TOP 200
PRESCRIPTION DRUGS
IN THE UNITED STATES

**RANKED BY NUMBER OF PRESCRIPTIONS DISPENSED
FROM JANUARY TO OCTOBER 1999**

(Generic products are followed by manufacturer name in parentheses.)

1. Premarin
2. Synthroid
3. Lipitor
4. Prilosec
5. Hydrocodone with APAP (Watson)
6. Albuterol (Warrick)
7. Norvasc
8. Claritin
9. Prozac
10. Trimox
11. Zoloft
12. Lanoxin
13. Glucophage
14. Prempro
15. Paxil
16. Zestril
17. Zocor
18. Zithromax Z-Pak
19. Prevacid
20. Augmentin
21. Hydrocodone with APAP (Mallinckrodt)
22. Celebrex
23. Coumadin
24. Amoxicillin trihydrate (Teva)
25. Vasotec
26. Furosemide (Mylan)
27. Levoxyl
28. Cephalexin (Teva)
29. Cipro
30. K-Dur
31. Prednisone (Schein)
32. Pravachol
33. Trimethoprim/sulfamethoxazole (Teva)
34. Acetaminophen with codeine (Teva)
35. Zyrtec
36. Propoxyphene-N with APAP (Mylan)
37. Ambien
38. Atenolol (Geneva)
39. Ortho-Tri-Cylen 28
40. Biaxin

41. Propoxyphene-N with APAP (Teva)
42. Amoxil
43. Cardizem CD
44. Alprazolam (Green-stone)
45. Ultram
46. Accupril
47. Prinivil
48. Glucotrol XL
49. Allegra
50. Triamterene/ HCTZ (Geneva)
51. Toprol-XL
52. Cardura
53. Flonase
54. Ibuprofen (Green-stone)
55. Procardia XL
56. Zithromax
57. Lotensin
58. Fosamax
59. Viagra
60. Ibuprofen (Par)
61. Depakote
62. Dilantin
63. Pepcid
64. Hytrin
65. Wellbutrin SR
66. Triamterene/HCTZ (Mylan)
67. Cozaar
68. Neurontin
69. Hydrochlorothiazide (Zenith Goldline)
70. Claritin-D 12-Hr
71. Diflucan
72. Atenolol (Lederle)
73. Alprazolam (Geneva)
74. Adalat CC
75. Atenolol (Mylan)
76. Relafen
77. Lorazepam (Mylan)
78. Monopril
79. Verapamil SR (Zenith Goldline)
80. Furosemide (Watson)
81. Risperdal
82. Xalatan
83. Triphasil 28
84. Hydrocodone with APAP (Qualitest)
85. Claritin-D 24-Hr
86. Clonazepam (Teva)
87. Propulsid
88. Levaquin
89. Cefzil
90. Ziac
91. Amitriptyline HCl (Mylan)
92. Lescol
93. Ortho-Novum 7/7/7
94. Buspar
95. Naproxen (Teva)
96. Hydrocholothiazide (Purepac)
97. Serevent
98. Imitrex
99. Veetids
100. Glyburide (Copley)
101. Atrovent
102. Ceftin
103. Flovent
104. Lotrisone
105. Metroprolol tartrate (Mylan)
106. Zyprexa
107. Effexor XR
108. Rezulin
109. Cyclobenzaprine HCl (Schein)
110. Warfarin (Barr)
111. Acetaminophen with codeine (Purepac)
112. Nasonex
113. Celexa
114. Ranitidine HCL (Geneva)

115. Singulair
116. Roxicet
117. Medroxyprogesterone (Greenstone)
118. Ranitidine HCl (Novo)
119. Lo/Ovral-28
120. Amaryl
121. Diazepam (Mylan)
122. Furosemide (Zenith Goldline)
123. Plavix
124. Diovan
125. Hyzaar
126. Potassium chloride (Ethex)
127. Imdur
128. Bactroban
129. Allegra-D
130. Vancenase AQ
131. Serzone
132. Amoxicillin trihydrate (Par)
133. Carisoprodol (Schein)
134. Verapamil SR (Mylan)
135. Ortho-Cyclen-28
136. Daypro
137. Zestoretic
138. Propranolol HCl (ESI)
139. Neomycin/Poly-myxin/HC (Bausch & Lomb)
140. Clonidine HCl (Mylan)
141. Azmacort
142. Miacalcin
143. Desogen-28
144. Detrol
145. Penicillin VK (Teva)
146. Evista
147. Furosemide (Geneva)
148. Cephalexin (Apothe-con)
149. Macrobid
150. Adderall
151. Nitrostat
152. Combivent
153. Lotrel
154. Cycrin
155. Temazepam (Mylan)
156. Alesse-28
157. Hydrochlorothiazide (Lederle)
158. Ery-Tab
159. Estrace
160. Necon 1/35 28
161. Axid
162. Avapro
163. Plendil
164. Klor-Con 10
165. Lorazepam (ESI)
166. Naproxen (Mylan)
167. Methylprednisolone (Duramed)
168. Arthrotec
169. Phenergan
170. Cyclobenzaprine (Mylan)
171. Lamisil
172. Mevacor
173. Oxycontin
174. Tamoxifen citrate (Barr)
175. Vioxx
176. Amitriptyline HCl (Geneva)
177. Alprazolam (Purepac)
178. Tobradex
179. Aricept
180. Gemfibrozil (Teva)
181. Metoprolol tartrate (Geneva)
182. Albuterol (Dey)
183. Tiazac
184. Isosorbide mononi-trate (Warrick)
185. Oxycodone with APAP (Mallinckrodt)
186. Proventil HFA
187. Trazodone HCl (Sidmak)

188. Alphagan
189. Ranitidine HCl (Mylan)
190. Climara
191. Altace
192. Glyburide (Green-
     stone)
193. Levothroid

194. Allopurinol (Mylan)
195. Folic acid (Schein)
196. Claritin Reditabs
197. Estradiol (Watson)
198. Elocon
199. Lorazepam (Purepac)
200. Flomax

Source: IMS Health, 1999.

Index of Generic and Brand-Name Drugs

How to Find Your Medication in *The Pill Book*

- *The Pill Book* lists most medications in alphabetic order by generic name because a medication may have many brand names but has only 1 generic name. Most generic medications produce the same therapeutic effects as their brand-name equivalents but are much less expensive. Drugs that are available generically are indicated by the Ⓖ symbol.

- When a medication has 2 or more active ingredients, it is listed by the most widely known brand name. In a few cases, pill profiles are listed by drug type (e.g., sulfonylurea antidiabetes drugs).

- *The Pill Book* includes the names of the top 100 brand-name drugs (cross-referenced to their generic name) in alphabetic order with the pill profiles.

- Most over-the-counter (OTC) medications are not included in *The Pill Book*. For complete information on OTC medications, refer to *The Pill Book Guide to Over-the-Counter Medications*.

- All brand and generic names are listed in the Index. Brand names are indicated by boldface.

- Sugar-free and alcohol-free brand-name drugs are indicated by the Ⓢ and Ⓐ symbols in the beginning of each pill profile.

ABOUT THE EDITOR

Educated at Columbia University, Dr. Harold Silverman has been a hospital pharmacist, author, educator, and pharmaceutical industry consultant. Currently, he is Vice Chairman of *Interscience,* a global health-care communications consultancy. Professionally, Dr. Silverman seeks to help people understand why medicines are prescribed and how to get the most from them. In addition to *THE PILL BOOK,* Dr. Silverman is coauthor of *THE VITAMIN BOOK: A No-Nonsense Consumer Guide* and *The MED FILE Drug Interactions System.* He is also the author of *THE PILL BOOK GUIDE TO SAFE DRUG USE, THE CONSUMER'S GUIDE TO POISON PROTECTION, THE WOMAN'S DRUG STORE,* and *TRAVEL HEALTHY.* Dr. Silverman's contributions to the professional literature include more than 70 articles, research papers, and textbook chapters. He is a member of many professional organizations and has served as an officer for several, including the New York State Council of Hospital Pharmacists, for which he served as president. He has taught pharmacology and clinical pharmacy at several universities and won numerous awards for his work. Dr. Silverman resides in a Washington suburb with his wife, Judith Brown, and their son, Joshua.

Create Your Own Medical Library with
BANTAM MEDICAL REFERENCE BOOKS

THE BANTAM MEDICAL DICTIONARY
by the editors of Market House Books

Offering the latest authoritative definitions in simple language, this exhaustive reference spans the entire domain of the health sciences, defining more than 10,500 medical terms and concepts in all the major medical and surgical specialties.

58189-9 $6.99/$8.99

THE VITAMIN BOOK
by Harold M. Silverman, Pharm.D., Joseph Romano, Pharm.D., and Gary Elmer, Ph.D.

Compiled by a team of eminent pharmacologists, this up-to-date comprehensive reference clearly separates the facts from the fiction regarding the overwhelming and often contradictory information about vitamins and minerals. THE VITAMIN BOOK also adds the latest benefits regarding the top ten herbal medicines and top five dietary supplements on the market today.

57975-6 $6.50/$9.99

THE PILL BOOK GUIDE TO OVER-THE-COUNTER MEDICATIONS
by Robert Rapp, Pharm.D.

Because you often treat yourself with over-the-counter medications without a physician's guidance, here is all the information you can get in choosing the product that is right for you and your family. With color photographs of brand-name medications, this guide includes complete profiles of each drug, including dosages, side effects, drug interactions, and more.

57729-8 $6.99/$9.99

THE PILL BOOK GUIDE TO CHILDREN'S MEDICATIONS
by Michael D. Mitchell, M.D. with Marvin S. Eiger, M.D.
This indispensable guide offers a pediatrician's expert advice on more than two hundred prescription and over-the-counter drugs for young children, plus reassuring suggestions for helping your child feel better fast.

56927-9 $6.50/$8.99

THE PILL BOOK GUIDE TO EVERYTHING YOU NEED TO KNOW ABOUT PROZAC
by Jeffrey M. Jonas, M.D., and Ron Schaumburg
This authoritative guide to America's most prescribed antidepressant separates the facts from the myths about the drug many doctors believe is the best medication available for the treatment of depression – an illness that affects fifteen million Americans.

29192-0 $5.50/$7.50

THE PILL BOOK GUIDE TO MEDICATION FOR YOUR DOG AND CAT
by Kate A. W. Roby, V.M.D., and Lenny Southam, D.V.M.
This one-of-a-kind guide provides important information about the most commonly prescribed and over-the-counter drugs for cats and dogs, plus the latest information on alternative therapies that will keep your pet healthy and happy.

57989-4 $6.99/$9.99